Care of the Trauma Patient

Care of the Trauma Patient

Second Edition

G. Tom Shires, M.D.

Lewis Atterbury Stimson Professor and Chairman
Department of Surgery
Cornell University Medical College
and
Surgeon in Chief
The New York Hospital

McGraw-Hill Book Company

New York St. Louis San Francisco Auckland Bogotá Düsseldorf
Johannesburg London Madrid Mexico Montreal New Delhi
Panama Paris São Paulo Singapore Sydney Tokyo Toronto

CARE OF THE TRAUMA PATIENT

Copyright © 1979, 1966 by McGraw-Hill, Inc. All rights reserved. Printed in the United States of America. No part of this publication may be reproduced, stored in a retrieval system, or transmitted, in any form or by any means, electronic, mechanical, photocopying, recording, or otherwise, without the prior written permission of the publisher.

234567890 VHVH 7832109

Library of Congress Cataloging in Publication Data

Shires, George Thomas, date
    Care of the trauma patient.

    Includes index.
    1. Wounds—Treatment. I. Title.
[DNLM: 1. Emergencies. 2. Patients. 3. Wounds and injuries—
Therapy. W0700 C271]
RD93.S5 1979   617'.1   78-10911
ISBN 0-07-056916-9

This book was set in Times Roman by Black Dot, Inc. (ECU).
The editors were J. Dereck Jeffers and Bob Leap;
the cover was designed by A Good Thing, Inc.;
the production supervisor was Milton J. Heiberg.
The drawings were done by Tek/Nek Inc.
Von Hoffmann Press, Inc., was printer and binder.

Contents

1

GENERAL PRINCIPLES

2

INITIAL DIAGNOSIS AND TREATMENT

3

SPECIFIC INJURIES: DIAGNOSIS, OPERATIVE TREATMENT, AND MANAGEMENT

4

MANAGEMENT IN THE POSTTRAUMATIC AND POSTOPERATIVE PERIOD: COMPLICATIONS

List of Contributors

WILLIAM D. ARNOLD, M.D.
Attending Surgeon (Orthopedic)
Cornell University Medical College

CHARLES R. BAXTER, M.D.
Frank H. Kidd, Jr., Professor of Surgery
The University of Texas Southwestern Medical
  School at Dallas

JAMES E. BERTZ, D.D.S., M.D.
Chief, Oral/Maxillofacial Surgery
Assistant Dean for Student Affairs
The University of Texas Medical School at
  Houston

THOMAS C. BRIGHT III, M.D.
Assistant Professor of Surgery (Urology)
The University of Texas Southwestern Medical
  School at Dallas

EARL Z. BROWNE, JR., M.D.
Associate Professor of Plastic Surgery
University of Utah College of Medicine

CHARLES J. CARRICO, M.D.
Professor of Surgery
University of Washington School of Medicine

W. KEMP CLARK, M.D.
Professor and Chairman
Division of Neurological Surgery
The University of Texas Southwestern Medical
  School at Dallas

WILLIAM A. COOK, M.D.
Boston, Massachusetts

P. WILLIAM CURRERI, M.D.
Johnson and Johnson Professor of Surgery
Director, Burn Center
Cornell University Medical College

PETER DINEEN, M.D.
Professor of Surgery
Cornell University Medical College

EUGENE P. FRENKEL, M.D.
Professor of Internal Medicine and Radiology

The University of Texas Southwestern Medical
  School at Dallas

WILLIAM A. GAY, JR., M.D.
Professor of Surgery
Cornell University Medical College

A. H. GIESECKE, JR., M.D.
Professor of Anesthesiology
The University of Texas Southwestern Medical
  School at Dallas

CHARLES F. GREGORY, M.D.
(Deceased) Formerly Professor and Chairman
Division of Orthopedic Surgery
The University of Texas Southwestern Medical
  School at Dallas

JOEL H. HOROVITZ, M.D.
Associate Professor of Surgery
Cornell University Medical College

LEONARD D. HUDSON, M.D.
Associate Professor and Chief
Respiratory Disease Division of Medicine
University of Washington School of Medicine

GARY R. HUNTER, M.D.
Salt Lake City, Utah

M. T. JENKINS, M.D.
Professor and Chairman
Department of Anesthesiology
The University of Texas Southwestern Medical
  School at Dallas

ROBERT F. JONES, M.D.
Professor of Surgery
University of Washington School of Medicine

JOHN H. LARAGH, M.D., F.A.C.C.
Master Professor of Medicine
Cornell University Medical College

JOHN R. LYNN, M.D.
Professor and Chairman
Department of Ophthalmology
The University of Texas Southwestern Medical
  School at Dallas

JOHN C. McCABE, M.D.
Assistant Professor of Surgery
Cornell University Medical College

ROBERT N. McCLELLAND, M.D.
Alvin J. Baldwin, Jr., Professor of Surgery
The University of Texas Southwestern Medical
  School at Dallas

ANDREAS P. NIARCHOS, M.D.
Assistant Professor of Medicine
Division of Cardiology
New York Hospital-Cornell University Medical
  Center

LOUIS H. PARADIES, M.D.
Professor of Orthopedic Surgery
The University of Texas Southwestern Medical
  School at Dallas

MALCOLM O. PERRY, M.D.
Professor of Surgery
Chief of Vascular Surgery
Cornell University Medical College

PAUL C. PETERS, M.D.
Professor and Chairman
Division of Urology
The University of Texas Southwestern Medical
  School at Dallas

GABRIEL A. SHAPIRO, M.D.
Associate Professor
Department of Internal Medicine
The University of Texas Southwestern Medical
  School at Dallas

G. TOM SHIRES, M.D.
Lewis Atterbury Stimson Professor and Chairman
Department of Surgery
Cornell University Medical College
Surgeon in Chief
The New York Hospital

CLIFFORD C. SNYDER, M.D.
Professor and Chairman
Division of Plastic Surgery
University of Utah College of Medicine
Chief of Surgery

Veterans Administration Hospital
Salt Lake City, Utah

ERWIN R. THAL, M.D.
Associate Professor of Surgery
The University of Texas Southwestern Medical
  School at Dallas

ROBERT V. WALKER, D.D.S.
Professor and Chairman

Division of Oral Surgery
The University of Texas Southwestern Medical
  School at Dallas

WATTS R. WEBB, M.D.
Professor and Chairman
Department of Surgery
Tulane University School of Medicine

Preface

Care of the Trauma Patient was originally the work of a department of surgery. The department received the impetus to write such a book from constant daily experience in the management of large numbers of injured patients. Parkland Memorial Hospital, immediately adjacent to The University of Texas Southwestern Medical School, is a 700-bed city–county general hospital which serves a county of approximately 1½ million people. The majority of patients from this population center who experience serious trauma are brought to the emergency room of this hospital.

A number of additional authors, nationally known for their work with injured patients, contributed to the second edition of *Care of the Trauma Patient*. These new authors, with their individual expertise, are welcome additions to the effort.

The magnitude of the problem of trauma in the United States is probably not adequately recognized. Trauma is the leading cause of death during the first 3 decades of life in this country. It ranks overall as the fourth leading cause of death in the United States today, and if arteriosclerosis is considered as a single entity, trauma is the third leading cause of death. Fifty million injuries occur annually in the United States; over 10 million of them are disabling. More than 100,000 deaths occur each year from accidents. Automobile accidents alone kill more Americans each year than were lost during the entire Korean War. Unlike some serious disease entities in the United States, the incidence of and mortality from injuries increases each year.

One lesson that has been learned in caring for large numbers of injured patients is not included in the text because it does not relate to a specific injury. This is the importance of the efficiency of emergency-room procedure. Technically, an emergency room which receives more than 100 patients per day should probably be divided into some major form of triage system. This has proved to be infinitely helpful in the initial management of the injured patient. More important is the quality of care which patients receive immediately after injury, the time when many patients' subsequent course and mortality are determined. We are indebted to a group of residents of high caliber who are constantly being trained, by surgeons of all disciplines, in the management and care of traumatized patients. To these residents must go a large share of the credit for the successful healing of many severely injured patients.

An attempt has been made to produce a useful text about the patient. More specifically, it is about the patient with single or multiple injuries of various types. Effort has been directed to avoid oversimplification. Similarly, our philosophy has been to avoid producing a lengthy reference text covering all injuries, all management schemes in use, and all related research. Many important aspects of the care of the trauma patient have, by necessity, been omitted. These include immediate rescue and transportation of the injured patient; intercommunication between fire department, police department, and ambulance service in emergency rooms, which is so critical; and different staffing patterns for emergency rooms in communities of various size. In addition, certain specific forms of trauma not generally encountered at the present time by the majority of physicians have been omitted, e.g., radiation injury. Therefore, the overall attempt has been to produce a practical guide to the principles, pathological physiology, and clinical care involved in treating the injured patient.

The authors, in addition to active daily participation in the management of injured patients, have research interests centered primarily on some phase of bodily injury. When practical, the results of such research are included in the chapters. Since the book has many authors, there are obviously a multitude of styles manifest in the writing. Although editing was done for content, little was attempted for individual author style.

Many questions concerning the future of research and care of injuries remain unanswered. Answers for clinical questions are still being sought, and it is hoped that a compilation such as this book will not only begin to answer some of these questions but also arouse interest to answer even more. Continuing research in the area of injuries is badly needed in the United States today. It has been estimated that accidents at the present time are costing our society over 18 billion dollars per year. It has further been estimated that an annual investment of 0.04 percent of the estimated cost of accidents is being spent on research in the realm of injuries at the present time. Consequently, it is also hoped that some impetus to stimulate research in the area of injuries and accidents may be given by the present work.

G. Tom Shires

Part One

General Principles

Chapter 1

Principles and Management of Hemorrhagic Shock

G. Tom Shires, M.D.

CLASSIFICATION AND CLINICAL AND PHYSIOLOGIC MANIFESTATIONS OF SHOCK

Definition and Working Classification

The scope of modern medicine is increasing steadily. As understanding of physiologic and biochemical derangements is broadened, so is the horizon of possibilities for the relief of illness. As more seriously ill patients are presented, shock is a symptom complex more frequently encountered by the physician.

Although shock has been recognized for over 100 years, a clear definition and dissection of this complex and devastating state has emerged only slowly. Many attempts have been made over the years to define adequately the entity known as shock. In 1872 the elder Gross defined shock as a "manifestation of the rude unhinging of the machinery of life."[57] Although the accuracy of this definition is

unquestioned, it is obviously far from precise. In 1942 Wiggers, on the basis of an exhaustive examination of available evidence at that time, offered the definition: "Shock is a syndrome resulting from a depression of many functions, but in which reduction of the effective circulating blood volume is of basic importance, and in which impairment of the circulation steadily progresses until it eventuates in a state of irreversible circulatory failure."[139] A definition which Blalock offered in 1940 was: "Shock is a peripheral circulatory failure, resulting from a discrepancy in the size of the vascular bed and the volume of the intravascular fluid."[17]

A more modern definition has been devised by Simeone.[123] He stated that shock may be defined as a "clinical condition characterized by signs and symptoms which arise when the cardiac output is insufficient to fill the arterial tree with blood under sufficient pressure to provide organs and tissues with adequate blood flow."

Shock of all forms appears to be invariably related to inadequate tissue perfusion. The low flow state in vital organs seems to be the final common denominator in all forms of shock.

For purposes of a working clinical classification, the etiologic classification offered by Blalock in 1934 is still a useful and functional one.[18] Blalock suggested four categories:

I Hematogenic (oligemia)
II Neurogenic (caused primarily by nervous influences)
III Vasogenic (initially decreased vascular resistance and increased vascular capacity)
IV Cardiogenic
  A Failure of the heart as a pump
  B Unclassified category (including diminished cardiac output from various causes)

It is now clear that shock invariably results from loss of function of one or more of four separate but interrelated functions. These are:

1 The pump (heart)
2 The fluid which is pumped (blood volume)
3 Arteriolar resistance vessels
4 The capacity of the venous bed (capacitance vessels)

In the context of Blalock's etiologic classification, these functions may be correlated:

I Cardiogenic shock. This implies failure of the heart as a pump and may be brought about by
  A Primary myocardial dysfunction from
    1 Myocardial infarction
    2 Serious cardiac arrhythmias
    3 Myocardial depression from a variety of causes
  B Miscellaneous causes would include mechanical restriction of cardiac function or venous obstruction such as oc-

curs in the mediastinum with
    1 Tension pneumothorax
    2 Vena caval obstruction
    3 Cardiac tamponade
II Reduction in the fluid which may be pumped, the blood volume. This loss of volume may be in the form of loss of whole blood, plasma or extracellular fluid in the extravascular space, or a combination of these three.
III Changes in resistance vessels may be brought about by specific disorders, which would include
  A Decrease in resistance
    1 Spinal anesthesia
    2 Neurogenic reflexes, as in acute pain
    3 Possibly the end stages of hypovolemic shock
  B Septic shock
    1 Change in peripheral arterial resistance
    2 Change in venous capacitance
    3 Peripheral arteriovenous shunting

Therapy of shock will obviously revolve around the etiologic type or combination of types of shock present in a given patient who has undergone trauma.

The signs and symptoms of hypovolemic shock, when they are well established, are classic and usually easy to recognize. Most of the signs of clinical shock are characteristic of low peripheral blood flow and are contributed to by the effects of excess adrenal-sympathetic activity. The signs and symptoms of shock in humans, according to the severity of the shock, were well described by Beecher et al., as summarized in Table 1-1.

On first inspection the patient in shock presents an anxious, tired expression, which early is that of restlessness and anxiety and later becomes a picture of apathy or exhaustion. Typically, the skin feels cool and is pale and mottled, and there is evidence of decreased capillary flow exhibited by easy blanching of the skin, particularly the nail beds.

Table 1-1: Grading of Shock

| Degree of shock | Blood pressure (approx.) | Pulse quality | Skin | | | Thirst | Mental state |
			Temperature	Color	Circulation (response to pressure blanching)		
None	Normal	Normal	Normal	Normal	Normal	Normal	Clear and distressed
Slight. . . .	To 20% increase	Normal	Cool	Pale	Definite slowing	Normal	Clear and distressed
Moderate .	Decreased 20-40%	Definite decrease in volume	Cool	Pale	Definite slowing	Definite	Clear and some apathy unless stimulated
Severe . . .	Decreased 40% to nonrecordable	Weak to imperceptible	Cold	Ashen to cyanotic (mottling)	Very sluggish	Severe	Apathetic to comatose, little distress except thirst

Source: H. K. Beecher, F. A. Simeone, C. H. Burnett, S. L. Shapiro, E. R. Sullivan, and T. B. Mallory: The internal state of the severely wounded man on entry to the most forward hospital, *Surgery*, **22**:672, 1947.

There are varying discrepancies in the classic picture of shock. In neurogenic shock, particularly that in response to spinal anesthesia, the pulse rate is normal or, more often, decreased; the pulse pressure is wide, and the pulse feels strong rather than weak. The rapid pulse characteristic of early hemorrhagic or wound shock may be absent, even if the patient has lost blood rapidly. This is also true if his position is supine or prone, in which case a rapid pulse may not appear until the patient is moved or elevated to a sitting position.[114]

In observing a large number of patients in hemorrhagic hypovolemic shock, one sees remarkably varied but typical responses of the sensorium to the shock episode. Most young, healthy patients who sustain hemorrhagic shock, when seen early, will appear to be restless and anxious and actually give the appearance of great fear. Shortly after being seen by a physician and started on treatment, this restlessness frequently gives way to great apathy, and the patient will appear sleepy. When aroused, the patient may complain of weakness or of a chilly sensation, although he or she does not actually have a chill. If blood loss is unchecked, the patient's apathy and sleepiness will rapidly progress into coma. In treating a large number of accident victims, it has been our experience that patients who have bled into frank coma from which they cannot be aroused, resulting simply from blood loss alone (unassociated with other injuries such as brain damage), have usually sustained lethal blood loss. This sign usually indicates rapid massive hemorrhage for which the compensations to shock are inadequate to maintain sufficient cerebral blood flow to sustain consciousness.

Another characteristic of the wounded person, described by many investigators, is thirst. Thirst seems to be a characteristic of the injured person and is found in most emergency room patients brought in acutely ill from trauma with or without shock. The studies carried out to elucidate the nature of the thirst are many and varied. Most of these patients have intense adrenal medullary stimulation from trauma, not necessarily accompanied by shock. Consequently, caution must be used in allowing water, since dangerous water intoxication may be induced by this intense stimulus to imbibe liquids in the face of altered renal function.

Another characteristic of the patient in hemorrhagic shock is the low peripheral venous pressure, which is manifested by empty peripheral veins on inspection. Indeed, the starting of a simple intravenous infusion in a patient in hemorrhagic shock can be quite difficult. Obviously there are exceptions, such as shock due to cardiac tamponade, in which there is restriction to inflow of blood to the right side of the heart. In this instance the peripheral veins, including the neck veins, will be distended.

Nausea and vomiting from hypovolemic shock are common. It is true that other causes should be sought, but shock alone may be first manifest in this manner.

Another classic finding in hemorrhagic hypovolemia is a fall in body "core" temperature. Whether this is due to a lowered metabolic rate or to lower perfusion in areas where body temperature is measured is debatable.

Physiologic Changes

Blood Pressure Arterial blood pressure is normally maintained by the cardiac output and the peripheral vascular resistance. Thus, when the cardiac output is reduced because of loss of intravascular volume, the blood pressure may remain normal so long as the total peripheral vascular resistance can be increased to compensate for the reduction in cardiac output. The vascular resistance varies for different organs and in different parts of the same organ, depending on the local conditions that determine the state of vasoconstriction or vasodilation at the time of the loss of intravascular volume. An example of the differential increase in peripheral resistance with reduction in cardiac output is seen in the change in distributional total blood flow to organs such as the heart and the brain as opposed to that to most other organs which are not essential for immediate survival. In hemorrhagic shock the

heart may receive 25 percent of the total cardiac output as opposed to the normal 5 to 8 percent. The great increase in peripheral resistance in such organs as the skin and the kidneys causes significant reduction in flow in these organs while providing a lifesaving diversion of the cardiac output to the brain and the heart.

Consequently, the blood pressure may not fall until the reduction in cardiac output or loss of blood volume is so great that the adaptive homeostatic mechanisms can no longer compensate for the reduced volume. As the deficit continues, however, there is a progressive hypotension.

Pulse Rate Characteristically, reduction of the volume in the vascular tree is associated with tachycardia. A fall in pressure within the great vessels results in excitation of the sympathicoadrenal division of the autonomic nervous system and, simultaneously, inhibition of the vagal-medullary center. Consequently, with hemorrhage or loss of circulating blood volume, the resulting fall in arterial blood pressure should cause an increase in heart rate.

However, this compensatory mechanism is variable in its effectiveness. Obviously, the degree of loss of intravascular volume, the amount of reduction in venous return, and other variables such as ventricular function may markedly influence the ability of Marey's phenomenon to compensate for the reduction in blood volume. Work with slow hemorrhage in normal, healthy volunteers by Shenkin et al.[114] has shown that, as long as the supine position is maintained, as much as 1000 mL of blood may be lost without significant increase in pulse rate. Similarly, the pacemaker system of the heart within the sinoatrial node is obviously influenced by other stimuli such as fear and anxiety that may also accompany the trauma producing the loss of intravascular volume.

Consequently, during the course of observation and treatment of shock, changes in pulse rate are of value only when followed over an extended period. Change in pulse rate may indicate response to therapy once other external sources that may have changed cardiac rate are diminished or removed.

Vasoconstriction Increase in peripheral vascular resistance by production of peripheral vasoconstriction rapidly becomes maximal in an effort to compensate for the reduced cardiac output. Vascular resistance can be measured only indirectly in humans and in animals. There is good evidence that early disproportionate reduction in vascular resistance in the heart occurs while there is still little change in vascular resistance in many organs. Subsequently, maximal vasoconstriction occurs in the skin, kidneys, liver, and, finally, in the brain.[123]

Concomitantly, there is generalized constriction of the veins in response to reduction in intravascular volume. Venoconstriction would be a necessary homeostatic mechanism since over half of the total blood volume may be contained within the venous tree.[123]

These vascular responses to hemorrhage are immediate and striking. Within seconds following the onset of hemorrhage there are unequivocal signs of sympathetic and adrenal activation. Serum catecholamine levels show prompt elevation indicative of action of the adrenal medullary function.[135] The adrenal cortical and pituitary hormones also show prompt increase in serum levels following shock. Many of the clinical signs associated with shock are simply signs of response of the sympathetic and adrenal medullary system to the insult sustained by the organism.

Hemodilution All the responses to reduction of intravascular volume eventually result in decrease in volume flow to tissues and initiation of compensatory mechanisms directed at correction of the low flow state. One such compensation is movement of fluid into the circulation, resulting in hemodilution. This fluid is commonly known as extravascular extracellular fluid; it has the composition of plasma, but a lower protein content.

It is now clear, however, that the hematocrit or hemoglobin concentration in shock is simply an index of the balance between the relative loss of whole blood or plasma and gain into the blood system of extravascular fluid. For example, in hemorrhagic hypovolemia there is generally progressive hemodilution, which increases with the severity of the shock state. Obviously, in this circumstance there has been a greater movement of fluid from the extravascular to the intravascular space with the progression of the shock. This is in contradistinction to shock associated with loss of intravascular volume primarily due to plasma loss. High hematocrit shock may occur with massive losses of plasma and extravascular extracellular fluid, such as is associated with peritonitis, burns, large areas of soft tissue infection, and the crush syndrome.

The mechanism of hemodilution following hemorrhage is probably on the basis of the Starling hypothesis; i.e., the reduction in hydrostatic pressure in the capillaries because of hypotension and arterial and arteriolar vasoconstriction results in a shift of the pressure gradient to favor the passage of fluid from the tissue extracellular space into the intravascular capillary bed.

It is worthy to note that the studies of Carey et al. do not demonstrate a significant reduction in serum protein content in patients following hemorrhagic shock and resuscitation.[29,34]

Biochemical Changes

The biochemically measurable changes that occur as response to the stress invoked by shock fall into three fairly well-defined categories. These are (1) the changes invoked by the pituitary-adrenal response to stress, (2) those changes brought about by a net reduction in organ perfusion imposed by a low rate of blood flow, and (3) those changes brought about by failing function within specific organs.

Pituitary-Adrenal The immediate effects seen from sympathicoadrenal activity are those associated with high circulating epinephrine levels. Characteristically, these include eosinopenia and lymphocytopenia along with thrombocytopenia. This doubtless represents the laboratory reflection of increased circulating epinephrine that, in itself, can be and has been measured to be elevated, as an early response to shock. These changes are nonspecific and are found early in a patient with shock or severe trauma. These phenomena usually disappear rapidly. Other evidences of the pituitary and hormonal response to shock are seen in the well-known stress reaction or metabolic responses so well described by Moore.[95] These include a striking negative nitrogen balance and retention of sodium and water, as well as a notable increase in the excretion of potassium.

Low Flow State Those changes incident to the low rate of blood flow during shock are now being better understood. More evidence is accumulating to support the observation that, as a result of a decreased blood flow or low rate of perfusion, there is a reduction in oxygen delivered to the vital organs and, consequently, a mandatory change in metabolism from aerobic to anaerobic. In the switch from aerobic to anaerobic metabolism, energy made available by the oxidation of glucose is greatly reduced during shock. The most striking example of a shift in metabolism is the production of the end product lactic acid instead of the normal aerobic end product of carbon dioxide. This is reflected in a metabolic acidosis with a reduction in the carbon dioxide combining power of the blood. The available buffer base is progressively decreased by combining with the increased lactic acid, and the respiratory compensation that occurs early in the course of hemorrhagic shock is frequently inadequate. Consequently the progressive decline in pH toward a striking acidosis is thereby hastened. Indeed, in several studies the ability of animals as well as humans to recover from shock has been found to correlate rather closely with the degree of lactic acid production and the decrease in the alkali reserve and pH of the blood.

In some cases determination of blood pH may not accurately reflect changes in pH at the cellular level. After the induction of hemorrhagic shock in experimental animals, skeletal muscle surface pH changes precede those in blood, and minimal changes may be masked by the efficient blood buffer systems.[81] Lactate and excess lactate levels correlate well with the clinical impression of the depth of shock, but the injuries producing the shock state have a much greater bearing on ultimate prognosis.[25]

Drucker pointed out that there is a consistent elevation of the blood sugar level in relation to the degree of blood loss and the severity of shock.[45] This was earlier observed in battle casualties studied in World War II, and has since been thoroughly confirmed by Simeone and others. It is Drucker's belief that this represents an increase in hepatic glycolysis by the change from aerobic to anaerobic metabolism, while Egdahl believes that there is decreased insulin secretion and decreased peripheral utilization of glucose.[65]

Other evidences of failure of different parameters of cell metabolism have been presented by Thal,[129] Schumer,[111] Mela,[90] and Baue.[7]

Organ Failure The biochemical changes that appear incident to organ failure seem to be dependent in large part on the duration and severity of the shock. The changes in renal function induced by hypovolemia may vary from simple oliguria with a concentrated and acid urine to high output renal failure with a urine of low specific gravity and high pH, or frank anuric renal failure. Similarly, the blood nonprotein nitrogen content will depend on the degree of impairment in renal function. This may vary from slight to no retention of nitrogenous products to a steep and progressive rise that may require therapy.

Changes in ion concentration, including a rise of serum potassium, are dependent on many things, among them adrenal cortical response, the change in metabolism from aerobic to anaerobic with resultant release of potassium, and also specific changes within tissues invoked by the shock. If renal function is maintained, the rise inevitably seen in serum potassium early after the onset of shock is short-lived, in that the renal excretion of potassium is high during recovery from hemorrhagic shock. If renal function is impaired, the concentration of potassium and magnesium as well as creatinine can rise to high levels in the serum.

RESPONSE OF THE EXTRACELLULAR FLUID

Experimental Studies

Early Results Hypovolemic shock is the most common form seen clinically and is also the form that has been studied most intensively both clinically and in the laboratory. Most of our own studies have been carried out using hypovolemic shock produced by external blood loss as the model. A method has been developed which allows the simultaneous measurement of total body red cell mass with the use of Cr^{51}-tagged red blood cells, and total body plasma volume with the use of I^{131}-and, later, I^{125}-tagged human serum albumin. In addition, total body extracellular fluid

can be measured simultaneously with the use of S^{35}-tagged sodium sulfate.[91] These three isotopes are simultaneously injected intravenously, and by the use of appropriate energy-differentiating counting instruments, all three isotopes can be determined after equilibration. Volumes are then determined by the dilution principle using multiple sampling.

In an early study the three spaces were measured; splenectomized dogs were then bled a sublethal, subshock amount of 10 percent of the measured blood volume. After hemorrhage the three spaces were again measured. The measured loss of red cells and plasma, removed during the hemorrhage, could be detected by the method used. It was shown that the decrease in extracellular fluid volume was only that which was lost as plasma removed during the hemorrhage.[118]

By use of the same model, spaces were measured before and after hemorrhage of 25 percent of the measured blood volume. This hemorrhage was again sublethal, but did produce hypotension. In this group of animals the loss of red cells and plasma could be measured by the method. In addition, however, the functional extracellular fluid volume as measured by the early S^{35}-tagged sodium sulfate space decreased by 18 to 26 percent of the original volume. Since there was no measurable external loss of S^{35} sulfate, this reduction was presumed to be an internal redistribution of extracellular fluid. Subsequent studies of external bleeding of 35 percent, 45 percent, and even above 50 percent hemorrhage always produced the same reduction in functional extracellular fluid, as long as the animal was in shock.

In subsequent studies splenectomized dogs were subjected to "irreversible" hemorrhagic shock according to a modified method of Wiggers, using a reservoir.[119] Return of shed blood in this severe preparation resulted in the return of blood pressure to near control levels followed by a fall in blood pressure within 1 to

16 h, with death in 80 percent of the dogs, a standard mortality rate.

In one group of animals the three volumes were measured; the dogs were then subjected to shock by the Wiggers method. The three spaces were remeasured by reinjection during the period of shock; then shed blood was returned. The decrease in blood volume was that which had been removed. Concurrently, the functional extracellular fluid exhibited a decided reduction. Immediately after the return of shed blood, the red cell mass returned to essentially normal levels, as did the plasma volume; however, there remained a deficit of functional extracellular fluid. In dogs treated with shed blood plus plasma (10 mL/kg), the losses during shock were again similar. After therapy with plasma, plus return of shed blood, there was a return of blood volume to normal. There remained, however, a decrease in functional extracellular fluid volume.

Dogs treated with an extracellular "mimic," such as a balanced salt solution plus shed blood, had comparable losses during shock. As in the previous groups, the blood volume returned essentially to normal after treatment. Dogs treated with salt solution plus shed blood exhibited return of functional extracellular fluid volume to control levels.

In this study only 20 percent of those treated with shed blood alone survived longer than 24 h. When plasma was used in addition to whole blood as therapy, 30 percent of dogs so treated survived. Of the animals treated with lactated Ringer's solution plus shed blood, 70 percent survived (Fig. 1-1). The 80 percent mortality of a standard "irreversible" shock preparation was reduced to 30 percent by restoration of functional extracellular fluid volume in addition to return of shed blood.

All these early studies on the measurement of the functional extracellular fluid were based on volume distribution curves of sulfate measured up to approximately 1 h. At any point in the course of the shock volume distribution curve, there will be a reduction in extracellular fluid in the untreated state of shock.

Subsequent work has followed these volume distribution curves out for many hours.[91] In true untreated hemorrhagic shock there is a reduction in the total extracellular fluid, or final diluted volume of radiosulfate, when compared with preshock volumes (Fig. 1-2).

Even when a less severe shock preparation is used, there will still be a reduction in every equilibrating extracellular fluid, or early available extracellular fluid, whereas the total anatomic extracellular fluid may remain normal. Subsequent studies have shown that if shock is not of sufficient duration to produce reduction in both functional and total extracellular fluid, then the reduction may be only in functional extracellular fluid. Furthermore, if therapy is instituted quickly and blood pressure is returned to normal, a long sulfate equilibration curve may fail to reveal the acute reduction which was corrected very early.

Consequently, the current status of sulfate as measure of the functional extracellular fluid must be interpreted in the light that early sulfate space measurement reveals *functional* or *available* extracellular fluid, and that prolonged measurement of these curves will give *total* extracellular fluid values. It must further be remembered that if therapy has been instituted or has been completed, then the total or even the available extracellular fluid reduction may not be measurable (Fig. 1-3).[68,120]

There is no question that some plasma, or transcapillary, refilling does occur in response to hemorrhage and to hemorrhagic shock. This response, however, is initially rather limited and, in severe hemorrhagic shock, is grossly inadequate to explain the reduction seen in interstitial fluid. Since there is no source for external loss, the question arose as to whether interstitial fluid might move into the cell mass in an isotonic fashion (Fig. 1-4).

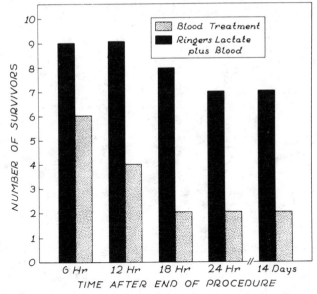

Figure 1-1 Acture hemorrhagic shock, survival study.

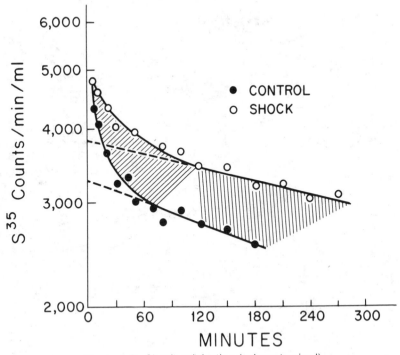

Figure 1-2 Shock, reinjection (splenectomized).

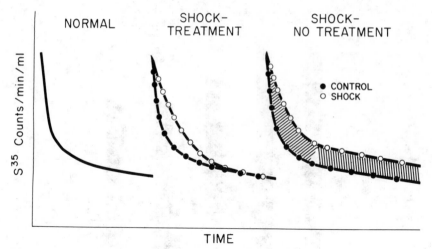

Figure 1-3 Radiosulphate equilibration curve; semilogarithmic plot, summary model.

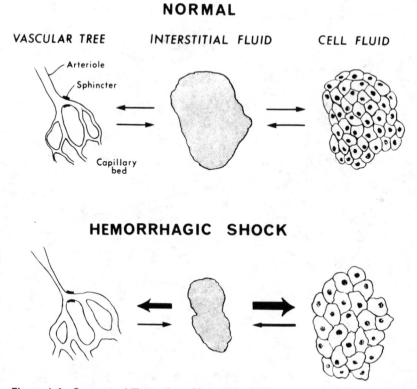

Figure 1-4 Conceptual illustration of interstitial fluid response to hemorrhagic shock.

Cellular Studies Subsequently, studies of ion transport across the cell membrane were undertaken in order to determine the possibility of intracellular swelling in skeletal muscle in response to hemorrhagic shock.[117] Using a Ling-Gerard ultramicroelectrode, intracellular transmembrane potential recordings were made with glass tip diameters of less than 1 μ (Fig. 1-5).[85] This electrode was modified to record intracellular transmembrane potentials in vivo before, during, and after shock.[23,31]

Skeletal muscle measurements in acute hemorrhagic shock demonstrate a constant and sustained fall in the normally negative intracellular transmembrane potential. This may represent a reduction in efficiency of the sodium pump induced by tissue hypoxia and is present only during shock producing hypotension. Additional studies in splenectomized dogs have shown that change in variables such as pH, P_{CO_2}, and bicarbonate have been shown not to influence the transmembrane potential in shock.[23] Even with progressive metabolic acidosis and its subsequent correction, the potential still follows the blood pressure and shock state (Fig. 1-6).

Additional studies have been reported utilizing the ultramicroelectrode measurement of transmembrane potential combined with direct skeletal muscle interstitial fluid aspiration by modification of the technique of Hagberg.[40,61] Using this technique, it can be seen that as blood pressure falls and transmembrane potential is reduced, plasma potassium rises slowly during the shock period (Fig. 1-7). However, the directly aspirated interstitial fluid potassium during the same period of time has risen to a height of above 15 meq/L of interstitial fluid. This study explained where potassium, moving out of skeletal muscle cells, was being sequestered as sodium chloride and water were moving into muscle cells.

Additional studies have now been performed in primates showing essentially the same phenomenon (Fig. 1-8). These same studies also reveal that this cellular membrane transport is a reversible phenomenon in that once the shock state is treated, transmembrane potential does recover. During these same studies in primates, concomitant muscle biopsies show clearly that muscle cells gain sodium and water and chloride while losing

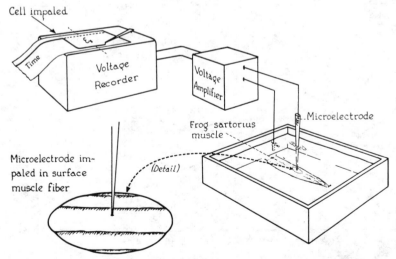

Figure 1-5 Schematic diagram of intracellular recording. (From Woodbury, in Ruch and Fulton (eds.): *Medical Physiology and Biophysics* 18th ed., W. B. Saunders Company, Philadelphia, 1960.)

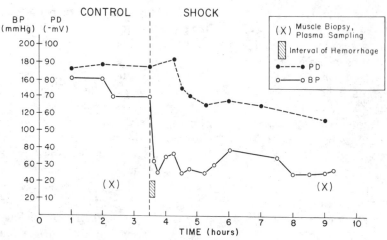

Figure 1-6 Changes in muscle membrane potential and blood pressure in response to hemorrhagic shock.

potassium. Consequently, the data reveal an isotonic swelling of skeletal muscle cells in response to shock injury (Fig. 1-9).

Studies that are currently being performed in humans reveal the same response to shock injury. Studies recently reported[115] have revealed interesting corroborative changes in action potentials of single cells in skeletal

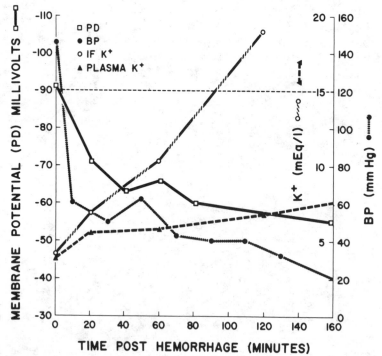

Figure 1-7 Changes in membrane potential and interstitial K[+] in rats with hemorrhagic shock.

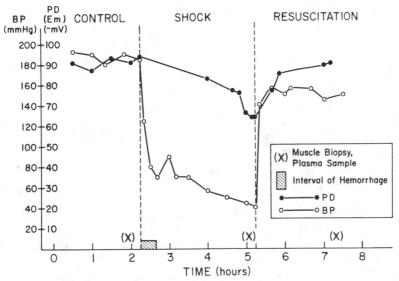

Figure 1-8 Changes in membrane potential and blood pressure during hemorrhagic shock and after resuscitation.

muscles in primates (Fig. 1-10). This study shows a decrease in resting membrane potential, a decrease in amplitude of action potential, and prolongation of both repolarization and depolarization times. Resuscitation reversed these changes acutely, except for repolarization time, which remained prolonged for several days. This study confirms in vitro the alterations in intracellular sodium and potassium concentrations which were measured by skeletal muscle biopsy and resting membrane potential measurements.

Interpretation of Experimental Studies Concisely stated, reduction in extracellular fluid in reversible hemorrhagic shock can con-

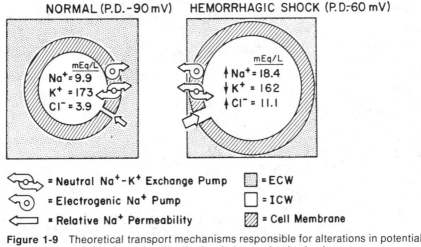

Figure 1-9 Theoretical transport mechanisms responsible for alterations in potential difference (PD) and fluid-electrolyte distribution in hemorrhagic shock.

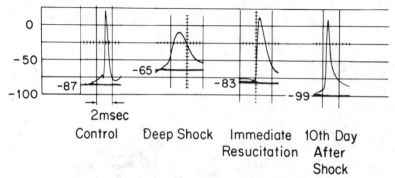

Figure 1-10 Action potentials in primates in hemorrhagic shock.

sistently be shown (1) with extracellular fluid markers that enter cells slowly or not at all in the shock state; (2) when reinjection of the extracellular fluid markers is utilized in the shock state; (3) when extracellular fluid markers or tracers are allowed sufficient time for equilibration; (4) when shock measurements are obtained while hemorrhagic shock is sustained; and (5) if the shock preparation is sufficiently severe and maintained until there is a change in cellular membrane transport.

The data obtained from prior experiments support the use of transmembrane potential measurements as an accurate indicator of cellular alterations resulting from the low flow state of hemorrhagic shock. Severe hypotension is associated with depression of transmembrane potential difference (PD) which is sustained in the presence of a continued shock state.[115]

Transmembrane potential difference is generally agreed to be the result of either an electrogenic sodium pump (with active outward extrusion of sodium from muscle cells by a redox system) or a coupled sodium-potassium exchange pump with diffusion of sodium and potassium down their respective chemical gradients.[37,53,67] In the latter theory the relative permeabilities of the membrane to the two ions must be considered, and the potential interpreted on the basis of the

Hodgkins-Katz-Goldman equation in which pNa^+ (relative sodium permeability) is 0.01. Since potassium permeability is assumed to be much greater than sodium permeability in the cell membrane, the PD is essentially a potassium diffusion potential.

The present data suggest, then, that skeletal muscle cells may be a principal site of fluid and electrolyte sequestration after severe, prolonged hemorrhagic shock. Adjunctive studies by Grossman et al. suggest that similar changes in the intracellular mass of neurons in the brain also occur in response to hypovolemic shock.[58] Furthermore, an increase in cellular water content of both cellular and connective tissue components following hemorrhagic shock has been demonstrated by Slonim and Stahl.[124] Fulton has suggested that connective tissue may be the site of some sodium and water sequestration.[51]

The exact mechanism for the production of electrolyte changes as well as the notable diminution in extracellular water which occurs after hemorrhagic shock is not known. It appears that they may well represent a reduction in the efficiency of an active ionic pump mechanism or a selective increase in muscle cell membrane permeability to sodium, or both (Fig. 1-9).

With a reset membrane potential, extracellular fluid electrolyte concentrations are unchanged. Consequently, from the Nernst equation, intracellular Cl^- must rise from 3.5 to 10 meq, and intracellular Na^+ from 10 to 22 meq (Fig. 1-11). For transposition of these data to the previously cited measurements in hemorrhagic shock, a model is shown (Fig. 1-12). This model shows a 10 percent isotonic swelling of muscle cells to explain the reduction in extracellular fluid measured in hemorrhagic shock. Studies are currently under way to determine the involvement of cell masses other than muscle during the course of hemorrhagic shock. One such study indicated that severe hemorrhagic shock of significant duration is associated with elevation of the internal sodium concentration of the red blood cells.[41] The magnitude of these changes appears to be a function of both the severity and duration of the shock process and seems to be well correlated with changes in clinical course when sequential sampling procedures are utilized.

Summary At present it appears that there is a measurable reduction in extravascular extracellular fluid in response to sustained hemorrhagic shock. It also appears that cellular response to hypovolemic hypotension demonstrates a consistent change in active transport of ions. The directly obtained evidence from living cells indicates that sodium and water enter muscle cells with resultant loss of cellular potassium to the extracellular fluid. The interstitial fluid holds the extruded potassium.

Replenishment of the depleted extracellular fluid has been shown to be of significant benefit in the cellular response to hypovolemic

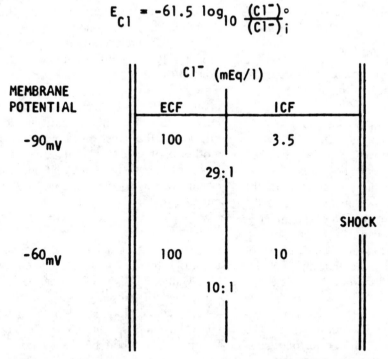

Figure 1-11 Changes in intracellular chloride in response to change in membrane potentials.

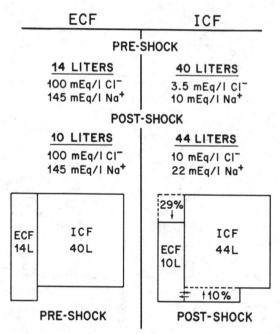

Figure 1-12 Schema of intracellular movement of extracellular electrolytes and water in response to hemorrhagic shock in man.

shock. It has also been shown to be of clinical benefit in large numbers of patients.

THERAPY OF HYPOVOLEMIC SHOCK

It is apparent from the previously described etiologic classification of shock that therapy will of necessity depend on detection of the causative mechanisms, while support of the patient is supplied. Correction of the underlying causative factors can then be carried out. Consequently one sees again the usefulness of a practical clinical classification that includes (1) oligemic shock; (2) cardiogenic shock; and (3) shock caused by changes in peripheral resistance and capacitance vessels (neurogenic shock and septic shock). In a patient who has undergone trauma, more than one causative factor may be operating. Once the diagnosis of shock has been made and supportive

therapy begun, a diligent search for the causative factor or factors can be made.

Treatment of shock, therefore, can best be thought of in relation to the type of shock that is present. As pointed out earlier, the pathogenesis of hypovolemic hypotension is varied. Recognition of deficits of total body water and electrolytes is usually subtle, and correction requires specific therapy with crystalloid solutions. Reductions in the extracellular fluid volume (plasma and interstitial fluids) primarily, such as occurs in burns, peritonitis, and some forms of crush injury, are more easily recognized. Specific therapy should be started with electrolyte solutions and rarely may require the use of plasma or some source of protein. External blood loss as seen in lacerations should be controlled immediately, as fluid therapy is begun. Similarly, an external loss, such as bleeding from a duodenal ulcer, should be treated with the usual measures, including decompression of the stomach, while supportive therapy is begun.

The only other immediate concern in addition to control of the causative wounds is maintenance of an open airway. Pulmonary insufficiency rarely occurs from shock alone, but concomitant injuries may include crush injuries of the chest, pneumothorax, and hemothorax or specific obstruction of the airway from injuries to the head and neck. In these circumstances adequate respiratory exchange must be restored promptly.

Volume

The treatment of hemorrhagic shock continues to be the adequate replacement of whole blood, since this is the fluid that has been lost. Early use of properly cross-matched, type-specific whole blood is still the primary therapy when shock is due to whole blood loss. When whole blood of the proper type and cross match is not immediately available, type-specific or Rh-negative "universal donor" type O blood with low anti-A titer can be administered.

Extracellular Fluid Replacement In view of the previously described changes in the peripheral circulation and interstitial fluid, an effective therapeutic regimen for the treatment of hemorrhagic shock has now been used successfully in several thousand patients.

When patients are admitted to the emergency room in hemorrhagic shock, a large-gauge needle or catheter is inserted into an appropriate vein (preferably in the arm) and an infusion of lactated Ringer's solution is begun immediately. At the same time, blood is drawn for type and cross matching. The lactated Ringer's solution is run at a rapid rate so that in a period of 45 min between 1000 and 2000 mL of lactated Ringer's solution has been given intravenously. This approach has several advantages.

1 This is a very effective therapeutic trial to determine the preexisting amount of blood loss or the presence of continuing blood loss. It is often observed that after infusion of 1 or 2 L of a balanced salt solution blood pressure will return to normal and remain stable in patients with severe hypotension. When such a response is correlated with measurements of red blood cell mass, plasma volume, and extracellular fluid volume, it has been shown that the preexisting blood loss was relatively minimal. If blood loss has been minimal and hemorrhage is not continuing, then hemorrhagic hypotension can be alleviated simply by the infusion of a balanced salt solution.

2 If blood loss has been severe or hemorrhage is continuing, then the elevation of blood pressure and decrease in pulse rate that occur with rapid intravenous infusion of lactated Ringer's solution will usually be transient. When this occurs, whole blood that has been accurately typed and cross matched is available and can be given immediately. Con-

sequently, the initial use of the balanced salt solution allows time for accurate typing and cross matching.

3 In view of the large, disparate reduction in the extravascular extracellular fluid as demonstrated in animals and humans, it is felt that even though blood is needed, as it is in the majority of patients admitted in hemorrhagic hypovolemia, alleviation of the reduction in functional extracellular fluid is desirable.

4 Lactated Ringer's solution as initial therapy, both from the standpoint of a therapeutic trial and as a therapeutic adjunct, is a procedure that has been found to be effective. This is understandable, since lactated Ringer's solution is isotonic, essentially free from side reactions, and virtually harmless from the standpoint of aggravation of other fluid and electrolyte imbalances that may be present.

Further, it appears that the use of a balanced salt solution in this fashion significantly reduces the requirement of whole blood in the patient with hemorrhagic hypotension. This is true not only from the standpoint of proper hemoglobin and hematocrit concentrations following therapy, but also from the standpoint of prevention of, or recovery from, renal failure.

A concern that Ringer's lactate solution may aggravate the existing lactate acidosis when used to treat patients in shock has been expressed by several investigators, but previous studies in both experimental animals and patients do not support this view.[8,28,73,130] The use of blood plus Ringer's lactate solution to treat hemorrhagic shock in experimental animals results in a more rapid return to normal of lactate, excess lactate, and pH than does treatment with return of shed blood alone. Recently, serial determinations of lactate, excess lactate, pH, and base excess have been obtained in 52 patients in hemorrhagic shock.[25] All patients received Ringer's lactate solution in addition to whole blood during the

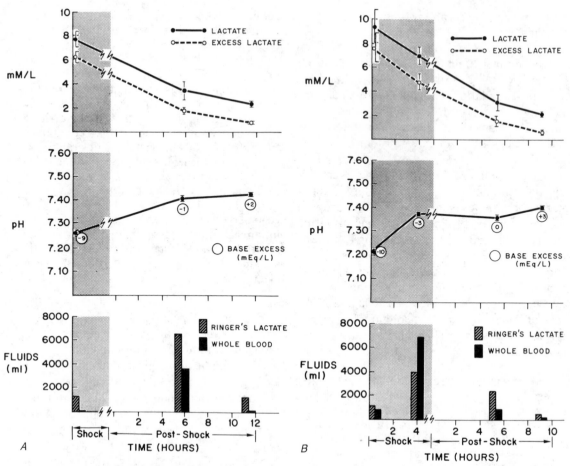

Figure 1-13 (*A*) Mean values (±SE) for 52 patients in hemorrhagic shock. Postshock values are the means for the 48 patients resuscitated from shock. The amount of fluids administered is indicated at the end of each interval. (*B*) Mean values (±SE) for 15 patients who had at least two determinations of lactate and excess lactate during the period of hemorrhagic shock.

period of resuscitation. There was a significant reduction in lactate and excess lactate levels and a return of pH and base excess values toward normal during the period of shock while Ringer's lactate solution was being infused. After resuscitation, all these values rapidly returned to normal levels Fig. 1–13.

Blood Transfusions The acceptability for transfusion of blood which has been stored in ACD (acid-citrate-dextrose) solution for up to 3 weeks is based on survival of at least 70 percent of the cells in the recipient's circulation. During this 3-week period, however, there is a rapid decline in erythrocyte 2, 3-diphosphoglycerate (DPG) and a progressive increase in hemoglobin-oxygen affinity (leftward shift of the oxygen dissociation curve).[15,22,42,43,133] After transfusion it requires 24 h or longer for the DPG levels to return to normal.[24,132] These findings indicate that oxygen delivery may be impaired after the administration of large quantities of stored blood and have led to a reevaluation of transfusion practices.

Obtaining a sufficient quantity of fresh blood for resuscitation of the patient in hemorrhagic shock is difficult, and attempts are being made to find a suitable storage medium that will maintain the level of organic phosphates in the red blood cells.[43,131,146] At present, storage of blood in CPD (citrate-phosphate-dextrose) solution seems to be the most practical alternative, since DPG is more stable in this medium than in ACD solution. The administration of limited quantities of older CPD-stored blood in acute situations is acceptable, although the capability of this blood to deliver oxygen fully may not be realized for several hours. When larger quantities of blood are administered, particularly in critically ill patients, the storage age of each unit should be recorded. If a significant portion of the blood administered is more than a few days old, every attempt should be made to obtain fresh blood for additional transfusion requirements.

Consideration of other factors that influence the position of the dissociation curve may also be important in the individual patient. For instance, the induction of a respiratory alkalosis may produce an abrupt increase in hemoglobin-oxygen affinity. This is a common occurrence during operation and in patients requiring ventilatory assistance in the postoperative period; coupled with other factors that limit oxygen transport, the capacity to maintain tissue oxygenation may be sharply reduced. Similarly, the sudden correction of an acidosis, whether metabolic or respiratory, may have undesirable effects. In this regard the indiscriminate use of sodium bicarbonate during resuscitation of patients in hypovolemic shock is discouraged. The presence of a mild metabolic alkalosis is a common finding after resuscitation, owing in part to the alkalinizing effects of blood transfusions and the administration of lactated Ringer's solution.

After infusion (and partial restoration of hepatic blood flow) the citrate and lactate contained in transfused blood and the lactate in lactated Ringer's solution are metabolized, and bicarbonate is formed. If excessive quantities of sodium bicarbonate are administered simultaneously, a severe metabolic alkalosis may result. The alkaline pH may be highly undesirable, particularly in patients with hypoxia or low fixed cardiac output. In combination with other factors incident to blood replacement which increase hemoglobin-oxygen affinity (low DPG concentration and hypothermia), significant interference with oxygen unloading at the cellular level may occur.

The immediate and direct pH influences on the curve (via the Bohr effect) are eventually offset by reciprocal changes in DPG concentration. There is a lag period, however, of approximately 4 h before any change in DPG concentration is noted, and the final level is not reached until 48 h after induction of acidosis or alkalosis.[14] The fact that the effects of sudden, large changes in pH may persist for several hours should be considered during therapy. Correction of a metabolic acidosis, therefore, is properly directed toward correction of the underlying disorder. Bicarbonate therapy may be reserved for the treatment of severe metabolic acidosis, particularly following cardiac arrest, when partial correction of pH is essential to restore myocardial function. Similarly, pH correction in more protracted states of metabolic acidosis may be indicated, but should be accomplished slowly.

Hematocrit   For many years the belief was held that hemorrhage and shock were separate entities, because hemorrhage was not accompanied by hemoconcentration, though shock was inevitably accompanied by a rise in hematocrit. As shown in Fig. 1-14 and as described previously in the pathologic physiology of shock, the hematocrit is not a differentiating

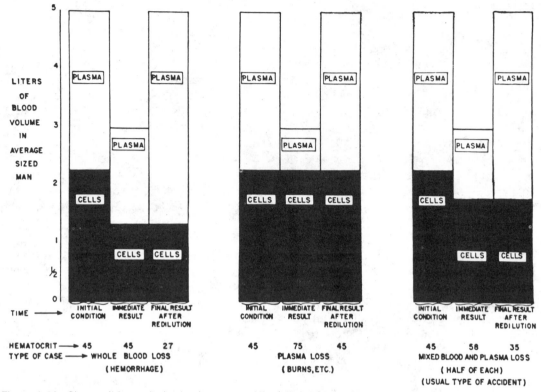

Figure 1-14   Six possible results in shock cases, and the fallacy of using hemoconcentration as the only guide to treatment. (From H. N. Harkins, Recent advances in the study and management of traumatic shock, *Surgery,* **9**:231–294, 1941.)

factor. The extent of concentration depends on the proportion of red blood cells and plasma lost in the hypovolemic episode, as well as on the compensatory adjustments that the interstitial fluid has been able to make to the intravascular volume reduction.

Blood Substitutes   In the absence of whole blood, many substances have been proposed as transient substitutes for the combination of red blood cells and plasma available in whole blood. The most popular and commonly used substitute had been human plasma. In some circumstances, e.g., battlefield conditions, plasma has been a highly serviceable substitute. An individual unit of plasma carries with it the same risk of viral hepatitis that whole

blood does.[2] A unit of pooled plasma, however, carries a greater risk of harboring and transmitting the infective viral hepatitis than a unit of blood. As shown by Allen, storage of fresh plasma at room temperature for 6 to 8 months significantly reduces the attack rate and infectivity of the virus infectious hepatitis.[2] In any event, the administration of plasma carries with it some risk of hepatitis as well as the poorly understood antigen-antibody reactions that frequently occur from homologous plasma. Further, the volume of plasma required is such that for all practical purposes restoration of blood volume is not generally feasible with plasma alone. Plasma contains no hemoglobin and, therefore, no oxygen-carrying capacity beyond that of any nonerythrocyte-containing liquid (physically dissolved oxygen in plasma constitutes only 0.3 percent by volume).

It should be pointed out that volume replacement with plasma is rapidly equilibrated into the total extracellular fluid. The albumin that remains in the vascular tree is easily degraded at a rapid rate. Moore estimates that plasma dispersal from the intravascular to extravascular phase may proceed at a rate approaching 500 mL, or 2 U/h.[94] Therefore plasma or albumin as a blood volume substitute is transient at best.

A number of other substances have been proposed for transfusion in hemorrhagic shock since early in World War I, when solutions of acacia were used. Several excellent review articles are available which summarize the problems with all these artifical solutions.[52] Suffice it to say that at present the only acceptable one of the entire group continues to be dextran. This substance has been shown to be effective clinically in the absence of a severe need for hemoglobin and its oxygen-carrying capacity. Nevertheless, like all other plasma or blood substitutes, this substance still causes occasional severe antigen-antibody reactions and, above all, regularly produces defects in the clotting mechanism. This has been shown in volunteers and patients when amounts greater than 1 L of clinical dextran with an average molecular weight of approximately 75,000 are used in humans.[69] The longest effect of dextran in maintaining an expanded plasma volume has been shown to be 24 to 48 h. Low-molecular-weight dextran in the average range of 35,000 to 40,000 has recently received renewed interest because of data suggesting its ability to lower the viscosity of blood and possibly to prevent agglutination of erythrocytes during the low flow state induced by hypovolemic shock.[5,55,82] But work by Replogle indicates that the effect of low-molecular-weight dextran on blood viscosity may be due entirely to

hemodilution or the change in blood volume.[106] When these parameters were controlled, no evidence for alterations in blood viscosity associated with infusions of low-molecular-weight dextran were observed. Although there are some theoretical advantages in using this plasma expander, investigative studies have indicated serious clotting mechanism defects with low-molecular-weight dextran, such as had been seen with the higher-molecular-weight dextrans.

Positioning

Positioning of the patient in shock has long been thought to be an adjunct in the treatment of hypovolemic shock. Most first-aid courses teach that the patient in shock should be placed in the head-down position. Although it is true that some forms of shock, particularly neurogenic shock, will respond to the head-down position, the effect of posture on the cerebral circulation in the face of true hypovolemia has not been defined. Frequently the patient with multiple trauma has sustained other injuries, within both the abdomen and the chest, so that the routine use of the Trendelenburg, or head-down, position may interfere with respiratory exchange far more than when the patient is left supine. The beneficial effect of the head-down position is probably the result of transient autotransfusion of pooled blood in the capacitance or venous side of the peripheral circulation. This beneficial effect can be obtained easily by elevating both legs while maintaining the trunk and the remainder of the patient in the supine position. This is probably the preferable position, then, for the treatment of hypovolemic shock.[60]

Pulmonary Support

In the past most writings on the treatment of hypovolemic shock stated that breathing high oxygen concentrations is probably of little value during a period of hypotension.[123] These conclusions were based on the concept that the principal defect is in volume flow to tissues and decreased cardiac output. The oxygen saturation in the majority of patients with uncomplicated hypovolemic shock is generally normal, and the small increase in dissolved oxygen in the blood contributed by raising the P_{O_2} above this level is insignificant, particularly in the face of a markedly decreased cardiac output. This concept continues to be valid in terms of improvement of the shock state or tissue oxygenation itself. Nevertheless, in the small but significant group of patients in hypovolemic shock in whom the oxygen saturation is not normal, the initial use of increased oxygen concentrations may be extremely important, since the fall in cardiac output accompanying hemorrhagic shock has been shown to compound existing defects in oxygenation.[103] This may occur in patients with preexisting defects, such as chronic obstructive lung disease, but more frequently problems in oxygenation arise directly from the patient's injury. Examples of this would be a coexisting pneumothorax, pulmonary contusion, aspiration of gastric contents or blood, and larger obstructive problems. Thus, although oxygen is not routinely administered to patients in shock, if any doubt exists as to the possibility of one of these circumstances or as to the adequacy of oxygenation of arterial blood, the initial administration of oxygen until diligent assessment of the injuries to the patient has been made is certainly justified. If oxygen is to be administered to patients under these circumstances, it should be delivered through loose-fitting face masks designed for this purpose. If a controlled airway is indicated for other reasons, an endotracheal tube is ideal. The use of nasal catheters, particularly those passed into the nasopharynx, is avoided because of potential complications of pharyngeal lacerations and gastric distention. Gastric rupture has been recorded secondary to such a catheter inadvertently placed into the esophagus.

Antibiotics

Antibiotics were used in the treatment of hypovolemic shock for many years and were thought to exert a protective mechanism against the ravages of hypovolemia. Subsequent data fail to support this hypothesis. The use of antibiotics in patients, however, who have open or potentially contaminated wounds continues to be sound practice, when combined with good surgical debridement and care. Consequently the use of wide-spectrum antibiotics, as well as specific coverage against the streptococcus and staphylococcus, is advisable as a preventive measure in the severely injured patient. Generally, penicillin is used in doses of 1 to 5 million units/24 h with parenteral administration of tetracycline in doses of 1 to 2 g for the first 24 h. These are started immediately on patients who have sustained hypovolemic shock from trauma.

Treatment of Pain

Treatment of pain in the patient with hypovolemic shock is rarely a problem from the standpoint of shock itself. If, however, the causative injury produces severe pain as in fracture, peritonitis, injury to the chest wall, and the like, then control of pain becomes mandatory. Generally, when the patient is moved to the emergency facility where physicians and care are available, simple restorative measures, administration of intravenous fluids, passing of catheters, and so forth, will give reassurance. The need for analgesics is greatly reduced, since the need to allay fear and anxiety becomes markedly less. If, however, the patient continues to have severe pain, then the observations made by Henry K. Beecher in World War II become extremely pertinent.[11] Beecher pointed out that many battle casualties received morphine or other narcotic agents by subcutaneous administration early after wounding. Since these analgesics were not put into the circulation immediately, the pain continued and the patient ultimately received several doses that were not absorbed. Once effective therapy was begun for shock, the doses previously administered were absorbed and profound sedation resulted. As a result, the recommendation was made that small doses of narcotics be given *intravenously* for the management of pain in the patient with shock. This has been standard practice for 20 years and relieves pain without contributing significantly to the potentiation of the shock syndrome.

Steroids

Adrenocorticoid depletion was commonly regarded as a contributory factor in shock after it was learned that the presence of hypovolemic shock could in itself deplete the adrenal cortex of adrenal cortical steroids. Subsequent studies, however, have shown that adrenal cortical steroid production is stimulated maximally by the presence of hypovolemic shock.[70] Steroid depletion with hypovolemic shock may possibly occur in the elderly patient or in patients who have specific adrenal cortical diseases such as incipient Addison's disease, postadrenalectomy patients, or patients who have had adrenal suppression with exogenous adrenal cortical steroids. In these specific instances the intravenous administration of hydrocortisone is desirable. In the general patient with hypovolemic shock, however, administration of adrenocorticoids is not indicated initially.[62] The use of steroids may be indicated in more complicated and unresponsive shock states, particularly when septic shock is suspected (see section on septic shock).

Digitalis

Digitalis has been advocated in the treatment of hypovolemic shock. There is no doubt that in some patients, particularly elderly ones, the stress of hypovolemic shock will in itself induce or aggravate cardiac failure. In these patients, digitalis is found to be helpful. Over the years many have investigated the role of the heart as a cause for the irreversible form of hemorrhagic shock, but experimental data obtained in patients indicate that heart failure in response to hypovolemic shock is merely a terminal event. Further evidence of this is supplied by the fact that the central venous pressure does not rise except terminally in hypovolemic shock.[123]

Intraarterial Infusions

Intraarterial infusions were advocated for many years for the rapid replacement of intravascular volume in hypovolemic hypotension and shock. The weight of evidence at present, supplied by Hampson, Scott, and Gurd,[63] and Harkins[64] and others, is that "the side of the circulation into which the blood is transfused is of no importance provided that the same rapid rate can be assured." Consequently the present-day usefulness of intraarterial transfusion resolves itself to a matter of convenience. If the operative procedure is in the area of a major artery, as in open-chest procedures, then a given quantity of blood may be delivered much faster via the intraarterial route. Otherwise, no specific advantage seems to be offered by the arterial route of transfusion.

Hypothermia

Since the basic defect during shock is inadequate perfusion to tissue for maintenance of normal metabolism, a logical approach to supportive therapy would include some mechanism, such as hypothermia, to lower normal tissue metabolism. To be sure, experimental results in animals have demonstrated that induction of hypothermia prior to the onset of hemorrhagic shock will in fact protect against the lethality of the shock.[101] Similarly, some experiments have shown that therapy of hemorrhagic shock with hypothermia has provided some beneficial effect. The available data for evaluation of hypothermia in humans with hypovolemic shock are meager. Since the induction of a hypothermic state is a serious undertaking, it is difficult to assess the effects on the severely injured patient. Some available data in humans would indicate that under some circumstances, hypothermia may be desirable. These circumstances need to be further elucidated, and are probably concerned with the later stages of prolonged hypovolemic or possibly septic shock.

Renal Hypothermia

Local or regional cooling is of proved benefit in protecting the kidney from damage during ischemic periods. Methods for local cooling have been developed in an attempt to reduce postoperative renal complications induced by the total ischemia necessary during renal artery repair, heminephrectomy, or stone removal,[35,112] as well as aorticorenal surgery.[98] Of far more common occurrence are the renal ischemia and resultant renal damage occasioned by hemorrhagic or hypovolemic shock. Since the kidney is rendered ischemic even in mild hypovolemic shock, rapid lowering of intrarenal temperature should afford protection during prolonged periods of ischemia.[39,79]

The effective methods of introducing local renal hypothermia previously described are limited for optimal use in emergency situations by requiring (1) the additional operative trauma of mobilization of the kidney; (2) cumbersome, special equipment that is not readily available or is difficult to sterilize and maintain; and (3) careful attention to prevent interference with other operative procedures within the abdominal cavity.[35,75,108]

The open peritoneal cavity affords a large surface area for heat exchange. Jaeger found that the introduction of a large volume of cold isotonic solution into the closed peritoneal cavity of dogs resulted in a rapid decrease in body temperature.[72] If intraabdominal organs, particularly the kidneys, which are apparently the most sensitive to hypoxia, can be effectively cooled by the direct introduction of cold solution, then a simple, expedient, practical method of cooling is readily available in every operating room. This consists in filling the

open abdominal cavity with isotonic salt solution that has been cooled in the operating room refrigerator (Fig. 1-15).

Experiments in animals were undertaken (1) to compare the temperatures obtained and the protection afforded the ischemic kidney by this method with that of direct surface hypothermia; (2) to evaluate the depth of cooling obtained in the ischemic versus the intact kidney; and (3) to determine the depth of cooling obtained in the kidney during hemorrhagic shock.[10] A summary of the results of these experiments follows.

1 Figure 1-16 shows the degree of protection afforded by surface cooling as opposed to formal hypothermia perfusion. Surface cooling provided significant protection from renal ischemia (100 percent survival rate). Lower intrarenal temperatures could be obtained by circulating coolant; however, the survival rate was lowered, probably because of the necessary extensive mobilization of the kidney.

2 A subsequent experimental study was designed to evaluate the effect of intact blood supply on the degree of hypothermia obtained by peritoneal cooling. The results of this study are shown in Fig. 1-17, and a comparison between esophageal temperatures with and without intact renal blood supply is also seen. These results demonstrate that there is some decrease in total body temperature, especially with intact blood supply to the kidneys, but that the intrarenal temperature even with intact blood flow is decreased at more than twice the rate of the general body temperature. Without blood flow, the depth of renal hypothermia achieved is 3 times that of the esophageal temperature as long as cooling is continued. An equally important observation is that the ischemic kidney rewarms only slowly as compared to the kidney with intact blood supply.

3 The results of the third study to determine the depth of cooling obtained during hemorrhagic shock are shown in Fig. 1-18. The depth of hypothermia obtained is seen to be approximately the same as that in the intact kidneys without hemorrhagic hypotension.

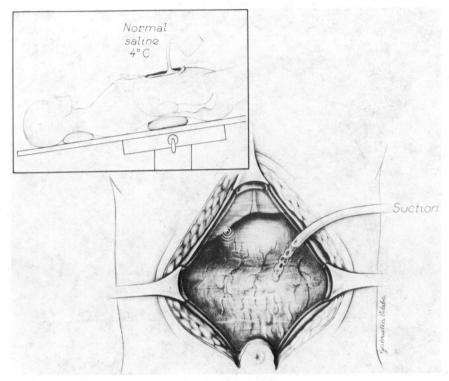

Figure 1-15 Technique of regional abdominal hypothermia.

Similarly, there was a concomitant lowering of the total body temperature to approximately 31°C. But after the chilled solution had been removed from the abdominal cavity, the intrarenal temperatures in the hypotensive animals continued to decline, reading 24°C in 30 min. Despite this, the total body temperatures did not reach significantly lower levels.

The studies indicate that intrarenal temperatures of approximately 25°C should furnish good protection, with only transient mild suppression of renal function.[20,76] Certainly 20°C offers complete protection to the ischemic kidney for periods extending to 6 h.[21,48] The effective cooling of the kidney with an intact blood supply versus the ischemic kidney emphasizes the importance of blood supply in determining the rate and depth of cooling.

Studies were then made in patients on the basis of the animal experiments. It was felt that this type of hypothermia could be used in patients with safety and could be expected to produce a sustained lowering of intrarenal temperatures during hypovolemic hypotension. Intrarenal hypothermia in patients was produced by filling the abdominal cavity with 2 L of refrigerated (3°C) isotonic salt solution. The solution was allowed to remain in contact with the peritoneal cavity for approximately 1 to 2 min. The bulk of this was removed by suction, and this was repeated several times, employing a total of 4 to 6 L of the cold solution during a 5-min period. Intrarenal temperatures were measured by sterilized needle prior to the induction of hypothermia and at intervals during and after cooling.

Figure 1-19 shows the intrarenal temperatures of 10 patients taken 5 min after the beginning of peritoneal hypothermia. It can be seen that in those patients who were normo-

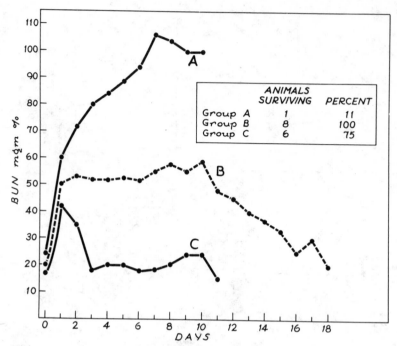

	ANIMALS SURVIVING	PERCENT
Group A	1	11
Group B	8	100
Group C	6	75

Figure 1-16 Blood urea levels after renal ischemia.

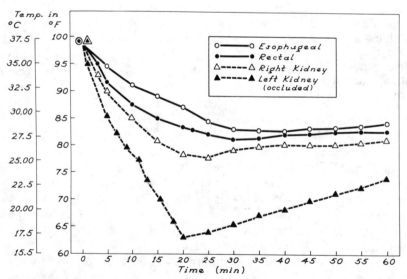

Figure 1-17 Peritoneal hypothermia by means of intraperitoneal iced saline solution at 2 to 3°C (left renal pedicle occluded).

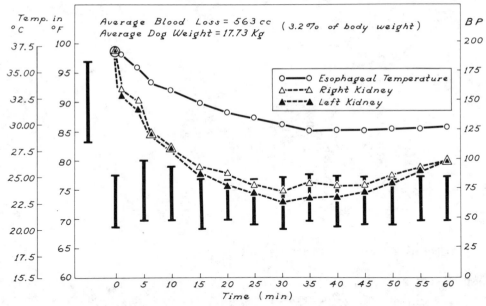

Figure 1-18 Peritoneal hypothermia by means of intraperitoneal iced saline solution at 2 to 3°C after blood loss shock (renal pedicle not occluded).

tensive, there was minimal lowering of the renal temperature. On the other hand, in patients with modest hypotension intrarenal temperatures were lowered to 31 to 32°C, and in the severely hypotensive patient the intrarenal temperature in 5 min had reached the level of 25°C.

Figure 1-20 depicts three patients in whom

intrarenal temperatures were measured prior to induction of renal hypothermia and at 1-min intervals thereafter. As would be expected from the studies just presented, the rate of fall in intrarenal temperature was directly proportional to the degree of hypotension present at the time of cooling.

Esophageal temperatures were monitored.

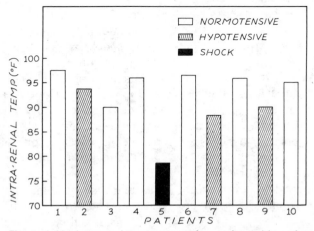

Figure 1-19 Intrarenal temperature after peritoneal hypothermia.

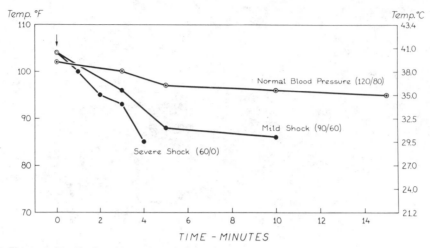

Figure 1-20 Regional hypothermia in patients.

In general, the fall in esophageal temperature was approximately half the fall in intrarenal temperatures in the first 10 min. The lowest temperature reached was 31°C in two patients. No untoward effects were noted other than a modest fall in blood pressure (less than 10 mmHg diastolic) in normotensive patients. There were no changes in cardiac rate or rhythm during this procedure.

The animal experiments show that an intrarenal temperature of 28 to 30°C is easily attainable in the ischemic dog kidney by sluice cooling of the peritoneal cavity. This moderate degree of hypothermia produced 100 percent survival, but with mild elevation of the blood urea nitrogen (BUN) for a period of 12 to 15 days. All these animals excreted normal or increased amounts of urine.

The preliminary data suggest that cooling by means of peritoneal irrigation (1) produces sufficient lowering of intrarenal temperatures to afford protection to the kidney with decreased blood flow; (2) offers a rapid means of lowering total body temperature; and (3) should produce a decrease in intrarenal temperature in a kidney completely deprived of blood comparable to that obtained by other local techniques.

In the past the chief objection to peritoneal irrigation was the introduction of infection. Peritoneal dialysis for uremia has proved to be a safe procedure on a short-term basis, infection occurring only after prolonged use.[44] In our experience the use of copious quantities of refrigerated salt solution in the operating room has been completely free from complications. Specifically, there have been no cases of peritonitis, abscess formation, wound disruption, or prolonged ileus in the patients studied.

Vasopressors

In the past the addition of substances that cause additional vasoconstriction in hypovolemic shock has been popular. These have largely been used because the blood pressure in humans can usually be elevated somewhat by the addition of one of a series of pressor agents. Although it is true that blood pressure can be elevated, the objective in treating hypovolemic shock is one of increasing tissue perfusion. By use of vasopressors the blood pressure is raised by increasing peripheral vascular resistance and decreasing tissue perfusion. Therefore the injurious effects of shock may well be aggravated.

As experience has accumulated with the use of vasopressors, it is obvious that the alpha- and beta-stimulating functions of the vasopressors must be separated during clinical evaluation (Fig. 1-21).[83] The vasopressors generally have a threefold action consisting of central inotropic and chronotropic effects as well as a peripheral vasoconstricting effect. In a recent evaluation of the comparative effects of a number of the catecholamines, Waldhausen et al. demonstrated significant differences.[134] Isoproterenol hydrochloride (Isuprel), levarterenol bitartrate (Levophed), epinephrine (Adrenalin), and phenylephrine hydrochloride (Neo-Synephrine) all produced a significant increase in contractility of the heart and an increase in heart rate. Isoproterenol had, in addition, a vasodilator effect on the peripheral vessels, while the other three amines were largely peripheral vasoconstrictors. Metaraminol (Aramine) produced a significant increase in myocardial contractility,

further increasing the efficiency of the heart beat while the heart rate fell; this amine was also a moderate vasopressor. Of the drugs tested, phenylephrine showed the least efficient inotropic effect and was predominantly a peripheral vasopressor.

In 1923 Cannon condemned the use of vasopressors on this physiologic basis: "Damming the blood in the arterial portion of the circulation, when the organism is suffering primarily from a diminished quantity of blood flow, obviously does not improve the volume flow in the capillaries."[26] In 1940 Blalock also condemned the use of vasopressors in treating shock.[3] Recent studies have more clearly defined the hazards of using vasopressors in hypovolemic shock. Close and his associates demonstrated a sharp increase in the mortality of dogs rendered hypotensive by hemorrhage when norepinephrine was administered in sufficient doses to raise the blood pressure from 40 mmHg to 100 mmHg.[33] Mortality in animals

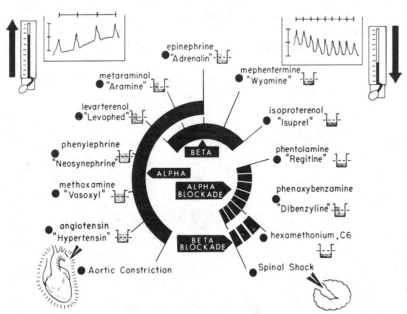

Figure 1-21 Adrenergic mechanisms. (From C. M. Lewis and M. H. Weil, Hemodynamic spectrum of vasopressor and vasodilator drugs. *J. Am. Med. Assoc.,* **208**:1391, 1969. Copyright, 1969, American Medical Association.)

so treated was 64 percent compared with 33 percent in the untreated controls. Catchpole et al., using a drip of norepinephrine after 30 min of hypotension and again before reinfusion of shed blood, obtained no improvement in survival.[32] Additionally, Hakstian, Hampson, and Gurd demonstrated no significant protection during hemorrhagic hypotension through the use of norepinephrine.[62] On the other hand, studies by Lansing and Stevenson suggest that the use of norepinephrine for the maintenance of blood pressure and cardiac output after normovolemia has been restored may be advantageous.[80] Simeone has similarly shown that the use of vasopressors after restoration of normal blood volume may be of some significant help if applied early.[122] Probably the beneficial effects of these experimental studies can be related more properly to their inotropic effect on the heart than to their vasoconstrictor properties. This is especially true since these studies show benefit only after volume has been restored.

There is other available evidence that the administration of vasopressors during hypovolemia will reduce the already depleted plasma volume. Our own data would tend to support this concept.[30,109]

The use of vasopressors in hemorrhagic shock is rapidly disappearing. Suffice it to say, as more and more data have become available, it is doubtful whether the use of vasopressors in the treatment of hypovolemic shock is ever warranted.

Vasodilators

In 1948 Wiggers and his associates predicted that a significantly increased survival rate in animals treated with an adrenergic blocking agent and subjected to hemorrhagic shock would indicate the detrimental influence of protracted vasoconstriction in shock.[140] Subsequently, in 1950, Remington and his associates reported an increased survival rate in dogs pretreated with Dibenamine before the induction of hemorrhagic shock. Zweifach, Baes, and Shorr[147] similarly found that Dibenamine protected rats against lethal graded hemorrhage if the animals were pretreated; and Boba and Converse[19] reported that ganglionic blocking agents increased the survival of experimentally shocked animals.

Webb et al. found that the administration of hydralazine during the hypovolemic hypotensive phase of experimental hemorrhagic shock was deleterious. In contrast, Hakstian, Hampson, and Gurd obtained 15 survivals out of 16 animals subjected to hemorrhagic shock and treated with hydralazine during the shock period.[62] Collins, Jaffee, and Zahony reported survival in a study of 396 patients treated with chlorpromazine; 186 of these patients were treated after the onset of shock, and the survival rate was said to be twice that of the control group.[36] Longerbeam, Lillehei, and Scott found that giving Dibenzyline (phenoxybenzamine) led to a remarkable improvement in the mortality rate of their animals.[86] In addition, Thal reported encouraging results with Dibenzyline in the treatment of refractory normovolemic endotoxic shock.[145]

Hemodynamic Measurements

A patient in hemorrhagic or oligemic shock may rarely fail to respond to vigorous management as outlined above. Such a patient usually presents a complicated clinical picture. Frequently, surgical procedures have been carried out for correction of the underlying causes of shock. Thus the problem is often compounded by massive fluid and blood administration, general anesthesia, and surgical trauma. At this point a comprehensive but rapid reevaluation of the patient must be carried out in order to institute effective therapy.

The basic defect underlying this "refractory shock" must be corrected. Possible causes are multiple: (1) continuing blood loss from the primary injury or disease or from another source must always be considered; (2) inadequate replacement of fluids; (3) massive trauma, and other derangements secondary to the trauma, must be considered, especially cardiac tamponade and pneumothorax; (4) myocardial insufficiency either as direct result of inadequate perfusion for a prolonged period or secondary to anesthetic agents may be present; and (5) even concomitant septic shock, as with intraperitoneal contamination from bowel perforation, may be a significant factor. The answer to this problem can best be obtained from careful clinical evaluation of the patient and evaluation of a few relatively simple hemodynamic parameters that may serve as a guide to satisfactory treatment.

Clinical evaluation includes a search for signs of bleeding, detection and correction of metabolic abnormalities, and reevaluation of the primary cause. Special attention must be paid to the adequacy of ventilation, with control of the airway and use of assisted respiration when necessary. In patients who have undergone prolonged surgical procedures requiring use of a muscle relaxant, subtle hypoventilation can be a significant problem.[116]

In order to be of value, hemodynamic measurements should include an evaluation of several parameters. First, some estimate of the amount of fluid available for circulation is imperative. Second, the ability of the cardiovascular system to circulate this fluid adequately must be evaluated. This includes an evaluation of the efficacy of the heart and of the resistance of the vascular system.

With reference to the amount of fluid available for pumping, direct measurement of the blood volume initially seemed to be the appropriate approach; however, for several reasons, acute blood volume measurements have proved to be unreliable as a guide for therapy of hemorrhagic shock.[138] If the plasma volume alone is measured, an estimate of the total blood volume requires the use of the hematocrit for calculation. These estimated volumes

are no more reliable than the hematocrit itself, which has been established to be erratic in hemorrhagic shock. Furthermore, the anatomic blood volume has little relation to that available for circulation if a large portion of this is involved at the site of injury or inflammation or is trapped in some vascular pool.

Determination of the extracellular fluid volume would seem extremely useful; however, this remains largely a research tool, since a rapid bedside method is not practical. Use of central venous pressure monitoring has recently been popularized.[141] This technique can be performed easily, and measurements can be repeated often. The central venous pressure has been shown to be a relatively reliable approximation of the efficacy of venous return. The information gained by this method is enhanced if the venous pressure response to rapid administration of fluids is assessed.[144]

The second of the two parameters requires evaluation of arterial blood pressure by either cuff or arterial cannulation, and some estimate of cardiac output. Cardiac output can be estimated by using arteriovenous oxygen difference as described by Wilson;[144] however, more rapid and direct measurements of cardiac output by the dye dilution principle are now available. These require only intraarterial cannulation in addition to the central venous catheter, and seem justified in these few critically ill patients.

With the use of these measurements the best method for treatment of the patient's hypotension can frequently be ferreted out of a complicated clinical picture. A depressed or normal central venous pressure that does not rise significantly with rapid administration of a balanced salt solution is usually indicative of a continuing hypovolemia. The diagnosis is supported by the presence of a measured decrease in cardiac output. If the hypovolemia is secondary to inadequate fluid replacement, a gradual and sustained rise in arterial pressure and cardiac output will result from the administration of appropriate fluids. If, on the other hand, continued fluid loss or acute bleeding is the cause, then fluid administration will produce either a transient rise or no rise in the blood pressure and cardiac output.

The presence of an elevated central venous pressure or a central venous pressure that rises with the rapid administration of fluids (and produces either no change or a decrease in cardiac output) is indicative of impairment of the pumping mechanism. Usually this represents primary myocardial deficiency and must be treated accordingly; however, the defect in the pumping mechanism may rarely be due to mechanical obstruction as with cardiac tamponade or mediastinal compression by intrapleural fluid or air. The possible presence of these surgically correctable lesions must be kept in mind, especially in the patient who has multiple injuries. Pulmonary embolism can produce a similar response, but is rarely seen early in the course of the injured patient.

A normal or slightly increased central venous pressure with a normal or high cardiac output and disproportionate hypotension is usually due to a loss of peripheral vascular resistance. Decreased peripheral resistance is rarely, if ever, seen in uncomplicated oligemic shock and, if present, should alert one to the possibility of a "septic" component. The converse is usually true in oligemic shock, since peripheral resistance is markedly increased; if this is accompanied by deficient myocardial function, the use of an inotropic agent (with minimal vasocontrictor or, preferably, with vasodilator effects) may be beneficial.[89] This should be done only after more direct measures such as adequate volume replacement or digitalization have been vigorously pursued. Hemodynamic measurements usually fail to show any indication for use of a vasoconstrictive agent in the therapy of hemorrhagic shock.

Several authors have questioned the value of central venous pressure measurements and pointed out that left ventricular overload and pulmonary edema can occur while right ventricular function (and the central venous pressure) remains adequate.[4,49,104] This is particularly true after myocardial injury and is discussed more fully in the section on cardiogenic shock.

In patients with normal cardiac reserve, however, *changes* in the central venous pressure with fluid infusion do indicate the ability of the myocardium to pump the volume presented to it. Thus, properly applied, the central venous pressure remains a useful clinical tool. Its interpretation can be augmented by measurement of pulmonary artery pressure and pulmonary wedge pressure, the latter approximating left atrial pressure. Such techniques are usually reserved for patients with more complicated problems, and use of a balloon-tipped Swan-Ganz catheter is necessary.

The ultimate hemodynamic criterion in the treatment of shock is the response of the patient. Two indications of adequate resuscitation are restoration of adequate cerebration and urine output. Although diuresis by any means may be beneficial when a large pigment load is presented to the kidneys, the object of treatment in hypovolemic shock is to reestablish urine flow by adequate restoration of circulation, and not to force urine flow in spite of inadequate resuscitation. The use of osmotic diuretics in the presence of uncorrected oligemic shock to produce "urine for urine's sake" would seem to have no physiologic basis and may, in fact, be detrimental by further depleting intravascular and extravascular extracellular fluid.

CARDIOGENIC, NEUROGENIC, AND SEPTIC SHOCK

Cardiogenic Shock

In this form of shock the heart fails as a pump. Consequently, primary therapy is directed toward the heart. Cardiac arrhythmias, whatever their origin, should be treated promptly. Cardiac tamponade, if this is the cause, should be relieved by pericardiocentesis. When the origin of the pump failure is myocardial infarction or myocarditis, then the primary therapy again is directed toward the myocardial damage. If the myocardial damage is sufficiently severe to produce reduction in blood pressure, and indeed in organ perfusion, to the point that organ functions begin to fall, then drugs with positive inotropic action may be efficacious.

Hemodynamic Measurements Hemodynamic measurements play an important role in the management of postoperative patients with this type of hypotension. As previously described, the classic findings are a central venous pressure that is elevated or rises briskly with fluid administration. This is accompanied by a cardiac output that is depressed and fails to respond to fluid administration. In evaluating postoperative hypotension, as after an extensive procedure in the elderly or especially after cardiac surgery, the measurement of hemodynamic parameters may be of great benefit in differentiating hypovolemic hypotension from hypotension due to depressed myocardial function.[50,103,137]

When hemodynamic measurements suggestive of deficient pumping action are found, myocardial insufficiency is usually at fault. It should be stressed again, however, that this can be due to mechanical obstruction (e.g., cardiac tamponade or mediastinal compression in the injured patient and pulmonary embolism in the postoperative patient), and treatment directed at primary myocardial insufficiency can lead to unnecessary delay and catastrophic results. Although identification of abnormalities causing mechanical obstruction to venous return or myocardial function must rest largely on clinical grounds, hemodynamic measurements may be of some benefit in that one may find a slow increase in cardiac output and arterial blood pressure accompanying the

rising venous pressure produced by rapid fluid administration. This is in contrast to the picture usually seen in pure myocardial insufficiency, in which the cardiac output frequently falls in the face of a rising venous pressure. The rise in cardiac output is probably because the rising venous pressure is partially effective in overcoming the obstruction and maintaining a nearer normal cardiac filling.

It has been demonstrated that with myocardial injury and after cardiac surgery, differences in functional reserve of the two ventricles occur and the central venous pressure alone loses a great deal of reliability.[96,104,107,113] Thus it is in these patients that the use of pulmonary artery pressure, pulmonary wedge pressure, and, when feasible, left atrial pressure have their greatest value.[50,128] Left atrial pressure (or left ventricular end-diastolic pressure) is not necessarily the same as right atrial pressure (or central venous pressure, or right ventricular end-diastolic pressure) under these circumstances.

In patients with low cardiac output from low blood volume who also have certain forms of heart disease, left atrial pressure may be considerably higher than right atrial pressure. Examples of such conditions are mitral stenosis and insufficiency, aortic stenosis and insufficiency, severe hypertension, and coronary artery disease. In such patients, unless actually measuring left atrial pressure, one should probably stop rapid infusion when right atrial or central venous pressure reaches 12 mmHg (150 mm saline). The relation between changes in atrial pressure and changes in stroke volume or cardiac output at relatively high atrial pressures is not known. In most patients, however, when atrial pressures are about 15 mmHg (230 mm saline), further increases do not seem to increase cardiac output. Thus, when central venous or right atrial pressure is less than 6 mmHg (80 mm saline), augmentation of blood volume is indicated. As the infusion proceeds, if central venous pressure rises rapidly and there is little evidence of increase in cardiac output, the infusion should probably be discontinued as being ineffective.

Abnormalities in Contractility In the condition in which there is low cardiac output and high atrial pressures, and tamponade and ventricular outflow obstruction have been ruled out, there is probably an acute reduction of myocardial contractility. Treatment must therefore be directed toward improving contractility.[27,47,59,99,134]

The drugs to be considered are:

Digitalis If time permits, digitalis is given, and digoxin is recommended. The estimated digitalizing dose given intravenously to a child or adult is 0.9 mg/m² of body surface area (1.5 mg for average adult). Half or two-thirds of this may be given initially intravenously. An effect can be seen in 10 to 20 min, and its peak effect is reached in about 2 h. After 1 to 3 h, if no contraindication develops and further effect is desired, an additional one-sixth of the estimated digitalizing dose is given. This may be repeated after another 2 to 3 h. In less acute situations the same drug may be given orally, and the digitalizing dose is then 1 mg/m². The estimated daily maintenance dose is one-quarter of the estimated digitalizing dose, and is usually given in divided doses.

Catecholamines Isoproterenol has a specific inotropic effect on cardiac muscle, and theoretically is the drug of choice when one needs a prompt and potent agent. It has also a peripheral vasodilating effect which may produce increased hypotension in a patient in shock. Because of a tendency to produce tachycardia and ventricular irritability, isoproterenol is particularly useful when the pulse rate is slow. It is administered by slow intravenous infusion drop by drop of a solution of 0.5 mg of isoproterenol in 250 mL of 5% glucose in water (2 μg/mL). The rate of infusion is regulated to obtain the desired hemodynamic effect.

Norepinephrine or epinephrine may be used when undue hypotension results from isoproterenol. They increase systemic venous tone and therefore can increase both right and left atrial pressures strikingly; thus caution is indicated, since pulmonary edema can result. These drugs are given intravenously by drop-by-drop infusion of solution containing 4 mg in 250 mL of 5% glucose in water.

A new and more specific inotropic agent, dopamine hydrochloride, may be used instead of isoproterenol. Dopamine is a naturally occurring catecholamine that is a biochemical precursor of norepinephrine. This drug has enjoyed recent popularity as a potent cardiac stimulant with few adverse effects.

Prior to treating patients with low cardiac output and high atrial pressures with these drugs on the basis that the cause is poor myocardial contractility, one must rule out pericardial tamponade. If high intrapericardial pressure exists in patients with high atrial and ventricular end-diastolic pressure, transmural pressure is low and the poor output is due to a decreased end-diastolic ventricular volume and fiber length. The treatment is relief of the pericardial tamponade, which is about the only acute cause of high atrial pressures and small end-diastolic ventricular volume. A clinical analysis and chest x-ray are helpful in establishing the diagnosis. The presence of a paradoxic pulse should suggest strongly the presence of tamponade, and needle aspiration or open pericardiotomy is indicated.

Ganglionic Blockade Some patients with low cardiac output and high atrial pressures have relatively high arterial blood pressure. Systemic arteriolar resistance is high (*afterload-load* resisting shortening of myocardial sarcomeres). In these circumstances systolic left ventricular pressure is relatively high, as is systolic ventricular wall stress. Theoretically, reducing arterial blood pressure and systolic ventricular wall stress increases cardiac output.[38,77] This can be done with an agent such as Arfonad. One should measure cardiac output before and during administration of this drug. The drug should be continued only if a significant increase in cardiac output accompanies the decrease in arterial blood pressure. Because of the present uncertainties with the use of this drug (such as the effect on coronary, cerebral, liver, and renal blood flow) in this situation, it should be given only under special circumstances.

Abnormalities in Rate Rapid ventricular rates (over 150 to 180 beats per minute) are usually deleterious to cardiac output. Ventricular end-diastolic pressure is small because of the short period of ventricular filling with tachycardia, and ventricular extensibility is probably decreased because ventricular relaxation is not complete by the end of the extremely short diastolic period. Both tend to reduce stroke volume more than can be compensated for by the rapid heart rate, and cardiac output falls. If atrial fibrillation is the cardiac mechanism, digoxin is the drug of choice. Atrial flutter is more difficult to treat, but should likewise be treated with digoxin. If no progress has been achieved with the drug after two-thirds of the digitalizing dose, consideration should be given to electroversion. Atrial tachycardia and premature atrial contractions as causes of excessively rapid heart rates are more difficult still to treat. A continuous intravenous infusion of a drug with pure peripheral vasoconstrictor properties may be helpful (Aramine, 500 mg in 500 mL of 5% glucose in water).

Premature ventricular contractions may on occasion cause fast ventricular rates. Their tendency to cause ventricular fibrillation is of even greater concern. Potassium chloride may be infused over a 10- to 20-min period. If this is not effective or if the permature ventricular contractions are frequent, lidocaine (Xylocaine) should be given intravenously in a single injection of 50 mg. If further lidocaine is needed, a solution containing 2 mg/mL of lidocaine can be given continuously. If it is used excessively, central nervous system irritability and depression of myocardial contractility may result. If protection against premature ventricular contractions is needed later, Pronestyl (procainamide hydrochloride) can be given orally in doses of 250 to 500 mg every 3 h.[6]

Low output associated with ventricular rates of less than 60 to 70 beats per minute may occur in patients in whom cardiac performance is impaired. Because the myocardium is impaired, stroke volume cannot increase sufficiently to compensate for the slow rate. Regardless of whether the mechanism is sinus rhythm, atrial fibrillation with slow ventricular rate (too much digitalis or too little potassium), or complete atrioventricular dissociation, electrical pacing of the heart at a rate of 80 to 110 beats per minute is advantageous. If there is a sinus mechanism, atrial pacing is preferred. Otherwise, direct ventricular pacing is indicated.[6]

Mechanical Assistance Effective support for cardiogenic shock may eventually depend on mechanical assistance. Assistive devices are currently available in several centers. At present their use is restricted to patients who do not respond to more conventional therapy.[100,107,127]

Neurogenic Shock

Neurogenic shock or, by the older classification, "primary shock" is that form of shock which follows serious interference with the balance of vasodilator and vasoconstrictor influences to both arterioles and venules. This is the shock that is seen with clinical "syncope," as with sudden exposure to unpleasant events such as the sight of blood, the hearing of ill tidings, or even the sudden onset of pain. Similarly, neurogenic shock is often observed with serious paralysis of vasomotor influences, as in high spinal anesthesia. The reflex interruption of nerve impulses also occurs with acute gastric dilation.

The clinical picture of neurogenic shock is quite different from that classically seen in oligemic or hypovolemic shock. While the blood pressure may be extremely low, the pulse rate is usually slower than normal and is accompanied by dry, warm, and even flushed skin. Measurements made during neurogenic shock indicate a reduction in cardiac output, but this is accompanied by a decrease in resistance of arteriolar vessels as well as a decrease in the venous tone. Consequently, there appears to be a normovolemic state with a greatly increased reservoir capacity in both arterioles and venules, thereby inducing a decreased venous return to the right side of the heart and, subsequently, a reduction in cardiac output.

If neurogenic shock is not corrected, there will eventuate reduction of blood flow to the kidneys and damage to the brain, and subsequently all the ravages of hypovolemic shock appear. Fortunately, treatment of neurogenic shock is usually obvious. Gastric dilatation can be rapidly treated with nasogastric suction. High spinal anesthesia can be treated effectively with a vasopressor such as ephedrine or phenylephrine (Neo-Synephrine), which will increase cardiac output as well as produce peripheral vasoconstriction. With the milder forms of neurogenic shock, such as fainting, simply removing the patient from the stimulus or relieving the pain will in itself be adequate therapy so that the vasoconstrictor nerves may regain the ability to maintain normal arteriolar and venular resistance.

There is rarely a need for a hemodynamic measurement in this usually benign and frequently self-limited form of hypotension. Correction of the underlying deficit usually results in a prompt resumption of normal cardiovascular dynamics. The exception to this occurs when this form of shock results from injury, as with spinal cord transection from trauma.

In this instance there may be significant loss of blood and extracellular fluid into the area of injury surrounding the cord and vertebral column. Considerable confusion can arise as to the relative need for fluid replacement, as opposed to the need for vasopressor drugs, under these circumstances. Similarly, if surgical intervention for any reason becomes necessary, hemodynamic measurements may be of great value in the management of these patients. In uncomplicated neurogenic shock, central venous pressure should be normal or slightly low with a normal or elevated cardiac output. On the other hand, as hypovolemia ensues, central venous pressure decreases, as does the cardiac output. Thus careful monitoring of the central venous pressure may be of great aid. Fluid administration without vasopressors in this form of hypotension may produce a gradually rising arterial pressure and cardiac output without elevation of central venous pressure, by gradually "filling" the expanded vascular pool; therefore caution must be utilized during fluid administration.

In the management of these patients in balancing the two forms of therapy, slight volume overexpansion is much less deleterious than excessive vasopressor administration. The latter compounds decrease organ perfusion in the presence of inadequate fluid replacement. This balance can best be obtained by maintaining a normal central venous pressure that rises slightly with rapid fluid administration (thus ensuring adequate volume) and using a vasopressor such as phenylephrine judiciously to support arterial pressure.[93]

Septic Shock

During the past several years there has been a progressive increase in the incidence of shock secondary to sepsis, and the mortality rate remains in excess of 50 percent. This has occurred despite a better understanding of this entity, use of newer treatment regimens, and development of more potent antimicrobial agents. The most frequent causative organisms are gram-positive and gram-negative bacteria, although any agent capable of producing infection (including viruses, parasites, fungi, and rickettsiae) may initiate septic shock. Because of effective antibiotic control of most gram-positive infections, the majority of septic processes that result in shock are now caused by gram-negative bacteria. Among other causes, Altemeier and associates attribute this rising incidence of gram-negative sepsis to (1) the widespread use of antibiotics with development of a reservoir of virulent and resistant organisms; (2) concentration in hospitals of large numbers of patients with established infections; (3) more extensive operations on elderly and poor-risk patients; (4) an increasing number of patients suffering from severe trauma; and (5) the use of steroids, immunosuppressive, and anticancer agents.[3]

Gram-positive Sepsis and Shock The shock state may be caused (1) by gram-positive infections that produce massive fluid losses (necrotizing fasciitis); (2) by dissemination of a potent exotoxin without evident bacteremia (*Clostridium perfringens* and *Clostridium tetani*); or (3) most often, by a fulminating infection from staphylococcus, streptococcus, or pneumococcus organisms. In the latter instance, shock is theoretically related to the release of exotoxins which many strains of staphylococcus and streptococcus (but not pneumococcus) are known to produce. The hemodynamic changes that occur are different from those seen in shock due to gram-negative organisms. Kwaan and Weil have noted hypotension of comparable severity in shock from both gram-positive and gram-negative infections, but their patients with gram-positive infections failed to show the other clinical manifestations of shock.[78] Arterial resistance fell, but there was little or no reduction in cardiac output even with progressive hypotension. Urine flow was normal, sensorium clear, and perfusion of other organs was not grossly impaired, since neither acidosis nor a significant increase in serum lactic acid concentration appeared.

Treatment consists of the use of appropriate antibiotics, surgical drainage when indicated, and correction of any existing fluid volume deficit. A rapid and favorable response may be anticipated in many patients, and survival is substantially better than with gram-negative infections.

Gram-negative Sepsis and Shock Gram-negative sepsis as a cause of shock is a more frequent and difficult problem. The highest incidence occurs during the seventh and eighth decades of life, and the response to treatment depends to a large extent on the age and previous health of the patient. There have been significant advances in the understanding of this entity, although much of the available information is still subject to controversy.

Source The most frequent source of gram-negative infections is the genitourinary system, and almost half of the patients have had an associated operation or instrumentation of the urinary tract.[3] The second most frequent site of origin is the respiratory system, and many of the patients have an associated tracheostomy. Next in frequency is the alimentary system, with diseases such as peritonitis, intraabdominal abscesses, and biliary tract infections; and then come diseases of the integumentary system, including burns and soft tissue infections. Indwelling venous catheters for monitoring and hyperalimentation are an increasing source of contamination, particularly with prolonged use. The reproductive system continues to be a significant source of infection (principally from septic abortions and postpartum infections), although the incidence is variable, depending on the hospital population.

The severity of septic shock varies considerably and appears to be a time-dose phenomenon, depending on the type and site of infection. For instance, mild hypotension following instrumentation of the genitourinary tract may represent nothing more than a transient bacteremia which is self-limited or responds to minimal therapy. In contrast, the patient with necrotizing pneumonia or multiple intraabdominal abscesses may have sepsis from an overwhelming number of organisms for a period of several days, and a much poorer prognosis. Similarly, the outlook is more favorable when the source of infection is accessible to surgical drainage, as in septic abortion, in which the infected products of conception can be removed readily. Variations in these factors must be considered when interpreting reported mortality rates and during the evaluation of new therapeutic regimens.

Associated Conditions The presence of underlying disorders which limit cardiac, pulmonary, hepatic, or renal function increases the susceptibility to gram-negative infections and adversely affects the response to treatment. In Altemeier's reported series of 398 patients with gram-negative sepsis, almost half of the patients had a serious associated disease, including diabetes mellitus, malignant neoplasms, uremia, cirrhosis, burns, and malignant hematologic disorders.[3] Of these conditions, cirrhosis of the liver appeared to have the most unfavorable prognosis. In addition, a small but significant number of patients were on corticosteroids or immunosuppressive agents, and corresponding mortality rates were 74 and 83 percent, respectively.

Bacteriology The common causative organisms are similar to those found in the human gastrointestinal tract and include (1) *Escherichia coli*, (2) *Klebsiella aerobacter*, (3) *Proteus*, (4) *Pseudomonas*, and (5) *Bacteroides* in decreasing frequency. Recently the Klebsiella-Enterobacteriaceae-Serratia groups have been isolated with increasing frequency,

and many are resistant to more conventional antibiotics.[125] There is also evidence to suggest that bacteroides species may be the predominant organisms in the fecal flora. These anaerobic organisms are difficult to culture, and may account for a far greater number of infections than was previously reported. The majority of infections are caused by a single gram-negative organism, although in 10 to 20 percent of cases more than one organism may be isolated.[3,125] The isolates may be two or more gram-negative organisms or mixed cultures containing both gram-negative and gram-positive bacteria.

Clinical Manifestations Gram-negative infections are often recognized initially by the development of chills and an elevated temperature above 101°F. The onset of shock may be abrupt and coincident with the signs and symptoms of sepsis or may occur several hours to days after recognition of an established infection. The complex hemodynamic abnormalities that follow are incompletely understood, but are probably initiated by endotoxins from the cell walls of gram-negative bacteria. Intravenous injection of this lipopolysaccharide-protein complex into experimental animals will produce a shock state, but the hemodynamic responses vary in different animal species. The use of experimental animal models has contributed to our understanding of this entity, but direct extrapolation of the findings to human septic shock is difficult. A single injection of endotoxin into dogs causes pooling of blood in the splanchnic circulation, decreased venous return to the heart, reduction in cardiac output, and an abrupt fall in blood pressure.[1,46] This initial response is transient and apparently due to hepatic venous outflow obstruction. Shortly thereafter the blood pressure rises toward normal, but then slowly declines over the next several hours until death of the animal. This pattern is different from that seen in the subhuman primate and in man. Injection of *E.*

coli endotoxin into human volunteers has been shown to produce either (1) no response;[102] (2) chills, fever, and vasoconstriction;[102] or (3) peripheral vasodilation and a rise in cardiac output.[56] These observations emphasize our lack of understanding of the effects of gram-negative infections and septicemia on the human circulation and the need for development of more realistic experimental animal models.

Clinically, the shock state may be characterized by a primary adrenergic response, as seen in hypovolemic shock, with hypotension, peripheral vasoconstriction, and cold, clammy extremities. Earlier in the course, however, there may be an absence of adrenergic effects, with warm, dry extremities and decreased peripheral resistance. These diverse responses, presumably to the same stimulus, have led to a considerable amount of confusion over the clinical manifestations of septic shock, although a recent report by McLean and associates tends to shed some light on this subject.[88] They have noted two distinct hemodynamic patterns, depending upon the existing volume status of the patient, and believe that the natural history of septic shock is one of progression from respiratory alkalosis to metabolic acidosis. A syndrome of early septic shock occurs in patients who are *normovolemic* prior to the onset of sepsis and exhibit a hyperdynamic circulatory pattern characterized by (1) hypotension, (2) high cardiac output, (3) normal or increased blood volume, (4) normal or high central venous pressure, (5) low peripheral resistance, (6) warm, dry extremities, (7) hyperventilation, and (8) respiratory alkalosis. A typical patient with this pattern is the young, previously healthy person with a septic abortion. The hemodynamic changes indicate an increased blood flow secondary to peripheral vasodilation or arteriovenous shunting. In either case the presence of oliguria, altered sensorium, and blood lactate accumulation reflect the need for a further increase in flow despite the high cardiac output. McLean suggests that treatment includes measures to increase the cardiac output even higher, combined with appropriate antibiotic therapy and early surgical drainage. In his series all but 4 of 28 patients with this hemodynamic pattern survived the episode of shock. If control of the infection is delayed or unsuccessful, the patient may pass into an acidotic phase with evidence of cellular damage (narrowing arteriovenous oxygen difference, decreasing oxygen consumption) and become refractory to further therapy.

In contrast, if septic shock develops in a patient who is hypovolemic a hypodynamic pattern emerges characterized by (1) hypotension, (2) low cardiac output, (3) high peripheral resistance, (4) low central venous pressure, and (5) cold, cyanotic extremities. This response is typically seen in a patient with strangulation obstruction of the small bowel and a moderate to severe extracellular fluid and plasma volume deficit. If seen early, these patients are also alkalotic and will respond favorably to treatment. In the absence of overt cardiac failure, prompt volume replacement will often increase cardiac output, and a more favorable hyperdynamic circulation may develop. If therapy to combat sepsis is delayed or unsuccessful, the patient will inevitably have cardiac and circulatory failure with a low fixed cardiac output and a resistant metabolic acidosis. At this point the patient may not be salvageable.

Our own experience in the treatment of septic shock tends to confirm McLean's findings, although the presence of a metabolic acidosis has not necessarily been an ominous finding. We have seen several patients with hypodynamic and hyperdynamic circulatory patterns and metabolic acidosis in the early phase who have responded satisfactorily to therapy. The clinical picture may also be influenced by the patient's ability to meet the increased circulatory requirements imposed by sepsis. The elderly patient with limited cardiac reserve may be unable to increase cardiac output and enter the hyperdynamic phase, even with prompt volume replacement and measures designed to increase cardiac efficiency. In this instance the typical adrenergic response may persist, and the patient may rapidly succumb to the disease process.

Progressive pulmonary insufficiency is characteristically seen in many patients with septic shock. Mild hypoxia with compensatory hyperventilation and respiratory alkalosis are commonly seen early in the course of shock in the absence of clinical or x-ray evidence of pulmonary disease. The arterial desaturation has been attributed to a variety of causes, including the presence of physiologic arteriovenous shunts in the pulmonary circulation secondary to perfusion of atelectatic or nonaerated alveoli. Regardless of the cause, the picture is frequently that of rapid deterioration of pulmonary function, development of patchy infiltrates which become confluent, superimposed bacterial infection, severe hypoxemia, and death.

Combining all these seemingly contradictory findings into a single unified concept is impossible at present, although Berk has recently suggested that excessive beta-adrenergic stimulation is the predominant response in septic shock and causes opening of splanchnic and pulmonary arteriovenous shunts.[12,13] This would produce a sudden drop in blood pressure and peripheral resistance and a compensatory increase in cardiac output. Shunting of poorly oxygenated pulmonary blood into the arterial circulation would lead to hypoxia, compensatory hyperventilation, and respiratory alkalosis. Arteriovenous shunting may also cause increased capillary hydrostatic pressure, stagnant hypoxia of the pulmonary capillaries, and a loss of pulmonary surfactant, leading to alveolar collapse and progressive pulmonary consolidation.

This attractive hypothesis lacks adequate supportive data, but deserves additional investigation because of its therapeutic implications.

Finally, it is worth emphasizing that development of mild hyperventilation, respiratory alkalosis, and an altered sensorium may be the earliest signs of gram-negative infection. This triad may precede the usual signs and symptoms of sepsis by several hours to several days. The exact cause is not known, although the condition is thought to represent a primary response to bacteremia. Early recognition of these findings followed by a prompt search for the source of infection may allow proper diagnosis prior to the onset of shock.

Treatment   The only effective way to reduce mortality in septic shock is by prompt recognition and treatment of the associated infection prior to the onset of shock. Once shock occurs, the control of infection by early surgical debridement or drainage and use of appropriate antibiotics represents definitive therapy. Other recommended measures, including fluid replacement, steroid administration, and the use of vasoactive drugs, represent adjunctive forms of therapy and are useful to prepare the patient prior to surgical intervention or to support the patient until the infectious process is controlled. This point deserves special emphasis, since death of the patient is inevitable if the infection cannot be adequately controlled.

As soon as gram-negative sepsis and shock are apparent, a prompt and thorough search for the source of infection is made while instituting other supportive measures. Because of the multiple complicating factors that may accompany endotoxemia, the patient is preferably treated in an intensive care unit. Careful monitoring of arterial pressure (preferably by a percutaneously inserted radial artery catheter), central venous pressure, urine output, and arterial and central venous blood gases may be essential for proper management.

If the infectious process is amenable to drainage, operation is performed as soon as possible after initial stabilization of the patient's condition. In some cases surgical debridement or drainage of the infection must be accomplished before the patient will respond, and may be performed under local or general anesthesia. For example, a patient with ascending cholangitis and shock secondary to sepsis may respond temporarily to supportive treatment. Improvement may be short-lived, however, unless prompt drainage of the biliary tract is accomplished. The importance of surgical drainage is emphasized by the experience of McLean et al. in their treatment of 53 patients; 48 percent of their patients with infections amenable to surgical drainage survived, while only 23 percent of those not amenable to surgical treatment survived.[88]

Antibiotic Therapy The use of specific antibiotics based on appropriate cultures and sensitivity tests is desirable when possible. The results may not be available for several days, but useful information may be gained from previous wound and blood cultures obtained during an earlier phase of the septic process. Generally, however, antibiotics may be chosen on the basis of the suspected organisms and their previous sensitivity patterns. These patterns are sufficiently diverse to preclude selection of a single antibiotic agent which will be effective against all the potential pathogens.

At present an effective combination of antibiotics in our hospital population includes the use of cephalothin (6 to 8 g/day intravenously in four to six divided doses) and gentamicin (1.2 to 1.6 mg/kg intramuscularly 4 times daily). These are average adult doses and should be reduced after initial control of the infection and modified in any patient with impaired renal function. This combination is effective against a majority of gram-negative organisms, with the notable exception of *Bacteroides species*. If presence of these organisms

is suspected, an antibiotic of known effectiveness (e.g., clindamycin or Chloromycetin) should be added to the regimen.

When culture and sensitivity reports are available, more specific antibiotic coverage may be initiated if the infection is not under control. Altemeier and associates reported a mortality rate of 54 percent from sepsis in patients receiving inappropriate antibiotics and 28 percent when appropriate antibiotics were given.[3]

Fluid Replacement Prompt correction of preexisting fluid deficits is essential. A majority of patients will incur fluid losses from the disease processes that initiate sepsis and shock. Third space losses with massive sequestration of plasma and extracellular fluid are characteristic of many surgical conditions, including peritonitis, burns, strangulation obstruction of the bowel, and extensive soft tissue infections.

The type of fluid used will vary, although most third space losses are properly replaced with a balanced salt solution such as Ringer's lactate. Blood replacement may be needed, depending on the hemoglobin and hematocrit levels, and plasma or albumin administration may be specifically indicated in an occasional patient. Although large quantities of replacement fluids may be required, every attempt is made to prevent volume overload. In addition to other measures, including response of the patient noted on frequent clinical observation, continuous monitoring of the central venous pressure may serve as a valuable guideline for fluid administration. The central venous pressure catheter may be inserted percutaneously into the subclavian or internal jugular vein (or by cut-down in an antecubital or the external jugular vein), threaded into the superior vena cava and connected to a saline manometer or other pressure-measuring device. Properly interpreted, the central venous pressure will give a reliable estimate of the ability of the right side of the heart to pump the blood delivered to it. It is best used as an upper limit guide; a rapid increase in central venous pressure, regardless of the initial level, may indicate that fluid is being administered too rapidly or that the heart is unable to handle additional volume. If central venous pressure is below 10 cm of water, fluids may be administered as rapidly as tolerated. If central venous pressure is above this level, fluids are still administered, but at a slower rate of infusion. The central venous pressure may fall as blood pressure rises, owing to better perfusion of the coronary arteries and improved myocardial function. An abrupt rise in the central venous pressure or a fall in arterial pressure may indicate inability of the heart to respond, and the use of drugs that increase myocardial performance may be considered.[9]

Many patients will respond favorably to fluid administration combined with prompt control of the infection with a rise in blood pressure, an increase in urine output, warming of the extremities, and clearing of the sensorium. In these instances no additional therapy may be indicated.

Steroids The use of pharmacologic doses of corticosteroids in the treatment of septic shock is controversial, but has become a common practice. There is no direct evidence that steroids are beneficial in these cases, although favorable responses with improvement in cardiac, pulmonary, and renal function, and better survival rates have been reported.[97,110,121,143] Large doses of steroids are known to exert a modest inotropic effect on the heart and produce mild peripheral vasodilation. Although these salutary effects may be desirable, there are other, more potent drugs available with similar actions. Others have suggested that steroids protect the cell and its contents from the effects of endotoxin, e.g., by stabilizing cellular and lysosomal membranes.[74]

Short-term, high-dose steroid therapy is associated with a minimal number of complications and is recommended in most cases that do not respond promptly to other measures. Steroids may be administered concomitant with volume replacement or reserved for use if the response to fluid administration is only temporary or produces a rapid rise in central venous pressure. Many dosage schedules have been recommended, and most stress the need for a large initial dose and cessation of therapy within 48 to 72 h. Our current regimen is based on guidelines suggested by Lillehei.[97] An initial dose of 15 to 30 mg/kg of body weight of methylprednisolone (or equivalent dose of dexamethasone) is given intravenously over a 5 to 10-min period. The same dose may be repeated within 2 to 4 h if the desired effects have not been achieved. If a beneficial response is obtained, additional injections are not given unless the effects are only short-lived. Used in this manner, there is rarely a need for more than two doses.

Vasoactive Drugs Vasopressor drugs with prominent alpha-adrenergic effects are of limited value in treatment of this type of shock, since artificial attempts to maintain blood pressure without regard to flow are potentially harmful. Further, they are probably contraindicated in hypovolemic patients with increased peripheral resistance in view of the known deleterious effects of prolonged vasoconstriction. Beneficial effects attributed to these agents are probably due to their inotropic effects on the heart, although better drugs are available for this purpose. Rarely, use of a vasoactive drug with mixed alpha- and beta-adrenergic effects (e.g., metaraminol) may be indicated in a patient with an elevated cardiac output and pronouned hypotension due to very low peripheral resistance. The increase in resistance (and slight increase in cardiac output) may produce a desired rise in blood pressure and improvement in flow.

Vasodilator drugs such as phenoxybenzamine have enjoyed some popularity, particularly when combined with additional fluid administration. Their use is based in part on improved survival of dogs when vasodilator drugs are given prior to the onset of endotoxic shock.[71,84] These observations probably represent a specific canine response and cannot be directly extrapolated to human septic shock. Vasodilator agents have also been used in conjunction with adrenergic agents (for their inotropic effects), but data on their usefulness are limited.[142]

Since the heart is frequently unable to meet the increased circulatory demands of sepsis, the use of isoproterenol (Isuprel) would seem ideal when volume replacement and other measures have failed to restore adequate circulation.[88] Isoproterenol has potent inotropic and chronotropic effects on the heart and produces mild peripheral vasodilation. It is a relatively safe drug, but close observation of the patient is necessary, since severe tachycardia or cardiac arrhythmias may occur, particularly in digitalized patients. One or two milligrams of isoproterenol diluted in 500 mL of 5% dextrose in water may be administered by slow intravenous drip at a rate of 1 to 2 μg/min, depending on the response. The infusion should be slowed or stopped completely if significant tachycardia or cardiac arrhythmias occur. In the absence of arrhythmias, a fall in blood pressure may result from the vasodilation induced by Isuprel and indicates the need for additional volume replacement to maintain cardiac filling pressure. This combination may effectively restore blood flow, even though blood pressure remains less than 100 mmHg. The response is often temporary, but occasionally the infusion may be continued for 2 to 3 days without loss of effect or known deleterious effects.[9]

A new and more specific inotropic agent, dopamine hydrochloride, may be used instead of isoproterenol. Dopamine is a naturally occurring catecholamine that is a biochemical precursor of norepinephrine. This drug has enjoyed recent popularity as a potent cardiac stimulant with few adverse effects.

In summary, a "polypharmacy" approach is discouraged, although proper selection and use of vasoactive drugs may offer the needed support until infection can be controlled or eradicated. If eradication is not possible, response to any of these drugs is only temporary. Determination of cardiac output combined with arterial and central venous pressure measurements can be of great benefit in establishing the nature of the hemodynamic alterations and evaluating responses to therapy.

Digitalis Digitalis is not routinely administered in the absence of specific indications. Gram-negative sepsis and shock frequently occur in older patients with congestive failure or may precipitate cardiac failure in patients with limited cardiac reserve. In these instances digitalis can be administered cautiously in full doses, although toxicity may occur if the patient is hypokalemic or receiving isoproterenol.

Recent work by Hinshaw et al. and Greenfield et al. have indicated that the heart failure which occurs 5 to 7 h after the injection of endotoxin into experimental animals can be prevented by the early administration of digoxin. Additionally, digoxin was shown to reverse the failure when used 5 to 7 h after endotoxin injection.[54,66]

Pulmonary Therapy Many patients with sepsis and shock will have significant pulmonary problems and may require maintenance of a controlled airway (via nasotracheal or endotracheal intubation) and assisted ventilation. Strict adherence to tracheobronchial hygiene is an important preventive measure in all patients, particularly those with limited pulmonary reserve. Encouraging deep breathing and coughing, use of humidified air to prevent inspissation of secretions, and avoidance of oversedation are all indicated. Proper management of the patient on a mechanical ventilator requires frequent measurements of blood gases and appropriate correction of the ventilatory pattern when indicated.

Since inadequate tissue oxygenation is a consistent feature of shock, attention to all components of the oxygen transport system is essential. Efforts to maintain a normal or rightward positioned oxygen-hemoglobin dissociation curve may be particularly important in view of reported reductions in red blood cell organic phosphates in late septic shock.[92] The use of hyperbaric oxygen has also been suggested and would appear to be an ideal therapeutic approach. Limited experience with its use has been disappointing, however.[16,88]

BIBLIOGRAPHY

1 Alican, F., M. L. Dalton, Jr., and J. D. Hardy: Experimental endotoxin shock, *Am. J. Surg.*, **103**:702, 1962.

2 Allen, J. G., H. S. Inouye, and C. Sykes: Homologous serum jaundice and pooled plasma-attenuating effect of room temperature storage on its virus agent, *Ann. Surg.*, **138**:476, 1953.

3 Altemeier, W. A., J. C. Todd, and W. W. Inge: Gram-negative septicemia: A growing threat, *Ann. Surg.*, **166**:530, 1967.

4 Azzoli, S. G., T. K. Shahinian, and C. Cha: Correlation among mean central venous pressure, mean pulmonary wedge pressure, and cardiac output after acute hemorrhage and replacement with Ringer's lactate solution in the dog, *Am. J. Surg.*, **123**:385, 1972.

5 Baker, R. J. et al.: Low molecular weight dextran in surgical shock, *Arch. Surg.*, **89**:373, 1964.

6 Ballet, S. and J. B. Kostis: "Recent Advances in the Therapy of Cardiac Arrhythmias," in J. Han (ed.), Cardiac Arrhythmias: A Symposium, Charles C Thomas, Springfield, Ill., 1972, p. 260.

7 Baue, A. E., M. A. Wurth, and M. M. Sayeed: The dynamics of altered ATP-dependent and ATP-yielding cell processes in shock, *Surgery*, **72**:94, 1972.

8 Baue, A. E., E. T. Tragus, S. K. Wolfson, Jr., A. L. Cary, and W. M. Parkings: Hemodynamic and metabolic effects of Ringer's lactate solution in hemorrhagic shock, *Ann. Surg.*, **166**:29, 1967.

9 Baue, A. E.: The treatment of septic shock: A problem intensified by advancing science, *Surgery*, **65**:850, 1969.

10 Baxter, C. R. et al.: A practical method of renal hypothermia, *J. Trauma*, **3**:349, 1963.

11 Beecher, H. K.: Preparation of battle casualties for surgery, *Ann. Surg.*, **121**:769, 1945.

12 Berk, J. L., J. F. Hagen, and J. M. Dunn: The role of beta adrenergic blockade in the treatment of septic shock, *Surg. Gynecol. Obstet.*, **130**:1025, 1970.

13 Berk, J. L., J. F. Hagen, W. H. Beyer, M. J. Gerber, and G. R. Dochat: The treatment of endotoxin shock by beta adrenergic blockade, *Ann. Surg.*, **169**:74, 1969.

14 Bellingham, A. J., J. C. Detter, and C. Lenfant: Regulatory mechanisms of hemoglobin oxygen affinity in acidosis and alkalosis, *J. Clin. Invest.*, **50**:700, 1971.

15 Beutler, E., A. Meul, and L. A. Wood: Depletion and regeneration of 2, 3-diphosphoglyceric acid in stored red blood cells, *Transfusion*, **9**:109, 1969.

16 Blair, E., R. Ollodart, W. G. Esmond, S. Attar, and R. A. Cowley: Effect of hyperbaric oxygenation (OHP) on bacteremic shock, *Circulation* (Suppl. I), **29**:135, 1964.

17 Blalock, A.: *Principles of Surgical Care, Shock and Other Problems*, The C. V. Mosby Company, St. Louis, 1940.

18 Blalock, A.: Shock: Further studies with particular reference to effects of hemorrhage, *Arch. Surg.*, **29**:837, 1937.

19 Boba, A. and J. G. Converse: Ganglionic blockage and its protective action in hemorrhage, *Anesthesiology*, **18**:559, 1957.

20 Bogardous, G. M. and R. J. Schlosser: Influence of temperature upon ischemic renal damage, *Surgery*, **39**:970, 1956.

21 Bounous, G., H. B. Schumacker, Jr., and H. King: Studies in renal blood flow. I. Some general considerations, *Ann. Surg.*, **151**:47, 1960.

22 Bunn, H. F. et al.: Hemoglobin function in stored blood, *J. Clin. Invest.*, **48**:311, 1969.

23 Campion, D. S. et al.: The effect of hemorrhagic shock on transmembrane potential, *Surgery*, **66**:1051, 1969.

24 Canizaro, P. C.: "Alterations in Oxygen Transport," in G. T. Shires, C. J. Carrico, and P. C.

Canizaro, *Shock*, W. B. Saunders Company, Philadelphia, 1973.

25 Canizaro, P. C., M. D. Prager, and G. T. Shires: The infusion of Ringer's lactate solution during shock, *Am. J. Surg.*, 122:494, 1971.

26 Cannon, W. B.: *Traumatic Shock*, Appleton-Century-Crofts, Inc., New York, 1923.

27 Carey, J. S. et al.: Cardiovascular function in shock: Responses to volume loading and isoproterenol infusion, *Circulation*, 35:327, 1967.

28 Carey, L. C., B. D. Lowery, and C. T. Cloutier: Hemorrhagic shock, *Curr. Probl. Surg.*, Jan. 1971.

29 Carey, L. C., B. D. Lowery, and C. T. Cloutier: Treatment of acidosis, *Curr. Probl. Surg.*, January 1971, p. 37.

30 Carrico, C. J., C. A. Crenshaw, and G. T. Shires: Effect of vasomotor drugs on the extracellular fluid volume during hemorrhagic shock, *Clin. Res.*, 10:288, 1962.

31 Carter, N. W. et al.: Measurement of intracellular pH of skeletal muscle with pH-sensitive glass microelectrodes, *J. Clin. Invest.*, 46:920, 1967.

32 Catchpole, B. N., D. B. Hackel, and F. A. Simeone: Coronary and peripheral blood flow in experimental hemorrhagic hypotension treated with L-norepinephrine, *Ann. Surg.*, 142:372, 1955.

33 Close, S. A. et al.: The effect of norepinephrine on survival in experimental acute hypotension, *Surg. Forum*, 8:22, 1957.

34 Cloutier, C. T., B. D. Lowery, and L. C. Carey: The effect of hemodilutional resuscitation on serum protein levels in humans in hemorrhagic shock, *J. Trauma*, 9:514, 1969.

35 Cockett, A. T. K.: The kidney and regional hypothermia, *Surgery*, 50:904, 1961.

36 Collins, V. J., R. Jaffee, and I. Zahony: Shock, a different approach to therapy, *Ill. Med. J.*, 122:350, 1962.

37 Conway, E. J.: Nature and significance of concentration relations of potassium and sodium ions in skeletal muscle, *Physiol. Rev.*, 37:84, 1957.

38 Cook, W. A., D. L. Schwartz, and B. G. Bass: Arfonad therapy: Hemodynamic responses and control, *Ann. Thorac. Surg.*, 7:322, 1969.

39 Corcoran, A. C., R. D. Taylor, and I. H. Page: Immediate effects on renal function of the onset of shock due to partially occluding limb tourniquets, *Ann. Surg.*, 148:156, 1957.

40 Cunningham, J. N., Jr., G. T. Shires, and Y. Wagner: Cellular transport defects in hemorrhagic shock, *Surgery*, 70:215, 1971.

41 Cunningham, J. N., Jr., G. T. Shires. and Y. Wagner: Changes in intracellular sodium and potassium content of red blood cells in trauma and shock, *Am. J. Surg.*, November 1971.

42 Dawson, R. B., Jr., W. F. Dockolaty, and J. L. Gray: Hemoglobin function and 2, 3-DPG levels of blood stored at 4°C in ACD and CPD: pH effect, *Transfusion*, 10:299, 1970.

43 Dawson, R. B., M. C. Edinger, and T. J. Ellis: Hemoglobin function in stored blood, *J. Lab. Clin. Med.*, 77:46, 1971.

44 Doolan, P. D. et al.: An evaluation of intermittent peritoneal lavage, *Am. J. Med.*, 26:831, 1959.

45 Drucker, W. R. et al.: Metabolic aspects of hemorrhagic shock. I. Changes in intermediary metabolism during hemorrhage and repletion of blood, *Surg. Forum*, 9:49, 1959.

46 Duff, J. H., G. Malave, D. I. Pertz, H. M. Scott, and L. D. MacLean: The hemodynamics of septic shock in man and in the dog, *Surgery*, 58:174, 1965.

47 Fitts, C. T.: Vasoactive drugs in treatment of shock, *Postgrad. Med.*, 48:105, 1970.

48 Fohrman, F. A.: "Oxygen Consumption of Mammalian Tissue of Reduced Temperatures," in *Physiology of Induced Hypothermia. Proceedings of a Symposium.* National Academy of Sciences Research Council, Washington, D.C., 1956.

49 Forrester, J. S., G. Diamond, T. J. McHugh, and H. J. C. Swan: Filling pressures in the right and left sides of the heart in acute myocardial infarction: A reappraisal of central-venous pressure monitoring, *N. Engl. J. Med.*, 285:190, 1971.

50 Freis, E. D., H. W. Schnaper, R. L. Johnson, and G. E. Schreiner: Hemodynamic alterations in acute myocardial infarction. I. Cardiac output, mean arterial pressure, total peripheral resistance, "Central" and total blood volumes, venous pressure and average circulation time, *J. Clin. Invest.*, 31:131, 1952.

51 Fulton, R. L.: Absorption of sodium and water

by collagen during hemorrhagic shock, *Am. Surg.,* **172**:861, 1970.

52 Gelin, L. E.: "Fluid Substitution in Shock," in *Shock: Pathogenesis and Therapy, An International Symposium.* Academic Press, Inc., Stockholm, 1962.

53 Goldman, D. E.: Potential, impedance and rectification in membranes, *J. Physiol.* **27**:37, 1943.

54 Greenfield, L. J., R. H. Jackson, R. C. Elkins, J. J. Coalson, and L. B. Hinshaw: Cardiopulmonary effects of cardio volume loading of primates in endotoxin shock, *Surgery,* **76**:560–572, October 1974.

55 Greenfield, L. and A. Blalock: Effect of low molecular weight dextran on survival following hemorrhagic shock, *Surgery,* **55**:684, 1964.

56 Grollman, A.: *Cardiac Output of Man in Health and Disease,* Charles C Thomas, Publisher, Springfield, Ill., 1932.

57 Gross, S. G.: A System of Surgery: Pathological, Diagnostic, Therapeutique and Operative, Lea & Febiger, Philadelphia, 1872.

58 Grossman, R.: Intracellular potentials of motor cortex neurons in cerebral ischemia, *Electroencephalogr. Clin. Neurophysiol.,* **24**:291, 1968.

59 Gunnar, R. M. and H. S. Loeb: Use of drugs in cardiogenic shock due to acute myocardial infarction, *Circulation,* **45**:1111, 1972.

60 Guntheroth, W. G., F. L. Abel, and G. L. Mullins: The effect of Trendelenburg's position on blood pressure and carotid blood flow, *Surg. Gynecol. Obstet.,* **119**:345, 1964.

61 Hagberg, S., H. Haljamas, and H. Rockert: Shock reactions in skeletal muscle. III. The electrolyte content of tissue fluid and blood plasma before and after induced hemorrhagic shock, *Ann. Surg.,* **168**:243, 1968.

62 Hakstian, R. W., L. G. Hampson, and F. N. Gurd: Pharmacological agents in experimental hemorrhagic shock, *Arch. Surg.,* **83**:335, 1961.

63 Hampson, L. G., H. J. Scott, and F. N. Gurd: A comparison of intraarterial and intravenous transfusion in normal dogs and in dogs with experimental myocardial infarction, *Ann. Surg.,* **140**:56, 1954.

64 Harkins, H. N.: "Shock," in *Surgery: Principles and Practice,* J. B. Lippincott Company, Philadelphia, 1961, pp. 104–125.

65 Hiebert, J. M., J. M. McCormick, and R. H. Egdahl: Direct measurement in insulin secretory rate: Studies of shocked primates and postoperative patients, *Ann. Surg.,* **176**:296, 1972.

66 Hinshaw, L. B., B. A. Archer, M. R. Black, L. J. Greenfield, and C. A. Gunther: Prevention in the reversal of myocardial failure in endotoxic shock. *Surg. Gynecol. Obstet.,* **136**:1, January 1973.

67 Hodgkin, A. L. and B. Katz: The effect of sodium ions on the electrical activity of the giant axon of the squid, *J. Physiol.,* **108**:37, 1949.

68 Horovitz, J. H.: The extracellular fluid space, Proceedings of the Workshop on Albumin, National Institutes of Health, February 12–13, 1975.

69 Howard, J. M. et al.: Studies of dextrans of various molecular sizes, *Ann. Surg.,* **143**:369, 1956.

70 Hume, D.: Discussion of some neurohumoral and endocrine aspects of shock, *Fed. Proc.* (Supp. No. 9.), pp. 87–97, 1961.

71 Iampietro, P. F., L. B. Henshaw, and C. M. Brake: Effect of an adrenergic blocking agent on vascular alterations associated with endotoxin shock, *Am. J. Physiol.,* **204**:611, 1963.

72 Jaeger, H. W.: "Panel Discussion on the Advantages and Disadvantages of Various Methods in Hypothermia," in *International Symposium on Cardiovascular Surgery,* W. B. Saunders Company, Philadelphia, 1955.

73 James, P. M., C. E. Bredenberg, R. N. Anderson, and R. M. Hardaway: Tolerance to long and short term lactate infusion in men with battle casualties subjected to hemorrhagic shock, *Surg. Forum,* **20**:543, 1969.

74 Janoff, A., G. Weissman, B. W. Zweifach, and L. Thomas: Pathogens of experimental shock. IV. Studies on lysosomes in normal and tolerant animals subjected to trauma and endotoxemia, *J. Exp. Med.,* **16**:451, 1962.

75 Jones, W. R. and V. A. Politano: Acute renal ischemia and regional renal hypothermia, *Surg. Forum,* **13**:497, 1962.

76 Karr, W. K. et al.: Renal hypothermia, *J. Urol.,* **84**:236, 1960.

77 Kouchoukos, N. T., L. C. Sheppard, and J. W.

Kirklin: Effect of alterations in arterial pressure on cardiac performance early after open intracardiac operations, *J. Thorac. Cardiovasc. Surg.*, **64**:563, 1972.

78 Kwaan, H. M. and M. H. Weil: Differences in the mechanism of shock caused by bacterial infections, *Surg. Gynecol. Obstet.*, **128**:37, 1969.

79 Lamport, H., in J. F. Fulton (ed.): *Howell's Textbook of Physiology*, 16th ed., W. B. Saunders Company, Philadelphia, 1949, p. 580.

80 Lansing, A. M. and J. A. F. Stevenson: Mechanisms of action of norepinephrine in hemorrhagic shock, *Am. J. Physiol.*, **193**:289, 1958.

81 Lemieux, M. D., R. N. Smith, and N. P. Couch: Surface pH and redox potential of skeletal muscle in graded hemorrhage, *Surgery*, **65**:457, 1969.

82 Lepley, D., Jr. et al.: Effect of low molecular weight dextran on hemorrhagic shock, *Surgery*, **54**:93, 1963.

83 Lewis, C. M. and M. H. Weil: Hemodynamic spectrum of vasopressor and vasodilator drugs, *J. Am. Med. Assoc.*, **208**:1391–1398, 1969.

84 Lillehei, R. C. and L. D. MacLean: Physiological approach to successful treatment of endotoxin shock in the experimental animal, *Arch. Surg.*, **78**:464, 1959.

85 Ling, G. and R. W. Gerard: The normal membrane potential of frog sartorius fibers, *J. Cell. Comp. Physiol.*, **34**:383, 1949.

86 Longerbeam, J. K., R. C. Lillehei, and W. R. Scott: The nature of hemorrhagic shock: A hemodynamic study. *Surg. Forum.* **8**:1, 1962.

87 McClelland, R. N., G. T. Shires, C. R. Baxter, C. D. Coln, and J. Carrico: Balanced salt solution in the treatment of hemorrhagic shock, *J. Am. Med. Assoc.*, **199**:830, 1967.

88 MacLean, L. D., W. G. Mulligan, A. P. H. McLean, and J. H. Duff: Patterns of septic shock in man: A detailed study of 56 patients, *Ann. Surg.*, **166**:543, 1967.

89 MacLean, L. D. et al.: Treatment of shock in man based on hemodynamic diagnosis, *Surg. Gynecol. Obstet.*, **120**:1, 1965.

90 Mela, L. M., L. D. Miller, and G. G. Nicholas: Influence of cellular acidosis and altered cation

concentrations of shock-induced mitochondrial damage, *Surgery*, **72**:102, 1972.

91 Middleton, E. S., R. Mathews, and G. T. Shires: Radiosulphate as a measure of the extracellular fluid in acute hemorrhagic shock, *Ann. Surg.*, **170**:174, 1969.

92 Miller, L. D. et al.: The affinity of hemoglobin for oxygen: Its control and in vivo significance, *Surgery*, **68**:187, 1970.

93 Moore, D. C.: "Complications of Regional Anesthesia," in J. J. Bonica (ed.), *Clinical Anesthesia*, F. A. Davis Company, Philadelphia, 1969, p. 218.

94 Moore, F. D.: The effects of hemorrhage in body composition, *N. Engl. J. Med.*, **273**:567, 1965.

95 Moore, F. D.: *Metabolic Care of the Surgical Patient*, W. B. Saunders Company, Philadelphia, 1959.

96 Moss, G. S., L. D. Homer, C. M. Herman, and H. J. Proctor: Right atrial and pulmonary artery pressure as indicators of left atrial pressure during fluid therapy following hemorrhagic shock in baboon, *Ann. Surg.*, **170**:801, 1969.

97 Motsay, G. J., R. H. Dietzman, R. A. Ersek, and R. C. Lillehei: Hemodynamic alterations and results of treatment in patients with gram-negative septic shock, *Surgery*, **67**:577, 1970.

98 Moyer, J. H. et al.: Hypothermia. III. Effect of hypothermia on renal damage resulting from ischemia. *Ann. Surg.*, **148**:156, 1957.

99 Mueller, H., S. M. Ayres, J. J. Gregory, S. Giannelli, Jr., and W. J. Grace: Hemodynamics, coronary blood flow, and myocardial metabolism in coronary shock: Response to I-norepinephrine and isoproterenol, *J. Clin. Invest.*, **49**:1885, 1970.

100 Mullins, C. B., W. L. Sugg, B. M. Kennelly, D. C. Jones, and J. H. Mitchell: Effect of arterial counterpulsation on left ventricular volume and pressure, *Am. J. Physiol.*, **220**:694, 1971.

101 Overton, R. C. and M. D. DeBakey: Experimental observations on the influences of hypothermia and autonomic blocking agents on hemorrhagic shock, *Ann. Surg.*, **143**:439, 1956.

102 Ollodart, R. M., I. Hawthorne, and S. Attar: Studies in experimental endotoxemia in man, *Am. J. Surg.*, **113**:599, 1967.

103 Pontoppidan, H., M. B. Laver, and B. Geffin:

"Acute Respiratory Failure in the Surgical Patient," in C. Welch (ed.), *Advances in Surgery*, Year Book Medical Publishers, Inc., Chicago, 1970, vol. 4.

104 Rahimtoola, S. H. et al.: Relationship of pulmonary artery to left ventricular diastolic pressures in acute myocardial infarction, *Circulation*, **46**:283, 1972.

105 Remington, J. W. et al.: Role of vasoconstriction in the response of the dog to hemorrhage, *Am. J. Physiol.*, **161**:116, 1950.

106 Replogle, R. L., H. Kundler, and R. E. Gross: Studies in the hemodynamic importance of blood viscosity, *J. Thorac. Cardiovas. Surg.*, **50**:658, 1965.

107 Sanders, C. A., M. J. Buckley, R. C. Leinbach, E. D. Mundth, and W. G. Austen: Mechanical circulatory assistance: Current status and experience with combining circulatory assistance, emergency, coronary angiography, and acute myocardial revascularization, *Circulation*, **45**:1292, 1972.

108 Schloerb, P. R., R. D. Waldorf, and J. S. Welsh: The protective effect of kidney hypothermia on total renal ischemia, *Surg. Forum*, **8**:633, 1957.

109 Schmutzer, J. J., E. Raschke, and J. V. Maloney, Jr.: Intravenous I-norepinephrine as a cause of reduced plasma volume, *Surgery*, **50**:452, 1961.

110 Schumer, W. and L. M. Nyhus: *Corticosteroids in the Treatment of Shock*, University of Illinois Press, Urbana, 1970.

111 Schumer, W., P. R. Erve, and R. P. Obernotle: Mechanisms of steroid protection in septic shock, *Surgery*, **72**:119, 1972.

112 Semb, C.: Partial resection of the kidney: Anatomical, physiological and clinical aspects, *Ann. R. Coll. Surg. Engl.*, **19**:137, 1956.

113 Sharefkin, J. B. and J. D. MacArthur: Pulmonary arterial pressure as a guide to the hemodynamic status of surgical patients, *Arch. Surg.*, **105**:699, 1972.

114 Shenkin, H. A. et al.: On the diagnosis of hemorrhage in man: A study of volunteers bled large amounts, *Am. J. Med. Sci.*, **208**:421, 1944.

115 Shires, G. T. et al.: Alterations in cellular membrane function during hemorrhagic shock in primates, *Ann. Surg.*, **176**:288, September 1972.

116 Shires, G. T. (ed.): *Care of the Trauma Patient*, McGraw-Hill Book Company, Inc., New York, 1966, Chap. 6.

117 Shires, G. T. and C. J. Carrico: Current status of the shock problem, *Curr. Probl. Surg.*, March 1966.

118 Shires, G. T., F. T. Brown, P. C. Canizaro, and N. Sommerville: Distributional changes in the extracellular fluid during acute hemorrhagic shock, *Surg. Forum*, **11**:115, 1960.

119 Shires, G. T., D. Coln, C. J. Carrico, and S. Lightfoot: Fluid therapy in hemorrhagic shock, *Arch. Surg.*, **88**:688, 1964.

120 Shires, G. T., C. J. Carrico, and P. C. Canizaro: *Shock*, W. B. Saunders Company, Philadelphia, 1973, Chap. 2.

121 Shubin, H. and M. H. Weil: Bacterial shock: A serious complication in urological practice, *J. Am. Med. Assoc.*, **185**:850, 1963.

122 Simeone, F. A., E. A. Husni, and M. G. Weidner, Jr.: The effect of I-norepinephrine upon the myocardial oxygen tension and survival in acute hemorrhagic hypotension, *Surgery*, **44**: 168, 1958.

123 Simeone, F. A.: "Shock," in *Christopher's Textbook of Surgery*, W. B. Saunders Company, Philadelphia, 1964, pp. 58–62.

124 Slonim, M. and W. M. Stahl: Sodium and water content of connective versus cellular tissue following hemorrhage, *Surg. Forum*, **19**:53, 1968.

125 Spink, W. W.: "The Ecology of Human Septic Shock," in Hershey, Del Guercio, and McConn (eds.), *Septic Shock in Man*, Little, Brown and Company, Boston, 1971.

126 Spodick, D. H.: Acute cardiac tamponade: Pathologic physiology, diagnosis and management. *Prog. Cardiovasc. Dis.*, **10**:64, 1967.

127 Sugg, W. L., M. J. Rea, W. R. Webb, and R. R. Ecker: Cardiac assistance (counterpulsation) in ten patients: Clinical and hemodynamic observations, *Ann. Thorac. Surg.*, **9**:1, 1970.

128 Swan, H. J. C. et al.: Catheterization of the heart in man with use of a flow-directed balloon-tipped catheter, *N. Engl. J. Med.*, **283**: 447, 1970.

129 Thal, A. P. and R. F. Wilson: Shock, *Curr. Probl. Surg.*, September 1965.

130 Trinkle, J. K., B. E. Rush, and B. Eiseman: Metabolism of lactate following major blood loss, *Surgery*, **63**:782, 1968.

131 Valeri, C. R. and N. L. Fortier: Red Cell 2,3-DPG, ATP, and creatine levels in preserved red cells and in patients with red cell mass deficits or with cardiopulmonary insufficiency, in George J. Brewer (ed.), *Red Cell Metabolism and Function*, Plenum Press, New York, 1970, p. 289.

132 Valeri, C. R. and N. M. Hirsch: Restoration in vivo of erythrocyte adenosine triphosphate, 2,3-diphosphoglycerate, potassium ion, and sodium ion concentrations following the transfusion of acid-citrate-dextrose-stored human red blood cells, *J. Lab. Clin. Med.*, **73**:722, 1969.

133 Valeri, C. R.: Viability and function of preserved red cells, *N. Engl. J. Med.*, **284**:81, 1971.

134 Waldhausen, J. A., J. W. Kilman, and F. L. Abel: Effects of catecholamines on the heart, *Arch. Surg.*, **91**:86, 1965.

135 Watts, D. T.: Arterial blood epinephrine levels during hemorrhagic hypotension in dogs, *Am. J. Physiol.*, **184**:271, 1956.

136 Webb, W. R., N. Shahbazi, and J. Jackson: Metabolic effects of vasopressors and vasodilators in the hypovolemia of standard hemorrhagic shock, *Surg. Forum*, **10**:378, 1960.

137 Weil, M. H., H. Shubin, and L. Rosoff: Fluid repletion in circulatory shock: Central venous pressure and other practical guides, *J. Am. Med. Assoc.*, **192**:668, 1965.

138 Welch, C. E. (ed.): "Blood Volume Measurement: A Critical Study," in F. J. Dagher, et al., *Advances in Surgery*, Year Book Medical Publishers, Inc., Chicago, 1965.

139 Wiggers, C. J.: Present status of shock problem, *Physiol. Rev.*, **22**:74, 1942.

140 Wiggers, H. C. et al.: Vasoconstriction and the development of irreversible hemorrhagic shock, *Am. J. Physiol.*, **153**:511, 1948.

141 Wilson, J. N. et al.: Central venous pressure in optimal blood volume maintenance, *Arch. Surg.*, **85**:563, 1962.

142 Wilson, R. F., R. Sukhnanden, and A. P. Thal: Combined use of norepinephrine and dibenzyline in clinical shock, *Surg. Forum*, **15**:30, 1964.

143 Wilson, R. F. and R. R. Fisher: The hemodynamic effects of massive steroids in clinical shock, *Surg. Gynecol. Obstet.*, **127**:769, 1968.

144 Wilson, J. N.: Rational approach to management of clinical shock, *Arch. Surg.*, **91**:92, 1965.

145 Wilson, R. F., D. V. Jablonski, and A. P. Thal: The usage of dibenzyline in clinical shock, *Surgery*, **56**:172, 1964.

146 Wood, L. and E. Beutler: Storage of erythrocytes in artificial media, *Transfusion*, **11**:123, 1971.

147 Zweifach, B. W., S. Baes, and E. Shorr: Effect of dibenamine against the fatal outcome of hemorrhagic and traumatic shock in rats, *Fed. Proc.*, **11**:7, 1952.

Chapter 2

Evaluation and Approach to the Bleeding Patient

Gabriel A. Shapiro, M.D.

Eugene P. Frenkel, M.D.

Critical to the correct evaluation of bleeding in an injured or surgical patient is the identification of a preexisting disorder of hemostasis or the advent of a de novo hemostatic derangement, either secondary to the trauma or iatrogenically induced. The presence of such an underlying bleeding diathesis will alter the interpretation of any acute bleeding and alter the therapeutic approach of not only the bleeding itself, but also the associated surgical or medical problems. In order to effectively evaluate the patient, the clinician must be aware of this possibility of a preexisting hemostatic disorder and be able to recognize the manifestations and complications of a systemic bleeding diathesis.

The ability to effectively institute a prompt and rational therapeutic program requires an understanding of the basic fundamentals of hemostasis. The clinician is often intimidated by the vast morass of studies available, with resultant confusion and unnecessary duplication. Employing a few rapidly performed and well-understood studies generally permits the physician to effectively identify and promptly deal with the basis for the hemorrhagic lesion. Subsequent to the acute crisis, other specific and sophisticated studies may be performed for more absolute delineation of the defect.

The Initial Clinical Evaluation

The most opportune time for a brief and expedient study of the hemostatic mechanism is during the initial clinical evaluation, since the data so derived can serve as the crucial basis for the decisions in management. While the first clue to an underlying hemostatic defect is often suggested by the magnitude of bleeding relative to that anticipated from the extent of injury, such data may not exist at the initial evaluation. Thus, as in any good clinical assessment, a complete evaluation of the patient is required.

The History

Although the past history is often sacrificed because of the tension of the moment, a careful but rapid inquiry into the patient's past may be richly rewarding and, in the long run, time saving. The most important questions relate to previous surgery, patterns of bleeding, family history, drug ingestion, and associated disease states.[17]

An excellent surgical challenge to hemostasis is a dental extraction. The history of an uneventful extraction usually rules out a clinically important inherited disorder, but an acquired defect may now have been superimposed. When patients relate that they have bled during surgery, one must ascertain the magnitude of the bleeding in relation to the surgery. For example, prolonged bleeding for a day or two from an incisor extraction is more indicative of an abnormality than similar bleeding from an impacted wisdom tooth.[13]

The type of bleeding is extremely important. A patient may claim to have "easy bruisability" or to be a "free bleeder," and careful questioning is necessary to resolve the issue. Bruising occurs often in normal people, especially in women. Large bruises (more than 5 to 6 cm in diameter) may be important, especially if they arise without trauma. Mucosal bleeding from the nose or gums may suggest a platelet defect, but is more commonly the result of local irritation. Spontaneous, deep soft tissue bleeding, hemarthrosis, or bleeding after circumcision are strongly suggestive of a coagulation disorder. Although previous gastrointestinal or urinary bleeding may be seen with disorders of either platelet or coagulation factors, these are most commonly due to anatomic lesions.

Family history may disclose an inherited disorder, but one must be leery of family "bleeders" whose defect has not been investigated. When one has evidence that a familial hemostatic defect has been characterized, the data is very valuable. Thus, previous studies of the patient's family should be explored.

Inquiry into prior drug ingestion is often overlooked, yet is extremely important. A surprising number of people take aspirin so routinely that they are often amnesic for its ingestion. Since aspirin may prolong the bleeding time in normal individuals, aspirin intake may have compromised previous surgical procedures such as tonsillectomy or dental extraction, confounding proper interpretation of excessive bleeding. A history of coumarin use should be sought, as well as details concerning other prescribed or proprietary drugs.

Associated disease states may be responsible for altered hemostasis. Uremic toxins inhibit platelet function, impairing primary hemostasis. Lupus erythematosus and lymphoma may be associated with immune thrombocytopenia. Severe liver disease may lead to multiple factor deficiencies. Malignancy, particularly when treated with chemotherapy, may be responsible for thrombocytopenia.

Initial Signs and Symptoms

The character of the bleeding in the patient often indicates the type of preexistent hemostatic defect. In a broad sense, such abnormalities can be divided into bleeding due to a platelet plug defect (recalling that the most crucial aspect of capillary integrity relates directly to platelet function) or bleeding due to a coagulation defect. Abnormalities in the platelets or vascular bed are manifested by excessive and prompt bleeding from small superficial cuts, evidence of petechiae, purpura, ecchymoses, or mucosal bleeding. With these abnormalities, stasis is easily achieved by compression. By contrast, when coagulation defects are present, small superficial cuts may not manifest bleeding until hours after the episode of trauma. Such defects are characterized instead by subcutaneous hemorrhages, hematomas, or hemarthroses. Compression yields transient stasis, but bleeding promptly recurs when pressure is removed.

Since the acquired lesion of disseminated intravascular coagulation (DIC) is a common sequela of many forms of injury (sepsis, hemorrhagic shock, burns, etc.), such underlying disturbances must be considered as potential etiologic factors of a generalized bleeding disorder.

Laboratory Evaluation

Although the precise biochemical and molecular mechanisms involved in hemostasis have not been elucidated, a general knowledge of the hemostatic factors is critical for prompt and accurate diagnosis and management of the bleeding patient.

Mechanisms of Hemostasis

Normal hemostasis is provided by (1) vessel integrity, (2) plasma coagulation factors, (3) platelets, and (4) a proteolytic (fibrinolytic) system capable of removing the clot as repair takes place.[7] Figure 2-1 schematically outlines the coagulation system, the formation of the platelet plug (primary hemostasis), and the interrelationship between the systems.

Certainly the activation of prothrombin to the catalytically potent thrombin is the most critical step in the coagulation mechanism. Thrombin is formed via two classical pathways, the intrinsic system and the extrinsic system. In the intrinsic pathway endothelial injury exposes the underlying collagen. Factor XII is activated, initiating a sequence of events which leads to the formation of activated factor X (Xa). Xa forms a complex (termed prothrombinase) with factor V, calcium, and phospholipid; prothrombinase converts prothrombin to thrombin. In the extrinsic pathway, tissue injury releases tissue factor which combines with factor VII and calcium to acti-

vate factor X; again, prothrombinase is formed for the conversion of prothrombin to thrombin. The thrombin so generated acts on the plasma substrate fibrinogen to produce fibrin and activates factor XIII, which covalently links the fibrin together to form a solid clot. Thrombin also ("auto") catalyzes its own formation by accelerating the activity of factors V and VIII, and contributes to platelet aggregation. Finally, thrombin activates a major compensatory system to thrombosis by triggering fibrinolysis.

Platelet plug formation, or primary hemostasis, is also initiated by vessel injury, with platelets initially adhering to exposed subendothelial collagen.[7,4] As the platelet changes its shape from a flat disk to a spiculated sphere, adenosine diphosphate (ADP) is released (with other vasoactive substances); this release reaction allows platelet aggregation with consequently more ADP release and more aggregation. The aggregates form the platelet plug, which undergoes consolidation, a process associated with a contractile protein (so-called "thrombosthenin"). Finally, the plug is stabilized by the fibrin mesh formed by ongoing coagulation triggered at the site of injury. While platelets contribute their membrane phospholipid (platelet factor 3) to coagulation and coagulation contributes to primary hemostasis, one system can usually operate normally if the other system is defective. This explains why the whole blood clot time is usually normal in thrombocytopenia, and why the bleeding time, which tests the platelet plug, is normal in classic hemophilia. If both systems are altered, a profound hemostatic defect may result. For instance, the patient with classical hemophilia who is given aspirin may have a significant increase in bleeding.[10]

Diagnostic Tests

The scheme outlined in Fig. 2-1 can be used to focus on the presence of a hemostatic defect. By simple screening tests one can decide

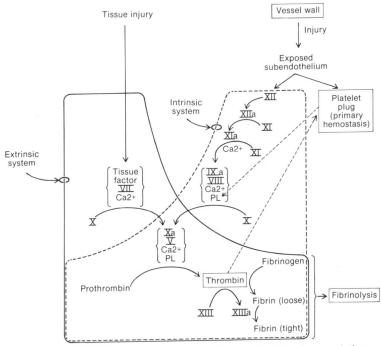

Figure 2-1 Schema of coagulation. International nomenclature for blood coagulation factors: I, fibrinogen; II, prothrombin; III, tissue thromboplastin; IV, calcium, V, labile factor, proaccelerin, Ac globulin; VI, not assigned; VII, stabile factor, proconvertin, SPCA, autoprothrombin I; VIII, antihemophiliac factor (AHF), antihemophiliac globulin (AHG); IX, plasma thromboplastin component (PTC), Christmas factor, autoprothrombin II; X, Stuart-Prower factor, autoprothrombin III; IX, plasma thromboplastin antecedent (PTA); XII, Hageman factor; XIII, fibrin-stabilizing factor.

whether the defect is in platelet plug formation (primary hemostasis), in a coagulation disorder, or in both.

Platelet plug formation can be evaluated by the platelet count and the bleeding time. Although actual platelet counting by phase microscopy or an electronic device is preferred, the platelet numbers (expressed as platelets per cubic millimeter) may be estimated at the microscope by multiplying the average number of platelets per oil immersion field by 20,000. The bleeding time may be properly performed either by the Ivy method or by the template method of Mielke.[11] In performing the Ivy time, a blood pressure cuff is applied to the upper arm and maintained at 40 mmHg. A hairless site midway on the outer surface of the forearm and not overlying superficial veins

is cleansed with alcohol and allowed to dry. Duplicate punctures about 1 cm apart are made with a disposable lancet, and every 30 s filter paper is used to scoop blood from the site without disturbing the wound. The timing begins with the puncture and ends when blood ceases to flow or when only serosanguineous fluid stains the filter paper. The normal bleeding time using this method is less than $5\frac{1}{2}$ min. The template bleeding time is performed in the same way except that, with a special kit, a Bard Parker No. 11 blade attached to a holder is preset to deliver an incision 1 mm deep. A template with a slit 1 cm long is pressed firmly against the skin, and duplicate incisions the length of the slit are made by the blade through the template. The normal template bleeding time is $2\frac{1}{2}$ to $9\frac{1}{2}$ min in most laboratories, and the test is more reliable than the lancet method. However, the lancet method, if done with consistency, is a quite satisfactory test for general screening purposes. Whichever method is used, each laboratory should establish its own normal range using healthy volunteers. The Duke method, utilizing the earlobe puncture, lacks accuracy, reproducibility, and sensitivity. Likewise, the Rumpel-Leede test has also been found too unreliable for meaningful use. Finally, microscopic evaluation of platelet morphology may be of value if sufficient time permits. When numerous large (hence, young) platelets are seen in the setting of thrombocytopenia, increased platelet consumption and turnover is suggested, a situation encountered in immune thrombocytopenia or in DIC.

When the platelet count is below 20,000/ mm,[3] the bleeding time is usually prolonged, although not necessarily if many of the circulating platelets are young and thus "active".[8] However, in profound thrombocytopenia the bleeding time is almost always prolonged. When the platelet count is normal (or increased) and the bleeding time is prolonged, one is dealing with a platelet functional defect. Platelet functional defects are usually acquired through either disease or drug. Once the platelet count and bleeding time separate a platelet functional defect from thrombocytopenia, one is well on the way to a diagnosis, and Fig. 2-2 outlines the major possibilities to be considered. Other platelet functional tests, such as platelet adhesion and aggregation, while useful for documenting inherited platelet functional defects, are usually not necessary in an acute situation and are usually invalid when thrombocytopenia is present.

Coagulation adequacy may be screened with three rapid procedures: the prothrombin time (PT), partial thromboplastin time (PTT), and the thrombin time (TT).

As seen in Fig. 2-3, the prothrombin time reveals defects in the extrinsic system (factor VII) and in the factors common to the extrinsic and intrinsic systems (X, V, prothrombin, and fibrinogen). The partial thromboplastin time reveals defects in the intrinsic system (XII, XI, IX, VIII) and in the factors common to both systems (X, V, prothrombin, and fibrinogen). The thrombin time measures only the conversion time of available fibrinogen to a loose fibrin clot. None of these tests measure factor XIII, since its fibrin stabilizing effects are preceded by the endpoint of the tests, clot formation. However, its measurement is only rarely relevent in a surgical or medical setting.

Table 2-1 provides a useful guide to possible coagulation disorders based on the initial screening tests, putting Fig. 2-3 into clinical relevance. An abnormal PTT in the face of a normal PT and TT would incriminate any of the first-stage clotting factors of the intrinsic pathway, usually factor VIII. Factor XII deficiency is almost never associated with clinically relevant bleeding. An abnormal PT with a normal PTT and TT suggests factor VII deficiency. An abnormal PT and PTT with a normal TT usually signifies multiple coagulation defects, most often in the setting of liver disease or coumarin ingestion, although in far advanced liver disease hypofibrinogenemia or the presence of fibrin split products may prolong the thrombin time as well. Abnormalities of all screening tests is usually seen in the setting of florid DIC or heparin therapy; in mild DIC, however, the tests are variable.

Once an abnormal test is demonstrated, one can gain considerable information by repeating the test with an admixture of the patient's plasma 1:1 with normal plasma. Correction to normal by this admixture strongly supports a deficiency of a clotting factor which was supplied by the normal plasma. Further testing, including other mixing tests or specific factor assays, may then be performed to pinpoint the defect. If the 1:1 dilution yields only partial or no correction, a circulating anticoagulant is strongly suspect. In a surgical setting the

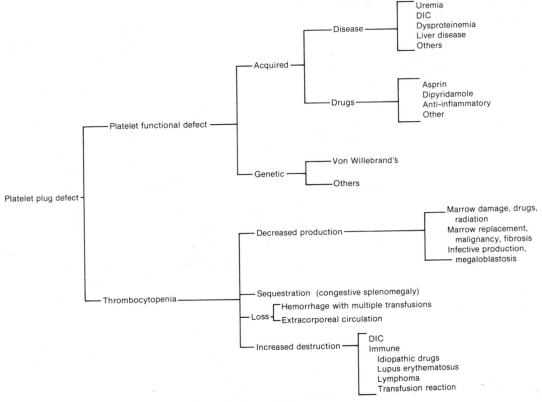

Figure 2-2 Platelet disorders. *(Modified from Harker, ref. 7)*

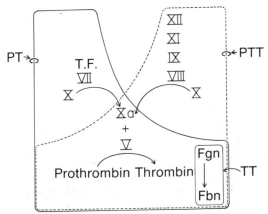

Figure 2-3 Assessment of coagulation abnormalities by simple laboratory screening. The aspects of the coagulation schema evaluated by each of the routine screening tests are encircled for clarity. The abbreviations Fgn for fibrinogen and Fbn for fibrin are used.

suspect circulating anticoagulant is usually fibrin degradation products or heparin. Occasionally, however, one encounters a circulating anticoagulant directed against a specific factor, most notably an acquired anti-factor VIII in a hemophiliac, and further special testing is required. It should be stressed that the 1:1 admixture method is only a rapid screening technique. It is by no means foolproof in separating factor deficiency from factor inhibition.

Table 2-2 summarizes the usual findings in most hemostatic disorders that the clinician will encounter. A combined clinical defect in both platelet plug formation and coagulation is most commonly seen in DIC. A combined defect is also seen in von Willebrand's dis-

Table 2-1: Coagulation Disorders Suggested by Screening Tests

PT	PTT	TT	Possible Defect
N	A	N	VIII, IX, XI, or XII defect; circulating anticoagulant (anti-VIII, etc.)
A	N	N	VII defect
A	A	N	Multiple factors: coumarin, liver disease, K deficiency Isolated defect: X, V, prothrombin
A	A	A	Multiple factors: DIC Isolated defect: fibrinogen Circulating anticoagulant: F.S.P., heparin, dysfibrinogenemia

PT = prothrombin time PTT = partial thromboplastin time
TT = thrombin time
N = normal FSP = fibrin split products
A = abnormal

ease, but this is obviously a much less common event.

THERAPY

General Considerations

When considering replacement therapy for the bleeding patient, a few general comments deserve mention. It is important to remember that the most common cause of bleeding in a surgical patient is a severed vessel and not an intrinsic platelet plug or coagulation defect. While transfusion may be required, restoring vessel integrity will allow hemostasis. Secondly, blood resources are always limited. By separating a single unit of blood into various components such as plasma, packed red cells, cryoprecipitate, platelets, and even granulocytes, the selected replacement needs of many may be met. Thus, the use of fresh whole blood is usually unnecessary and, in fact, wasteful. While fresh whole blood may be used in the previously massively transfused patient (at a ratio of 1 fresh/2 banked), the combination of fresh-frozen plasma and packed red cells will substitute for fresh blood and can be used in the same ratio with banked blood. This helps prevent an immediate major stress on a blood bank's phlebotomy and crossmatching resources. If platelets are dangerously depleted in the course of multiple transfusions, platelet concentrates may be supplied. Packed red cells are often given instead of whole blood when the possibility of circulatory overload exists. Many clotting factors, particularly the prothrombin complex (prothrombin, VII, IX, X) are quite stable in banked plasma. Thus, judicious employment of component therapy will be beneficial to the patient and to the nation's blood resources.

Specific Considerations

Platelets The identification of a quantitative platelet deficiency raises the question of the significance of any given numerical platelet level (Fig. 2-4). In general terms, 40,000 to 50,000 platelets/mm^3 are adequate for hemostasis. Yet clinically there often is a poor correlation between the presence of bleeding and the specific platelet numbers. Thus, prolongation of the bleeding time serves as a better criterion of the potential clinical significance of the platelet depression than any absolute platelet numbers. When the Ivy time is prolonged in the face of clinical bleeding, platelet transfusions (usually 4 to 6 platelet packs) will usually return the bleeding time to a safe range unless the platelets are consumed or otherwise rendered ineffective in the patient's blood stream. Platelet concentrates must be infused through a special platelet recipient filter; if a standard blood filter is

Table 2-2: Usual Laboratory Results in Hemostatic Abnormalities

Diagnosis	BT	Plt. count	PT	PTT	TT	Other Possible Tests
Uremia	A	N	N	N	N	Abnormal platelet aggregation, adhesion
Aspirin ingestion	N or A	N	N	N	N	Abnormal platelet aggregation
von Willebrand's disease	A	N	N	N or A	N	Abnormal platelet adhesion, low factor VIII activity
Immune thrombocytopenia	N or A	$\downarrow\downarrow$	N	N	N	Large platelets on smear, marrow megakaryocytes present, platelet antibodies detected, shortened platelet survival
Marrow hypoplasia, marrow invasion	A	$\downarrow$	N	N	N	Abnormal bone marrow and peripheral blood
Congestive splenomegaly	N	50,000–100,000	N	N	N	Relatively normal platelet survival
Hemophilia A	N	N	N	A	N	Low factor VIII activity, in vitro correction with normal or absorbed plasma, no correction with aged plasma
Coumarin or liver disease	N	N	A	A	N	In vitro correction with normal plasma
Disseminated intravascular coagulation*	A	$\downarrow$	A	A	A	Elevated FSP, fibrinogen level often low, poor in vitro correction with normal plasma
Multiple transfusions (banked blood)	N	50,000–100,000	A	A	N	In vitro correction of PT, PTT, with normal plasma

BT = bleeding time
N = normal
Plt. = platelet
A = abnormal

PT = prothrombin time
FSP = fibrin split products
PTT = partial thromboplastin time
TT = thrombin time

*Abnormalities may vary widely with severity.

used, the platelets will adhere to the meshwork, resulting in reduced in vivo recovery. If platelet separations are not available, fresh whole blood may be used, but this is a less desirable choice. Again, a postplatelet transfusion bleeding time is the best means of evaluating the adequacy of repair. Platelet transfusions may be used in a similar fashion preoperatively, but the amount should be doubled in the face of fever or sepsis. In immune thrombocytopenia, platelet transfusions are of less value because of their rapid in vivo destruction, but they are indicated adjunctively in life-threatening bleeding while other measures (e.g., adrenal cortical steroids) are being instituted.

The management of platelet functional defects must be individualized. In uremia the platelet defect may be improved after peritoneal dialysis or hemodialysis.[16] In the acute situation, platelet transfusions may be lifesaving until dialysis is accomplished. In von

Willebrand's disease, both the platelet defect and reduced factor VIII activity may be corrected by cryoprecipitate.

Prothrombin Complex All the factors of the prothrombin complex (prothrombin, VII, IX, and X) are synthesized in the liver and require modification by vitamin K for coagulation activity.[15,12] Thus, selectively decreased prothrombin complex activity is seen in coumarin administration and vitamin K deficiency. Administration of vitamin K_1 (Aqua mephyton) will allow the prothrombin complex activity to rise, but since an effect is not seen for several hours one may need plasma to manage severe bleeding. Administration of 500 to 1000 mL of plasma will rapidly return the prothrombin time toward normal. Since the prothrombin complex is stable in banked plasma, fresh or fresh-frozen plasma is not required.[5] Prothrombin complex concentrates may also be given, especially if the patient cannot tolerate the plasma volume load, but their use carries a high incidence of hepatitis and a possible risk of thromboembolic phenomena.

Liver Disease In hepatocellular disease, the synthesis of most clotting factors is impaired, including the prothrombin complex.

Vitamin K_1 is often given, but prothrombin complex activity will not respond to vitamin K_1 unless there is an obstructive component. In addition, factor V, which is also made in the liver, is labile in banked blood, so the mainstay of therapy in this type of bleeding must be in the form of fresh or fresh-frozen plasma.

Hemophilia In classic hemophilia factor VIII is present but is nonfunctional, resulting in markedly reduced activity.[14,2] The use of whole plasma has largely been replaced by cryoprecipitate or commercial lyophilized concentrates, thus assuring high activity without volume overload. For simple hemarthroses or small hematomas the reliable patient may be given a single infusion of factor VIII (20 to 30 U/kg) which will raise the factor VIII level to between 40 and 50 percent.[9] The patient may be followed closely as an outpatient, but if pain or swelling has not lessened after 12 to 24 h, the patient should be admitted for more intensive therapy.[1] For intraabdominal or retroperitoneal bleeding, head injuries, and bleeding in the floor of the mouth, an initial dose is given to raise the factor VIII level to between 80 and 100 percent; then half this dose is given every 12 h for at least 5 to 7 days after bleeding has ceased. Head injuries should be treated in this manner even if bleed-

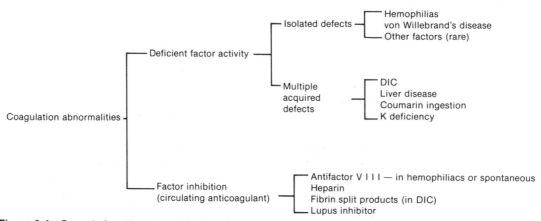

Figure 2-4 Coagulation disorders. *(Modified from Harker, ref. 7)*

ing is not apparent. For patients requiring surgery or extractions of adult teeth the same initial dose is given, and the same maintenance levels should be given for 10 to 14 days.

Disseminated Intravascular Coagulation (DIC) This is a complicated syndrome, in which there is widespread clotting factor and platelet consumption, secondary fibrinolysis, and platelet dysfunction.[3] DIC is always the result of an underlying trigger mechanism. In a surgical setting the trigger is commonly sepsis, hemorrhagic shock, massive crush injury, burns, thoracic procedures, transfusion reactions, and abruptio placentae. Therapy should be vigorously directed toward the underlying process. Replacement therapy in the form of plasma and platelets is usually not beneficial, but in abruptio placentae large doses of fibrinogen have been given when bleeding is severe. In most cases of DIC, heparin therapy is not necessary, but if bleeding is generalized and life-threatening, or if thrombosis occurs, heparin is administered in full dose.

BIBLIOGRAPHY

1 Abildgaard, C. F.: Current concepts in the management of hemophilia, *Semin. Hematol.,* **12**: 223, 1975.

2 Bennett, R., W. C. Forman, and O. D. Ratnoff: Studies on the nature of antihemophilic factor (factor VIII): Further evidence relating the AHF-like antigens in normal and hemophilic plasmas, *J. Clin. Invest.,* **52**:2191, 1973.

3 Deykin, D.: The clinical challenge of disseminated intravascular coagulation, *N. Engl. J. Med.,* **283**:636, 1970.

4 Deykin, D.: Emerging concepts of platelet function, *N. Engl. J. Med.,* **290**:144, 1974.

5 Deykin, D.: Warfarin therapy, *N. Engl. J. Med.,* **283**:801, 1970.

6 Garg, S. K., E. L. Amorosi, and S. Karpatkin: Use of the megathrombocyte as an index of megakaryocyte number, *N. Engl. J. Med.,* **284**: 11, 1971.

7 Harker, L. A.: *Hemostasis Manual,* F. A. Davis Company, Philadelphia, 1974.

8 Harker, L. A. and S. J. Slichter: The bleeding time as a screening test for evaluation of platelet function, *N. Engl. J. Med.,* **287**:155, 1972.

9 Honig, G. R., E. N. Forman, C. A. Johnson, et al.: Administration of single doses of AHF (factor VIII) concentrate in the treatment of hemophilic hemarthroses, *Pediatrics,* **43**:26, 1969.

10 Kaneshiro, M. M., C. H. Mielke, Jr., C. K. Kasper, and S. I. Rapaport: Bleeding time after aspirin in disorders of intrinsic clotting, *N. Engl. J. Med.,* **281**:1039, 1969.

11 Mielke, C. H., M. M. Kaneshiro, I. A. Maher, J. M. Weiner, and S. I. Rapaport: The standardized normal Ivy bleeding time and its prolongation by aspirin, *Blood,* **34**:204, 1969.

12 Nelsestuen, G. L., T. H. Zytkovicz, and J. B. Howard: The mode of action of vitamin K, *J. Biol. Chem.,* **249**:6347, 1974.

13 Owen, C. A., E. J. Bowie, P. Didisheim, and J. A. Thompson: *The Diagnosis of Bleeding Disorders,* Little, Brown and Company, Boston, 1969, p. 274.

14 Shapiro, G. A., J. C. Andersen, S. V. Pizzo, and P. A. McKee: The subunit structure of normal and hemophilic factor VIII, *J. Clin. Invest.,* **52**:2198, 1973.

15 Stenflo, J.: Vitamin K and the biosynthesis of prothrombin, *J. Biol. Chem.,* **247**:8167, 1972.

16 Stewart, J. H. and P. A. Castaldi: Uraemic bleeding: A reversible platelet defect corrected by dialysis, *Q. J. Med.,* **36**: 409, 1967.

17 Williams, W. J.: "General Effects of Disorders of Hemostasis," in W. J. Williams et al. (eds.), *Hematology,* McGraw-Hill Book Company, New York, 1972, p. 1120.

Chapter 3

Metabolic Response to Trauma

Malcolm O. Perry, M.D.

Trauma acutely and often extensively alters the delicate integration of endocrine and metabolic systems in the patient. However, a wide range of response is noted which correlates with the magnitude of the injury and the metabolic adjustments of which the patient is capable. The acute sympathicoadrenal discharge producing a pale, sweating, apprehensive patient needs only hypotension to result in the classic picture of shock. These dramatic responses evoke further adjustments and are replaced by less apparent, though no less important, endocrine and metabolic aberrations. Moore has divided the metabolic response into four phases:[44]

1 The initial injury reaction with a duration of 2 to 4 days
2 The turning point, requiring 1 to 2 days
3 An anabolic period, characterized by protein synthesis and lasting 2 to 5 weeks

4 A period of several months of final adjustment in which "fat gain" is preponderant

There is, of course, a subtle and occasionally undetectable blending of these artificial divisions; but in general they form a basis which facilitates logical examination of the complex interrelationships which characterize response to trauma.

THE ENDOCRINE RESPONSE

Pituitary

The anterior pituitary produces a variety of trophic hormones which appear to act directly on target organs.[20,21] Of these endocrine organs responding to the trophic influence of the anterior pituitary hormones, the adrenal cortex would appear to be the most important. Adrenocorticotropic hormone (ACTH) is a low-molecular-weight protein hormone or hormones. Stimuli arising as a result of injury or stress reach the cerebral cortex and apparently release the inhibition of the reticular formation upon hypothalamic centers located in and around the median eminence and the tuberoinfundibular nucleus. Corticotropin releasing factor (CRF) is a polypeptide hormone mediator which is then released by large neurons in the area. The elaboration of ACTH, and its subsequent action on the adrenal cortex, result in a rise in the blood cortisol level, which in turn partially suppresses the output of corticotropin by the anterior pituitary. The result of this feedback inhibitory effect is to maintain the level of circulating plasma cortisol within relatively narrow limits, but the impact of trauma will induce an increase in corticotropin irrespective of the level of circulating hydrocortisone. Measurements of blood ACTH reveal a diurnal variation, with more secretion of corticotropin during the morning hours. Injury, however, results in an absolute increase in these levels.[5,20,21,43,46]

Somatropin, or growth hormone, is also produced by the anterior pituitary and has a profound effect on body metabolism, particularly skeletal growth and the synthesis of protein. Normal growth and development would seem to be directly related to its presence. There is, however, no evidence that this hormone is necessary for normal convalescence since following total hypophysectomy, patients recover without the administration of any somatropinlike substances. At the present time, the exact role of somatropin and the reaction to injury remain unclear.[43,45,47]

Antidiuretic hormone (ADH) apparently is produced by areas in the hypothalamus and then transmitted through the pituitary portal circulation to its ultimate storage area in the posterior pituitary gland. The often-noted antidiuresis subsequent to injury or operation is related to the production of ADH and its effect upon the renal tubules. A detailed discussion of the interrelationships of ADH, al-

dosterone, and translocation of fluid attendant upon injury and trauma is found in Chap. 1.

Adrenal Cortex

The adrenal cortex occupies a central role in the response to trauma; and more than 50 different steroids have so far been isolated from the adrenal cortex. The majority of these compounds are intracellular intermediates in the production of the few steroids which are normally secreted into the blood stream. These may be divided into five groups.[21]

The glucocorticoids are characterized by the presence of an 11-hydroxyl group and include cortisol or hydrocortisone, which has, in addition, a 17-hydroxyl group. Cortisol represents over 80 percent of the total 17-hydroxycorticoids, and approximately 15 to 20 mg is secreted daily in adults under basal conditions. In addition, 2 to 5 mg of corticosterone is secreted daily. The mineralocorticoids include aldosterone and 11-desoxycorticosterone, with the former being the most important of the electrolyte active hormones. Approximately 75 to 125 μg of aldosterone is secreted each day.

The remainder of the active steroid hormones include those with androgenic and estrogenic activity and are characterized by the 17-ketosteroids. About 75 percent is present in the form of dehydroepiandrosterone which is secreted in quantities of 20 to 35 mg/day.

Blood levels of 17-hydroxycorticoids, when measured in the posttraumatic state, reveal acute and very significant increases. After a suitable latent period, these are reflected by various products in the urine. Normal blood levels of 17-hydroxycorticoids are between 5 and 15 μg per 100 mL. Within a few minutes after the initiation of anesthesia or physical trauma, this level may reach 70 to 80 μg per 100 mL.[23,24,35,43,51]

The exact mode of action of the adrenal steroids is unknown, but the effects have been variously described as "permissive" or "normalizing" and in some instances even synergistic with that of other hormones, notably the catecholamines.[31] The action of the glucocorticoids can be divided into several phases. Gluconeogenesis is fundamentally a catabolic process characterized by the deamination of amino acids with nitrogen loss and a rise in blood sugar followed by a rise in liver glycogen.[9,56,63] In the presence of large amounts of glucocorticoids, this abnormal protein breakdown reduces the production of bone matrix. There is a secondary resorption of calcium following the loss of bone matrix, which is further aggravated by a reduction in calcium absorption from the intestine because of an antagonism to vitamin D by hydrocortisone.[21] Similarly, total body fat may be increased at the expense of body protein.

Although aldosterone is the most important adrenal corticoid influencing sodium reabsorption, both cortisol and cortisone affect water metabolism and ion exchange.[5,21,26] These substances enhance water diuresis, and this apparently is related to an increased glomerular filtration rate and antagonism of ADH. The effect on sodium reabsorption is relatively minor, but is associated with a consequent loss of potassium and hydrogen ions.[21]

The reduction in circulating lymphocytes and eosinophils exhibits some temporal relationship to the actual metabolic effects produced by these hormones. This lymphopenia is related to both increased destruction of cells and sequestration in the lungs and spleen.[26,44,63]

The antiinflammatory properties of the glucocorticoids constitute a prominent part of their therapeutic usefulness. The initial action of prevention of excessive granulation tissue and scarring is followed by the less desirable effects of inhibition of reparative changes and delayed wound healing.

The 17-ketosteroids illustrated by the weak androgens exhibit two primary actions: an acceleration of protein metabolism and an accentuation of secondary sex characteristics. The retention of nitrogen following administration of androgen may be in part due to the increased synthesis of protein from amino acids, but may reflect only protein sparing by increased utilization of fat for caloric needs. In contrast to the previously noted action of cortisone on calcium, androgens improve bone development and increase the utilization of calcium.[21]

The androgenic effects are primarily those of stimulation of the male features, but only in the situations of very excessive production, such as the adrenogenital syndrome, are the effects on secondary sex characteristics of significance.[26]

Specific Relations to Trauma

Many of the metabolic changes noted following injury are similar to those induced by the administration of excessive amounts of cortisone or hydrocortisone; similarly, the excretion of conjugated steroids in the urine shows an increase in the posttraumatic state.[24,43] Normally 10 to 20 mg of 17-hydroxycorticoids is secreted in a 24-h period, and this is often doubled or tripled for the first 3 to 4 days following an injury of moderate severity.[23,43,44,66] In the absence of shock or impaired liver function, the peak blood levels of 17-hydroxycorticoids are attained about 6 h after the trauma. This reaction appears to be nonspecific and is related more to the severity of injury than the specific type of injury.[30,31,44,57] Many of these changes cannot be demonstrated in an adrenalectomized animal.[7,19] In addition, the increases in urinary nitrogen and in urinary corticoids are related and parallel the degree of severity of the injury. There is, however, a less exact correlation between this increased nitrogen excretion and increasing levels of corticoid production.[35,67] In adrenalectomized rats, urinary nitrogen excretion after fractures will be increased if the animals are maintained on constant amounts of adrenocortical extracts.[31,64] Similar findings have been reported by numerous other workers, suggesting that the metabolic changes which are attendant upon injury are not directly related to the absolute level of the corticoids which are produced.[16,57] This would be in accord with the permissive or supporting action which has been advanced as the primary purpose of these hormones; or as previously described by Selye, a "conditioning action."[58]

Aldosterone

Aldosterone is one of the most important hormones produced by the adrenal cortex and by itself can sustain life in the adrenalectomized animal. The exact mechanism regulating the secretion of aldosterone is unclear, but appears to be independent of pituitary action. Ablation of the pituitary gland practically abolishes the secretion of hydrocortisone, but reduces the secretion of aldosterone by only 60 to 80 percent.[16] Administration of ACTH does increase the secretion of aldosterone, but only minimally. In contradistinction, a fall in blood volume may result in a 30-fold increase in the secretion of aldosterone.[5,20]

Aldosterone, by its action on the distal renal tubules, strongly promotes the reabsorption of sodium and excretion of hydrogen and potassium. The subsequent increased reabsorption of water is related to the reabsorption of the sodium ion. The rate of transport at these ions is influenced by the amount of aldosterone present. The sweat glands and salivary glands also respond to aldosterone and secrete less sodium and more potassium as the levels of aldosterone rise.[5]

The increase in plasma volume due to reabsorption of sodium and water following the secretion of aldosterone will tend to increase blood pressure, but there is evidence that aldosterone also has a direct effect upon the vasculature and acts in a synergistic fashion with the catecholamines. A further relationship exists in that another pressor substance, angiotensin II, strongly stimulates the adrenals to increase the excretion of aldosterone.[5]

A decrease in blood volume is a very potent stimulus to the production of aldosterone, but following bilateral nephrectomy this response is lost. The increased retention of sodium and water postoperatively is thought to be related to the production of aldosterone and antidiuretic hormone.[14,15,41] This effect can be obviated by treatment schedules in which balanced salt solutions are administered to prevent a volume deficit created by translocation of functional extracellular fluid.[60,61] The relationship between plasma or blood loss and secretion of aldosterone is discussed in Chap. 1.

Adrenal Medulla

The chromaffin cells of the adrenal medulla produce the catecholamines, epinephrine, and norepinephrine. The sympathetic stimuli emanate from the tenth thoracic to the first lumbar spinal cord levels and reach the adrenal glands via the preaortic ganglia. The average amount of catecholamines found in the normal human adrenal medulla is 2 to 4 mg/g. About 70 to 80 percent of this is epinephrine and the remainder norepinephrine. Norepinephrine, however, is the predominant catecholamine found in extramedullary tissues.[21]

Although norepinephrine and epinephrine differ considerably in the degree of their pharmacologic actions, they tend to produce the same effects. One of the most important of these is the temporary elevation of blood pressure. Norepinephrine is the more potent in producing a sustained arteriolar contraction and a positive ionotropic effect on the heart. Epinephrine stimulates the central nervous system, dilates the bronchi, and has a more pronounced chronotropic effect on the heart. The metabolic effects of epinephrine are more predominant than those of norepinephrine. Hyperglycemia is produced by the degradation of liver glycogen to glucose following activation of the liver enzyme phosphoralase. Both hormones have an equal effect in the liberation of nonesterified fatty acids from the neutral lipids present in fat depots.[21]

Following injury, the urinary excretion of epinephrine and norepinephrine and their metabolic products are elevated for 1 to 2 days. The measurement of blood levels, however, does not always correlate well with this finding.[27] Sympathicoadrenal activity reveals itself clinically as tachycardia, sweating, and vasoconstriction in a pale, apprehensive patient. This clinical picture may also be evoked by psychologic stimuli, anesthesia, anoxia, and, of course, hemorrhage.[44] Thus, it is seen that the primary findings of sympathicoadrenal action are noted during the early phases of the initial stage of injury and pass rather rapidly if no complications supervene.[45]

Changes in Other Endocrine Glands

The exact relationship between injury and the functions of the thyroids, parathyroids, gonads, and pancreas remains unclear at this time.[25,28,67] The increase in oxygen consumption and carbon dioxide production following injury tempts one to postulate that the thyroid gland plays an essential role, but these factors can be produced by a variety of influences in the absence of trauma. The measurements of various parameters, such as protein-bound iodine and radioactive iodine uptake, which would indicate increased thyroid function, do not correlate well with these energy changes, nor have they been consistently altered in any one direction. Similarly, increased excretion of calcium upon injury can be related quite well to immobilization and may not be directly related to parathyroid function at all. Although androgenic hormones produce an anabolic effect, gonadal function does not have a direct important effect on the metabolic response to injury, but does appear to be decreased after major trauma.[67]

THE CATABOLIC RESPONSE

As noted in the preceding sections, catabolism is increased following injury. This has some correlation with adrenal cortex activity, but the exact relationships are somewhat obscure. There is dissolution of body protein as reflected by increased urinary nitrogen excretion, which may reach 15 to 20 g/day, or even higher after the extensive trauma of burns, widespread soft-tissue injury, or multiple fractures.[5,31,64] A similar response will occur in the event of infection which may complicate an initial traumatic episode. These increased rates of excretion may persist for 3 to 5 days in the uncomplicated case but can be reduced by the administration of exogenous protein and other compounds which supply calories, thus reducing the effect of starvation.[18,53] The inability to obviate these nitrogen losses completely is indicative of a definite catabolic effect.[2,47,55]

The classic approach to this evaluation of catabolism revolves around nitrogen balance, and zero balance is indicative of neither absolute gain nor loss of protein. The normal urinary excretion of nitrogen is 7 to 8 g daily, predominantly as urea. It is possible to administer protein substances at a rate exceeding the excretory ability of the kidney, and thus falsely indicate a positive nitrogen balance.[54]

Careful monitoring of weight change reveals a loss of body tissue if water gain or loss is kept at minimal rates. The oxidation of fat, as previously noted, also results in weight loss. Approximately 1 g of nitrogen is liberated by dissolution of 6.25 g of protein; thus a urinary loss of 10 g of nitrogen represents about 62 g of protein lost, or about 300 g of wet lean muscle. The protein in bone, connective tissue, and the plasma protein less readily reflect these changes in body protein. There can be, in fact, large losses or gain of protein without detectable changes in the concentration of plasma proteins.[29,65]

As the initial responses to injury dissipate, a rather abrupt change toward normal occurs in urinary nitrogen excretion. It is at this point that, in the presence of sufficient caloric intake, protein balance is restored. In the absence of subsequent complications, net protein gain is prominent and recovery proceeds. The gain, however, is usually much slower than the initial loss. A negative nitrogen balance does not necessarily interfere with wound healing. The concept of primacy of the wound is real and is demonstrated by the ability of even cachectic patients to attain wound healing, but at the expense of other tissues.[44]

Attempts to alter this catabolic response and perhaps accelerate convalescence have not been consistently successful. There is, to be sure, the real benefit of adequate dietary intake in minimizing protein breakdown. Replacement of protein mass may be demonstrated by careful weight measurements. During protein synthesis, a 70-kg man may gain 100 to 120 g/day, and metabolic studies indicate that this is predominantly a gain in lean body tissue. It will thus require three to six times as long to repair the protein deficit as it took to create it. The eventual level obtained, however, is quite close to that prior to the loss. Subsequent metabolic efforts will restore body fat, and the patient will have completed his recovery.[44]

Energy

Variable periods of starvation almost inevitably follow severe trauma, particularly since interdiction of oral intake is often necessary. Nevertheless, the traumatized patient has increased caloric requirements. A normal person at rest may require 2000 cal per day, but a febrile, severely injured patient may utilize 4000 cal in a single day.[3] Obviously the administration of 2000 mL of a 5 % dextrose and water solution, an amount customarily given, will not meet these demands. Weight loss in excess of water loss may reach as high as 500 g daily as the energy demands are met by the utilization of body tissue.[51,52]

The initial energy need is supplied by the limited stores of body carbohydrate, 300 to 500 g, mostly present as liver and muscle glycogen. This supply is exhausted within 14 to 18 h after severe trauma, and subsequent energy requirements are predominantly supplied by the oxidation of stored fat, which will yield 9 cal/g.[4] In the postinjury period, 200 to 500 g of fat may be oxidized daily to yield 1800 to 4500 cal. This is greatly in excess of the 1000 to 1300 cal liberated by the oxidation of 100 to 150 g of fat per day in starvation. It is thus apparent that factors other than starvation influence the energy requirements in the postinjury period.[44,54,55]

Although the major contribution to energy needs comes from the oxidation of fat, protein catabolism yields a significant number of calories. Normal daily intake of 75 g of protein results in the urinary excretion of some 10 g of nitrogen daily. Following extensive injury, urinary nitrogen may reach levels as high as 20 g/day, and this represents the liberation of more than 500 cal.

The intravenous administration of carbohydrate-containing solutions may supply a significant portion of the caloric needs and exert a protein "sparing" effect, thus reducing the dissolution of lean body tissue.[3] Approximately 100 g of carbohydrate appears to be adequate to obtain maximum protein sparing. As the first phase of injury passes, parenteral feeding is replaced by oral intake, caloric requirements are supplied, and anabolic processes approach normal. There is often a continued need for increased caloric supplies. Moore indicates that approximately 0.1 g of nitrogen and 20 cal/kg per day are necessary to ensure restoration of body tissues during early convalescence.[44] It can be seen that these levels are relatively low and can be met easily if the patient is capable of taking oral nutrients.

The final common pathway as regards energy production is the oxidation of metabolites via the Kreb's tricarboxylic acid cycle.[34] Figure 3-1 illustrates the cellular energetics which must obtain for the output of cellular work. The 2-carbon fragments, "active acetate" or coenzyme A (CoA), assume a pivotal position in this important process. It is seen that acetyl CoA combines with oxalacetic acid to form citric acid which is subsequently degraded stepwise eventually to yield eight hydrogen atoms, two molecules of carbon dioxide, and oxalacetic acid. The eight electrons which are thus liberated by specific dehydrogenases are

then introduced into the electron transport chain for transfer to oxygen. In a process known as oxydative phosphorylation, the energy of foodstuffs is converted to adenosine triphosphate (ATP), which is the ultimate driving force for most of the energy reactions within the cells. The hydrolysis of the ATP produced in this manner results in the performance of chemical, mechanical, and osmotic work within the cell and is correlated with the production of heat as a waste product.[50]

Carbohydrates

The monosaccharide glucose occupies a very important position in body metabolism. Although present in relatively small amounts, its

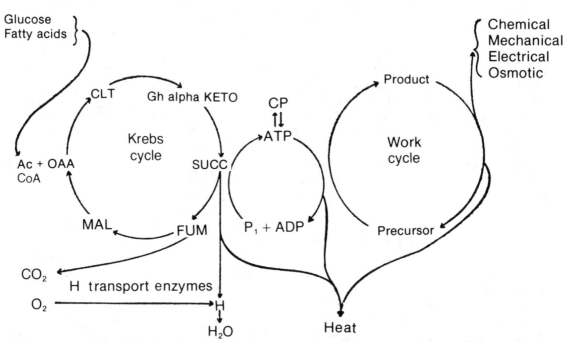

Figure 3-1 Diagram illustrating mechanism of energy produced within the cell. Schema of energetics in the cell. OAA, oxalacetic acid; CIT, citric acid; a-KETO, a-ketoglutaric acid; SUCC succinic acid; FUM, fumaric acid; MAL, malic acid; ADP, adenosine diphosphate; P_i, inorganic phosphate; ATP, adenosine triphosphate; CP, creative phosphate. (Reproduced with permission from Robert E. Olson, M.D., J. Am. Med. Assoc., **183**(6):471, 1963.)

ready availability for energy is quite important. The more recent concepts which describe active acetate (the 2-carbon fragments) as an intermediate in fatty acid metabolism and energy production further emphasize this importance. Stetten, using isotopes, has demonstrated a rapid conversion of glucose to fat.[62] Via transamination reactions, as first suggested by Needham, various intermediate compounds in glucose metabolism may eventually be converted to amino acids and proteins.[4] Thus, glucose is an important precursor to fat and protein, as well as a supplier of oxidative energy.

Approximately 55 percent of absorbed carbohydrate is rapidly introduced into the Kreb's cycle and converted into energy, carbon dioxide, and water. A portion of the remaining carbohydrate is converted to fat or protein, and about 5 percent reaches storage as liver and muscle glycogen.[4] The carbohydrate present in muscle is not readily available for use save by the muscle itself. Liver glycogen, on the other hand, can readily be broken down and utilized elsewhere in the body. This is rapidly utilized in periods of starvation, and in less than 5 h may be exhausted if gluconeogenesis is interdicted.

Without supplemental carbohydrate, body tissues must be utilized if energy requirements are to be met. This resultant loss in protein mass and fat has been described.[52] The restoration of normal oral intake permits the reversal of these processes and the subsequent repair of the deficit incurred during the first two phases of injury.

Fat

The oxidation of fat to yield energy proceeds rapidly during starvation. From 75 to 100 g daily is mobilized under these conditions, but after extensive injury as much as 500 g/day may be used.[52] In addition to energy, free water is obtained. Although neutral fat contains little free water, oxidation of a kilogram of fat liberates more than 1000 mL of water. This fact assumes some importance in the management of the fluid status of injured patients who, in addition, may not be able to eat.

Carbohydrate deprivation, which initiates oxidation of body fat, may result in less desirable effects. Ketosis occurs during fasting and can be traced to the lack of glucose in adipose tissue. Subsequent release of nonesterified fatty acids will increase the rate of delivery to the liver and may exceed the rate at which the liver can utilize or dispose of these fatty acids.[50] Acetoacetate is then produced and released into the blood. When glucose becomes available for metabolism, this flow of nonesterified fatty acids will cease, and ketosis also will cease. During the initial period following trauma, fat stores are thus reduced. With the return of a normal diet, repair of this deficit begins. The time required to restore this tissue will vary, but with adequate caloric intake, the rate of fat gain ranges from 75 to 150 g daily.

Previous attempts to reverse this depletion of fat stores by the intravenous administration of fat and protein solutions were not entirely satisfactory. As alluded to previously, starvation is not the single and may not be even the most important factor in the loss of body tissue following extensive trauma. Recent developments in hyperalimentation have been shown to be very effective in these patients. Those principles originally presented by Dudrick and Rhodes and Wilmore and their coworkers have been extremely important.[17] Previous studies demonstrated that fat emulsions caused impaired liver function and coagulation defects and, although in these preparations could be shown to exert a beneficial effect in certain situations, they were not suitable in most cases. The technique presented by Dudrick et al. is an extremely important and innovative approach to the metabolic management of these seriously ill patients, and the importance of the effects achieved with these solutions cannot be over-emphasized.

Vitamins

The National Research Council Committee on Nutrition has suggested that the daily requirements of vitamins may be satisfied by the following therapeutic regimen: niacin, 100 mg; thiamine, 5 mg; riboflavin, 5 mg; calcium pantothenate, 20 mg; pyridoxine, 2 mg; folic acid, 1.5 mg; vitamin B$_{12}$, 1 μg; vitamin C, at least 200 mg.[3] The exact vitamin requirements in the injured patient are not known, but it is probable that vitamin C requirements are increased out of proportion to that of the other vitamins. As Lowry has noted, there is a great individual variability in requirements for ascorbic acid in healthy adults, and this has been confirmed by the studies of Kline and Eheart.[33,37] It has also been observed that when body stores are extremely low, determinations of blood levels or buffy-coat levels of vitamin C do not necessarily accurately reflect the magnitude of the deficit.[13] In experimental human scurvy, these measured plasma values reach extremely low levels in about 6 weeks. In such cases with low ascorbic acid stores, a smaller dose may be required to sustain or elevate blood levels. As Coon has pointed out, the size of the dose, the route of administration, and the timing of administration are important in any effort to raise the body stores and plasma levels of ascorbic acid.[10] If vitamin C is given in high levels intravenously, the renal threshold is soon exceeded and a large portion of the administered dose is lost in the urine. It is for this reason that the subcutaneous injection of vitamin C has been reported to be more efficacious than the intravenous administration. Moore believes that the failure of wound healing and subsequent dehiscence is related more to lack of vitamin C than it is to actual caloric starvation. It would certainly appear that the intake of vitamin C required

for the maintenance of normal body functions, especially in the posttraumatic patient, is considerably higher than those amounts which will prevent scurvy.

Most patients who are on parenteral therapy for short periods following surgical procedures or trauma do not require supplemental vitamins A and D; but in addition to C, certainly thiamine is needed. The rapid depletion of body stores of thiamine after the administration of large amounts of glucose has been documented by Coon and Wolfman. The final common pathway of energy production is the Kreb's tricarboxylic acid cycle, and one of the important coenzymes necessary for the oxidative decarboxylation of pyruvate to acetyl coenzyme A is cocarboxylase, or thiamine pyrophosphate. The further studies of Coon and Wolfman would suggest that a defect in oxidation of pyruvate may be related to a preexisting thiamine deficiency in some patients.[11] As is true of the other vitamins, the exact amount of thiamine necessary to prevent this defect has not been determined, but requirements appear to be in excess of those necessary in a normal healthy individual.

Management

Most patients will reach the operating room in good nutritional status, but this desirable goal is not easily attained after extensive trauma. Thus, preexisting nutritional and vitamin deficits may further complicate the severe catabolic response which follows trauma, and in such instances, it is desirable to ensure adequate postoperative nutritional supplementation. Patients with hypoproteinemia may exhibit diminished tolerance to blood loss and lack the ability for adequate antibody production, with subsequent reduced resistance to infection.[3] Some investigators indicate that there is impaired wound healing, delayed union of fractures, and perhaps fatty infiltration of the liver with subsequent liver dysfunction.

The normal patient at bed rest can be maintained fairly easily with approximately 1 g of protein and 25 to 30 cal/kg of body weight. After extensive trauma, these requirements are increased, and following a large body surface third-degree burn, they may reach as much as 3 g of protein and 90 cal/kg of body weight. With the development of hyperalimentation techniques these requirements can be met, although the ability to obviate all nitrogen losses is not yet possible. Nitrogen losses in the injured patient exceed those found in starvation; but the studies by Elman, Holden, and Peden and coworkers reveal that parenteral protein replacement may adequately balance these losses.[17,18,29,53] These studies would suggest that nitrogen wasting is greatly increased by protein starvation.

Parenteral nutrition, used alone or in combination with oral feeding, has proved to be of immense value in many clinical situations, and this may especially be true in patients who have massive tissue destruction as a result of burns or other injuries. Because of the metabolic gains which may be achieved with intravenous hyperalimentation, reconstructive surgery in certain trauma cases may be delayed to achieve better nutritional status before other operations are performed. Hyperalimentation has enabled these patients to receive not merely the normal nutritional needs, but also additional therapeutic requirements.

The success obtained with parenteral hyperalimentation is largely the result of newer techniques to insert and maintain for long periods an indwelling intravenous line for the safe administration of these solutions. In addition, rapid improvement in the types of solutions available, and emphasis on the administration of essential amino acids and other constituents, have permitted the physician to supply these severely injured patients with adequate amounts of protein, carbohydrate, minerals, and associated nutrients.[17] Many of the problems encountered following extensive trauma are now successfully managed with hyperalimentation, and this subject is dealt with in greater detail elsewhere.

Although protein may be supplied by the intravenous administration of blood, plasma, or albumin, the protein hydrolysates appear to be more useful.[18,53] The former solutions are expensive and require considerable metabolic work for their assimilation. Additionally, caloric values are quite low.[2] Although 1 g of protein hydrolysates is only equivalent to 0.75 g of protein, this solution contains amino acids and small peptides. The urinary losses noted following intravenous administration consist mainly of the peptide fraction, thus allowing the metabolic use of the amino acids. Others have found that even in stress these substances may be utilized in protein synthesis. Maximum use of these solutions will probably not be obtained if caloric equilibrium cannot be induced.

Caloric demands continue to occupy a pivotal position in posttraumatic patients, and it has long been recognized that lipids provide the richest source of calories. Abbott demonstrated that the nitrogen deficit in postoperative patients could be reduced to one-fourth by administration of fat emulsions and adequate nitrogen.[1] Other studies testify to the efficacy of these solutions as a supply of calories.[3,9,36,53] Furthermore, newer techniques of production of these cottonseed oil emulsions have reduced the side effects.

Clinical and pathologic studies reported by Lehr et al. indicate that late deleterious effects are uncommon, and the earlier milder reactions are insignificant. If a patient tolerates the initial infusion, the probability of a later reaction seems remote. It would appear that if these solutions are given, initial administration rates should be slow and the patient carefully monitored for a rise in temperature. Subsequently, changes in liver function and coagulation defects may appear. The administration of these solutions has certain inherent problems which have been alluded to in the preceding sections, but with proper precautions they can be used in specific instances where protein and caloric requirements are quite high and convalescence is prolonged. Certainly adequate vitamin, fluid, and electrolyte intake can be maintained without difficulty. A discussion of the fluid and electrolyte requirements in the posttraumatic or postoperative patient is found in Chap. 1.

SUMMARY

A patient who has sustained severe trauma exhibits both endocrine and metabolic responses to this insult. The earlier endocrine changes are due to sympathicoadrenal discharge and are reflected clinically by tachycardia, vasoconstriction, and diaphoresis. Metabolically, epinephrine and norepinephrine result in hyperglycemia by mobilizing liver glycogen. There is an increase in the blood level of nonesterified fatty acids, and the pituitary adrenal axis may be activated by catecholamines. In the absence of continuing trauma or complications, this initial picture passes fairly rapidly and is replaced by more profound metabolic and endocrine changes. The adrenal cortical hormone levels are increased both in the blood and urine, and there is some loose correlation between the level of these hormones and the increase in caloric requirements and protein catabolism which appears within 1 to 2 days after injury. Urinary nitrogen excretion levels may be doubled or tripled, and caloric requirements may increase by two to two and one-half times. There is an early depletion of body stores of carbohydrate, and with interruption of oral intake, energy demands are met by the utilization of body protein and fat. Weight loss becomes prominent as caloric requirements following injury exceed those found in starvation alone. Following moderately extensive trauma, this picture persists for 3 to 5 days,

and then a rather rapid change occurs in which improvement is noted clinically and is reflected further by a return to normal nitrogen balance and an increase in strength exhibited by the patient. With the restoration of normal oral intake, protein synthesis and rebuilding begin. These continue for variable periods, but the deficit may require several times as long to repair as it took to create it. The subsequent and final phase of convalescence reveals the total restoration of protein and fat tissue which was lost during the initial injury and, barring the advent of complications, will be reached within a period of several months.

BIBLIOGRAPHY

1 Abbott, W. D. et al.: Effect of I.V. administered fat on body weight and nitrogen balance in surgical patients, *Metabolism,* 6:691, 1957.
2 Alnight, F., A. P. Forbes, and E. C. Reiferstein, Jr.: Fate of plasma protein administration I.V., *Trans. Assoc. Am. Physicians,* 59:221, 1946.
3 Artz, C. P.: Newer concepts of nutrition by the I.V. route, *Ann. Surg.,* p. 841, 1959.
4 Best, C. H. and N. B. Taylor: *Physiological Basis of Medical Practices,* The Williams & Wilkins Company, Baltimore, 1961.
5 Biglieri, E. G.: *Aldosterone,* Clinical Symposium, Ciba, 1963, vol. 15, No. 1.
6 Blocher, T. G., Jr., W. C. Lewis, W. W. Nowinskin, S. R. Lewis, and V. Blocker: Nutrition studies in the severely burned, *Ann. Surg.,* 141:589, 1955.
7 Campbell, R. M., G. Sharpe, A. W. Boyne, and D. P. Cuthbertson: Cortisone and the metabolic response to injury, *Br. J. Exp. Pathol.,* 35:566, 1954.
8 Cannon, P. R.: The problem of the metabolic response to injury, *Mil. Med.,* 117:222, 1955.
9 Cohn, I., S. Singleton, Q. L. Harterj, and M. Atile: New I.V. fat emulsion, *J. Am. Med. Assoc.,* 183:755, 1963.
10 Coon, W. W.: Ascorbic acid metabolism in postoperative patients, *Surg. Gynecol. Obstet.,* vol. 534, May 1962.
11 Coon, W. W and E. F. Wolfman: Limiting factors in maximal utilization of I.V. glucose by

the postoperative patient. I. Thiamin deficiency, *Surg. Forum,* **10**:3227, 1959.

12 Coon, W. W. and E. F. Wolfman: Thiamin deficiency in surgical patients, *Ann. Surg.,* vol. 115, December 1961.

13 Crandon, J. H., B. Landan, S. Mikal, J. Blmanno, M. Jefferson, and N. Mahoney: Ascorbic acid economy in surgical patients as indicated by blood ascorbic acid levels, *N. Engl. J. Med.,* **258**:105, 1958.

14 Cuthbertson, D. P.: Further observations on the disturbance of metabolism caused by injury, with particular reference to the dietary requirements of fracture cases, *Br. J. Surg.,* **23**:505, 1936.

15 Dudley, H. A. F.: The neuro-endocrine response to surgery, *J. R. Coll. Surg. Edinburgh,* **4**:132, 1959.

16 Dudley, H. A. F., J. S. Robson, M. Smith, and C. P. Stewart: The relationship of aldosterone excretion to the metabolic response to adrenalectomy, *Clin. Chim. Acta,* **2**:461, 1957.

17 Dudrick, S. J. and J. E. Rhodes: "Metabolism in Surgical Patients: Protein, Carbohydrate and Fat Utilization by Oral and Parenteral Routes," in D. C. Sakiston, Jr. (ed.), *Textbook of Surgery,* W. B. Saunders Company, Philadelphia, 1972.

18 Elman, R.: Amino acid mixtures on parenteral protein food, *Am. J. Med.,* **5**:760, 1948.

19 Engel, F. L.: The endocrine control of metabolism, *Bull N.Y. Acad. Med.,* **29**:819, 1953.

20 Ezrin, C.: *The Pituitary Gland,* Clinical Symposium, Ciba, 1963, vol. 15, No. 3.

21 Forsham, P. H.: *The Adrenal Gland,* Clinical Symposium, Ciba, 1963, vol. 15, No. 1.

22 Frankson, C., C. A. Gemryell, and U. von Euler: Cortical and medullary adrenal activity in surgery and allied conditions, *J. Clin. Endocrinol.,* **14**:608, 1954.

23 Gold, J. J.: Blood corticoids: Their measurement and significance—A review, *J. Clin. Endocrinol.,* **17**:296, 1957.

24 Gold, J. J., E. Singleton, D. A. MacFarlane, and F. D. Moore: Quantitative determination of the urinary cortisol metabolites, "Tetrahydro F," "Aldo-tetrahydro F" and "Tetrahydro E": Effects of adrenocorticotropin and complex trauma in the human, *J. Clin. Invest.,* **37**:813, 1958.

25 Goldenberg, I. S., L. Sutwak, P. J. Rosenbaum, and M. A. Hayes: Thyroid activity during operation, *Surg. Gynecol. Obstet.,* **102**:129, 1956.

26 Goodall, M., C. Stone, and B. W. Haynes, Jr.: Urinary output of adrenalin and noradrenalin in severe thermal burns, *Ann. Surg.,* **145**:479, 1957.

27 Halme, A., A. Pekkarmian, and M. Turonen: On the excretion of noradrenalin, adrenalin, 17-hydroxycorticoids and 17-ketosteroids during the postoperative stage, *Acta Endocrinol.,* vol. 24 (Suppl. 32), 1957.

28 Hardy, J. D.: *Surgery and the Endocrine System: Physiologic Response to Surgical Trauma—Operative Management of Endocrine Dysfunction,* W. B. Saunders Company, Philadelphia, 1952.

29 Holden, W. D., H. Krieger, S. Levey, and W. E. Abbott: The effect of nutrition on nitrogen metabolism in the surgical patient, *Ann. Surg.,* **146**:563, 1957.

30 Ingle, D. J.: Permissive action of hormones, *J. Clin. Endocrinol. Metab.,* **14**:1272, 1954.

31 Ingle, D. J., E. O. Ward, and M. H. Kuizega: The relationship of the adrenal glands to change in urinary NPN following multiple fracture in the force-fed rat, *Am. J. Physiol.,* **149**:510, 1947.

32 Jordan, P. H.: Use of I.V. fat emulsion in management of surgery patients, *Arch. Surg.,* **76**:794, 1958.

33 Kline, A. B. and M. S. Eheart: Variations in the ascorbic acid requirements for saturation of nine normal young women, *J. Nutr.,* **28**:413, 1944.

34 Krebs, H. A. and J. M. Lowenstein: "Tricarboxylic Acid Cycle, Metabolic Pathways," vol. 1, Academic Press, Inc., New York, 1960.

35 Kriegler, H., W. D. Abbott, S. Levey, and W. D. Holden: Re-evaluation of the role of the adrenal and other factors in the metabolic response to injury, *Surgery,* **44**:138, 1958.

36 Lehr, H. B., J. E. Rhoads, O. Rosenthal, and W. S. Blakemore: The use of I.V. fat emulsion in surgical patients, *J. Am. Med. Assoc.,* **181**:745, 1962.

37 Lowry, O. H.: Biochemical evidence of nutritional status, *Physiol. Rev.,* **32**:431, 1952.

38 Madden, S. C., P. M. Winslow, J. W. Howland, and G. H. Whipple: Blood plasma protein regeneration as influenced by infection, digestive disturbances, thyroid and food proteins; defi-

ciency state related to protein depletion, *J. Exp. Med.,* **65**:431, 1937.

39 Marshall, W. N.: Clinical use of I.V. fat in surgical patients, *Arch. Surg.,* **78**:851, 1959.

40 Mason, A. S.: Metabolic response to total adrenalectomy and hypophysectomy, *Lancet,* **2**:632, 1955.

41 Mirsky, I. A., M. Stein, and G. Panlisch: The secretion of an antidiuretic substance into the circulation of adrenalectomized and hypophysectomized rats exposed to noxious stimuli, *Endocrinol.,* **55**:28, 1953.

42 Moore, F. D., I. S. Edelman, J. M. Olney, A. H. Jarvis, L. Brookes, and E. M. Wilson: Body sodium and potassium. III. Interrelated trends in alimentary, renal and cardiovascular disease: Lack of correlations between body stores and plasma concentration, *Metabolism,* **3**:334, 1954.

43 Moore, F. D.: Hormones and stress-endocrine changes after anesthesia, surgery and unanesthetized trauma in man, *Recent Prog. Horm. Res.,* **13**:511, 1957.

44 Moore, F. D.: *Metabolic Care of the Surgical Patient,* W. B. Saunders Company, Philadelphia, 1959.

45 Moore, F. D. and M. R. Ball: *The Metabolic Response to Surgery* American Lecture Series, No. 132, Charles C Thomas, Publisher, Springfield, Ill., 1952.

46 Moore, F. D., R. W. Steinbreng, M. R. Boll, G. M. Wilson, and J. A. Myrden: Studies in surgical endocrinology. I. The urinary excretion of 17-hydroxycorticoids and associated metabolic changes in cases of soft tissue trauma of varying severity and in bone trauma, *Ann. Surg.,* **141**:145, 1955.

47 Moore, F. D.: Systemic mediators of surgical injury, *Can. Med. Assoc. J.,* **78**:85, 1958.

48 Nell, E. R. and M. L. Gerbe: Administration of I.V. fat emulsion to surgical patients, *U.S. Armed Forces Med. J.,* **10**:811, 1960.

49 Nicholas, J. A. and P. D. Wilson: Adrenocortical response in operative procedures upon the bones and joints, *J. Bone J. Surg.,* **35A**:559, 1953.

50 Olson, R. E.: The two-carbon chain in metabolism, *J. Am. Med. Assoc.,* **183**:471, 1963.

51 Paquin, A. J., Jr.: Insensible body weight loss following uniformly severe surgical trauma, *Ann. Surg.,* **148**:937, 1958.

52 Paquin, A. J.: The rate of body weight loss following surgical stress of uniform intensity, *Ann. Surg.,* **141**:383, 1955.

53 Peden, J. C., A. Olin, P. T. Williams, and H. Weathers: I.V. protein hydrolysates, *Arch, Surg.,* **87**:59, 1963.

54 Peters, J. P.: Effect of injury and disease on nitrogen metabolism, *Am. J. Med.,* **5**:100, 1948.

55 Peters, J. P.: Nitrogen metabolism in acute and chronic diseases, *Ann. N.Y. Acad. Sci.,* **47**:327, 1946.

56 Pincus, G. and K. V. Thimarm: *The Hormones,* Academic Press, Inc., New York, 1955.

57 Robson, J. S., H. A. F. Dudley, D. B. Horn, and C. P. Stewart: Metabolic response to adrenalectomy, *Lancet,* **2**:325, 1955.

58 Selye, H.: "Conditioning" vs. "permissive" actions of hormones, *J. Clin. Endocrinol. Metab.,* **13**:122, 1954.

59 Selye, H.: *The Story of the Adaptation Syndrome, Told in the Form of Informal Illustrated Lectures,* Acta, Inc., Montreal, Canada, 1952.

60 Shires, G. T., J. Williams, and F. Brown: Acute changes in extracellular fluids associated with major surgical procedures, *Ann. Surg.,* **154**:803, 1961.

61 Shires, G. T. and D. E. Jackson: Postoperative salt tolerance, *Arch. Surg.,* **84**:703, 1962.

62 Stetten, D. W.: Metabolic effects of insulin, *Bull. N.Y. Acad. Med.,* **29**:466, 1953.

63 Thom, G. W., D. Jenkins, and J. C. Laidlow: Adrenal response to stress in man, *Recent Prog. Horm. Res.,* **8**:171, 1953.

64 Toby, C. C. and R. J. Nolk: The role of the adrenal cortex in protein catabolism following trauma, *J. Clin. Endocrinol.,* **7**:461, 1947.

65 Weil, P. G.: The plasma proteins: Clinical significance, *Am. Pract. Dig. Treat.,* **9**:1499, 1958.

66 Williams, R. H.: *Textbook of Endocrinology,* W. B. Saunders Company, Philadelphia, 1962.

67 Zimmerman, L. M. and R. Levine: *Physiologic Principles of Surgery,* W. B. Saunders Company, Philadelphia, 1957.

Chapter 4

Cardiac Arrest: Resuscitation

Watts R. Webb, M.D.

Sudden cardiac arrest constitutes one of the most dramatic and frequent causes of death during surgical procedures. Approximately one out of every 3000 patients receiving general anesthesia will develop cardiac arrest. Even if, as has been estimated, approximately one-half of the patients developing cardiac arrest are saved, it is likely that between 6000 and 8000 patients die annually of sudden cardiac arrest which might have been prevented or corrected.[11] If one includes the sudden deaths associated with myocardial disease, this figure probably jumps to over 300,000 per year in the United States alone. As cardiac arrest is experienced only rarely by the average physician, he must be prepared to meet its sudden reality. Also the training for cardiopulmonary resuscitation (CPR) should be extended to every possible layman, including those in the teen-age groups.

ETIOLOGY

Most cases occurring following trauma or during a surgical procedure can be traced to overt hypoxia, inadequate coronary perfusion due to hypovolemia and hypotension, or overdosage of or sensitivity to drugs. Hypoxemia is almost always the common denominator, though in many cases the precipitating factors are obscure. Other observers have suggested that hypercapnia with its associated metabolic derangements, including increased plasma levels of potassium, may be one of the further responsible factors. Certainly, the combination of hypoxia and carbon dioxide retention (suffocation) is experimentally the best background on which to produce profound cardiac arrhythmias.[9,10] Another most important factor in resuscitation from hemorrhage is the use of large quantities of old, cold acidotic blood leading to high potassium levels and cardiac hypothermia, both of which lead to arrhythmias or arrest.

PREVENTION

The most important aspect of prevention is the maintenance of an adequate respiratory exchange at all times to prevent hypoxia and hypercapnia. In addition, one should allay anxiety, maintain the circulating blood volume, and probably reduce the number of anesthetic agents administered. Corrective steps can be taken at the onset of premonitory signs of cardiac arrhythmia, which nearly always appear before actual cessation of the heart. Runs of arrhythmia or a failing pulse are best treated by improving the ventilatory exchange of the patient utilizing pure oxygen and by intravenous injections of lidocaine or of procaine amide (Pronestyl) in a dosage of 100 to 200 mg. Lidocaine seems to be the best drug available at the amount for reducing excess irritability of the heart and stopping extraventricular contractions. By preventing the release of acetylcholine, injections of atropine in large dosage may prevent the occasional lethal vagal reflex. The vagovagal reflex has probably been overstressed, as experimentally at least vagal stimuli cannot cause cardiac standstill in the absence of anoxia and/or hypercapnia.[10]

Unfortunately in the patients with coronary disease, only a small percentage of the episodes of ventricular fibrillation or sudden death are preceded by prodromal symptoms adequate to forewarn the patient or to provoke a patient's call for help.[3,8]

DIAGNOSIS

It is not always easy to know exactly when the heart has stopped functioning effectively as a pump. The sudden loss of blood pressure or pulse always puts the burden of proof on the physician to demonstrate that the heart's pumping action is adequate, and these signs, when associated with sudden cessation of respiration, are pathognomonic of cardiac arrest. Listening for heart sounds, looking for cyanosis, or sticking needles in the chest are all only a waste of valuable time. Unquestionably, closed massage or even thoracotomy has been performed when the heart was still beating with a certain though limited degree of efficiency. There can be no justifiable condemnation of this, but only severest criticism of any hesitation to act under these circumstances as all these patients with feebly beating hearts can be saved, whereas indecision might allow irreversible cerebral changes to occur. Once resuscitation has been started, an electrocardiogram can be obtained for confirmation of the diagnosis without loss of valuable time.

Equipment. For immediate resuscitation, no equipment whatsoever is absolutely essential. Rapidly available apparatus should include (1) equipment for artificial respiration including oxygen and endotracheal tubes and (2) basic surgical instruments for thoracotomy. There should also be readily available drugs such as sodium bicarbonate, atropine, lidocaine, epinephrine, norepinephrine, morphine, and calcium chloride with syringes and needles and an adequate defibrillator or electroshock apparatus.

Treatment. The basic treatment is composed of three simple elements: speed, pumping the heart, and ventilating the lungs. These are aimed at preserving the viability of the individual, particularly the brain, until cardiac function can be restored. Effective circulation of oxygenated blood must be restored within 3 or 4 minutes after the onset of cardiac arrest.

Mouth-to-mouth or mouth-to-nose insufflation should be started immediately. Expired air, particularly during hyperventilation, will contain about 18% O_2 and only about 2% CO_2, and so constitutes a very acceptable respiratory gas. Tidal volumes up to 1000 cm³ can easily be achieved. Nonetheless, artificial respiration utilizing pure oxygen should be started as soon as possible. This is most readily accomplished through an endotracheal tube, and since the patient is completely flaccid the insertion of the tube takes only a few seconds. However, perfectly adequate respiration can be maintained by a tight-fitting face mask and a rebreathing bag or bellows.

Circulation can be restored immediately by external cardiac massage which compresses the heart between the sternum and the vertebral column.[5,7] The heel of one hand with the other hand superimposed is placed over the lower sternum of the supine patient (Fig. 4-1). Rhythmic compression at 60 to 80 strokes/min should produce a strong, palpable peripheral (carotid) pulse at near normal blood pressure. If the technique is correctly applied, failure

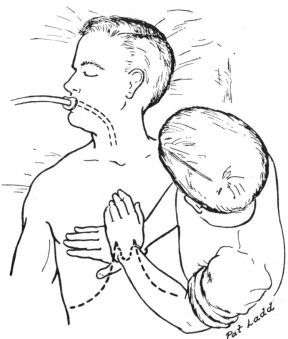

Figure 4-1 Position of hands in closed-chest massage. Only the heel of the palm touches the chest over the distal sternum. For infants, two fingers are used instead of the hand.

indicates some mechanical difficulty such as cardiac tamponade and is an indication for a rapid thoracotomy in order to use open massage. Even though some patients will suffer fractured ribs, sternum, or even liver and spleen,[2] the more rapid restitution of circulation under almost any circumstances at any site inside or outside the hospital has provided a much-improved survival rate that has more than justified the complications.

When there is only a single rescuer, two quick lung inflations should be performed after each 15 chest compressions (15:2 ratio), using a rate of 80 compressions/min. If there are two operators, one should compress the chest about 60 times/min and the other interpose one quick breath for each five compressions (5:1 ratio).

OPEN MASSAGE

When external cardiac massage fails to restore a normal carotid pulse, a thoracotomy must be done without delay in order to start open massage. The incision is preferably made just below the breast in the left fourth interspace, extending from the sternum to the midaxillary line (Fig. 4-2). Bleeding is no problem as the heart is not pumping, and the incision may be extended into the thoracic cavity with one or two strokes of a knife. A rib spreader is helpful but not necessary as the ribs can be spread sufficiently with the fingers, or if necessary, by incising one of the anterior cartilages to admit the hand easily. No delay should be allowed in an attempt to achieve asepsis unless such conditions already exist. Infection will seldom be a problem if at the time of closure of the chest adequate hemostasis is obtained and the thoracic cavity is drained with a catheter attached to a water-seal system to ensure complete expansion of the lung and evacuation of all pleural fluid. If the abdomen is open, one should likewise open the diaphragm, as intermittent cardiac com-

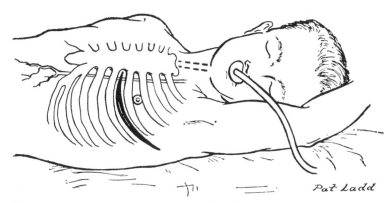

Figure 4-2 Site of incision beneath the breast through the fourth or fifth interspace for emergency thoracotomy. Open massage must be used when closed massage is not effective, such as with cardiac tamponade, following pneumonectomy, etc.

pression cannot be efficiently performed through the intact diaphragm. It should be remembered that this produces an open pneumothorax and requires positive-pressure anesthesia both during the procedure and while closing the diaphragm.

Cardiac compression is usually most efficiently performed with the fingers behind and the thumb in front of the heart (Fig. 4-3). A large heart, however, may be better pumped by one hand in front and one hand behind or alternately by massage from behind, using the sternum as the anterior buttress. The optimum is about 90 compressions/min, there being no need to wait for cardiac filling.[4] This procedure will markedly improve the circulation to the dilated cyanotic heart and maintain a satisfactory blood pressure. It is often helpful to place the patient in the Trendelenburg position during this procedure or even to clamp the thoracic aorta just above the diaphragm.

Very adequate stroke volumes can be maintained without opening the pericardium, which by its tough envelope and the lubricating pericardial fluid minimizes trauma to the myocardium. Even should ventricular fibrillation be present, the pericardium need not be opened for application of electrodes for defibrillation.

DEFIBRILLATION

Once adequate cardiac compression and respiratory exchange are attained, there is no further need for haste as little or no deterioration will occur during the brief time required to obtain desired drugs or a defibrillator. In fact, it is axiomatic that the hypoxic heart cannot be defibrillated or restarted, and time must be taken to obtain a pink heart with good tone before attempting electric shock.[12] The use of an external pacemaker is rarely successful if asystole has been present for as long

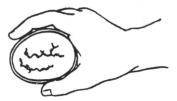
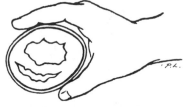

Figure 4-3 Method of one-hand open massage. The pericardium should *not* be opened. Note that the fingers and thumb are kept flat to prevent digging into or even through the myocardium. Also, the hand must be opened widely to allow maximal filling of the heart.

as 30 s and, of course, the heart will be found in fibrillation in about 10 percent of the cases of "cardiac arrest." If the chest is open, fibrillation is best treated by an electric shock applied through two metal electrodes, one on either side of the heart (Fig. 4-4).

If the chest has not been opened and fibrillation has been demonstrated by the electrocardiogram, external defibrillation should be used. A single defibrillator shock does not cause serious functional damage to the myocardium, so it should be tried in the unconscious, pulseless adult patient even though the patient is unmonitored. This must not delay the prompt application of basic life support measures. Closed-chest massage is interrupted long enough to apply the electrodes and initiate a shock. One electrode is placed at the right of the upper sternal region and the other beneath the left breast. The electrodes are applied firmly by the operator, who should wear gloves and be well grounded to prevent electrocution. A large adult will require 480 V, and children will need 240 V or less. Work by Lown and his coworkers[6] has demonstrated

that a dc defibrillator is safer and more effective than ac equipment. The dc apparatus using a capacitor discharge delivers up to 400 W/s—which may represent several thousand volts—in less than 2.5 ms. Lower settings are frequently effective in converting ventricular fibrillation or ventricular tachycardia. Damage resulting from defibrillar shocks is directly proportional to the energy used, and maximal settings, when not required, may further impair a damaged myocardium.

DRUGS

The various drugs are far less important than adequate ventilation with oxygen and intermittent cardiac compression. Lidocaine and quinidine are the preferred drugs for reducing cardiac irritability. Epinephrine must be used with caution as it may cause fibrillation in the presence of myocardial cyanosis. It has its greatest value in increasing the tone of the flaccid, sluggish heart, and the intracardiac dosage should rarely exceed 1 mL of a 1:10,000 solution. Calcium chloride in dosages of 5

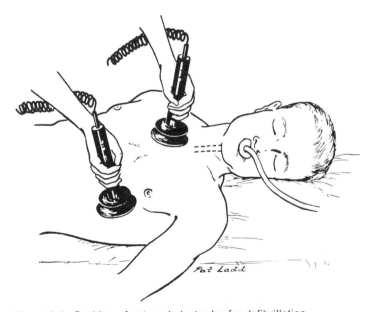

Figure 4-4 Position of external electrodes for defibrillation.

mL of a 10% solution given into the ventricle is of great value in producing the same effect as epinephrine without the dangers. If good cardiac action has not been restored within 5 min, sodium bicarbonate in dosages of approximately 1 meq/kg should be given repeatedly to reverse the metabolic acidosis of inadequate tissue perfusion. Isuprel (0.2 mg in 200 mL of saline solution) has a very beneficial positive inotropic effect on the myocardium. At times a potent peripheral vasopressor may also be required.

HYPOTHERMIA

Reduction of the patient's body temperature causes a reduction in cerebral metabolic needs, blood flow, brain volume, and intracranial pressure. The physiologic changes are of particular importance in preventing the edema usually seen following severe cerebral hypoxia, which would be self-perpetuating. If the patient responds to the arrest measures immediately with full consciousness, hypothermia is not necessary. If not, hypothermia to about 32°C (89.6°F) should be induced with a cooling blanket, an ice bath, or ice packs. Promethazine (Phenergan) or chlorpromazine may be necessary to prevent shivering, which would raise the body temperature. As the patient's central nervous system function returns, the hypothermia can be discontinued. At times the temperature may have to be raised to differentiate cold narcosis from central nervous system damage.

Extreme medical vigilance is necessary during hypothermia, particularly with regard to ventilation, adequate but not excessive hydration, and frequent turning of the patient. Urea in doses of 1 to 1.5 g/kg of body weight administered as a 30% solution at the rate of about 60 drops/min may aid in controlling the cerebral edema and increased intracranial pressure, but it has the disadvantage of a severe rebound effect on discontinuance.

Constant infusions of glucose solution (50%) may be of greater value by supporting cerebral metabolism and having less rebound effect and being readily available and almost equally effective in controlling cerebral edema. Perhaps of greatest value is the use of steroids such as dexamethasone phosphate in doses of 4 to 8 mg every 6 h.

Since there is a period of hypercoagulability of the blood following arrest, heparin given intravenously is often used if the clinical situation permits.

PROGNOSIS

Where the above resuscitative procedures have been made a part of the physician's armamentarium, the results have been extremely encouraging (Fig. 4-5). We experienced 17 cases in one specialized chest hospital; one was due to Pontocaine sensitivity and each of the others occurred during a general anesthesia. Five occurred during induction of the anesthetic, and the others during a thoracotomy. It was possible to reestablish a normal cardiac rhythm in all, with complete recovery in all but two. Most of the episodes followed a period of recognized inadequate respiratory exchange with attendant hypoxia and probably hypercapnia. Each of these was in cardiac standstill, none having demonstrated fibrillation.

The use of closed-chest massage has offered new hope for the patients suffering cardiac arrest outside the operating room or even outside the hospital.[8] Our total recovery rate for arrests occurring on the hospital wards has approximated 25 percent. Jude has reported recovery rates for cardiac arrest of 96 percent in the operating room, 70 percent following cardiac surgery, and 46 percent in other areas of the hospitals.[5]

Utilization of mobile intensive care/coronary care units can achieve excellent results, such as the successful resuscitation,

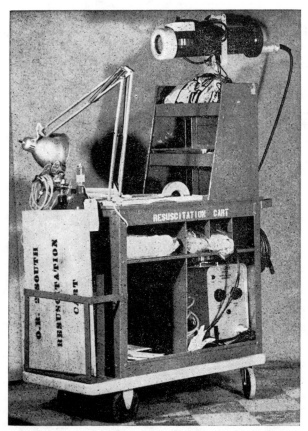

Figure 4-5 Resuscitation cart which is kept in the operating room to be taken by a nurse and anesthesiologist to the site of a cardiac arrest. It contains emergency drugs, syringes, O_2, masks, laryngoscopes, and endotracheal tubes, Ambu rebreathing bag, defibrillator, ECG monitor oscilloscope, bed board, and a set of instruments for emergency thoracotomy. Note the light. Various adaptors are included so that the electrical power cord can be plugged into any type of outlet. At each nursing division only resuscitube plastic airways are kept, since mouth-to-mouth ventilation and closed-chest massage are all that is needed, at least until arrival of the resuscitation cart.

defibrillation, hospitalization, and discharge of some 234 patients in 51 months in the Seattle area. This represented a resuscitation rate of 43 percent of out-of-hospital patients found in ventricular fibrillation with a long-term survival rate of 26 percent.[8] The frequency of fibrillation and sudden death in patients recovering from acute myocardial infarctions can be reduced by chronic beta-adrenergic blockage.[13]

Damage to the heart is relatively rare.

Though the possibility of coronary thrombosis during the period of hypotension is always present, postoperative electrocardiograms rarely show changes. Cerebral complications are the most feared and can lead to complete decerebration. Severe neurologic sequelae, however, may completely clear during the early postoperative period, and hope should not be abandoned for several days.

An episode of cardiac arrest does not necessarily prevent the continuation of an operation even if it occurs during induction of anesthesia. Great care must be taken at this point, however, to ascertain that the arrest was due to some extrinsic and correctable factor and not to an intrinsic heart defect such as a myocardial infarct. Similarly, a necessary operation need not be unduly delayed if the patient makes an uneventful recovery from the arrest without residual cardiac or cerebral damage.

SUMMARY

Cardiac arrest still constitutes one of the most common causes of death during surgical procedures. Studies on resuscitation have demonstrated that most such episodes can be prevented and when they occur can be successfully treated. The basic requisite of prevention involves the maintenance of adequate respiratory exchange and circulating blood volume. Treatment has as its primary aim the immediate reestablishment of an adequate volume of circulating oxygenated blood by intermittent cardiac compression and artificial respiration until a normal cardiac rhythm is reestablished.

BIBLIOGRAPHY

1 American Heart Association Committee on Cardiopulmonary Resuscitation: Standards for cardiopulmonary resuscitation (CPR) and emergency cardiac care (ECC), *J. Am. Med. Assoc.,* **227**:837, 1974.

2 Clark, D. T.: Complications following closed-chest cardiac massage, *J. Am. Med. Assoc.,* **181**:127, 1962.

3 Fulton, M., B. Duncan, W. Lutz, et al.: Natural history of unstable angina, *Lancet,* **1**:860, 1972.

4 Johnson, J. and C. K. Kirby: An experimental study of cardiac massage, *Surgery,* **26**:472, 1949.

5 Jude, J. R., W. B. Kouwenhoven, and G. G. Knickerbocker: A new approach to cardiac resuscitation, *Surgery,* **154**:311, 1961.

6 Lown, B., J. Neuman, R. Amarashingham, and B. V. Berkovits: Comparison of alternating current with direct current electroshock across the closed chest, *Am. J. Cardiol.,* **10**:223, 1962.

7 Mathews, D. H., M. E. Avery, and J. R. Jude: Closed-chest cardiac massage in the newborn infant, *J. Am. Med. Assoc.,* **183**:964, 1963.

8 Schaffer, W. A. and L. A. Cobb: Recurrent ventricular fibrillation and modes of death in survivors of out-of-hospital ventricular fibrillation, *N. Engl. J. Med.,* **293**:259, 1975.

9 Sealy, W. C., W. G. Young, Jr., and J. S. Harris: Studies of cardiac arrest: The relationship of hypercapnia to ventricular fibrillation, *J. Thorac. Surg.,* **28**:447, 1954.

10 Sloan, H. E.: The vagus nerve in cardiac arrest: Effect of hypercapnia, hypoxia and asphyxia on reflex inhibition of heart, *Surg. Gynecol. Obstet.,* **91**:254, 1950.

11 Stephenson, H. E., Jr., L. C. Reid, and J. W. Hinton: Some common denominators in 1,200 cases of cardiac arrest, *Ann. Surg.,* **137**:731, 1953.

12 Wegria, R., C. W. Frank, H. Wang, G. Misrahy, R. Miller, and P. Kornfield: A study of the usefulness and limitations of electrical countershock, cardiac massage, epinephrine and procaine in cardiac resuscitation from ventricular fibrillation, *Circulation,* **8**:1, 1953.

13 Wilhelmsson, C., J. A. Vedin, L. Wilhelmsen, et al.: Reduction of sudden deaths after myocardial infarction by treatment with alprenolol: Preliminary results, *Lancet,* **2**:1157, 1974.

Chapter 5

Anesthesia Considerations

A. H. Giesecke, Jr., M.D.

M. T. Jenkins, M.D.

Civil trauma occurs in a cross section of the population. Healthy adults and children, pregnant women, and victims of the entire host of human afflictions are all subject to civil trauma.

Prior to choosing premedication and selecting anesthetic agents and techniques, an effort must be made to evaluate factors which may influence the anesthetic management of the acutely traumatized patient. These factors include the extent of injuries, the degree of hemorrhage and fluid replacement, the adequacy of ventilation, preexisting diseases, prior drug therapy, time of last meal, and intoxication.[31]

The anesthetic management should continue into the recovery room, where the patient must be monitored through emergence from anesthesia while being checked for evidences of occult multiple injuries. A significant number of traumatized patients return to the operating room at least once for secondary surgery, and they present special problems uncommon in the usual elective procedure.

PREMEDICATION

The moral obligation of the anesthesiologist is to relieve pain, but in recent years this aspect of the management of the traumatized patient has been relegated to secondary importance, preempted by the need for immediate and effective restoration of respiration and circulation. Nevertheless, the preanesthetic suppression of pain should not be ignored if the patient's general physical condition is such that the judicious administration of analgesic drugs will neither further depress cardiac or respiratory function nor mask evidences of increasing intracranial pressure.

For maximum safety, analgesic drugs should be given in small doses intravenously, and repeated if necessary after the full effect of the preceding dose has been observed. In general, barbiturates are not used in preoperative medication if the patient is in pain. In this circumstance, they tend to produce the paradoxical response of excitement rather than sedation. If the patient is unconscious or disoriented, analgesic drugs are contraindicated as preanesthetic medications.

However, the anticholinergic drugs, such as atropine, are indicated for the suppression of undesirable reflexes and of cardiac dysrhythmia and for the depression of secretions from glands in the airway. In the atropinized adult patient, the pulse rate seldom exceeds 120 beats/min, and so the use of an anticholinergic drug should not mask a tachycardia secondary to hypovolemic shock. The desired effect may be achieved by the intravenous administration of the atropinelike drug a few minutes before anesthesia is started.

CHOICE OF ANESTHESIA

The anesthetic management of the traumatized patient may involve the use of regional or general anesthetic techniques. In many cases, the choice of technique is not critical, but in other instances specific advantages may be attributed to a particular technique.

The concept that any anesthetic agent can be used successfully (if used judiciously) for any kind of case should be abandoned. Sound pharmacologic knowledge of the various modern anesthetic agents should enable the anesthesiologist to select an agent for a particular patient which will facilitate the patient's compensatory responses and enhance other therapeutic resuscitative efforts.

Spinal anesthesia may be the choice for patients with traumatized lower extremities if the central nervous system is not involved, if the blood volume has been replaced, and if the patient is not intoxicated or otherwise unmanageable. Spinal anesthesia is generally contraindicated in problems associated with severe hypovolemia.

Local anesthesia has been recommended in many poor-risk patients, but care must be exercised in the selection of dose and technique of the block. Regional blocks, such as sciatic-femoral blocks for lower extremity work or brachial plexus blocks for upper extremity operations, may be utilized if the patient is cooperative or if the patient's physiologic state is such that sedation may be used without undue adverse effect.

However, general anesthesia is preferred where trauma is of a severe nature, or where the head, neck, or trunk is involved. When general anesthesia is selected, many factors may influence the choice of anesthetic technique to be employed. Of these factors, the most important are:

1 The physical status of the patient
2 The sites of injury and the nature of the anticipated surgery
3 The presence of specific contraindications to a particular technique
4 The experience and competence of the anesthesiologist

Often, a debate arises over whether to proceed at once with an indicated operation, or whether to delay while assessing the full extent of the patient's deranged physiology. Uncontrolled hemorrhage, unresolved airway obstruction, compound fractures, and penetrating wounds of the abdomen, neck, or axilla are usually indications for immediate surgery. Anesthetic problems may be minimized, however, if a definitive surgical procedure for most other trauma is delayed, usually not over a maximum of 6 h, while reestablishing cardiovascular or respiratory dynamics, obtaining adequate diagnostic information, and initiating treatment of associated conditions.

The patient in shock needs oxygen and volume expansion. The patient has a dulled appreciation for pain, and profound anesthesia will further depress the cardiovascular and respiratory systems. Thus, anything but the most judicious administration of anesthetic agents may be called "misguided humanitarianism." One should remember that complete suppression of sensation is not necessary and may be harmful if achieved by deep anesthesia. Extensive surgical procedures can be accomplished in *analgesic* planes of anesthesia, achieved with nitrous oxide, or with low concentrations of a volatile agent, or by an appropriate combination of light general plus local anesthesia. Neither can one forget that muscle relaxants are not anesthetics and significant awareness, pain, and postoperative neuroses have occurred in patients who were curarized but conscious.[14]

THE EXTENT AND DURATION OF INJURIES

In the emergency management of the patient with multiple injuries, medically correct decisions must be made based on the sum total of one's pertinent knowledge, experience, and skill. Deliberation and equivocation are often out of the question. Many of the decisions made intuitively at this critical state of the patient's care have serious legal implications. We must therefore know the common combinations of injuries occurring in the trauma patient. We must recognize that all injuries may not be diagnosed at the time of anesthesia induction. We must realize that the associated injury may be a greater threat to life than the primary target of the surgical procedure, and, above all, we must maintain that degree of suspicion that will lead us to search for occult explanations for serious alterations in vital signs. For example, the average anesthesiologist has the ability, knowledge, and tools at hand to diagnose a pneumothorax, pericardial tamponade, or intraabdominal hemorrhage. One must, however, train oneself to suspect these common associated injuries in the patient with maxillofacial or extremity trauma. In an inventory of all trauma, 20 percent of those patients have multiple injuries.[30] However, where motor vehicle accidents are the cause, injuries involving more than one body area are found in 65 percent of patients.[57] Beware of the undetected injuries associated with head trauma. Head trauma results in varying degrees of concussion, unconsciousness, memory loss, and interference with neurological function. These signs may be confused with or dismissed as alcohol intoxication. The patient may not be able to describe the pain in his or her neck, chest, or abdomen. Seven percent of motor vehicle accident victims have neck and cervical spine injuries. Unrecognized cervical spine injuries are significant because manipulation of the patient in positioning for operation or tracheal intubation may injure the spinal cord. Rubsamen[48] reports three cases of quadriplegia which developed during ambulance or hospital care in patients with head injuries and unsuspected fracture dislocations at the cervical spine. Courts found in favor of the injured patients in all three cases.

Head injuries are also commonly associated with intrathoracic and intraabdominal trauma. Patients with combinations of head and abdominal injuries are difficult to evaluate. As reported by Tovee.[56] Initial examination revealed no abdominal findings in 8 of 16 patients with combined head and abdominal injury; 12 of the 16 patients had persistent shock after what should have been "adequate resuscitation." Decreasing blood pressure is rarely a manifestation of closed head injury. Hypotension in head-injury patients should alert the anesthesiologist to look for abdominal or chest bleeding, pneumothorax, cardiac tamponade bleeding, severe fractures, or transected spinal cord.

Head injury is not a contraindication to general anesthesia when necessary. Anesthetic management is directed principally toward preventing further rise in intracranial pressure by utilizing a technique which allows smooth induction and intubation, unobstructed airway, and controlled hyperventilation to produce hypocarbia with resultant reduction in volume of the cerebral contents. Thiopental, in generous doses, reduces intracranial pressure. Although succinylcholine produces a rise in intracranial pressure, this may be prevented by a small dose of nondepolarizing muscle relaxant previously administered to control muscle fasciculations. Reduction of cerebral edema by the use of corticosteroids or diuretic agents such as urea, mannitol, or furosemide is adjunctive to the basic anesthetic technique. Ketamine should be avoided if a probability of increased intracranial pressure exists.[29] Halothane can increase intracranial pressure unless used with previously established hyperventilation.[1]

Damages to the chest wall or to the myocardium may not appear significant until a pneumothorax becomes apparent or until arrhythmias develop during an operation for associated trauma. Major cardiovascular injuries can occur in motor vehicle accidents without external evidence of serious trauma to the chest wall. Cardiac injury is said to occur in 10 to 75 percent of cases with trauma to the chest.[24] This may range from minor subpericardial hemorrhage to rupture of the heart or great vessels. Signs include electrocardiographic (ECG) alterations, arrhythmias, congestive heart failure, tamponade, and hemothorax.

THE EXTENT OF HEMORRHAGE AND REPLACEMENT

The extent of hemorrhage and adequacy of replacement is obviously one of the most important factors influencing the choice of anesthetic agent and technique. Techniques of anesthetic care for the patient will differ according to whether bleeding develops during the progress of a corrective surgical procedure, or whether it eventuates postoperatively as a cause of continued deterioration of the traumatized patient's inherent vital functions.

The signs of hypovolemia should be sought and an assessment made of the degree of shock. Some or all of the following may be present: pallor; tachycardia; hypotension; pale, cold, and sometimes cyanosed extremities; low central venous pressure; and oliguria or anuria. Hypovolemia may also cause confusion, restlessness, air hunger, and coma. These signs result from a loss of over 40 percent of blood volume in a previously healthy patient. The same signs may appear with smaller blood losses in geriatric or previously anemic patients; in those who have received narcotics and tranquilizers; or in those who have been badly transported. Normovolemic patients may mimic the signs of shock as a result of injury to the cervical spinal cord, cardiac tamponade, or pneumothorax. In practice, three types of patients emerge and their anesthetic requirements differ distinctly according to volumes of blood lost.

Minor Trauma with Minor Amounts of Blood Loss Surgical intervention is not an urgent necessity and may be deferred until a thorough preanesthetic evaluation and laboratory workup has been completed. Regional anesthesia or anesthesia under mask is perfectly acceptable in many cases. Endotracheal anesthesia is indicated where a suspicion of a full stomach exists; where surgical access demands it; where controlled ventilation is planned; or where any doubt whatsoever exists concerning the integrity of the patient's airway. The range of anesthetic techniques is as wide as in elective surgery, but a few are suggested here.

1 Under the action of the dissociative agent, ketamine, minor surgical procedures

may be performed on infants and children. Given either intravenously or intramuscularly, ketamine is eminently suitable for reduction of fractures, suturing of lacerations, or the application of splints or dressings. The early claims that ketamine preserves laryngeal reflexes have now been largely disproved.[22] To use this agent alone in the presence of a full stomach is inadvisable.

2 Reduction of simple forearm fractures has been successfully performed using diazepam intravenously in a dose of about 0.3 to 0.5 mg/kg.[18] The success of this technique is based on the combined hypnotic, muscle relaxant, and amnesic properties of diazepam.

3 Intermittent administration of an intravenous barbiturate may also be used to provide adequate surgical conditions for brief, minor procedures. Where this technique is being used for outpatient surgical procedures, methohexital is preferred to thiopental because recovery is expected to be more rapid.[27]

4 Where anesthesia is expected to last for more than a few minutes, more conventional anesthetic techniques are required, e.g., rapid induction as described under Endotracheal Intubation below and maintenance with nitrous oxide and oxygen (70:30) supplemented by a volatile agent such as halothane or enflurane. Spontaneous respiration is permitted after return from the succinylcholine.

5 The increasing anxiety concerning the possible toxic effects of the volatile anesthetic agents on both the patient and the operating room personnel[4] have made the use of Innovar, a neuroleptanalgesic agent, increasingly popular.[38] One technique using Innovar is as follows: Initially, Innovar is administered intravenously in divided doses up to 0.1 ml/kg body weight. If necessary, this is followed by a "sleep" dose of thiopental. After topical application of 4% lidocaine to the larynx, endotracheal intubation is performed. Intravenous succinycholine may or may not be required to facilitate intubation. Anesthesia is maintained using nitrous oxide and oxygen (70:30) with the patient breathing spontaneously. Supplemental analgesia is obtained using intravenous increments of 0.05 mg fen-

tanyl. The aim is to maintain a respiratory rate of 8 to 10 respirations/min. The same effect may be achieved by adding fentanyl, 10 to 12 ml to 250 ml of IV fluid, and adjusting the rate of infusion until the desired respiratory rate is obtained.

6 Probably the simplest and safest technique in longer surgical procedures is controlled ventilation with oxygen and nitrous oxide, using a muscle relaxant and a narcotic agent (the so-called "nitrous oxide–relaxant technique").

Greater Trauma with Loss of 10 to 30 percent of the Patient's Blood Volume This patient will have an increased pulse rate, decreased blood pressure, decreased venous pressure, peripheral vasoconstriction, reduced urinary output, mild respiratory distress, decreased Pa_{O_2} and Pa_{CO_2}, and a normal to disoriented mental status. By the time the patient reaches the operating room, the patient may have vital signs that are nearly normal due to partial blood and fluid replacement and partial vasomotor compensation. General anesthesia may render the patient severely hypotensive by abolishing vasomotor tone.

Surgical intervention for patients in this category is frequently urgent, although rarely of an immediate lifesaving nature. Time is usually available to perform adequate preanesthetic evaluation and to correct deficiencies. Once circulating blood volume has been adequately restored, the patient's physical status may be upgraded and anesthesia administered accordingly. If operation is urgent, the patient's unstable cardiovascular condition must be suspected and the nitrous oxide/oxygen–relaxant technique chosen. The patient is preoxygenated and anesthesia is induced using methohexital in a dose up to 1.5 mg/kg. Methohexital is preferred over thiopental because of the lesser incidence of hypotension associated with its use.[27] Succinylcholine is preferred for endotracheal intubation, although relaxation should be maintained with pancuronium, 1 to 2 mg repeated, as muscle tone recurs. Pancuronium is chosen over d-tubocurarine because of the greater degree of cardiovascular stability associated with its use.[35] Anesthesia is maintained using nitrous oxide and oxygen (70:30) by controlled ventilation plus an intravenous narcotic agent; whether controlled hyperventilation with its concomitant lowered Pa_{CO_2} enhances the anesthetic effect and reduces the requirement for narcotic is controversial.[11] Choice of narcotic usually lies between morphine, meperidine, and fentanyl.

Reversal of muscle relaxation is achieved at the end of the procedure using atropine 0.04 mg/kg and neostigmine 0.07 mg/kg. The endotracheal tube is removed when the patient's respiratory function is judged adequate and when protective laryngeal and pharyngeal reflexes have returned. Techniques utilizing potent volatile agents (halothane, enflurane, or methoxyflurane) or vasodilating intravenous drugs such as droperidol must be used with great care to prevent serious hypotension.

Major Trauma with Loss of 50 percent or Greater of Blood Volume This patient is expected to be severely hypotensive and to evidence tachycardia, low venous pressure, severe respiratory distress, marked vasoconstriction, and advanced hypoxia. Pa_{CO_2} may be elevated or decreased. The only urine is that which was in the bladder when the shock commenced. This patient is usually semiconscious, but may be comatose.

Surgical intervention becomes an urgent and lifesaving necessity for the more severely traumatized patients. Such patients are frequently thrust upon the anesthesiologist when the bare minimum of data are available, and the anesthesiologist is obliged to accept all the risks involved in the management of such a case. Nevertheless, some attempt must be made prior to induction of anesthesia to correct the hypovolemia by rapid infusion of a balanced salt solution and type-specific blood or equivalents in component therapy.

These patients need no anesthetic agent at all. The use of potent intravenous or inhalational anesthetic agents, even in small dosage, may be sufficient to precipitate complete and irreversible cardiovascular collapse. Severely hypovolemic patients are so critically ill that their pain appreciation and basic reflexes are obtunded, and they offer little resistance to procedures such as endotracheal intubation. Despite severe trauma, if blood loss has not been great, the patient may still maintain a recordable blood pressure and have some degree of awareness which may require some minimal doses of anesthetic agents or adjuvants.

Maintenance of anesthesia may vary depending on the condition of the patient, such as when anesthetic management consists of controlled ventilation using 100% oxygen with no anesthetic or analgesic agents but with muscle relaxation provided by intravenous pancuronium, using increments of 1 to 2 mg as required. Where evidence of inadequate analgesia exists using this technique, nitrous oxide/oxygen (50:50) may be initiated, supplemented as the patient's general condition improves by small doses of ketamine or fentanyl. Thus, a technique utilizing pancuronium, ketamine, controlled ventilation, and either undiluted oxygen or nitrous oxide and oxygen (50:50) has gained wide popularity in the management of the adult patient in extremis.

Fluid Resuscitation

Principles in the management of shock are dealt with in Chap. 1, and discussion here is limited to the intraoperative use of intravenous infusions. Current concepts indicate that an internal redistribution of functional extracellular fluid (FECF) exists incident to the necessary trauma of the surgical procedure. The magnitude of redistribution (internal shift) reflects the magnitude of trauma or of surgical manipulation. A patient with a burn or crush injury has wound edema that can be seen. This edema is an obligatory response to tissue trauma, and can be measured by an isotope equilibration curve of several hours duration. The sequestered fluid is nonfunctional in that it is not available to perform the physiologic duties of normal extra-cellular fluid, and it does not enter into the dynamics of the circulation. Infusion of balanced salt solutions (BSS) during surgery and following trauma are intended to restore this deficit of FECF.

The characteristics of the loss of FECF during and after hemorrhagic hypovolemic shock are different. Patients who have unreplaced blood loss will partially restore their vascular volume with a buffered saline of their own manufacture from their interstitial fluid. The thoughtful anesthesiologist will perform this restoration for the patient rather than expose the patient to the hazards of hypovolemia while transferring fluid from one compartment to another. Some studies suggest that in addition to a movement of FECF into the vascular space, a movement of FECF into the cells occurs during and following hemorrhagic shock.[53] Because the loss of FECF is isotonic, the repair solution should have a composition of electrolytes which approaches that of the lost fluid. Such solutions are referred to as balanced salt solutions. Lactated Ringer's, a solution commonly infused, will move freely between the intravascular and interstitial compartments and will expand the entire extracellular fluid compartment. The distribution of the infused solution into the two compartments occurs within 30 to 60 min in accord with the Starling hypothesis governing the movement of isotonic solutions.[23]

By contrast, infusions of plasma, albumin, and dextran-70 will sustain elevations of plasma volume up to 5 h, and plasma volume expansion with dextran-40 lasts about 2½ h. The use of balanced salt solutions is not meant to be a substitute for whole blood.[49] Limitations exist to restoration of blood loss with BSS, though they can be used alone to replace volume losses of up to 20 percent of blood volume.[41] Quantities up to 3 to 4 L in the average adult can be used safely as initial resuscitation of hemorrhagic shock while type-specific whole blood or components are being prepared. The ultimate volume of BSS required depends on the condition of the patient, the severity of tissue injury, and the severity and duration of shock. Patients with cardiac or renal disease deserve special consideration and care in fluid therapy, although in general they tolerate a mild overload better than a deficit, even a mild deficit.

All practicing anesthesiologists have been caught in a situation where rate of bleeding exceeded the ability of the blood bank to supply whole blood for transfusion. A report of one such circumstance shows that massive hemorrhages in humans can be successfully replaced with lactated Ringer's solution,[17] although anemia, hypoproteinemia, and pulmonary and peripheral edema are a few of the expected limitations.[50] Human blood losses up to 50 percent of blood volume have been successfully resuscitated with balanced salt solutions.[58] In experimental animals blood losses up to 85 percent of blood volume have been replaced with Ringer's lactate alone;[19] however, volumes up to 25 times the shed blood are required to produce survival.[43] Serial measurements of hematocrit during surgery with transfusion of blood whenever the hematocrit falls below 28 percent have been proposed as a practical method to balance fluid and blood therapy.[51]

Many recent studies show BSS to be as effective as the dextrans in the resuscitation of hemorrhagic shock and to be devoid of some of the undesirable side effects of the dextrans.[20,51] Both forms of currently used dextrans produce increased bleeding when given in volumes that exceed 10 ml/kg per 24 h. If dextrans are to be used at all, most patients in shock require more volume than this limit imposes. Resuscitation with balanced salt solutions in massive quantities leads to transient hypoproteinemia. In one experimental study, animals bled to 73 percent depletion of red cell mass were given 12.2 volumes of salt solution per final volume of blood shed to effect resuscitation.[23] This huge volume of electrolyte solution reduced the hematocrit from a control value of 40 percent to a postresuscitation value of 11 percent and reduced the total serum protein from 5.3 g per 100 ml to a postresuscitation value of 1.4 g per 100 ml. Twenty-four hours following resuscitation, the hematocrit remained at 11 percent, but total serum protein had spontaneously recovered to 4.4 g per 100 ml.

Carey[21] used albumin solutions with whole blood in the resuscitation of 10 soldiers wounded in the Vietnam war. He stated that the clinical course of these patients was much less satisfactory than that of 20 patients resuscitated with balanced salt solutions and blood. Those patients given albumin required almost twice as much total volume to stabilize vital signs, but urine output was half that of patients given salt solutions. Preoperative lab studies suggested that injury severity and blood loss were similar in both groups. In spite of vigorous albumin therapy, the patients did not have significantly higher postresuscitation total protein or albumin levels than those receiving salt solutions and blood. Vigorous albumin therapy failed to maintain a significantly higher plasma protein concentration than resuscitation with salt solutions and blood. However, plasma protein concentrations will fall significantly if massive blood loss is resuscitated with packed cells and saline. In order to prevent severe hypoproteinemia and dilutional thrombocytopenia, our routine is to give 2 U of fresh-frozen plasma and 2 U of platelets with every 10 U of packed cells.[34]

Urine Formation

Evidence of the efficacy of fluid replacement will depend not only upon the restoration of an acceptable blood pressure level and pulse rate but also upon the evidence of urine excretion. Usually urine flow is quickly reestablished and readily sustained using balanced salt solution and blood in resuscitation of hemorrhagic shock.[21] Urine flow is maintained during major surgical procedures when sufficient balanced salt solutions are given despite the renal depressant effects of anxiety, premedication, anesthesia, dehydration, stress, and bleeding. Admittedly, adequate urine flow does not always mean that renal function is adequate.[3,46] The alterations of renal function associated with trauma and hemorrhage are related to the severity and duration of shock. Renal failure can be separated into oliguric and polyuric (high-output) types. Balanced salt solutions have been reported to reduce the incidence of oliguric renal failure following major trauma,[7] extensive vascular surgery,[54] and hemorrhagic shock.[52] Renal failure which occurs in the presence of adequate urine output carries a lower mortality rate (18.5 percent) than does oliguric renal failure (50 to 70 percent).[7] Infusion of Ringer's lactate adequate to maintain the urine output over 100 ml/h has been shown to protect against expected renal complications in 16 patients with documented hemolytic transfusion reactions.[8]

Other factors may alter urine flow from the traumatized patient. Many popular antibiotics and drugs, including anesthetics, affect renal function. Complications such as fat embolism and hemolytic transfusion reactions can lead to renal failure.

When urine flow remains below 25 ml/h in spite of volume replacement which is judged to be clinically adequate, an intravenous diuretic agent may be given to distinguish prerenal from renal cause of oliguria. Either mannitol, 25 g, or furosemide, 40 to 80 mg, may be used for this purpose. Prerenal oliguria may be distinguished from renal oliguria by the measurement of urinary sodium and creatinine and plasma creatinine.[5] Urinary sodium concentrations are less than 20 meq/L in prerenal failure and above 20 meq/L in renal failure. The ratio of urinary to plasma creatinine is normally 20:1. In prerenal failure the ratio is elevated to 25 or 30:1. In renal failure the ratio is depressed to 10:1 or less. Urine output can generally be maintained without the use of diuretics if blood and fluid replacement are adequate and if the anesthesia is maintained at light levels.

Hypotension during Anesthesia

Even for the nontraumatized patient a variety of causes of hypotension exist in the conduct of anesthesia. Unintentional hypotension is not an acceptable response to anesthesia, even though it is not entirely unexpected. The cardinal principle of management for the patient who becomes hypotensive during the operation is that the administration of all anesthetic agents should be stopped and inhalation agents remoded from the breathing circuit by flushing with oxygen and from the patient by vigorous ventilation with oxygen. The other basic principles of treatment of hypotensive patients should be followed as discussed in Chap. 1 (Principles in the Management of Shock). The application of these treatment modalities should follow a brief but thoughtful differential diagnosis based on the classification (cardiogenic, vasogenic, neurogenic, or hematogenic), which is useful from a clinical therapeutic viewpoint.

Cardiogenic hypotension with normal blood volume should be treated with inotropic drugs. Inappropriate volume therapy or vasoconstrictors can be fatal. Vasogenic hypotension resulting from loss of peripheral resistance may be treated with vasopressors or volume. Neurogenic hypotension from spinal anesthesia, quadriplegia, or simple syncope are classified by modern authors in the vasogenic group. Hematogenic hypotension is usually caused by oligemia, and is the primary indication for volume therapy with crystalloids, colloids, and/or blood. Hypotension due to inadequate venous return has a diversity of causes besides hypovolemia. Other common causes include the supine hypotensive syndrome of pregnancy, pneumothorax, and cardiac tamponade (Chap. 1).

Adjunctive Therapy in Shock

Warming of the infused blood and fluids is strongly recommended. The greater the volume of infusions required, the more imperative the need to warm. Both wet and dry warmers are commercially available and are probably safe, but microwave warmers have been shown to induce excessive hemolysis.[39] Microfilters with a pore size of 20 to 50 μ should be used in those situations where rapid or massive transfusions are necessary.[40]

Alkalinizing agents are frequently necessary to correct the acidosis consequent to the low flow state and transfusion of large quantities of whole blood. Sodium bicarbonate is most commonly used. The dosage should be guided by blood gas analysis using the formula: $0.3 \times$ body weight in kg $\times$ base deficit in meq/L = $NaHCO_3$ required. Unmonitored or empiric use of alkalinizing agents may result in severe metabolic alkalosis.[6]

Reportedly, large doses of steroids given intravenously produce a beneficial effect in the shocked patient, but the exact mechanism of this effect has not been fully determined. The mode of action may be a direct myocardial inotropic effect combined with a peripheral vasodilator mechanism. Regardless of mechanism, an increased blood pressure and a decreased peripheral resistance are known to occur.[44] The "antistress" action of the corticosteroids may also be of importance. Dose requirements are in the order of 1 to 2 g of methylprednisolone administered intravenously. The precise benefit derived from inotropic drugs in hemorrhagic shock has not been established. Isoproterenol is the agent most widely used. Its potent stimulation of beta-adrenergic receptors combined with its tendency to lower peripheral vascular resistance benefits cardiac output, venous return, and peripheral perfusion. Isoproterenol is contraindicated in the presence of an existing tachycardia, which may occur in hypovolemia. Isoproterenol is probably best administered in an infusion containing 2 mg/500 ml of 5% dextrose and with careful ECG monitoring.

Digitalis may be used to benefit patients, particularly when fluid replacement has been massive. The positive inotropic actions of calcium may similarly be of value. For rapid IV digitalization, digoxin 0.25 to 1.0 mg may be used, its onset of action occurring within 20 min of injection. Where very rapid digitalization is required, ouabain 0.25 to 0.5 mg can be used, and its action is expected to commence within 3 to 10 min.

The administration of 1 g of calcium gluconate with every 4 or 5 U of blood infused should prevent the citrate intoxication which will occur if the patient's ability to mobilize ionized calcium from the bones is impaired. Also, the administration of calcium will correct the calcium-potassium imbalance imposed by transfusion of hyperkalemic banked blood. Potassium is released into the serum from the red cells of stored bank blood because of increasing hemolysis in aging blood. Concomitantly, potassium may be released from the liver stimulated by norepinephrine secreted in response to shock. Tolerance of the heart muscle to hyperkalemia is decreased if traumatic or anoxic myocardial damage has already occurred. Overuse of calcium also has its hazards. The dangers of hypercalcemia are primarily those of cardiac arrhythmias, particularly if some degree of hypothermia of the myocardium exists. Likewise, the administration of calcium to a digitalized patient may result in digitalis intoxication. An electrocar-

diographic monitor should be in use during calcium administration to detect early evidence of arrhythmias.

The use of vasodilator drugs is sometimes advocated in order to improve the peripheral circulation. Since the use of such drugs in the presence of hypotension is still the subject of much debate, we rarely administer them. The most commonly used of these agents are phenoxybenzamine, methylprednisolone, chlorpromazine, and droperidol. To use phenoxybenzamine, a dose of 1.0 mg/kg body weight is diluted in 250 to 500 ml of IV solution and infused over a period of about 1 h.

Transfusion Reactions

Significant morbidity is associated with transfusions which are administered in haste to a deteriorating patient. Historically, a unit of incompatible blood administered rapidly results in a severe hemolytic reaction from which only one patient in four will survive. Careful checking of the patient's identity against the identity of the blood is absolutely mandatory. Under anesthesia a hemolytic reaction is recognized early by the onset of hypotension, skin flush, hyperpyrexia, and tachycardia. Hemoglobinuria and hemoglobinemia can be observed at this point. Later unexplained, disproportionate hemorrhage may indicate the occurrence of disseminated intravascular coagulation associated with a hemolytic reaction.

With the diagnosis of a hemolytic transfusion reaction, the anesthesiologist should stop the administration of the incompatible blood, speed the infusion of lactated Ringer's solution to promote diuresis, and alkalinize the patient with sodium bicarbonate until the urine becomes alkaline. Hemoglobin is less likely to precipitate and obstruct the renal tubules if the urine is alkaline.[8]

Febrile and allergic reactions can occur under anesthesia, but do not carry the same serious prognosis as hemolytic reactions. Parenteral antihistamines will usually relieve the urticaria and bronchospasm associated with the allergic responses.

Monitoring

Monitoring of the patient's condition has been facilitated by the development of modern and complex devices which complement the more traditional methods. The patient's clinical condition will determine the extent of monitoring which is required. Some or all of the following methods may be utilized:

1 Palpation of the pulse will give information on heart rate and rhythm, and pulse volume may give some indication of cardiac output. Capillary pulse monitors utilizing the photoelectric cell are available, but offer little advantage over simple palpation.

2 Observation of capillary refill time is a useful indicator of peripheral circulation.

3 Arterial blood pressure may be measured by use of the sphygmomanometer cuff and stethoscope. The oscillotonometer tends to give a greater degree of accuracy at lower levels of blood pressure. Direct measurement of arterial blood pressure may be performed using an indwelling cannula. This method is the only practical one during cardiopulmonary bypass where pulsatile circulation is not present. The catheter, which must be regularly flushed by a heparinized solution, is connected by a fluid column to a transducer or to a simple manometer. The system must be accurately calibrated before use, and care must be taken in choosing the length and diameter of tubing used since these factors may affect the accuracy of readings. In the severely hypovolemic patient, peripheral pulses may be impalpable, so that arterial puncture is difficult. Arterial damage and thrombosis following catheterization has been reported.[9,26]

4 Monitoring of the patient's respiratory function may be performed clinically by noting the color of the skin and blood for signs of oxygen desaturation and by observing respiratory movements for evidence of airway obstruction, pneumothorax, or paradoxical respiration. Auscultation of breath and heart sounds using a precordial or esophageal stethoscope is also important. Use of an esophageal stethoscope may give valuable additional evidence of the occurrence of air embolism. A stethoscope on each hemithorax is useful in diagnosing unilateral chest pathology.

5 Central venous pressure monitoring is essential where significant blood loss has occurred and massive fluid infusion is required. Serial measurements of central venous pressure are of greatest value in the evaluation of fluid replacement, since a single reading is of little value. Several routes for placement of a central venous catheter are available. Usually, one of the veins of the antecubital fossa, preferably the basilic vein[61] is cannulated with a long catheter which is advanced centrally to the superior vena cava or to the right atrium. Percutaneous cannulation is satisfactory, but occasionally a cut-down may be required. The external jugular vein can be cannulated using a 14 cm, 16 gauge around the needle catheter. The sigmoid portion of the external jugular vein can be negotiated with a 35-cm-long, 0.089-cm-diameter flexible angiographic wire (J wire) with a 3 mm radius of curvature.[15] The internal jugular and subclavian veins may also be used, although risk of multiple complications exists with these approaches. The inferior vena cava may be cannulated via the femoral vein and the catheter threaded centrally. This route may lead to development of thrombosis and pulmonary embolism. In addition, where there are abdominal injuries present, it is best to avoid this route because of a possible ruptured or compressed inferior vena cava.

6 Measurement of urinary output is useful as a guide to fluid replacement. Urinary flow of 0.5 to 1.0 ml/kg per hour is considered satisfactory. All trauma patients except those with minor injury should have a urinary catheter in place.

7 Electrocardiographic monitoring is recommended in all cases since it provides evidence of cardiac arrhythmias, myocardial ischemia, and electrolyte changes. In the event of cardiac arrest, it is the only method of distinguishing asystole from ventricular fibrillation and of assessing the response to treatment.

8 Temperature monitoring is recommended in all traumatized patients under general anesthesia. Temperature elevations due to febrile or hemolytic transfusion reactions, sepsis, or malignant hyperpyrexia must be detected early in order to institute appropriate therapy. Inadvertent hypothermia due to air-conditioned operating rooms and fluid infusions must be detected in order to avoid overdosage with inhalation or parenteral anesthetic agents. Esophageal temperature will reflect the temperature at the heart, and a typmpanic or nasopharyngeal temperature probe will give an indication of brain temperature.

9 Assessment of intraoperative blood loss is an additional guide to fluid replacement. Simple observation of surgical sponges and suction is notoriously inaccurate, even to the experienced anesthesiologist. Weighing of blood soaked swabs and colorimetric methods are somewhat more accurate.

10 Laboratory assistance is required to monitor some of the patient's parameters. Frequent blood gas analysis and assessment of acid-base status are essential in severe trauma cases. In addition, where massive fluid and blood replacement is occurring, intermittent assessment of hematocrit and plasma electrolytes may be of value. Defects of blood clotting occasionally complicate massive fluid replacement. Consultation from a hematologist may be required to determine the nature of the clotting defect, although simple clinical tests may be adequate.[30] Intraoperative bleeding is most commonly due to thrombocytopenia, labile factor deficiency, fibrinolysis, or hypofibrinogenemia. Refer to Chap. 3 for specific diagnostic and therapeutic scheme for coagulopathies.

ADEQUACY OF AIRWAY AND VENTILATION

One of the most cherished platitudes in anesthesiology, "maintain a clear airway," is interpreted differently by various practitioners of medicine. However, proper care of airway problems in the acutely traumatized patient may be the significant factor in achieving successful resuscitation and avoiding morbidity related to the patient's respiratory or nervous systems.

Airway problems may be compounded by food in the stomach not easily removed by gastric tube. The tracheobronchial tree may already have been transgressed by silent aspiration during a period of hypotension and nonresponsiveness. Injuries specifically affecting the upper airway, as in maxillofacial trauma, may readily encroach upon the patient's ability to breathe without added effort.

Although many alternatives have been proposed in the past, tracheostomy and endotracheal intubation are the techniques most available to "maintain a clear airway" in the trauma patient.

Tracheostomy

Patients with injuries of the larynx or cervical portion of the trachea should have a tracheostomy. Patients with combined injuries of the maxilla and mandible should have tracheostomies, for when the jaws are wired and the nasal passages are obstructed by blood clots or edema, the patient can breathe only with conscious, concentrated effort. Even though a surgical indication for a tracheostomy exists, the patient's physical status can be improved by endotracheal intubation prior to tracheostomy.

If a tracheostomy is to be done for the patient with such severe maxillofacial damage that introduction of an endotracheal tube from above would be inadvisable, oxygenation of the patient can be accomplished by high flows of oxygen (up to 20 L/min) through an 18- to 15-gauge needle introduced into the tracheal lumen through the cricothyroid membrane. The lung will not be overly expanded by this maneuver.

If an endotracheal tube can be introduced, and if the need is not immediate, the tracheostomy is better deferred until the corrective operation for the primary trauma has been accomplished. Although good hemostasis may have been established during the performance of the tracheostomy, slow drainage of blood and serum may occur into the trachea around the tube, adding to the airway problems during the operative procedure.

Endotracheal Intubation

Preparedness is essential before induction of anesthesia for the traumatized patient. Anesthesia machine, suction, monitors, drugs, laryngoscope with an assortment of blades, all with good batteries and bulb, and tubes of various sizes and styles should be at hand ready for use for the average case. A rapid-acting antacid such as milk of magnesia 15 to 30 ml is given orally to all patients who do not have injuries of the gastrointestinal tract. Preliminary evidence indicates that milk of magnesia will increase the pH of gastric contents above the critical level of 2.5 from 10 to 80 min after the oral dose has been given. The incidence and severity of acid aspiration pneumonitis is expected to be greatly reduced should regurgitation and aspiration occur during this interval.[62] The patient's mouth, teeth, neck, and quality of respiration should be noted and a decision made as to the type of intubation to be performed. Generally these fall into two categories: rapid controlled intubation and awake intubation. The *rapid controlled intubation* is a specific series of events designed to reduce the time from loss of the patient's protective reflexes to absolute airway security by the anesthesiologist. First, the awake patient is preoxygenated with 100% oxygen. Preoxygenation replaces alveolar nitrogen with oxygen and can add several minutes before hypoxia supervenes in the apneic patient should the intubation prove difficult. Nasogastric tubes are suctioned and then removed as they prevent good mask fit and interfere with competence of the cardia. Atropine 1 mg is administered intravenously. Atropine decreases the effects of vagal stimulation associated with intubation and blocks the

bradycardia associated with repeated administrations of succinylcholine.

d-Tubocurarine (DTC) 3 mg is given intravenously 2 to 3 min before induction to prevent fasciculations of the diaphragm and muscles of the abdominal wall and diminish the likelihood of regurgitation. Anesthesia is induced with either thiopental (3 to 4 mg/kg IV) or ketamine (2 mg/kg IV) depending on the cardiovascular status of the patient. Thiopental is avoided in hypovolemic patients. The induction agent is *immediately* followed by succinylcholine (1 to 1.5 mg/kg IV). Waiting to make sure that the patient is asleep before paralyzing him or her may lead to aspiration.

Cricoesophageal compression (Fig. 5-1) applied after the loss of consciousness will help prevent regurgitation into the pharynx. An assistant applies forceful posterior pressure on the cricoid cartilage, compressing the cervical portion of the esophagus between the broad posterior aspect of the cricoid cartilage and the anterior surface of the body of the sixth cervical vertebrae. Care must be taken to press on the cricoid cartilage and not on the thyroid cartilage. The pressure must be applied as soon as the patient loses consciousness and must be maintained while the patient becomes sufficiently relaxed for laryngosco-

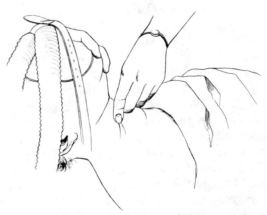

Figure 5-1 Cricoesophageal compression (Selleck maneuver). See text for explanation.

py, insertion of the endotracheal tube, and inflation of its cuff. Only after the airway is secure can the assistant relax pressure on the cricoid cartilage. The anesthesiologist can now use any method indicated for maintenance of anesthesia. At no time during this induction is the patient given positive pressure ventilation by mask unless it is required to prevent hypoxia in the patient in whom initial attempts at intubation have failed. The risk of further inflating the stomach, causing regurgitation, or of forcing regurgitated fluid from the pharynx into the trachea is too great.

Awake intubations are considered to be indicated in patients with distended bowel (especially high obstruction) and airway malformations which may make laryngoscopy difficult (especially those who already have partial airway obstruction). That the patient is voluntarily controlling the airway and has the protective reflexes intact is the principal advantage of awake intubation. Either an oral or nasal route can be used.

For an oral intubation lidocaine 4% is applied topically to the tongue, gently advancing the curved laryngoscope blade posteriorly to gain exposure. The cords are not anesthetized. Care must be taken to stay below the toxic levels of lidocaine. Once the cords are visualized, the tube is inserted during inspiration and the cuff is inflated. Usually tachycardia ensues and will resolve when anesthesia is induced. Occasionally vagally induced bradycardia may result, which will respond to atropine. Thiopental is given immediately after cuff inflation. This technique requires a cooperative patient, so some sedation may be necessary. Sedation means that the patient is awake with full reflex control but calm and cooperative. This state may be accomplished with diazepam or small doses of thiopental. Diazepam induces anterograde amnesia, a benevolent side effect in circumstances in which awake intubation is necessary.

Nasal intubation must be preceded with some agent to shrink and anesthetize the nasal mucous membranes. Either cocaine 4% or a combination of oxymetazoline (Afrin) nasal spray and lidocaine 4% is sufficient. The tube is guided in its passage to the pharynx by passing a small suction catheter through the tube so that it protrudes about 3 cm beyond the end of the tube. This catheter bends easily and acts as a guide through the nose, preventing mucosal injury, submucosal tunneling, or entry of debris into the tube. Once the tube has negotiated the curve and has passed into the oropharynx, the suction catheter should be removed. A small whistle to magnify breath sounds may be used to aid proper positioning of the tube (Waldhaus Tracheal Indicator, Ohio). While listening, one advances the tube during inspiration. If the esophagus is intubated or if the tube enters either pyriform sinus, breath sounds through the tube cease. Once the trachea is intubated and the cuff inflated, the anesthesiologist may proceed with indicated methods of any anesthetic induction and maintenance. Blind intubations are not indicated in maxillofacial trauma, and the nasal intubation should be performed under vision.

Fiberoptic Intubation

Fiberoptic laryngoscopy by both oral and nasal routes has been described by Raj.[45] This instrument enables performance of intubation in otherwise nearly impossible situations, such as for the patient with cervical trauma whose neck cannot be moved but for whom blind nasal intubation has failed. This technique is not quick and requires either extensive topical anesthesia, including transtracheal instillation of lidocaine, or a spontaneously breathing patient under general anesthesia. The topical anesthesia technique is preferred for patients with a full stomach.

The fiberoptic laryngoscope is a flexible, fiberoptic device, the tip of which may be deflected 120° in a single plane by means of a knob on the handle. Illumination is provided at the endoscopist's end of the scope by either an external, ac power source or by a bulb and battery contained in the handle. Both the fiberscope and the endotracheal tube (size 8 mm or larger) are lubricated with a local anesthetic ointment. The tip of the fiberscope must be covered with an antifogging compound or soaked in warm water.

The nasotracheal tube is inserted through the nares into the nasopharynx as previously described. The fiberscope is passed through the tube and past the epiglottis by flexing or extending the scope's tip in the saggital plane. Once past the epiglottis, the glottis is visualized. The scope is advanced through the glottis into the trachea where tracheal rings and the carina may be seen. Transillumination of the larynx and trachea provides external confirmation of placement. The light is visible as a glow when the tip passes the glottis. The glow is not visible with the tip in the esophagus. The fiberscope positioned in the trachea acts as a guide for the nasotracheal tube, which is now advanced through the larynx into the trachea. Endobronchial intubation is avoided if visualization of the carina is maintained. The endotracheal tube is held in place as the fiberscope is withdrawn. The fiberscope may be used for oral intubation.

Catheter-guided Intubation

Another technique for blind nasotracheal intubation is illustrated in Fig. 5-2.[37] This method is used when all other methods are predicted to be too difficult or too traumatic or impossible.[16] In the awake patient a topical anesthetic agent is injected into the trachea through the cricothyroid membrane after infiltration of the skin with local anesthetic. A Tuohy needle (17-gauge Huber point) is inserted into the tracheal lumen with its bevel pointing cephalad. A plastic epidural catheter is then advanced between the vocal cords into the pharynx (Fig. 5-2A).

Next, after spraying the nose with 4% co-caine to provide topical analgesia and to shrink the mucosa, a small rubber catheter is advanced to the nasopharynx. The patient is instructed to deliver the loops of the catheters from the mouth using the tongue (Fig. 5-2B). When both catheters are outside the mouth, the proximal end of the epidural catheter is tied to the distal end of the rubber catheter (Fig. 5-2C) so the epidural catheter can then be brought out of the nose (Fig. 5-2D). An endotracheal tube can now be threaded over the small, plastic epidural catheter and advanced into the trachea (Fig. 5-2E). When the tube is in the proximal trachea, the plastic tubing is cut near the skin overlying the cricothyroid membrane and removed from the lumen of the nasotracheal tube at its connector end (Fig. 5-2F). The endotracheal tube is simultaneously advanced a few centimeters into the trachea, and the cuff is inflated.

Maxillofacial Trauma

When inserting endotracheal tubes in patients having maxillofacial injuries, particular care must be taken that bone fragments of either the maxilla or mandible which contain teeth are not further dislodged. The teeth may remain viable after jaw reconstruction if the tooth-bearing bones are not further dislocated. To protect these, a tracheostomy may be performed first unless orotracheal intubation is needed for immediate resuscitative efforts.

For the patient who has had trauma to the face, neck, or chest, for whom there is no clear indication for tracheostomy, the anesthesiologist should consider leaving the endotracheal tube in place until the patient is sufficiently wide awake postoperatively to maintain his or her own airway. Even though the endotracheal tube is not removed until the patient is awake and responsive, the one removing the tube should be prepared to replace it or to perform a tracheostomy should the patient manifest airway obstruction. The pres-

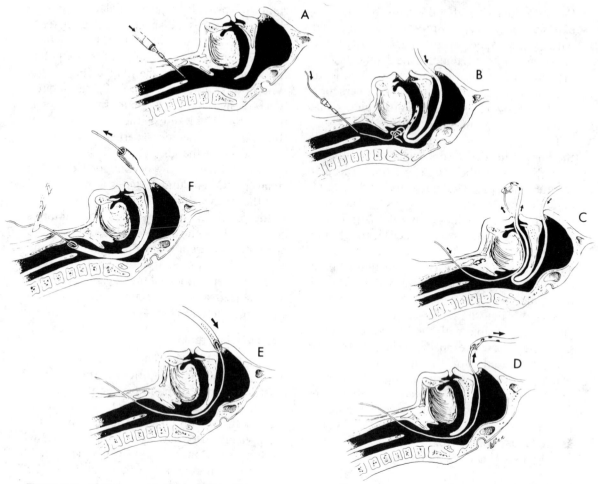

Figure 5-2 Catheter-guided nasotracheal intubation. See text for explanation. (From G. Lopez and N. R. James.[37])

ence of the tube in the trachea does not diminish the responsibility for vigilance in its care. If an endotracheal tube is to remain in place for a prolonged period, adequate humidification is imperative to prevent inspissation of secretions and airway obstruction. Saline 2 to 5 ml should be instilled prior to periodic suctioning using sterile technique. Manual sighs equal to 5 times tidal volume should be delivered at hourly intervals following suctioning. Chest physiotherapy consisting of postural drainage, percussion, and vibration performed at intervals will prevent atelectasis. Bronchodilator drugs may be aerosolized as needed. Managed in this way, endotracheal tubes may stay patent and trouble-free indefinitely.

Airway Trauma

Bronchoscopy is often necessary in patients with suspected airway injury. A potent inhalational agent delivered in oxygen with the patient breathing spontaneously is probably safest. Paralyzing the patient would require the use of positive pressure ventilation either by means of a ventilating bronchoscope or a jet injection ventilator.[32] If the airway is truly torn, the risk of mediastinal or subcutaneous emphysema is great with positive pressure ventilation. In the presence of mediastinal emphysema, nitrous oxide should not be given, as it will dramatically expand the volume of gas in the tissues. A ventilating broncho-scope may be used with the spontaneous respirations. The fresh gas delivery tube is attached to the side arm with an appropriate adaptor to deliver high flows (6 to 10 L/min) of oxygen and halothane.

Double-lumen tubes (Robertshaw) may be used to isolate the injured segment during surgery in order to allow use of relaxants and intermittent positive pressure breathing during thoracotomy. This may be especially necessary with a large bronchopleural fistulae, tracheoesophageal fistulae, and open chest wall injuries.

Extubation

The anesthesiologist should be certain at the end of the reparative procedure that no foreign bodies remain anywhere in the respiratory tract. Particularly for patients with maxillofacial injuries and missing teeth, a search of the hypopharynx and nasopharynx may recover one or more teeth. If the breath sounds are not clear on auscultating the chest, indication exists for radiographic studies in search of foreign bodies which may require bronchoscopic removal. One should leave the tube in place until the patient is fully awake, has reflex control, and has finished whatever reflex vomiting will be done on emergence. Vigilance combined with careful technique can provide safety for the patient who has a compromised airway but must be anesthetized.

Chest Trauma and Associated Injuries

Thirty-seven percent of motor vehicle accident victims have thoracic and thoracic spine injuries. Possible injuries include fractured sternum and ribs, flail chest, tension pneumothorax, lung contusion, major vascular tears, myocardial contusion, ruptured diaphragm, and bronchial tear. In one study the diagnosis of flail chest was missed in 25 of 180 cases.[13] Most of these patients had multiple organ injuries.

Chest injuries may be classified as mild, moderate, or severe. Mild injuries include one or two fractured ribs. These patients can breathe and cough adequately and have no ventilatory impairment. They need only pain relief. Those patients with moderate injury cannot handle secretions and have altered arterial blood gases, even with adequate pain relief. They need intubation or tracheostomy. Patients with severe injury cannot ventilate adequately even with a tracheostomy. They may have a flail chest or contused lung and require intermittent positive pressure breathing (IPPB) or even continuous positive pressure breathing. Lung contusion has been estimated to occur in 70 to 75 percent of major chest trauma. In one study, 45 of 180 cases of flail chest had lung contusion. The incidence is highest with crush injuries.[13]

Characteristically, the patient with a flail chest as a result of trauma has associated injuries which require priority surgical treatment. Endotracheal intubation and controlled ventilation plus chest tubes, if needed for control of pneumothorax and/or hemothorax, should be sufficient to stabilize the chest and restore respiratory dynamics while making the surgical approach to other emergency trauma, such as bleeding intraabdominal injuries.

Of special concern to the anesthesiologists is the occasional emergency patient who is using accessory muscles of respiration prior to the beginning of anesthesia. The accessory respiratory muscles are active when there is partial airway obstruction, such as by external pressure of a hematoma or internal pressure from damaged tissue or foreign bodies in any part of the airway. The accessory muscles of respiration may be considered volitional. A patient who is using these muscles to breathe will become completely apneic when sedated or when any form of general anesthesia is started. Apnea at the beginning of anesthesia, when sensory reflexes have not been obtunded and airway anatomy is distorted, will pose problems to the anesthesiologist attempting to establish an airway.

PAST MEDICAL HISTORY AND DRUG THERAPY

Depending upon the severity of the injury, the reliability of the patient, and the urgency for beginning a corrective operation, a history of preexisting diseases, allergies, or the nature of chronic drug therapy may be difficult to obtain. The presence of preexisting illness adversely influences the prognosis of injuries. The mortality following trauma is highest in patients with preexisting cardiovascular, central nervous system, and hematologic diseases.[25]

A careful history and physical examination should reveal preexisting diseases of the respiratory system, cardiovascular system, endocrine system, liver, and kidneys. Special attention should be paid to the detection of such disease entities as diabetes mellitus, hyperthyroidism, emphysema, asthma, coronary artery disease, treated hypertension, cirrhosis, and chronic renal failure. One should also have a history of allergies and chronic drug therapy. Patients in shock may not produce a wheal response to skin testing with tetanus antitoxin, although they may be highly allergic. When taking the history, emphasis should be placed on chronic therapy with antihypertensives, such as reserpine and guanethidine; diuretics, such as chlorothiazide and its analogues; tranquilizers, especially the phenothiazine family of drugs; steroids; and antibiotics.

Previous therapy with cardiac drugs such as quinidine and digitalis may be the only overt indication of an otherwise unknown cardiac disease and may alter a patient's response to anesthesia.

THE TIME OF THE LAST MEAL

The problem of the nonemptied stomach in the emergency patient deserves emphasis because aspiration pneumonitis remains a major cause of anesthetic morbidity and mortality. Since gastrointestinal motility ceases under the stimulus of either somatic or visceral pain or as the result of hypotension, the stomach is not likely to empty normally by propelling food through the pylorus, even if the operative procedure is delayed. Patients who have sustained injury within 1 or 2 h of eating will still have a full stomach 8 to 10 h later unless they have actively vomited. Consequently, in considering the problem of the full stomach, the interval between the last meal and the time of accident is more important than the interval between the last meal and the induction of anesthesia.[42]

One must decide which to do first: empty the stomach or insert an endotracheal tube. Both decisions carry possible disadvantages. One method is to introduce orally a large gastric tube, No. 34 French, with an inflatable esophageal cuff. This tube, or a similar cuffed double-lumen tube, will allow for gastric lavage and may prevent the active regurgitation of stomach contents around the tube and into the pharynx. Drawbacks to this approach include: lack of skill and experience on the part of the physician or nurse introducing this large tube, possible damage to the esophagus, violent retching by the patient. Retching is particularly undesirable in patients with abdominal visceral injuries, for extensive peritoneal contamination may occur, or in patients with penetrating eye injuries, for the vitreous may be extruded. Premature ventricular contractions may occur on inflation of the esophageal cuff.

A sump-type nasogastric tube should be inserted prior to induction of anesthesia in all trauma patients. Although this tube is not usually effective in removing large food particles, it will relieve gastric distention caused by fluids or swallowed air provided that it has not been clamped off after its insertion. Unless the stomach is decompressed, the patient will regurgitate when anesthesia is induced, seriously obstructing the airway at a time when it is difficult to cleanse the pharynx without stimulating reflexes such as laryngospasm, breath holding, and coughing. Simple introduction of a tube into the stomach is an occasional cause of gastric dilatation if the tube is clamped immediately after insertion. The conscious patient does not become acclimatized to the nasogastric tube readily; so in response to the foreign body in the pharynx, the patient may involuntarily swallow air around the tube. If the tube is clamped, the stomach may become quite distended.

Unless the patient vomits or is in a state of shock, the superior esophageal sphincter usually prevents contents from gaining access to the hypopharynx. The presence of a nasogastric tube is said to interfere with the integrity of the cardiac sphincter. Consequently, a gastric tube may serve as a wick around which stomach contents may flow into the hypopharynx undetected by the patient. The proximity of a stomach tube to the posterior aspect of the arytenoids obtunds laryngeal sensitivity, so that the patient may be unaware of aspirating small quantities of thin secretions from the pharynx.

It is axiomatic that the patient who has anything in the stomach will vomit upon awakening from anesthesia. The anesthesiologist must maintain airway control until this episode of vomiting has taken place postoperatively. Usually this is done by leaving the cuffed endotracheal tube in place until the patient is fully awake.

The use of antacids prior to induction of anesthesia raises the pH of gastric contents and renders them less harmful in the event of aspiration. Milk of magnesia mixes quickly with stomach contents, promptly neutralizes the acid, and is probably preferred for this purpose. No antacid should be given to a patient who is suspected of having a perforating injury of the gastrointestinal tract.

ASPIRATION SEQUELAE

Aspiration of acid gastric contents (pH of 2 or lower) into the trachea may set up a bronchospasm of such severity that effective ventilation cannot be accomplished, even with high inspiratory pressures applied to the breathing bag. If aspiration has occurred, tracheobronchial cleansing can be accomplished by suctioning through the endotracheal tube while the operative procedure is continuing. In repeated sequences, the patient should have assisted ventilation with 100% oxygen, instillation of 2 to 5 ml of isotonic saline solution through the endotracheal tube, positive pressure ventilation again for a few breaths, and suction by a catheter introduced through the endotracheal tube. For such a complication the anesthesiologist cannot be overly conscientious in attempting to cleanse the tracheobronchial tree. Care must be exercised, however, since hypoxia may be produced by suctioning for periods of more than 10 to 15 s. The lungs should be inflated again several times with oxygen before the next suctioning. Positive pressure ventilation should be continued, and consideration should be given to the administration of 30 mg/kg methylprednisolone sodium succinate or its equivalent intravenously to suppress the mucosal inflammatory response.

INTOXICATION

All too commonly, when brought to the hospital the traumatized patient is inebriated, engorged, and in shock. Two aspects of this triad have been discussed. The third, inebriation, is no less important. More than half of the trauma in this country (motor vehicle accidents) directly involves intoxicated drivers.[47,59] One study of drinking drivers revealed that 21 percent had been simultaneous users of other drugs.[28] The acutely intoxicated patient is pharmacologically modified by a potent respiratory, cardiovascular, and central nervous system depressant. The patient may also be the victim of widespread pathology in numerous organ systems as the result of chronic alcoholism. Ethanol intoxication not only increases the incidence of traumatic injuries, but also may influence the type of complication. For example, in a series of 575 traumatized patients, Lee found that the incidence of preoperative respiratory complications correlated with blood alcohol level.[36] His data suggested, however, that if the patient reaches the operating room alive for definitive surgery, mortality and morbidity are not adversely influenced by the intoxicated state.

No set procedure exists for coping with the problems of the inebriated patient who is scheduled for an emergency definitive surgical procedure; however, a number of useful guidelines can be recommended for the patient acutely intoxicated with drugs or alcohol.[60]

1 Because of the decreased ability of intoxicated patients to withstand hemorrhage, blood replacement therapy should probably be instituted earlier than in the nonintoxicated patient.
2 Because the chronic alcoholic may actually be isoosmotically overhydrated, fluid therapy must be planned with care.
3 Because of the tendency to hypoglyce-

mia, glucose should be added to the fluid management regimen.
4 Because of the enzyme induction effect of chronic ethanol ingestion, anesthetic agents that are in part metabolized (methoxyflurane, halothane, fluroxene) are perhaps best avoided. Increased biotransformation of inhalation anesthetic agents appears to be associated with their toxicity.
5 Because ethanol is a central nervous system depressant and tends to induce a lack of recall, supplementation of the nitrous oxide–relaxant technique with narcotics or other depressant drugs should be reduced or eliminated in the acutely intoxicated patient.
6 Because acutely intoxicated individuals are more prone to hypothermia, their core temperature should be monitored intraoperatively. All intravenous fluids should be warmed and a warming blanket should be employed, if necessary, to maintain body temperature.

POSTOPERATIVE CARE

The effects of massive trauma may not all be apparent at the same time. Following the successful definitive operative correction of injuries in one or more areas, the patient must be closely observed for evidences of occult damage in other sites or for progressive neurocardiorespiratory deterioration.

Gentleness and care must be exercised in moving the patient from the operating table to the recovery cart. A patient with a precariously maintained blood pressure can be thrown into a severe state of hypotension if roughly handled in transportation. Continued hemorrhage may be the reason for the redevelopment of shock postoperatively, depending upon the nature of the patient's injury and the magnitude of the operative procedure. Those caring for the patient in the postoperative period should be aware of the cardinal signs of hypovolemic hypotension. The dosage of sedatives or analgesics should be adjusted for the patient whose vital signs are not well stabilized.

The usual principles of recovery room care must be applied. These include oxygen and mist by mask for 2 to 6 h; periodic use of IPPB with wetting agents and bronchodilators; frequent turning; monitoring vital signs; recording intake and output; noting progressive emergence; and assessing blood loss. Delayed emergence from anesthesia may result from many conditions, including head or spinal cord injury, cerebral damage from shock or hypoxia, residual anesthetic or relaxant activity, myasthenia gravis or myasthenic syndrome, hypothyroidism, hypoglycemia, hypothermia, and persistent narcosis with alcohol. Uncommon causes for failure to awaken include sickle-cell crisis, intermittent porphyria, severe metabolic acidosis of methyl alcohol intoxication, and hyperosmolar nonketotic coma.

Hypoventilation in the postoperative period is difficult to assess and diagnose clinically. Its detection depends on an alert nurse and a suspicious, attentive physician. Its cause can be one or a combination of several perplexing conditions. A list of the reasons for hypoventilation includes most of those in the differential diagnosis of delayed emergence from anesthesia plus anesthetic overdosage or idiosyncrasy; relaxant overdosage or idiosyncrasy; overdosage of narcotics given for postoperative pain relief; endocrinopathies, including myasthenia gravis and hypothyroidism; fluid overload; shock; intraperitoneal antibiotics such as neomycin or streptomycin; upper and/or lower airway obstruction; respiratory restriction by dressings or casts; pneumothorax or hemothorax; abdominal distention; and pain.

An informed suspicion may lead to the early diagnosis of hypoventilation since the classical syndrome of hypoventilation appears late and may be masked. Signs include restlessness, auditory and/or visual evidences of airway obstruction, air hunger, disorientation or stupor, diminution of respiration (volume and/or frequency), hypertension which progresses to hypotension, tachycardia changing to bradycardia, and pallor or cyanosis. Chest roentgenograms may show atelectasis, pneumonitis, pneumothorax, or hemothorax. Spirometer measurements will confirm diminished tidal ventilation. Arterial blood gas analysis will show hypercarbia, acidosis, and arterial unsaturation.

The proper treatment of hypoventilation is directed primarily at ventilatory support with a mechanical respirator. Other measures will be indicated, depending upon the suspected diagnosis. Atropine and neostigmine to reverse curare effects; naloxone or levallorphan to reverse narcotics; and analeptics all are useful but must be secondary to good ventilatory support.

SECONDARY SURGERY IN TRAUMA

Having survived the initial traumatic episode and the early surgical care, many patients must face one or more secondary procedures for staged correction of cosmetic defects, bowel surgery, or neurological explorations. They may have fluid and electrolyte disturbances, acid-base imbalance, and weight loss. On these occasions dangerous arrhythmias including cardiac arrest have been reported following succinylcholine. Belin and Karleen[10] noted that patients receiving succinylcholine for dressing of burns around the sixth week after injury were particularly liable to develop a severe arrhythmia. A dramatic rise in serum potassium was thought to be the precipitating cause. Birch et al.[12] have convincingly shown that serum potassium increases from normal to as high as 15 meq/L in crush injuries when given succinylcholine from 10 to 120 days after injury. Another occasion in which serum potassium dramatically rises is in patients with paraplegic injury.[55] Succinylcholine should be avoided and other relaxants selected as anesthetic adjuncts during the hazardous interval for trauma patients having secondary operations. Small doses of a nondepolarizing muscle relaxant given IV 3 min before the succinylcholine may modify the release of potassium and help prevent arrhythmias,[12] although evidence to the contrary exists.[33] Premedication with magnesium sulfate 1 to 2 qIM has also been reported to abolish the hyperkalemic response to succinylcholine.[2]

BIBLIOGRAPHY

1 Adams, R. W., G. A. Gronert, T. M. Sundt, and J. D. Michenfelfer: Halothane hypocapnia and cerebrospinal fluid pressure in neurosurgery, *Anesthesiology,* 37:510, 1972.

2 Aldrete, J. A., A. Zahler, and J. K. Aikawa: Prevention of succinylcholine induced hyperkalemia by magnesium sulfate, *Can. Anaesth. Soc. J.,* 17:477, 1970.

3 Anonymous: Administration of crystalloids in shock and surgical trauma, *Lancet,* 1:1298, 1969.

4 Anonymous: Pollution in the operating theatre, *Br. Med. J.,* 2:123, 1972.

5 Ballinger, W. F., R. B. Rutherford, and G. D. Zuidema: *The Management of Trauma.* W. B. Saunders Company, Philadelphia, 1973.

6 Barcenas, C. G., T. J. Fuller, and J. P. Knochel: Metabolic alkalosis after massive blood transfusion, *J. Am. Med. Assoc.,* 236:953, 1976.

7 Baxter, C. R. W. H. Zedlitz, and G. T. Shires: High output acute renal failure complicating traumatic injury, *J. Trauma,* 4:567, 1964.

8 ——— and D. R. Maynard: Prevention and recognition of surgical renal complications, *Clin. Anesth.,* 3:322, 1968.

9 Bedford, R. F. and H. Wollman: Complications of percutaneous radial-artery cannulation, *Anesthesiology,* 38:228, 1973.

10 Belin, R. P. and C. I. Karleen: Cardiac arrest in the burned patient following succinyldicholine administration, *Anesthesiology,* 27:516, 1966.

11 Bendixin, H. H. and K. Suwa: "The Ventilation Requirement," in T. C. Gray and J. F. Nunn, *General Anesthesia,* 3d ed., Appleton-Century-Crofts, New York, 1971.

12 Birch, A. A., G. D. Mitchell, G. A. Playford, and G. A. Lang: Changes in serum potassium response to succinylcholine following trauma, *J. Am. Med. Assoc.,* 210:490, 1969.

13 Blair, E., C. Tapuzlu, and J. H. Davis: Delayed or missed diagnosis in blunt chest trauma, *J. Trauma,* 11:129, 1971.

14 Blatcher, R. S.: On awakening paralyzed during surgery, *J. Am. Med. Assoc.,* 234:67, 1975.

15 Blitt, C. D., W. A. Wright, W. C. Petty, and T. A. Webster: Central venous catheterization via the external jugular vein, a technique employing the J-wire, *J. Am. Med. Assoc.,* 229:817, 1974.

16 Bourke, D. and P. LeVesque: Modification of retrograde guide for endotracheal intubation, *Anesth. Analg.,* 53:1013, 1974.

17 Bridenbaugh, P. O., R. I. Balfour, D. C. Moore, and L. D. Bridenbaugh: Limitations of lactated Ringer's solution in massive fluid replacement, *J. Am. Med. Assoc.,* 206:2313, 1968.

18 Bultitude, M. I., J. M. Wellwood, and R. P. Hollingsworth: Intravenous diazepam: Its use in the reduction of fractures of the lower end of the radius, *Injury,* 3:249, 1972.

19 Butcher, H. R. and A. Braitberg: Hemorrhagic shock in rats: A method of therapeutic bioassay, *Arch. Surg.,* 98:685, 1969.

20 Carey, J. S., R. S. Brown, N. W. Woodward, S. T. Yao, and W. C. Shoemaker: Comparison of hemodynamic responses to whole blood plasma expanders in clinical traumatic shock, *Surg. Gynecol. Obstet.,* 121:1059, 1965.

21 ———, B. D. Lowery, and C. T. Cloutier: "Hemorrhagic Shock," in *Current Problems in Surgery,* Year Book Medical Publishers, Inc., Chicago, 1971.

22 Carson, I. W., J. Moore, J. P. Balmer, J. W. Dundee, and T. G. McNabb: Laryngeal competence with ketamine and other drugs, *Anesthesiology,* 38:128, 1973.

23 Cervera, A. L. and G. Moss: Crystalloid distribution following hemorrhage and hemodilution, *J. Trauma,* 14:506, 1974.

24 Chambers, A. A.: Traumatic aortic rupture, *J. Am. Med. Assoc.,* **229**:463, 1974.

25 Crighton, H. C. and A. H. Giesecke: One year's experience in the anesthetic management of trauma, *Anesth. Analg.,* **45**:835, 1966.

26 Downs, J. B., A. D. Rackstein, E. F. Klein, Jr., and I. F. Hawkins, Jr.: Hazards of radial-artery catheterization, *Anesthesiology,* **38**:283, 1973.

27 Dundee, J. W.: Comparative analysis of intravenous anesthetics, *Anesthesiology,* **35**:137, 1971.

28 Finkle, B. S., A. A. Biasotti, and L. W. Bradford: Occurrence of some drugs and toxic agents encountered in drinking driver investigations, *J. Forensic Sci.,* **13**:236, 1968.

29 Gardner, A. E., F. J. Dannemiller, and D. Dean: Intracranial pressure in man during ketamine anesthesia, *Anesth. Analg.,* **51**:741, 1972.

30 Giesecke, A. H., R. M. H. Hodgson, and P. P. Raj: Anesthesia for severely injured patients, *Orthop. Clin. North. Am.,* **1**:21, 1970.

31 ——— and J. F. Lee: Anesthetic management of the severely traumatized patient, *J. Okla. State Med. Assoc.,* **69**:464, 1969.

32 ———, H. U. Gerbershagen, C. Dortman, and D. Lee: Comparison of the ventilating and injection bronchoscopes, *Anesthesiology,* **38**:298, 1973.

33 Gronert, G. A.: Potassium response to succinylcholine, *J. Am. Med. Assoc.,* **212**:300, 1970.

34 Jenkins, M. T. and A. H. Giesecke: Fluid therapy in the traumatized patient, *Clin. Anesth.,* **11**:57, 1976.

35 Kelman, G. R. and B. R. Kennedy: Cardiovascular effects of pancuronium in man, *Br. J. Anaesth.,* **43**:335, 1971.

36 Lee, J. F., R. J. Samuelson, T. D. Watson, and A. H. Giesecke: Anesthesia for trauma: Is blood alcohol a factor? *Tex. Med.,* **70**:84, 1974.

37 Lopez, G. and N. R. James: Mechanical problems of the airway, *Clin. Anesth.,* **3**:8, 1968.

38 McDowell, S. A. and J. W. Dundee: Neuroleptanesthesia: A comparison with a conventional technique for major surgery, *Can. Anaesth. Soc. J.,* **18**:541, 1971.

39 McCullough, J., H. F. Polesky, C. Nelson, and T. Hoff: Iatrogenic hemolysis, a complication of blood warmed by a microwave device, *Anesth. Analg.,* **51**:102, 1972.

40 Miller, R. D.: Complications of massive blood transfusions, *Anesthesiology,* **39**:82, 1973.

41 Moore, F. D. and G. T. Shires: Moderation, *Ann. Surg.,* **166**:300, 1967.

42 Morris, R. E. and G. W. Miller: Preoperative management of the full stomach, *Clin. Anesth.,* **11**:25, 1976.

43 Moss, G. S.: Fluid distribution in prevention of hypovolemic shock, *Arch. Surg.,* **98**:281, 1969.

44 Novak, E., S. S. Stubbs, C. E. Seckman, and M. S. Hearron: Effects of a single large intravenous dose of methylprednisolone sodium succinate, *Clin. Pharmacol. Ther.,* **11**:711, 1970.

45 Raj, P. P., J. Forestner, T. D. Watson, R. E. Morris, and M. T. Jenkins: Technics for fiberoptic laryngoscopy in anesthesia, *Anesth. Analg.,* **53**:708, 1974.

46 Roth, E., L. C. Lax, and J. V. Maloney: Ringer's lactate solution and extracellular fluid volume in the surgical patient: A critical analysis, *Ann. Surg.,* **169**:149, 1969.

47 Rubin, E. and C. S. Lieber: Alcoholism, alcohol and drugs, *Science,* **172**:1097, 1971.

48 Rubsamen, D. S.: Head injury with unsuspected cervical fracture, a malpractice trap for the unwary physician, *J. Am. Med. Assoc.,* **229**:576, 1974.

49 Rush, B. F. and P. Bosomworth: Buffered saline solutions: A definition of moderation, *Surgery,* **66**:461, 1969.

50 ———, J. B. Richardson, P. Bosomworth, and B. Eiseman: Limitations of blood replacement with electrolyte solutions, *Arch. Surg.,* **98**:49, 1969.

51 ——— and R. Morehouse: Volume replacement following acute bleeding compared to replacement after hemorrhagic shock, effectiveness of dextran and buffered saline, *Surgery,* **62**:88, 1967.

52 Saltz, J. J.: Shock and the extracellular fluid space, *Am. J. Surg.,* **117**:603, 1969.

53 Shires, G. T., J. N. Cunningham, C. R. F. Baker, S. F. Reeder, H. Ilner, I. Y. Wagner, and J. Maher: Alterations in cellular membrane function during hemorrhagic shock in primates, *Ann. Surg.,* **176**:288, 1972.

54 Thompson, J. E., L. H. Hollier, R. D. Patman, and A. V. Persson: Surgical management of

abdominal aortic aneurysms, *Ann. Surg.,* **181**: 654, 1975.

55 Tobey, R. E.: Paraplegia, succinylcholine and cardiac arrest, *Anesthesiology,* **32**:359, 1970.

56 Tovee, E. B.: Blunt abdominal trauma, *J. Trauma,* **10**:72, 1970.

57 Trowbridge, A. M. and A. H. Giesecke: Multiple injuries, *Clin. Anesth.,* **11**:79, 1976.

58 Trudnowski, R. J.: Hydration with Ringer's lactate solution, *J. Am. Med. Assoc.,* **195**:545, 1966.

59 Waller, J. A.: Holiday drinking and highway fatalities, *J. Am. Med. Assoc.,* **206**:2693, 1968.

60 Watson, T. D. and J. F. Lee: Intoxication and trauma, *Clin. Anesth.,* **11**:31, 1976.

61 Webre, D. R. and J. F. Arens: Use of cephalic and basilic veins for introduction of central venous catheters, *Anesthesiology,* **38**:389, 1973.

62 Wheatley, R. G., F. T. Kallus, R. C. Reynolds, and A. H. Giesecke: Milk of magnesia is an effective preinduction antacid in obstetrical anesthesia, in preparation.

Chapter 6

Surgical Infections in Trauma Patients: Management and Prevention

Peter Dineen, M.D.

INTRODUCTION

Clinical infection in any patient is dependent on two factors. The first is the nature of the invading agent; the second is defense mechanisms of the host. The prevention and management of surgical infections in trauma patients is dependent on inhibiting the former and bolstering the latter.

Obviously one of the most important aspects of the management of infection is the appropriate use of antimicrobial agents. Much has been written about the use of prohylactic antibiotics. However, strictly speaking, prophylaxis implies the delivery of antimicrobial agents to the tissue before the bacteria have arrived on the scene. This situation, for all practical purposes, never occurs in the trauma patient; so in actuality one is in a position of using antimicrobial agents from a therapeutic rather than a prophylactic standpoint from the beginning.

Some of the basic principles involved in the management of the bacterial complications of trauma should be discussed first.[6] One of the most important factors in the problem of infection is the nature of the parasite. Pathogenic bacteria may be classified by the degree of invasiveness. This may be considered as a spectrum. At one end there is botulism, a disease caused entirely by the toxin of the *Clostridium botulinum,* in which the parasite does not even enter the host. Next in line is *Clostridium tetani,* which causes disease by a small nidus of infection in the host which elaborates large quantities of toxin. Those organisms which reside in the gastrointestinal tract are for convenience's sake lumped under the title of the enteric group of organisms.

These include gram-negative organisms such as the enterobacteriaceae, pseudomonas, proteus, aerobic and anaerobic bacteroids, streptococci, and clostridia. This group of organisms as a whole are able to invade devitalized tissue, but usually are limited to that area by the host defenses. For the most part they have no active proteolytic enzymes of their own in their more dormant state. Consequently, it is necessary for their survival in vivo to have a source of these enzymes. In necrotic tissue these are available from the autolysis of cells, particularly leukocytes. It is for this reason that infections caused by these organisms are seen in association with necrotic material. Also these organisms can obtain the needed enzymes when these infections are in association with staphylococci or streptococci. The latter organisms do possess the proteolytic enzymes.

Two of the most important organisms which are involved in infections are the *Staphylococcus aureus* and the beta-hemolytic streptococcus (group A). These two organisms rank high on the spectrum of invasiveness, and in the wake of their infection the enteric organisms may come.

The *S. aureus* is able to invade living tissue, to survive in living tissue, and even to destroy it. This is obviously a much more virulent opponent than the enteric organisms. The *S. aureus* is usually associated with a local inflammatory response and tends to stimulate the formation of a purulent exudate.

The group A streptococcus (beta-hemolytic type) is one of the most virulent of all organisms. It can invade and multiply in normal healthy tissue and is very little hampered by the host attempts to limit the area of infection. Within a very short period of time a few bacteria can cause an overwhelming infection.

From the above it is obvious that a knowledge of the various potentialities of the different microorganisms suggests which ones should be given the first priority in the matter of antimicrobial therapy.

Another important principle which must be considered is the response of the host to trauma and infection. When chemotherapy is started in the presence of an established infection, the drugs may be of little efficacy because they either cannot reach the organisms or the organisms are able to elaborate a protective enzyme. For example, this is seen when a well-established abscess with organization of the walls has occurred. However, in the case of a sudden trauma where organisms have recently been inoculated, there is no barrier to the drugs. Therefore while the bacteria are going through the lag phase in their growth curve (a matter of a few hours usually), adequate blood and tissue levels of chemotherapeutic agents can be obtained. It has been established experimentally and observed clinically that trauma or other stress per se has a deleterious effect on the host's ability to combat infection. Since it is known that trauma reduces the body's capacity to combat infection and since the parasite is not protected initially from the blood-borne drugs, early use of antimicrobial agents in trauma is definitely indicated.

The selection of appropriate antibiotic agents in any case of trauma is difficult. If one is to wait for the results of sensitivity testing, the time from the point of injury to the start of therapy is much too long. Therefore, the selection must be made on a clinical basis, and frequently this is to use one's best judgment and a knowledge of the source of contamination.

A wound classification[2] based on a clinical estimation of bacterial density, contamination, and risk of subsequent infection is contained in Table 6-1, which is now widely accepted as a standard classification of operative wounds. It is recommended for use in collating information concerning infections and relating them to sources of contamination and degree of risk to infection.

Therefore the management and prevention of infection related to trauma is dependent on

Table 6-1: Classification of Operative Wounds in Relation to Contamination and Increasing Risk of Infection

Clean

    Nontraumatic
    No inflammation encountered
    No break in technique
    Respiratory, alimentary, genitourinary tracts not entered

Clean-Contaminated

    Gastrointestinal or respiratory tracts entered without significant spillage
    Appendectomy
    Oropharynx entered
    Vagina entered
    Genitourinary tract entered in absence of infected urine
    Biliary tract entered in absence of infected bile
    Minor break in technique

Contaminated

    Major break in technique
    Gross spillage from gastrointestinal tract
    Traumatic wound, fresh
    Entrance of genitourinary or biliary tracts in presence of infected urine or bile

Dirty-Infected

    Acute bacterial inflammation encountered, without pus
    Transection of "clean" tissue for the purpose of surgical access to a collection of pus
    Perforated viscus encountered
    Traumatic wound with retained devitalized tissue, foreign bodies, fecal contamination and/or delayed treatment, or from dirty source

two principles: (1) to combat the invading organisms and (2) to strengthen host defense mechanisms. The latter are more appropriately discussed with the various trauma, but the general principle of locally debriding wounds to remove all foreign body, necrotic material, and hematoma is essential. The systemic management of shock and its concomitant effects on host defenses are mentioned earlier in this volume.

MINOR TRAUMA ASSOCIATED WITH SERIOUS INFECTIONS

In this group of infections the trauma associated with the introduction of the bacteria is usually quite minimal and the resulting infection is a serious one. These infections, to a very large extent, depend on the virulence of the organism and for the most part are associated with the group A beta-hemolytic streptococci and *S. aureus*. (Clostridial infections will be discussed separately.)

Streptococcal Infections

The vast majority of streptococcal infections are caused by the group A beta-hemolytic aerobic streptococci. A few are caused by viridans streptococci and some nonhemolytic and microaerophilic streptococci.

The characteristics of streptococcal infections are twofold: the rapid and virulent progression of the disease and its lack of localization. The primary manifestation is usually a diffuse inflammation characterized by cellulitis, lymphangitis, and, not infrequently, extension along fascial planes. The development of a purulent reaction on the part of the host is infrequent, and abscess formation is quite rare. Thin, watery pus and gangrene of the overlying skin are frequently seen. Bacteremia is common, and intravascular hemolysis is often seen as an accompaniment.

Cellulitis This occurs following small puncture wounds or superficial injuries and is characterized by local pain, redness, edema, and heat. The superficial lymphatics are the next area of spread.

Erysipelas This is an acute, spreading cellulitis and lymphangitis and is seen predominantly about the face and neck. It occurs following minor injury or a small break in the skin, and the incubation period is usually less than 24 h. The onset is abrupt, with the infected skin becoming fiery red, tender, and with swollen, raised, irregular margins. High fevers, prostration, chills, and tachycardia are frequently seen.

Lymphangitis This condition is associated with the development of red streaks, usually emerging from an area of cellulitis and running toward the local lymphatic bed. The lymph nodes in the drainage area are usually involved, so that with lymphangitis there is almost always a lymphadenitis.

Wound Infection Wound infections caused by the beta-hemolytic streptococcus is not common, but occasionally (in about 3 percent of cases) postoperative or posttraumatic wounds may become infected with this organism. The characteristic here is of a rapid onset, usually within 24 h, with shaking chills and high fever. Aspiration of the wound on Gram's stain will reveal gram-positive streptococci in chains. This is the one type of wound infection which does not usually result in the development of a purulent exudate.

Treatment The treatment of streptococcal infections is primarily by the use of antimicrobials (see Table 6-2). Since there is not the development of a necrotic central area and a purulent exudate, rapid treatment with appropriate agents will reverse the condition quite promptly. The use of penicillin in high doses intravenously is the treatment of choice, usually 2 to 6 million units per day intravenously, until all evidence of infection has been gone for a period of 48 h.

Staphylococcal Infections

These infections are usually localized, although the process may become invasive and may be associated with lymphangitis, lymphadenitis, or thrombophlebitis. The typical lesion demonstrates an area of cellulitis with a central area of necrosis or abscess formation which contains odorless, creamy pus. The symptoms include swelling, erythema, and local pain. The area is generally tender to palpation, and the pain may be throbbing and synchronous with the heartbeat. Folliculitis, furuncles, and carbuncles are local staphylococcal infections which are commonly seen and are usually a result of a very minor trauma to the skin. The management of these is essentially incision and drainage, and antibiotics are used only when there is a specific indication of spread beyond the localized area.

Acute Streptococcal Gangrene

This relatively uncommon infection may be confused with several others. Nevertheless it appears to be a distinct entity. Hemolytic streptococci are usually obtained in pure culture.

Typically, there is a history of relatively minor trauma such as a puncture wound or an insect bite. Most commonly this occurs on an extremity. The systemic response is usually

Table 6-2: Summary of the Major Surgical Infections

Infection	Cause	Rate of spread	Clinical features	Primary treatment
Cellulitis	Streptococcus	Hours	Redness, edema, pain	Antibiotics
Erysipelas	Streptococcus	Hours	Redness, edema, pain raised irregular margin	Antibiotics
Lymphangitis	Streptococcus	Hours	Red streaks which follow lymphatics, lymphadenopathy	Antibiotics
Furuncles, carbuncles	Staphylococcus	Days	Pus formation	Incision and drainage
Streptococcal gangrene	Hemolytic streptococcus	Hours to days	Bleb formation and gangrene of the skin, dark serous drainage	Extensive incision and drainage beyond gangrenous areas (multiple, often)
Necrotizing fasciitis	Hemolytic streptococcus, hemolytic staphylococcus	Usually days	Necrotic fascia outstanding, cutaneous gangrene, extensive undermining, pus formation infrequent	Radical incision and drainage
Streptococcal myositis	Anaerobic streptococcus	Hours to days	Severe local pain, foul odor, edema, crepitation of muscle which is still viable	Incision and drainage, occasional excision of necrotic muscle
Progressive bacterial synergistic gangrene	Microaerophilic streptococcus, aerobic hemolytic staphylococcus	Days to weeks	Central necrosis, surrounding purple zone, outer zone of cellulitis	Wide excision and antibiotic, local and systemic

not severe, but there is tachycardia and temperature elevation.

The affected skin region is hot, red, edematous, and often quite painful. If there is no treatment, there is a development of a dusky hue over the skin after a few days, with the formation of blebs and devitalization of the skin. The treatment consists of emergency drainage with longitudinal incisions, thereby releasing skin tension and decreasing the ischemia. The incisions should extend beyond the obviously involved gangrenous area. This is done in conjunction with high-dose penicillin or erythromycin therapy, but it is essential to treat this infection promptly by surgical intervention so that there is a minimal loss of skin.

After incision and drainage through the superficial fascia, the wound is treated in the usual method by rest, elevation, and moist dressings (Fig. 6-1).

Necrotizing Fasciitis

This condition often follows tissue trauma, whether operative or external. It is often confused with acute streptococcal cutaneous gangrene, and indeed there may be some overlap. Therefore, once the diagnosis of streptococcal cutaneous gangrene has been made, it is obligatory to make the incisions down to the superficial fascia and inspect it thoroughly.

The prime lesion in necrotizing fasciitis is

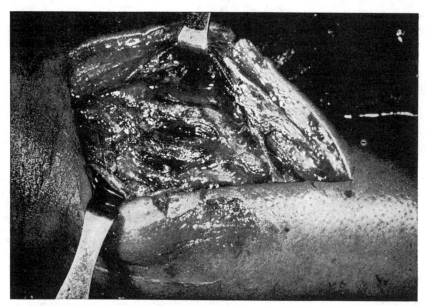

Figure 6-1 Wide local incision and drainage of deep dissecting abscess. Note that glistening viable tissue remains.

the necrosis of the superficial fascia. This is usually caused by the hemolytic streptococcus, but occasionally can be caused by hemolytic staphylococci (Fig. 6-2). Necrotizing fasciitis is characterized by an undermining of an area of cutaneous gangrene, or there may be no evidence of gangrene at all. The liquefaction of the subcutaneous fat is profound, and the fascia is swollen, stringy, and necrotic. The involvement of the fascia extends or undermines considerably farther than the skin or subcutaneous involvement which may be present (Fig. 6-3). Pus formation is infrequent, but there is a serosanguineous exudate.

The treatment consists of radical and extensive incisions past the areas of skin and subcutaneous involvement until a good normal fascia is obtained. As long as the fascia seems to give way to normal manipulations, the overlying skin and subcutaneous tissue must be incised. Not until normal, stout fascia has been observed at all limits of the incisions can the surgical treatment be considered adequate. Once the incisions have been performed, the

wounds should be held open loosely and local treatment with saline dressing should be initiated. The use of topical antimicrobial agents is probably of little value. Systemic antimicrobial agents should be used in high doses; from 2 to 6 million units IV per day of penicillin or one of the cephalosporins may be used. Lincomycin, clindamycin, chloramphenicol, and tetracycline should not be employed unless there is a specific indication. If the patient is allergic to penicillin, then the cephalosporins or erythromycin are probably the drugs of choice.

In necrotizing fasciitis it is frequently possible to save a great deal of skin which eventually can be put back down after the infection has been controlled. Therefore it is not necessary to excise viable skin if the disease is in the fascia. The fascia is the area that needs to be incised widely.

Streptococcal Myositis

This is a relatively rare, anaerobic streptococcal infection and progresses more slowly than

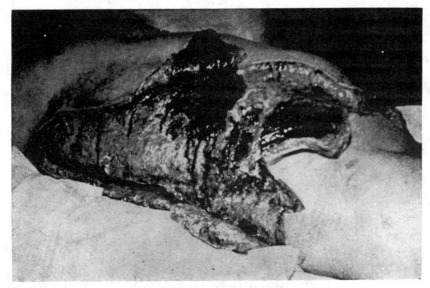

Figure 6-2   Necrotizing fasciitis, demonstrating marked undermining of tissues.

other streptococcal infections. It is characterized by severe local pain and generalized toxemia. It is difficult to distinguish from clostridial myositis, but Gram's stain should be done and will be helpful. The management consists of primary incision and drainage of the abscesses, fasciitis, and infected muscle groups. The treatment is essentially a radical surgical debridement. There is usually much less necrotic material than in clostridial myo-

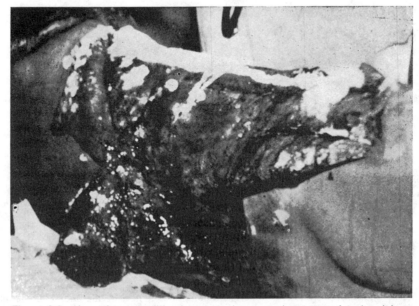

Figure 6-3   Necrotizing fasciitis, demonstrating posterior extent of undermining.

sitis. Antimicrobial therapy is indicated, usually high-dose penicillin or cephalothin. In this particular instance the antibiotics sensitivity tests are most helpful.

Progressive Bacterial Synergistis Gangrene (Meleney's Ulcer)

This infection is rarely seen now, but is usually a complicating factor in the operative treatment of purulent infections of the peritoneal cavity. It is caused by the synergistic action of a microaerophilic nonhemolytic streptococcus and an aerobic hemolytic *S. aureus.*

The disease is a relatively slow one in its development and progress. The surrounding skin about the ulcer becomes edematous, red, and usually tender. It usually becomes demarcated into three zones: the peripheral wide area of fiery red cellulitis, which is where the actual infection is progressing; the middle zone of purplish, tender skin (Fig. 6-4); and finally the central necrotic black area. Untreated, this can be a fatal disease. Recognition is extremely important because conserva-

tive and local debridement fail to halt the progressive infection. The synergistic action of the bacteria in the peripheral red zone is left untreated by central necrotic debridement. The treatment of choice is twofold. One is radical excision of all necrotic and undermined skin to an area which includes the red cellulitis area. Antibiotics, both local and parenteral, are important. It is in this disease state that bacitracin was first brought into use. Frequently the staphylococcus is penicillin-resistant, so that this is not the drug of choice. High doses of cephalothin or nafcillin are indicated. The local use of bacitracin solution is also indicated.

Human Bite Infections

Reasonable initial care is more effective in the prevention of this type of infection. Adequate excision of the wound as soon as the patient is seen, followed by copious irrigations with sterile saline solution, is the treatment of choice. The wound should be left open to allow adequate drainage. Only a rare wound

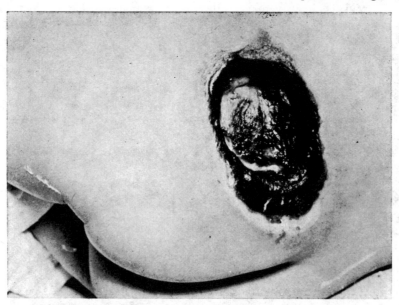

Figure 6-4 Progressive bacterial synergistic gangrene, demonstrating characteristic three zones of central necrosis, surrounding purple zone, and outer zone of cellulitis.

should be sutured for cosmetic purposes. Immobilization and antibiotic therapy (usually penicillin) are necessary adjuvants. If infection does develop, it is usually polymicrobic and consists of spirochetes, staphylococci, anaerobic streptococci, and gram-negative rods.

INFECTIONS FOLLOWING BLUNT TRAUMA

This includes infection which may follow any type of crushing or gross impact injury.[7] These would be seen in automobile injuries, etc. Microbial infection in impact and crushing injuries is of secondary importance to the original injury at the time of the occurrence. In a severe trauma such as an automobile injury there may be multiple injuries to the head, chest, and abdomen as well as fractures of the extremities and crush injuries. The surgeon's first concern is to maintain survival of the patient, and action is directed against stopping hemorrhage, restoring airway, and maintaining vital functions. Frequently, because of the severity of the injury, the host defense mechanisms are severely impaired, and the stage is set for subsequent serious infection if the patient lives. There are two possible sources of microbial contamination at this time. The first is from the bacteria resident in and on the host. These include bacteria of the gastrointestinal and respiratory tracts, which may find egress to a new environment from lacerations or disruptions of either tract. A very common example is an esophageal tear from a steering wheel injury. Microorganisms of the esophagus can enter the mediastinum and, frequently, the pleural cavity. Rupture of any hollow viscus in the abdomen is followed by bacterial seeding of the peritoneal cavity. Therefore, the first and most common method of developing infection secondary to blunt trauma is a break in the mucosal barrier, which gives bacteria ready access to the peritoneal or pleural cavities.

The second route by which bacteria can enter the tissues of the host and cause infection is by secondary invasion. The development of a large hematoma, hemothorax, or any area of impaired blood supply creates a favorable medium for bacterial growth. Microorganisms delivered to such areas either by lymphatics or bloodstream may then proliferate. A second source of bacterial contamination in crushing injuries is exogenous—the microorganisms of the environment in which the victim is found. Exogenous bacteria are usually not prime pathogens and cause disease only if the local wound is not properly treated.

An open fracture with a crushed extremity forms an ideal nidus for the development of serious infection. Bacteria resident on the skin (*S. aureus, S. epidermidis,* diphtheroids) and in the gastrointestinal tract and which could not multiply in normal healthy tissue begin to grow luxuriantly in such wounds. When proteolysis occurs, a reducing environment is achieved in necrotic tissue and hematomas. Then foreign bodies, such as bits of clothing or dirt, may also be present. In such circumstances even pathogens of low virulence may proliferate and cause a progressive infection to develop. The diagnosis and management of injuries of both intrathoracic and intraabdominal types are discussed in detail in other chapters in this volume. This section is confined to discussing the management of the established contamination and infection following perforation of a hollow viscus of the chest or abdomen or crush injury secondary to blunt trauma.

The treatment of gastrointestinal perforation requires prompt correction. The specific surgical procedure is dictated by the location of the defect. When the alimentary tract is perforated (and this includes the biliary tract as well), chemical peritonitis develops immediately. Edema of the bowel wall results and is associated with paralytic ileus; bacteria proliferate rapidly in the boggy bowel and then migrate through the bowel wall into the peritoneal cavity. The entire process requires about 12 to 24 h. Even if the original contamination was sterile, the peritoneal cavity soon becomes contaminated with microorganisms which migrate by this mechanism. Successful localization of infection from impact injury may not be manifest for a week or more after the original trauma, and it is an indication for surgical intervention. Empyemas must be drained, and intraabdominal abscesses must be evacuated.

When one is dealing with a crush injury of the extremities, it is absolutely essential that adequate and complete debridement and irrigation be carried out.

Antimicrobial therapy is indicated in the patient who sustains a crushing or gross impact injury. The rationale for the use of antimicrobial agents is not one of prophylaxis but of treatment. Whenever the skin barrier is broken by impact, there is bound to be gross contamination. Also, when the gastrointestinal tract has been broached, a similarly massive contamination has occurred. Even the best surgical debridement leaves some microorganisms behind. It is reasonable to attempt to eradicate such bacteria with parenterally administered antimicrobial agents. Early treatment, before proliferation can lead to additional tissue injury or abscess formation, is more likely to be effective than when treatment is delayed. Thus the initial selection of agents is based on clinical judgment. On the assumption that wounds may be contaminated with various kinds of streptococci, staphylococci, anaerobes, and enteric bacteria, a combination of penicillin 4 to 10 million units in divided doses per day intravenously and gentamicin 3.0 to 5.0 mg/kg of body weight per day given intramuscularly in divided doses is recommended. The gentamicin can be given intravenously if the patient is in shock. In several large series penicillin and tetracycline have proven effective.[1] Doxycycline can be used instead of tetracycline. Antimicrobial

therapy should be adjusted in the light of culture and susceptibility studies and in accordance with the patient's clinical state. It is desirable during all procedures in debridement, drainage, etc., to obtain material for culture and susceptibility testing so that this information will be available as soon as possible.

The prevention of infection in crushing and impact injuries depends on the adequacy of debridement of the wound, because the removal of all dead tissue, evacuation of hematomata, removal of foreign bodies, reestablishment of the blood supply, and obliteration of all dead spaces are necessary. Anesthesia and operating room facilities are almost always required.

INFECTIONS FOLLOWING PENETRATING INJURIES

Penetrating injuries may occur in any part of the body and are caused by a variety of agents, ranging from high-velocity bullets and shrapnel to such protean objects as knives, pins, splinters, and nails.[8] The common distinguishing features of penetrating injuries is the small area of laceration of the skin relative to the depth of the tract beneath. The true extent of the injury is very often completely masked. It is therefore essential to know the physical characteristics of the object that caused the wound.

The major differentiating feature of penetrating injuries is the extent of tissue injury that surrounds the tract of penetration. In general, this zone of injury reflects the quantity of kinetic energy delivered to the tissues. High-velocity agents are associated with zones of trauma much greater than the visible tract of the missile. It is of the utmost importance to regard the break in the skin as a view through a small end of a long cone. The entire length of the lesion must be evaluated, especially at the end distal to the initial penetration.

Many kinds of microorganisms cause infection following a penetrating injury. What is carried into the wound by the penetrating agent is important, as is the location of the wound and the organs that are perforated. Although almost any combination may occur, microorganisms from the gastrointestinal and respiratory tracts predominate.

The original injury may be as minor as a splinter through the skin or as severe as a knife wound of the abdomen. The basic problem is the same. The wounding agent inevitably causes tissue destruction, usually carries in some foreign matter, and is associated with some degree of bleeding in the tract of penetration. A culture medium suitable for microbial replication is established. With or without foreign matter, necrotic tissues and hematomas provide ideal conditions for growth. There is protection from phagocytes and humoral antibodies. Oxygen is depleted, and the growth of microaerophilic and anaerobic microorganisms is enhanced. When the penetrating wound enters the gastrointestinal tract, urinary tract, or respiratory tract, there is the serious further complication of contamination by microorganisms resident in the host.

Infections from penetrating wounds vary in manifestations according to the location of the injury. There are two broad types of infection. More immediately serious are those arising from lacerations of hollow viscera or the respiratory tract. These result in peritonitis or mediastinitis.

When the injury involves only soft tissues, several days may pass before the development of local pain, swelling, and tenderness. Fever, leukocytosis, lymphangitis, and septicemia may occur in more severe cases.

The diagnosis of infection from penetrating injuries is straightforward. The history of injury, the location of the wound, and the subsequent course are usually sufficient to make the diagnosis. However, there are occasions when this is not the case. Perforations with sharp, thin objects, especially when the patient has been under the influence of alcohol or other drugs, may go entirely unnoticed. The patient may subsequently have a high fever, leukocytosis, and very little in the way of localizing signs. This is common in rectal perforations resulting from implementation. A very careful history and thorough physical examination are essential.

Perforation of either the gastrointestinal or respiratory tract must be diagnosed quickly. When the trachea or the lung is injured, there are almost immediate signs of respiratory distress, with pneumothorax and mediastinal and subcutaneous emphysema developing quickly. Perforation of an abdominal hollow viscus may be less apparent during the first hour. Diagnosis may frequently be made by exploration of the tract under local anesthesia. Injection of radiopaque material in the tract has been utilized, but this has not proved very reliable. The latter has been less successful in our experience than local exploration of the tract. Diagnostic paracentesis is of great value, and is described elsewhere in this volume.

The basic treatment of penetrating wounds is surgical. The location of the wound and the degree of injury determine the extent of the surgical procedure. The objectives of the local surgical treatment are fourfold: (1) to stop hemorrhage and repair arteries and nerves; (2) to close all perforations; (3) to repair and reduce skeletal injury; and (4) to remove all necrotic tissue, hematomas, and foreign bodies. Debridement of a tract is often best accomplished by excising the tract in toto. Adequate drainage should be established, and most wounds should not be closed completely.

Despite the best debridement, microorganisms are left behind. For this reason, treatment with antimicrobial agents is recommended. The severity, location, and extent of the wound determines the kinds of agents and dosage that should be employed. Because it is unlikely that a clear-cut bacteriologic diagnosis will be available for at least 24 h, antimicrobial therapy is directed against group A *Streptococcus pyogenes,* anaerobic streptococci, enterococci, *S. aureus, Escherichia coli* and other enteric bacilli, and anaerobic organisms including clostridium. Penicillin G 5 to 12 million units intravenously per day plus gentamicin 3 to 5 mg/kg of body weight either intramuscularly or intravenously per day are the drugs most commonly used under these circumstances. An alternate and proven effective regimen is penicillin and tetracycline intravenously. The prevention of infection is important and depends on the care of the wound at the time of the original treatment. The skin around the penetrating wound should be carefully washed with a germicidal soap or detergent and then wet thoroughly with a germicidal solution. The nature of the surgical procedure then carried out is determined by the perforating wound or wounds. Perforating wounds of the peritoneum require a complete and thorough examination of the gastrointestinal tract.

The treatment of established infections from penetrating wounds is also essentially surgical. If the patient has survived such an injury and has not had peritonitis or empyema or meningitis, the patient may develop a local abscess in the tract of the penetration. Usually located at the depths of the penetration, such abscesses, like all others, require surgical drainage. Antimicrobial agents are not necessary unless there is evidence of dissemination under the latter circumstances.

CLOSTRIDIUM INFECTIONS

Gas Gangrene

Gas gangrene is a necrotizing infection of the soft tissue that occurs after trauma or surgery.[9] It is caused by several species of clostridium and is frequently fatal. The clostridium species most frequently associated with gas gangrene are the capsulated, nonmotile *Clostridium perfringens* and the noncapsulated

motile *Clostridium oedematiens, Clostridium septicum,* and *Clostridium histolyticum.* All are anaerobic, gram-positive bacilli that measure 0.5×1 to $5 \mu m$. As bacillary or vegetative forms, they are destroyed by a variety of chemical and physical agents; they are moderately susceptible to penicillin G and some other antimicrobial agents. It is also in the vegetative form that the powerful exotoxins (tissue necrosins and hemolysins) are liberated. One or more of the group normally inhabits the gastrointestinal and female genital tracts of humans and many nonhuman species. All clostridium organisms sporulate, producing a structure that is highly resistant to heat, cold, sunlight, drying, and many chemical agents. Spores are widely distributed in the environment and are especially prevalent in fertile soil. In wounds of violence, clostridium organisms capable of producing gas gangrene have been recovered in up to 40 percent of war wounds and 14.7 percent of civilian wounds. Nevertheless, the incidence of postoperative wounds and civilian trauma in which spores of gas gangrene bacteria enter wounds either from the soil or from the patient's own gastrointestinal tract is probably significantly higher. Clostridium infections cannot develop unless conditions within a wound are conducive to the germination of implanted spores. Foreign bodies and devitalized tissues are essential to the induction of anaerobic conditions. Once a suitable focus obtains, toxins formed by multiplying bacilli perpetuate and extend anaerobiosis by causing thrombosis in regional vessels and the necrosis of surrounding tissues. As the infection progresses, CO_2 and H_2 are liberated as metabolic byproducts and are readily palpable in the tissues. The combination of gas and local edema produces intense swelling. The infection spreads rapidly until an overwhelming sepsis occurs. The areas most frequently affected are the extremities, abdominal wounds, and the uterus. No organ or area is exempt however.

Disease states caused by infection with this

group of clostridia take one of three clinical forms: (1) anaerobic cellulitis, (2) anaerobic myositis (true gas gangrene), or (3) anaerobic puerperal sepsis (true uterine gangrene).

Of the three, anaerobic cellulitis is the least severe. Multiplication with the production of gas in the subcutaneous tissues results in the destruction of these tissues with rapid spread of the process. Some local pain, crepitation in the tissue, and moderate fever are common. Prostration and anuria, hemolysis and delirium are unusual. In persons debilitated from leukemia or metastatic carcinoma, clostridia, like other enteric bacteria, escape from the gut into the blood. If they lodge in the neoplastic tissues, a clostridial cellulitis may result.

True gas gangrene (anaerobic myositis) is an acute illness which has an abrupt onset and a rapid progression. This leads to early death if untreated. The time from the initial injury or surgery to the first symptom may actually be only 4 to 6 h. However, in most instances the onset of gas gangrene occurs within 72 h of the time of wounding or operation. The most consistent and obvious symptom is pain in the area of the wound. The severity of the pain is out of proportion to that normally found in an uninfected wound of identical extent. Tenderness or swelling of the area of the wound are also present, but usually there is no crepitation at this early stage (Fig. 6-5). Despite the relative paucity of local signs, toxemia and hypovolemia develop in the next few hours and give rise to tachycardia, hypotension, and rapid respiration. There is a moderate fever of 1 to 2°C. During the first 6 h, progressive edema of the wound area stretches the skin, which produces a tense, shiny, dusky appearance. Bullae form, and the skin around the wound becomes necrotic. The whole sequence may require less than 36 h until the skin ruptures, revealing pallid, necrotic muscle. One of the most unique and characteristic findings in true gas gangrene is the toxic delirium that appears quite early in the disease. Several hours before any changes are

visible in the wound area, the patient becomes incoherent, disoriented, and obstreperous. Restraints may be required to prevent the patient from getting out of bed. As the disease progresses, there is overwhelming prostration, toxemia, and, frequently, a bacteremia (Fig. 6-6).

Anaerobic puerperal sepsis is secondary to instrumentation of the genital tract and usually the result of attempts at criminal abortion. Prolonged labor, premature rupture of the membranes, and instrumentation are also predisposing events. The clinical course and findings are essentially those of anaerobic myositis, which are simply transposed to the uterus. There is a foul-smelling, watery discharge, extreme prostration, and marked intravascular hemolysis. This course is again characterized by sudden onset and rapid progression.

Because of the gravity of the illness and the fulminant course that may ensue, a working diagnosis must be made on clinical grounds. Treatment cannot be withheld pending laboratory verification of the diagnosis, although Gram's stain may be of immediate value. The essential clinical features include (1) kind and location of injury or operation (contamination with soil or feces is particularly important), (2) appearance of the wound (edema, discoloration, evidence of spreading, and discharge), (3) pain referred to the wound area (time of onset and severity), (4) affect of the patient (disorientation, delirium), and (5) crepitation. In anaerobic cellulitis, severity, extent, and speed of evolution of the manifestations are much less than in other forms of infection with clostridia.

Laboratory data are necessary, and specimens must be collected before therapy is undertaken. However, one should not wait to initiate therapy for the results of the laboratory tests. Early in the course of gas gangrene, there will be leukocytosis, gram-positive bacilli in smears of wound exudate, and roentgenographic evidence of gas in the tissues may

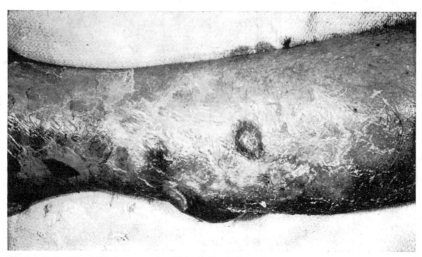

Figure 6-5 Clostridial gangrene. This patient demonstrated marked crepitation of tissues.

be present, but this sometimes is a late occurrence. Late in the illness, hemolysis is prominent, and cultures will have yielded clostridium. There are other conditions which feature wound-associated gas formation. Actually the incidence of gas present in gangrenous extremities associated with peripheral vascular disease is probably higher with gram-negative organisms (particularly *E. coli* and *Klebsiella*

aerogenes) than with clostridia. The presence of gas alone in the tissue does not mean that a clostridial infection is present. Gas in the wound can also occur with the synergistic gangrene (Meleney's gangrene) and with necrotizing fasciitis. Both of these have been discussed previously.

If left untreated, clostridial myositis, puerperal sepsis, and cellulitis are fatal diseases.

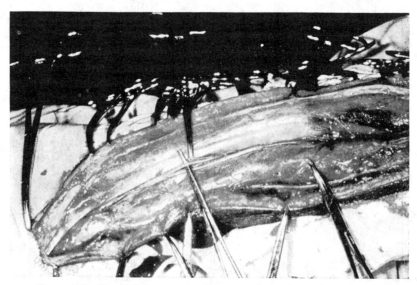

Figure 6-6 Clostridial gangrene, demonstrating pale necrotic muscle.

The unrelenting course of the infection (especially myositis), even with ideal treatment, is still associated with a high mortality. The true mortality rate is difficult to assess because many cases are called clostridial gangrene without bacteriologic proof. With prompt treatment, four of every five patients with gas gangrene of the extremities should survive.

The basic principles of treatment in all clostridial infections are the surgical excisions of infected tissues and high-dose antimicrobial therapy. Polyvalent antitoxin should not be used. Hyperbaric oxygen may be of some value, but this is unproven.

Although clostridial cellulitis is less severe than clostridial myositis, the suggestion that less radical surgery is required is a trap for the unwary. Multiple openings are made into the affected subcutaneous tissue by incisions carried into unaffected tissue. Necrotic tissue is also excised, which enables oxygen to reach the areas of infection. Penicillin G should be given in a dose of 6 to 12 million units intravenously as a continuous drip over a 24-h period.

Hyperbaric oxygen should never be used as a substitute for surgery. Its effectiveness has never been clearly established, and its use is certainly not mandatory. After adequate debridement, the patient can be placed in a hyperbaric chamber and exposed to 3 atm of pressure for periods of 1 to 3 h every 6 to 8 h.

Clostridial myositis should be treated in the same way as clostridial cellulitis, except that therapy is decidedly more urgent. Once the clinical diagnosis is made, immediate energetic extensive surgical treatment is mandated. Either delay or a limited surgical excision are fatal mistakes. The only thing that a surgeon can do that is wrong in this situation is to equivocate. All involved tissue must be excised. Dead muscle must be removed (Fig. 6-6). Involved extremities should be amputated. In the abdominal wall, the whole area of involvement must be removed.

Penicillin G should be given in the same dosage as mentioned above for clostridial cellulitis. Only after surgical excision has been carried out may the patient be placed in a hyperbaric chamber. If a hyperbaric chamber large enough to contain an operating room is available, surgical treatment can be carried out in it. But again, the value of this is open to question.

Clostridial puerperal sepsis requires the same principles of treatment. The gynecologist must decide early in the disease whether a dilatation and curettage is likely to be sufficient or whether a hysterectomy should be performed. In most instances the latter is indicated and is lifesaving.

Polyvalent gas gangrene antitoxin should not be used because it is ineffective. The gas gangrene group of clostridium produces several antigenically distinct toxins. *Clostridium perfringens* alone produces at least five and probably eight different toxins. Commercially available antisera neutralize only a small portion of the spectrum of toxins.

The key to the prevention of gas gangrene lies in rendering wounds unsuitable to the growth of clostridium. That is, all foreign bodies must be removed and devitalized tissues excised. Wounds that are closed must not have dead spaces and must be adequately drained. Every traumatic wound or surgical wound should be treated the same. The surrounding skin should be washed with a germicidal detergent or soap. Traumatic wounds should be irrigated with saline. The wound should be thoroughly explored under adequate anesthesia.

In the past, operating rooms were closed for 48 h after a patient with gas gangrene had been treated to allow some unexplained process to take place that purified the room and made it safe for use once again. There is no rationale for this.

Tetanus

This is a disease caused by the tetanal toxin which is secreted by the organism. The infection is usually small and well localized, and the disease is a true toxemia. The tetanal toxin probably spreads by two mechanisms.[3] One is by lymphatic and blood stream and the second is by migration through perineural tissue spaces of nerve trunks to the central nervous system. The toxin (tetanospasmin) becomes bound to gangliosides within the central nervous system.

The organism *C. tetani* is an obligate anaerobe which requires a low oxygen reduction potential for conversion to a vegetative state and for the multiplication of the organism and secretion of tetanospasmin. The organism is a large spore-forming gram-positive bacillus which is often present in the intestinal contents of humans and animals.

The causative agent is carried into human tissue by contamination of a wound. A variety of lesions may offer a suitable site for the growth of clostridial organisms. These include penetrating lesions produced by nails, splinters, thorns, gunshot wounds, burns, bedsores, and open fractures.

As mentioned previously, the mere presence of *C. tetani* in the wound does not mean that tetanus will develop. The local conditions in the wound must be favorable to its growth. *Clostridium tetani* will thrive only in the presence of an oxidation reduction potential far lower than that existing in normal living tissue. A fall of potential may occur as a result of the presence of necrotic tissue, soil, bits of cloth, metal, wood, or of tetanus toxin. Once the organism begins to grow, it produces toxin and can maintain the conditions necessary for continued multiplication.

The incubation period for the disease varies from 48 h to several months. The severity of the disease is inversely proportional to the length of the incubation period. The majority of cases fall in the period of between 1 and 2 weeks of incubation.

The diagnosis of tetanus is usually not difficult in the later stages; in wounds related to trauma the possibility of tetanus should always be remembered in order to diagnose it at its early stage.

There are two forms of tetanus: local and general. Local tetanus is confined to a muscle group in the area of the injury. This is a mild disease and will respond promptly to treatment. General tetanus involves a systemic spread of the toxin and is the more serious and more common manifestation of the disease. In general tetanus the usual first symptom is associated with spasm of the masseter muscles (lockjaw). From this the disease can spread to generalized facial involvement (risus sardonicus) and finally to generalized involvement with convulsions, respiratory paralysis, and death.

The typical paroxysms of tetanus left untreated occur more and more frequently with associated opisthotonos. These can be triggered by very minor environmental stimuli, so that the patient must be kept in a very quiet, sound-restricted, darkened area.

The diagnosis of tetanus is usually not difficult once the clinical manifestations are present. However, one must be extremely cautious in diagnosing tetanus in any person who has been immunized even only to a partial degree.

In the treatment of tetanus there are three general facets: (1) to remove the source of tetanospasmin, (2) to neutralize circulating toxin, and (3) to render supportive care until the toxin that is fixed to the tissue has been metabolized.

To eradicate the source of the toxin, the area of the wound must be adequately debrided to remove all necrotic material. This may require amputation of a digit on occasions, but in general a wide excision is sufficient. The wound then should be irrigated with hydrogen peroxide on a regular basis. The patient should also receive antimicrobial therapy, usually penicillin G in high doses (6 to 12 million units intravenously over a 24-h period). The purpose of this is to kill or inhibit any *C. tetani* that may remain in the tissues. The antimicrobial agents are of no use in the treatment of the disease caused by the circulating or fixed toxin, but they may be of value in the management of secondary bacterial complications, in the respiratory tract particularly.

The second factor of importance in the management of tetanus is the neutralization of circulating toxin. This is best done by administering tetanal immune globulin of human origin; 3000 U is injected, usually 1000 U in each of three sites intramuscularly. This produces a peak of immunity at about 48 h and lasts in a decreasing manner for about 25 days. It is not necessary to repeat the doses of tetanal immune globulin after the initial medication has been given.

The supportive care is, of course, most necessary in full-blown tetanus. This involves management of the respiratory tract, maintaining adequate oxygenation of the patient; sedation to prevent convulsions and paroxysms; and hyperalimentation to maintain nutrition. Meprobamate, diazepam, and muscle relaxants in association with small doses of phenobarbital are probably the most effective medications to use. The details of respiratory support are covered in other areas of this volume.

The prevention of tetanus depends on two things. (1) In those wounds which are so-called "tetanus-prone," complete, thorough debridement should be carried out. Theoretically, tetanus-prone wounds are in reality almost any wound that an individual can suffer, but particularly those that have the potential of necrotic material, foreign body, devitalized tissue, and similar type of circumstances. The adequate treatment of the wound is the single most important factor in preventing tetanus in unimmunized individuals. (2) Preventing tetanus in unimmunized individuals who have sustained a potentially dangerous wound requires that they be treated with tetanus immune globulin. The administration of a single 250- to 500-U dose IM of tetanus immune globulin is sufficient to be protective.

In conjunction with any passive immunization, active immunization should be started.

Tetanus prophylaxis by active immunization should be accomplished in childhood. Active immunization with: (1) diphtheria-tetanus-pertussis in infants and children under 6 years of age, or (2) tetanus toxoid or "adult-type" diphtheria-tetanus toxoid in adults and children over 6 years of age.

I "Depot" (alum precipitated, aluminum hydroxide or aluminum phosphate absorbed)

  A Advantages

    1 Induces more prolonged immunity.

    2 Is less likely to produce systemic reactions because of lower protein content and slower absorption.

  B Dosages

    1 Infants and small children: three 0.5-mL doses 4 to 6 weeks apart, intramuscularly, and at sites away from previous injections.

    2 Older children and adults: two 0.5-mL injections 4 to 6 weeks apart. In both groups, the injections may be as long as 6 to 12 months apart and still be effective. A reinforcing dose is recommended 1 year after the basic immunization, with a booster dose approximately every 4 years thereafter. The booster dose is usually 0.5 mL, but may be 0.25 mL in those who have had at least one prior booster.

II Tetanus toxoid "plain" (fluid, nonabsorbed)

  A Advantages

    1 Has slightly greater speed in producing antibodies.

    2 Is less likely to cause local reactions.

  B Dosage: three 0.5-mL injections subcutaneously (at sites away from previous injections) 3 to 4 weeks apart. They may be given as close as 10 days apart if necessary to achieve rapid protection. A reinforcing dose and subsequent boosters are given in the same time interval and same volume as above.

For the prevention of tetanus in the event of injury:

I In previously immunized individuals whose last booster was over 1 year but less than 10 years prior to the injury
  A Treat the injury as required. Adequate debridement is essential.
  B Give 0.5 mL tetanus toxoid (depot or plain) or one of the combined toxoids.
II In unimmunized individuals or those who have not had a booster within 10 years
  A If in the judgment of the physician the injury is tetanus-prone (such as compound fracture, deep puncture, crushing injury, extensive burn, gunshot wound, soil- or dirt-contaminated wound, expecially if over 24-h old), human tetanus antitoxin is given.
  B Now that human tetanus immune globulin has become more widely available, it is considered by many to be the agent of choice for passive immunization. The dosage is variously recommended as 200 to 500 U for adults, with 200 to 250 U recently suggested as being adequate. For children a dose of 5 U/kg of body weight (2.3 U/lb) to a total of 100 to 200 U has been recommended.

ASPLENIC HOST

It has become apparent in the literature in the past few years that the absence of the spleen may result in overwhelming sepsis, particularly in infants and young children. The offending organism is usually pneumococcus. Dickerman[5] refers to this problem in a review of bacterial infections in patients who have had splenectomy primarily for trauma. Because of this potential, Burrington[4] has reported the successful surgical repair of a ruptured spleen in children. Because of these reports it should be kept in mind that in rupture of the spleen,

particularly in children, the surgical repair of the spleen may be indicated rather than splenectomy. Although this concept has not received wide acceptance, it bears further study and evaluation.

Many pediatricians maintain young splenectomized patients on penicillin prophylactically for indefinite periods of time—frequently many years. Also, pneumococcal poly-valent vaccine is now available.

OTHER INTRAABDOMINAL INFECTIONS

Intraabdominal abscesses continue to present serious and important problems in the practice of clinical surgery. These abscesses occur as complications of injury, disease, and operations on the genitourinary and gastrointestinal tracts. Because the onset of intraabdominal abscesses is often insidious, their presence obscure, and their diagnosis and localization difficult, surgical management is filled with hazards. Moreover, the associated pathophysiologic effects may become life-threatening and lead to extended periods of morbidity and hospitalization. The need for additional nursing care, diagnostic procedures, and, often, multiple operations may lead to increased cost to the patient, the hospital, and to society.

Clinical Features of Intraabdominal Abscesses

The formation and progression of an intraperitoneal abscess are often not dramatic and become apparent only gradually. The patient who had seemed to be recovering from peritonitis or an abdominal operation stops improving and begins to regress; the patient becomes pale and weak, is anoretic or easily filled, is distended, and begins to experience nausea and vomiting. Temperature, heart rate, and white blood count are elevated. Fever is generally of an intermittent, spiking variety, but is often progressive and continuous. Chills are common.

In many patients the abscess resolves with

conservative treatment, which includes intravenous fluids, nasogastric suction, and antibiotics.

There are certain times in the genesis of an intraabdominal abscess when the condition really can be considered as a local area of cellulitis. This can be in the subdiaphragmatic area or pelvis, or indeed in the lateral gutters. At this time, the appropriate use of antimicrobial therapy may abort the development of an abscess. The use of intravenous penicillin 10 to 12 million units a day, and doxycycline 200 mg a day, or gentamicin 3 and 5 mg/kg/day, may be successful in preventing the development of an abscess. If the clinical situation warrants, it is certainly worth a clinical trial.

Administration of antibiotics may suppress but not extinguish the abscess, which then smolders for weeks or months before becoming manifest. Therefore, it is frequently preferable to discontinue antibiotics in order to expedite the diagnosis. The hazards of a nonoperative approach must be kept in mind. An undrained abscess may erode into a blood vessel and cause serious bleeding or generalized dissemination of the infection; it may create an internal or external fistula; or it may rupture into the general peritoneal cavity. Patients receiving antibiotic therapy should be closely observed and evaluated frequently. Indefinite postponement of surgical drainage is rarely possible.

Subphrenic Abscesses

Because these abscesses are so deeply located, there are usually few local signs of inflammation. Occasional symptoms are pain in the upper abdomen and lower chest, sometimes referred to the shoulder, and respiratory difficulty.

Physical examination may reveal a combination of signs highly suggestive of subphrenic abscess: an elevated, fixed hemidiaphragm and a smooth, sharp liver edge beneath the costal margin.

Radiographic examination reveals a pleural effusion or platelike atelectasis above the affected diaphragm in about 80 percent of patients, and elevation and reduction in motion of the diaphragm in two-thirds of patients. An air-fluid level, which is separable from the gastrointestinal tract, is present in about 25 percent of patients and is diagnostic of subphrenic abscess. Scout films of the abdomen in three positions—flat plate, upright, and lateral decubitus—are helpful in diagnosis; an abnormal gas pattern is present in 25 percent of patients. Barium enema, an upper gastrointestinal series with special views of the area in question, abdominal sonography, "CCT scan," and a combined liver-lung scan are also helpful in establishing the diagnosis.

Other than septicemia, the principal danger of an undrained subphrenic abscess is the probability of rupture into the abdomen, or rupture through the diaphragm to produce an empyema, a bronchopleural fistula, or necrotizing bronchopneumonia.

Right Subhepatic Abscesses

Of the upper abdominal spaces, the right subhepatic space is most commonly involved by abscess formation because it is the watershed of the appendix, duodenum, and biliary tract. Abscesses here usually originate from a duodenal stump leakage (following gastrectomy), a perforated duodenal ulcer or gallbladder, or a perforated lesion of the right colon, including the hepatic flexure. Diagnosis in these patients is more dependent on physical examination and much less dependent on x-ray studies than is diagnosis in patients with subphrenic abscess, because no lung or diaphragmatic abnormalities are usually demonstrable in patients with right subhepatic abscess. However, recent use of an upper gastrointestinal series with selective spot films ("abscess series") has enabled the physician to diagnose the condition more readily.

In addition to an enlarging, ill-defined tender mass, tenderness to palpation in the right upper quadrant and right flank pain are often found in patients with right subhepatic abscess. A high index of suspicion in a patient with such symptoms who fails to do well postoperatively may be an important factor in the early diagnosis and treatment of right subhepatic abscess.

Pelvic Abscesses

Pelvic abscesses most often follow pelvic inflammatory disease, a ruptured appendix, or diverticulitis, but they may also result from drainage into the pelvis from an upper abdominal peritoneal effusion. Symptoms include fever, lower abdominal pain, diarrhea, urinary urgency and frequency, and dysuria.

Pelvic abscesses are readily palpated as tender masses that bulge into the anterior rectal wall. The anterior rectal mucosa becomes thick and edematous, and the rectal sphincter becomes lax. It is important to distinguish between a pelvic inflammatory mass and a pelvic abscess so that an attempt at drainage does not cause a small bowel fistula. In general, an inflammatory mass does not cause the rectum to bulge, has ill-defined limits, and becomes smaller and less tender over a period of a day or two. An abscess is a discrete bulge that grows larger each day, and this growth is associated with a continuing or worsening illness.

Lesser Sac Abscesses

Abscesses in the lesser omental cavity deserve special mention because undiagnosed abscesses in this region have been found at autopsy. The possible presence of such an abscess should be considered if there are suggestive clinical findings following pancreatitis or the perforation of a gastric or duodenal ulcer.

Treatment of intraabdominal abscesses is primarily surgical. Appropriate drainage should be carried out. In general, for subdiaphragmatic abscesses, the transperitoneal approach has been used in this institution most commonly. It has the advantage of giving the operator the opportunity to explore the area more carefully and to see any subhepatic extension; however, if the abscess is very posterior or lateral, the extraperitoneal or posterior approach is acceptable. Pelvic abscesses can be drained either through the rectum or vagina, or abdominally. If the abscess is large and diffuse, abdominal drainage is probably more satisfactory.

The use of antimicrobial therapy in the management of intraabdominal abscesses is essentially supportive. It should be used, as mentioned earlier, in an attempt to abort the development of an abscess. However, when an abscess is fully developed, antimicrobial drugs are used primarily to prevent systemic extension. If one selects antimicrobial therapy, a combination of penicillin and tetracycline or doxycycline, as mentioned earlier, is probably the treatment of choice. However a combination of cephalin and gentamicin, and in some instances the addition of clindamycin, may be indicated. Each case should be individualized, and use of the antimicrobial drugs may well depend on the sensitivity studies which have been obtained at the time of the original operation preceding the development of the abscess.

BIBLIOGRAPHY

1 Altemeier, W. A. and J. H. Wulsin: Antimicrobial therapy in injured patients, *J. Am. Med. Assoc.*, **173**:527, 1960.

2 Altemeier, W. A.: *Manual of Control of Infection in Surgical Patients*, American College of Surgeons, J. B. Lippincott Company, Philadelphia, 1976.

3 Bennett, J.: in Paul D. Hoeprich (ed.) *Infectious Diseases*, 2d ed., Harper & Row Publishers, Incorporated, New York, 1977, Chap. 120.

4 Burrington, J. D.: Surgical repair of a ruptured spleen in children, *Arch. Surg.*, **112**:417–419, April 1977.

5 Dickerman, J. D.: Bacterial infection and the asplenic host: A review. *J. Trauma*, **16**(8):662–668.

6 Dineen, P.: "Antibiotics in Trauma," in Preston A. Wade, M.D. (ed.), *Surgical Treatment of Trauma*, Grune & Stratton, Inc., New York 1960, Chap. 7.

7 ———: in Paul D. Hoeprich (ed.), *Infectious Diseases*, 2d ed., Harper & Row Publishers, Incorporated, New York, 1977, Chap. 147.

8 ———: in Paul D. Hoeprich (ed.), *Infectious Diseases*, 2d ed., Harper & Row Publishers, Incorporated, New York, 1977, Chap. 148.

9 ———: in Paul D. Hoeprich (ed.), *Infectious Diseases*, 2d ed., Harper & Row Publishers, Incorporated, New York, 1977, Chap. 149.

Part Two

Initial Diagnosis
and Treatment

Chapter 7

Initial Care of the Injured Patient

G. Tom Shires, M. D.

The patient with multiple injuries is best managed when the overall responsibility for his care rests with one physician. Division of responsibility may decrease awareness of delayed complications and evaluation of the patient's overall problems. Nursing care of the patient is simplified if all orders are written by one physician or service. Consultation is obtained from other services to manage individual problems. This procedure is certainly of inestimable value. Meticulous and detailed attention to total patient care cannot be overemphasized.

Priority by Injury Patients may be placed in one of three categories according to the immediacy of their injury:

Those with injuries which interfere with vital physiologic functions. These patients have

sustained injuries which involve an immediate threat to life: airway inadequacy, hemorrhage, or shock. The primary treatment is establishment of an airway and control of bleeding. No time is wasted in getting the patient into "operative condition" or in attempting to establish a definitive diagnosis by laboratory means.

Those with injuries which are severe but offer no immediate threat to life. These patients have had an injury to the abdomen, chest, or extremities which will obviously require surgical intervention, but their vital signs are stable. Here there is time to obtain x-rays to determine the course of the missile and the extent of possible associated injuries such as fractures or a ruptured bladder. If the patient has hematuria, bilateral renal function may be assessed. The majority of injured patients are in this category, and although they are taken to surgery within 1 to 1½ h, much additional information is obtained.

Those with injuries which produce occult damage. This group of patients includes those with injuries which may require surgical intervention, although the exact nature of the injury is not apparent. The end result may be observation or it may be a surgical procedure, depending on additional physical findings, x-rays, and laboratory studies. Surgical intervention in this group may be delayed hours, days, or weeks, as in the case of delayed rupture of the spleen. These patients should be observed in the hospital and not as outpatients.

EMERGENCY SURGICAL CARE

Adequate Airway The first emergency measure in the management of the severely injured patient is to establish an effective airway. The easiest and quickest method is usually by means of an endotracheal tube. This rapidly establishes an airway and simultaneously allows endotracheal suction for removal of secretions or aspirated blood. When an endotracheal tube cannot readily be inserted, a tracheostomy may be rapidly done. (See Chap. 12.) An intermittent positive pressure breathing machine should be available in the emergency area to assist respiration.

Shock and Hemorrhage The next most important measure is the control of shock. This may be accomplished while another person is managing the patient's airway problem. Internal hemorrhage will usually require immediate surgical intervention. Prevention of shock is best accomplished by starting intravenous infusions in at least two extremities, utilizing 18-gauge needles. At least one upper extremity should be chosen for intravenous infusion

for abdominal wounds, since inferior vena cava injuries will deprive the heart of an infusion coming from the lower extremity. Extremities with possible vascular injuries should not be used for infusions. A balanced salt solution such as Ringer's lactate solution is started until blood is available. (See Chap. 1.)

Blood for typing and cross matching is drawn at the time the intravenous fluids are started. Hemostasis is most easily accomplished by utilizing simple finger pressure or packing a wound with gauze and applying steady pressure with the hand. Tourniquets are usually not effective and may be dangerous if forgotten. Not infrequently the venous flow is occluded with a tourniquet but not the arterial, causing increased hemorrhage. Ligation of superficial vessels may be done if vessels are readily seen; however, wounds should not be probed in an attempt to blindly place a hemostat on a vessel. As soon as bleeding is controlled, the wound is covered with a sterile dressing and the patient is taken to the operating room, where visualization of the wound is more adequate and proper instruments are available. The needless probing of wounds in the emergency room will frequently lead to severe infection, which can be avoided by proper irrigation and care in the operating room. (See Chap. 6.)

Tracheostomy After an airway is established and bleeding is controlled, a tracheostomy, if required, may be done with greater ease. If the patient has aspirated vomitus or blood from facial or oral injuries, he or she should be bronchoscoped when feasible. (See Chap. 12.) This may be delayed until the surgical procedure if there is a thoracic or abdominal injury requiring emergency surgical intervention. When bronchoscopy is done, the bronchial tree is irrigated with copious amount of saline solution. Antibiotics are administered to the patient who has aspirated vomitus or blood since pneumonia is a frequent complication. Shock may not be due to blood loss, as may be thought on initial observation, but rather to chest injuries with impaired respiration. The differentiation may be difficult until emergency measures are instituted.

Chest Injuries If the patient does not ventilate normally after an endotracheal tube inserted or a tracheostomy has been performed, a ruptured bronchus, pneumothorax, hemothorax, cardiac tamponade, or flail chest should be considered.

Ruptured Bronchus The patient with a ruptured bronchus will be in respiratory distress, probably cyanotic, and may often be seen with hemoptysis. This injury is managed with intercostal closed chest drainage and will subsequently require an open thoracotomy with repair of the bronchus. (See Chap. 12.)

Pneumohemothorax When the injured patient is first seen in the emergency room, the chest is examined to determine whether a pneumothorax is present. If there is doubt as to the existence of a pneumothorax, an 18-gauge needle may be inserted in the anterior axillary line and aspiration done to reveal the presence of air. If the patient is on the emergency room stretcher, the needle may be inserted in the eighth interspace in the posterior axillary line and aspiration done to reveal the presence of a hemothorax. The patient with a pneumothorax or hemothorax is treated with closed chest drainage and observed. Thoracotomy may be indicated, depending on the rate of bleeding or bronchus injury. (See Chap. 12.)

Flail Chest Patients sustaining blunt trauma to the chest resulting in a flail chest are best treated with tracheostomy and intermittent positive pressure breathing. This immediately expands the lungs and gives adequate ventilation. It eliminates the problems of a suspension apparatus and greatly decreases the incidence of pneumonia following such injury. A less desirable method of treatment is with a suspension apparatus utilizing towel clips around the ribs. This method does not ventilate the lungs nearly as well since the patient splints the chest on the affected side because of pain. This form of treatment is completely ineffective should the towel clips slip from beneath the ribs. Sandbags are of little value in the management of the patient with the flail chest and lead to the development of pulmonary complications. (See Chap. 12.)

Open Chest Wounds The patient with a chest injury which results in a sucking chest wound is best managed by immediately covering the open wound with whatever material is available. Covering the opening prevents further shifting of the mediastinum and allows ventilation of the opposite lung. Immediate surgical intervention is indicated. Chest tubes are inserted following the surgical procedure but are of occasional value preoperatively. (See Chap. 12.)

Cardiac Tamponade During inital observation, the patient may develop an unsuspected cardiac tamponade secondary to a blunt or penetrating trauma. This is manifest by decreased pulse pressure and respiratory distress with or without cyanosis. The emergency treatment is aspiration of the pericardial sac with an 18-gauge spinal needle through the sternocostal angle at the level of the xiphoid process. As little as 20 mL of aspirated blood may make a remarkable difference in the patient's vital signs. Should a second aspiration be necessary, the patient may require an emergency thoracotomy. When a patient arrives in the emergency room in shock without evidence of blood loss, this diagnosis should be suspected. A pericardial tap is indicated without a chest film if such an injury is likely. (See Chap. 12.)

The Unconscious Patient Patients with severe closed or open head injuries who are unconscious must have an airway established immediately. This may be done as previously described. Since a history is not available and the patients are often comatose, they must be observed for evidence of thoracic or abdominal injury. This may be determined by utilizing an 18-gauge needle for abdominal and chest taps, which may reveal the presence of nonclotting blood. The absence of blood does not rule out an intraabdominal or a thoracic injury. Patients who are unconscious with evidence of intracranial injury and hypotension should certainly be observed for the possibility of acute blood loss occurring either in the abdomen or in the chest. Hypotension from closed head injury is usually only a terminal finding. (See Chap. 11.)

IMMEDIATE NONOPERATIVE SURGICAL CARE

After the airway, hemostasis, and initial care have been attended to, a further history and physical examination should be done. Portions of the usual thorough physical examination may have to be omitted when the patient has massive internal bleeding. The operating room is alerted to the possibility of an emergency surgical procedure when a patient is admitted to the emergency room. Blood for typing and cross matching is drawn and blood is made available if there is any possibility that the patient will require surgical intervention. If vital signs are stable, x-rays may be taken. These are particularly helpful in locating a missile and determining its course of injury. Because patients with penetrating and blunt abdominal injuries may develop shock at any moment, a physician must be in constant attendance. Patients who suddenly go into

shock are immediately taken to the operating room.

Hematuria The presence of gross hematuria is evidence of urinary tract injury. Hematuria may clear rapidly and indicate only contusion. An intravenous pyelogram may be done to determine whether or not the patient has two normally functioning kidneys prior to surgical intervention. A single film at 15 min is usually adequate to determine function as well as indicate extravasation in most instances. If time is not available for an intravenous pyelogram, a cassette may be placed under the patient prior to his being placed on the operating table. Should a nephrectomy be required during the laparotomy, pyelography may be obtained on the table. A kidney should not be removed until there is evidence of a functioning kidney on the opposite side. In addition to the intravenous pyelogram, a cystogram is done in patients with a fractured symphysis to rule out extravasation from the bladder. Failure to demonstrate extravasation does not rule out the possibility of a ruptured bladder or kidney. (See Chap. 14.)

Fractures Fractures of the extremities are best managed with splints, such as a Thomas splint for the lower extremities and an arm board for the upper extremities. These prevent additional nerve and blood vessel injury as well as avert conversion of a closed to an open fracture. The presence or absence of pulses in the fractured extremity should be noted on initial examination.

X-rays of fractures are taken preoperatively if the patient's vital signs are stable. Massive bleeding takes precedence over fractures unless there is an accompanying arterial injury of such magnitude that there is danger of loss of limb. In such instances, it is often necessary to have two surgical teams working simultaneously. Necessary x-rays can be obtained in the operating room with a portable x-ray machine while the thoracic or abdominal bleeding is being controlled. (See Chap. 16.)

The management of pelvic fractures is usually conservative and may consist of a pelvic binder, traction, or only bed rest. A Foley catheter is routinely inserted, particularly with blunt trauma to the abdomen, to determine the presence of hematuria as well as to follow the urinary output during and immediately following surgical intervention. Pelvic fractures associated with hematuria may indicate the presence of a urethral injury. This injury may prevent the passage of a catheter into the bladder, thus establishing the diagnosis of a urethral injury. (See Chap. 14.)

Prophylactic Antibiotics   Prophylactic antibiotics are utilized in patients with gunshot wounds and shotgun wounds of the abdomen, chest, and extremities or in patients with penetrating injuries which enter the colon or other segments of the gastrointestinal tract and cause spillage of its contents. Antibiotics are not routinely used in patients with stab wounds. Tetanus-prone wounds are treated with antibiotics, and an attempt is made to convert them to open wounds when feasible. (See Chap. 6.)

DIAGNOSIS AND MANAGEMENT OF UNAPPARENT INJURIES

All penetrating injuries which can conceivably enter the abdomen, either as a stab wound or a gunshot wound, and injuries to the extremity which are near major blood vessels or nerves are routinely explored. X-rays are usually not of value except to determine the course of injury. These may reveal that a missile has gone from the chest into the abdomen. Films of extremities will be of value in determining whether or not the missile struck bone, fractured bone, or failed to pass near vital structures if it has remained in the extremity. A thorough neurologic evaluation is done when the patient is first observed. Blunt as well as penetrating injuries to the abdomen may transgress the retroperitoneal space and injure the spinal cord or cause fracture of vertebrae with a surrounding hematoma. This may produce progressive neurologic changes and require immediate decompression. (See Chap. 11.)

Thoracoabdominal injuries usually take precedence over neurologic injuries unless a rapidly expanding intracranial hematoma is obvious and the abdominal or thoracic injury is minor.

Blunt Trauma   Blunt trauma to the abdomen may produce severe retroperitoneal injury with minimal physical findings. Bowel sounds may not be lost for several hours, and evidence of retroperitoneal or intraabdominal injury may not become apparent for as long as 18 h. An abdominal tap may reveal the presence of nonclotting blood. A negative tap does not rule out the presence of an intraabdominal injury. A technique which has been used in recent years to augment diagnostic accuracy in blunt trauma to the abdomen has been peritoneal lavage. This procedure has proven to be a safe and reliable adjunct procedure. (See Chap. 13.)

Nasogastric Intubation   A Levin tube is routinely inserted in a severely injured patient. This may cause the patient to vomit and empty the stomach of large particles while awake, thus preventing aspiration during anesthesia. An unrecognized stomach injury from a penetrating or blunt trauma may be revealed by finding bright red blood in the drainage. This measure also prevents gastric dilatation during intubation and aids in the prevention of postoperative distention of the small bowel. (See Chap. 27.)

X-rays   These are taken when a patient's vital signs remain stable, but are omitted in patients in severe shock. These latter may be x-rayed by portable machines in the operating room if necessary.

X-rays are usually not informative in stab wounds except to demonstrate a pneumohemothorax and to rule out foreign bodies, such as a part of a knife blade, in the wounds. Patients sustaining gunshot wounds should have x-rays when possible in an attempt to trace the course of the missile. These are extremely useful in injuries to the extremities where fractures may be present secondary to the gunshot. Patients sustaining blunt trauma require many x-rays to rule out obscure frac-

tures such as those of the cervical spine and vertebral column.

Management of the Injured Patient

1 Adequate airway
2 Initial appraisal of shock
3 Intravenous fluids
4 Assessment of chest injuries
5 History and physical
6 Splint fractures
7 Levin tube
8 Bladder catheter
9 X-rays
10 Special procedures and observation

Part Three

Specific Injuries: Diagnosis, Operative Treatment, and Management

Chapter 8

Burns

P. William Curreri, M.D.

Major thermal injury is almost always associated with complex pathophysiological alterations which challenge the diagnostic and therapeutic capabilities of the medical staff. However, rapid progress in the development of new treatment modalities during the past two decades has resulted in marked improvement in clinical results. Preservation of function and increased survival of patients with greater than 50 percent total body surface burns has resulted from the development of comprehensive treatment centers where sophisticated, multidisciplinary teams have attained the capability of monitoring the rapidly changing physiological responses to burn injury and quickly responding with a large number of specialized therapeutic modalities.

Over 2.5 million persons require treatment for burns annually in this country, of whom 75,000 require hospitalization resulting in 9 million disability days. Hospital and medical costs alone for the treatment of burn injuries are estimated at over 1 billion dollars a year. Burn injury is exceeded only by motor vehicle accidents and falls as the primary cause of accidental death. As in other types of trauma, thermal injury frequently afflicts children and young adults. Prolonged morbidity, as well as temporary or permanent disability, is often associated with large financial obligations incurred by the families of patients, hospitals, insurance companies, and other social resources in order to defray expenses associated with prolonged hospitalization, loss of family income sources, and replacement of lost manpower within the labor force.

ETIOLOGY OF BURNS

Burn injury is caused by the application of heat to viable cellular elements. The depth of cutaneous burns is dependent on the intensity and duration of the applied heat. The source of heat may include open flame, hot liquid, hot metal, toxic chemicals, or high-voltage electrical current. Whatever the source, cell injury results from denaturation of protein when temperatures exceed 50°C.

In a civilian population, chemical burns are most frequently associated with industrial mishaps, laboratory accidents, civilian assaults, or inexpert application of medicinal agents.[30] In contrast to thermal injury, in which cellular damage ceases shortly after removal of the heat source, chemicals often cause tissue damage for prolonged periods until inactivated by chemical reaction with tissue protein. Therefore, a major consideration in the emergent treatment of chemical burns is effective removal of the toxic agent by dilution with large quantities of water or saline.[27] During the first several postburn days, the full-thickness chemical burn may appear deceptively superficial, exhibiting only mild bronze discoloration of intact skin.[21]

Electrical burns frequently cause only minimal destruction of skin, usually limited to sites of entrance and exit (grounding point) of the current. However, deep tissue injury is frequent and is proportional to the magnitude of current passing through the various organs. Since nerve, blood, and muscle offer least electrical resistance to electrical current, these organs sustain the most severe injury.[22,40] In addition to the cutaneous injury noted at the entrance and exit sites, small areas of cutaneous injury may be noted on flexion surfaces of extremity joints. Because electrical resistance of skin is markedly reduced by moisture, e.g., perspiration, current traveling through deeper tissue within the extremity may arc across the joint surface. When present, arc burns are nearly always associated with extensive muscular damage. Thermal injury to muscles often results in the release of hemochromagens into the bloodstream, which must be subsequently secreted via the urinary tract, resulting in port wine-colored urine containing myoglobin.

EMERGENT THERAPY

With the exception of chemical injury, in which tissue damage is minimized if the toxic agent is rapidly diluted and physically removed with water, the burn wound is of secondary importance during the first several hours following the injury. Rather, initial efforts should be directed toward restoration of normal physiological parameters and prevention of life-threatening complications.

Maintenance of Airway

Thermally injured patients may exhibit immediate pulmonary complications including carbon monoxide poisoning and upper airway obstruction. Carbon monoxide intoxication is manifest by signs and symptoms of hypoxia, which may range from pronounced tachypnea and agitation to respiratory arrest and coma.[57] Increased blood carboxyhemoglobin concentration confirms the clinical diagnosis, and treatment is effected by administration of 100% oxygen with appropriate ventilatory support as required. The syndrome is usually reversible if hypoxic damage to distant organs has not occurred prior to treatment, since carbon monoxide has virtually no toxic effects on pulmonary tissue itself. The advanced training of paramedical personnel, allowing immediate endotracheal intubation and initiation of ventilatory support at the scene of the accident, has resulted in greater salvage of patients with severe carbon monoxide poisoning during the last 5 years.

Exposure of the posterior and pharynx and the vocal cords to hot gases may induce upper airway obstruction during the first 2 postburn days. This syndrome is usually heralded by tachypnea, progressive hoarseness, and anxiety. The patient often exhibits progressive difficulty in clearing bronchial secretions as the tracheal orifice is decreased by edematous vocal cords. Examination of the posterior oral pharynx and cord via a fiberoptic bronchoscope allows early confirmation of impending obstruction. At the same time, the tracheal epithelium may be viewed beyond the cords, and assessment of smoke inhalation (to be discussed later) may be accomplished.

Immediate endotracheal intubation should be performed when impending upper airway obstruction is diagnosed. Since soft tissue edema following burn injury is maximal between 24 and 48 h, extubation is not usually attempted prior to the third postburn day.

Fluid Resuscitation

Following major thermal injury, fluid and electrolytes move from the intravascular and interstitial fluid space into the cells, resulting in marked extracellular hypovolemia with associated cardiovascular alterations. If hypovolemic shock is prevented, spontaneous movement of sodium and water back into the extracellular fluid space begins within 24 and 48 h.[9]

Initial loss of fluid from the extracellular fluid is proportional to the extent and depth of burn. Therefore, the appropriate treatment of postburn hypovolemia requires accurate assessment of the magnitude of the burn injury.

Burns are classified as first, second, or third degree. When only superficial layers of the epidermis are destroyed, resulting in cutaneous erythema, the burn is classified as first degree. The water barrier of the skin (located in the dermis) is preserved in such burns, and therefore it is of little clinical or physiologic significance. Rapid healing is normally observed, unless conversion to deeper second-degree burn occurs as a result of further exposure to a heat source, e.g., the ultraviolet light of the sun. Because systematic cardiovascular disturbances are rarely observed after first-degree injury, areas of first-degree burns are *not* included when estimating the magnitude of burn injury for purposes of planning intravenous fluid replacement.

On the other hand, second- and third-degree burns are of equal physiological significance and should be added together when estimating total body surface injury. Second-degree, or partial-thickness, burns retain viable epithelial elements from which reepithelialization of the cutaneous surface may occur. Only a few epithelial cells associated with sweat glands or subcutaneous portions of hair follicles are capable of regenerating epithelium following deep second degree injury.

Third-degree, or full-thickness, burns are characterized by total irreversible destruction of all epithelial elements within the skin. Spontaneous regeneration of epithelium is not possible, and healing occurs with deposition of scar tissue (collagen) by fibroblasts unless skin grafting is performed.

The depth of burn injury, following application of the same intensity of heat over a given time period, will vary, depending on the location of the burn. Skin thickness, as well as the existence and degree of development of the dermal appendages (sweat glands and hair follicles) and dermal papillae, will be influential in determining the severity of the burn. In infants, in whom dermal papillae and appendages are not yet fully developed, and in the aged, in whom they are atrophic, less heat intensity is necessary to produce full-thickness burn than in the middle-aged adult. Skin over the back, palms, and soles is very thick; thus, full-thickness injury is less common in these areas, as compared with skin overlying the inner arm and dorsum of the hand, where brief exposure to a heat source often results in third-degree burn injury.

The magnitude of burn injury is expressed as the percent of the total body surface area displaying either second- or third-degree burn injury. The total body surface burn may be estimated by utilizing the "rule of nines" (Fig. 8-1) which takes advantage of the fact that the adult body may be divided anatomically into eleven areas, each comprising 9 percent of the total surface area. After estimating the proportion of each area with second- or third-degree burn, the sum of these estimates represents the magnitude of burn injury. The rule of nines yields inaccurate results in infants and young children, since the surface area of the head and neck is significantly greater than 9 percent, and the surface area associated with the anterior and posterior aspects of each lower extremity is less than 18 percent. At birth, the surface area of the head constitutes 19 percent of the total body surface area, and each lower extremity only 13 percent. Therefore, the magnitude of burn injury in children is best estimated by the utilization of specialized body surface diagrams which relate regional body surface to age (Fig. 8-2).

The ideal formula for fluid resuscitation of patients with major burn injury would rapidly restore normal hemodynamic function while maintaining normal concentration of plasma proteins and electrolytes. Although many formulas have been developed during the past two decades to achieve rapid initial resuscitation of postburn hypovolemia, most have been derived empirically from observation of clinical response (primarily renal function). Few human studies have documented the rate and composition of extracellular fluid loss or attempted to establish the efficiency with which various volume expanders restore an effective extracellular volume. Although most formulas recommend a combination of crystalloid and colloid, they differ widely in regard to the recommended crystalloid-to-colloid ratio and in the suggested rate of administration.[16]

Most experimental investigation has supported the need for both crystalloid and colloid fluid administration. The selection of a specific formula to initiate resuscitation is of

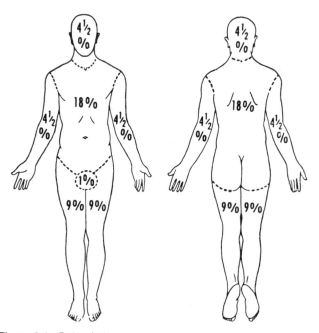

Figure 8-1 Rule of nines.

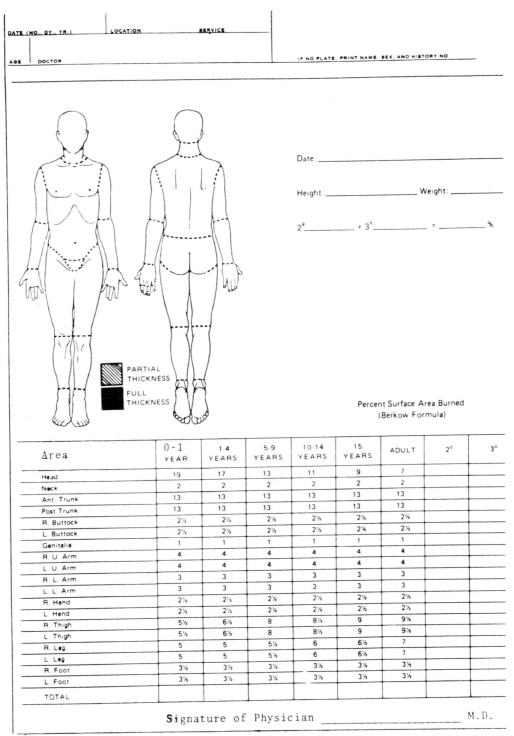

Date: _____

Height _____ Weight: _____

$2°$ _____ + $3°$ _____ = _____ %

PARTIAL THICKNESS

FULL THICKNESS

Percent Surface Area Burned
(Berkow Formula)

Area	0-1 YEAR	1-4 YEARS	5-9 YEARS	10-14 YEARS	15 YEARS	ADULT	2°	3°
Head	19	17	13	11	9	7		
Neck	2	2	2	2	2	2		
Ant. Trunk	13	13	13	13	13	13		
Post. Trunk	13	13	13	13	13	13		
R. Buttock	2½	2½	2½	2½	2½	2½		
L. Buttock	2½	2½	2½	2½	2½	2½		
Genitalia	1	1	1	1	1	1		
R. U. Arm	4	4	4	4	4	4		
L. U. Arm	4	4	4	4	4	4		
R. L. Arm	3	3	3	3	3	3		
L. L. Arm	3	3	3	3	3	3		
R. Hand	2½	2½	2½	2½	2½	2½		
L. Hand	2½	2½	2½	2½	2½	2½		
R. Thigh	5½	6½	8	8½	9	9½		
L. Thigh	5½	6½	8	8½	9	9½		
R. Leg	5	5	5½	6	6½	7		
L. Leg	5	5	5½	6	6½	7		
R. Foot	3½	3½	3½	3½	3½	3½		
L. Foot	3½	3½	3½	3½	3½	3½		
TOTAL								

Signature of Physician _____ M.D.

Figure 8-2 Body surface diagram relating regional body surface to age of patient.

less importance than frequent modification of the rate of fluid delivery to accommodate the individual patient's changing requirements during the first 48 h postburn. The formula shown in Table 8-1 has been popularized by Baxter and is known as the Parkland formula.[10,11] Currently, it is utilized by many burn units and remains the standard against which new formulas must be compared as they are developed. Both fluid volume and the sodium ion appear critical for achieving satisfactory reversal of hypovolemic burn shock. Crystalloid administration at rapid rates of delivery provides early expansion of depleted extracellular fluid volume and return of cardiac output to nearly normal levels. After 24 h, colloid has been shown to more efficiently maintain plasma volume without further increasing edema formation. By simultaneously measuring red cell, plasma, and extracellular fluid volume, as well as cardiac output, in both animals and humans with burn shock, Baxter was able to observe the specific beneficial effects of both colloid and crystalloid over the immediate postburn course.[9] Furthermore, the rates of

Table 8-1: Fluid Resuscitation of Burned Patients (Parkland Formula)

First 24 hours

Electrolyte solution (lactated Ringer's): 4 mL/kg body wt./% 2° & 3° burn

Administration rate: 1/2 first 8 h, 1/4 second 8 h, 1/4 third 8 h

Urine output: 30–70 mL/h

Second 24 hours

Glucose in water (D$_5$W): To replace evaporative water loss maintaining serum sodium concentration of 140 meq/L

Colloid solution (plasma): To maintain plasma volume in patients with greater than 40% 2° & 3° burns

Urine output: 30–100 mL/h

---

fluid administration required over time could be estimated by calculating the rates of extracellular fluid loss. His formula advocates the administration of 4 mL of lactated Ringer's solution/kg of body weight per percent of body surface area burn during the first 24 h following injury. During the second 24 h, free water (as dextrose 5% in water) is given in quantities sufficient to maintain a normal serum sodium concentration of 140 meq/L (approximately 3 to 4 L in a 70-kg man with a 50 percent burn). In addition, in order to sustain adequate organ perfusion, colloid may be required to maintain normal plasma volume (approximately 3 mL/kg body weight for each 10 percent total body surface burn over 20 percent). Providing urinary output has remained satisfactory, additional potassium should be administered after the first 24 h to replace urinary losses associated with the early postburn catabolic state.

Initial resuscitation fluids should be delivered at a rate which corresponds as closely as possible with estimated extracellular fluid loss. Since extracellular deficits following burn injury occur rapidly (within 6 to 12 h), one-half of the required total calculated fluid volume should be delivered during the first 8 h *from the time of injury,* and the remaining fluid at a constant rate over the next 16 h.

Patients with major thermal injury must be closely monitored during the initial period of resuscitation in order to assess the adequacy of treatment. Restoration of normal vital signs, urinary output, mentation, and central venous pressure should be quickly obtained and preserved. Hourly urine outputs in the adult should be maintained between 30 and 100 mL/h. Oliguria during the early postburn period is nearly always an indication of hypovolemia secondary to inadequate fluid resuscitation, and increased administration of crystalloid should be the treatment of choice.[12] Acute tubular necrosis, with resultant renal failure, is rare in the adequately resuscitated patient. Occasionally, electrical injury with extensive muscular damage results in the release of hemachromagens and intratubular protein precipitation causing subsequent renal failure, despite vigorous fluid administration.

Analgesia

A major therapeutic error in the treatment of extensively burned patients is the intramuscular administration of narcotics in large doses. Intrinsic sensory nerve endings in areas of full-thickness burn have been destroyed, and the wound itself is anesthetic. On the other hand, partial-thickness injury is often associated with severe pain. Therefore, requirements for analgesic administration are inversely proportional to the depth of injury.

Since most sedatives also depress cardiopulmonary function, the initial administration of narcotics should be minimized to allow appropriate hemodynamic response. Furthermore, narcotics often interfere with accurate evaluation of sensorium, a valuable indicator of the adequacy of fluid resuscitation. Marked peripheral vasoconstriction usually is associated with the hypovolemic state, resulting in decreased regional flow to muscles and skin. Therefore, analgesic agents should be administered intravenously in multiple small doses to ensure that predictable concentrations of the drug reach the central nervous system within a reasonable time interval.

Systemic Antibiotics

In the absence of topical chemotherapeutic agents, bacteria contaminating the surface of the burn wound and persisting in the depth of the skin appendages begin to proliferate rapidly. Characteristically, gram-positive organisms initially colonize the wound. Therefore, most clinicians prophylactically administer penicillin for 3 to 4 days to patients with major burn injury. The penicillin prevents overgrowth of the gram-positive organisms and has virtually eliminated streptococcal burn wound sepsis, a common cause of early postburn death three decades ago.[29] Since full-thickness burn is almost completely avascular by the fourth postburn day, antibiotics delivered parenterally or enterally after this time do not reach the wound in substantial enough concentration to play an effective role in control of delayed gram-negative bacterial colonization. It is not surprising, therefore, that administration of systemic antibiotics after the fourth postburn day has not been associated with decreased morbidity from infection. In fact, systemic administration of antibiotics is probably contraindicated after the fourth postburn day unless a specific distant bacterial infection (e.g., pneumonia) or systemic sepsis has complicated the burn.

Tetanus Prophylaxis

Burn wounds, like other forms of soft tissue trauma, must be considered contaminated, and therefore appropriate action must be taken to prophylactically protect the patient from tetanus. Patients that have been actively immunized within the year prior to injury will not require additional immunization. Adequate protection is afforded patients immunized within the previous 10 years by the intramuscular administration of 0.5 mL of absorbed tetanus toxoid. In the presence of a high-risk, heavily contaminated burn wound, or when no active immunization has been received within 10 years prior to injury, 250 to 500 u of tetanus immunoglobulin (human) should be simultaneously administered at another site, utilizing a different syringe and needle, in order to prevent inadvertent inactivation of the immune globulin by toxoid.

Blood Flow to Extremities

A principal characteristic of human skin is a remarkable degree of elasticity allowing significant stretching with only minimum applied force. As a result, considerable soft tissue edema may be present without increasing central limb pressure to a point which would result in a decrease of either venous outflow or arterial inflow. Although these elastic properties of the skin are retained following second-degree injury, full-thickness burns are characterized by nearly complete loss of elasticity. As a result, circumferential third-degree burns of the extremity are often associated with a severe decrease in peripheral blood flow as fluid resuscitation, accompanied by soft tissue edema, is administered. Without prompt intervention, unnecessary loss of distal tissue may result.

Decreased peripheral blood flow in the circumferentially burned extremity is diagnosed clinically by a decreased rate of capillary refill (usually observed in the nail beds) and by the development of motor or sensory deficits. Findings may be reliably confirmed by evaluation of venous and arterial flow in digital vessels with the ultrasonic Doppler. Diminished peripheral pulses by palpation and decreased skin temperature (the principal clinical signs associated with decreased blood flow to an extremity in the nonburned patient) are relatively poor indicators of blood flow in the burned extremity. Virtually all patients with major burns initially exhibit cool extremities as a result of hypovolemia with peripheral vasoconstriction, and peripheral pulses frequently disappear as soft tissue edema prevents satisfactory palpation of the underlying artery.

Initial treatment should be directed toward maintaining patency of small, low pressure venules. Active exercise of the extremity and elevation of the extremity promotes venous and lymphatic drainage, thus minimizing soft tissue edema under the unyielding eschar. However, if vascular impairment becomes manifest despite these preventive measures, immediate escharotomy should be performed.[18] Escharotomies (linear incisions through the full depth of the skin) allow spontaneous separation of the eschar and,

therefore, relieve underlying pressure on the central arteries and veins. No anesthesia is required for the procedure, since third-degree burns render the damaged skin anesthetic. Escharotomies are usually performed on the lateral and medial aspects of the extremity and should be extended across the joints, since skin is most tightly adherent to the underlying fascia around joints, and local vascular obstruction is most likely to occur in these areas. The escharotomies should extend through all areas of circumferential full-thickness burn down to and including eschar over thenar and hypothenar spaces of the hand and the lateral borders of the foot, in order to preserve distal intrinsic musculature.

In contrast, fasciotomy (linear excision of the deep fascia surrounding muscle) is rarely required in *thermally* burned extremities. On the other hand, after electrical injury, when extensive muscular damage beneath the deep fascia has occurred, fasciotomy may prevent irreversible necrosis of edematous muscle.[12]

Gastrointestinal Function

Although gastrointestinal motility usually is present for 6 to 10 h following burn injury, patients with greater than 20 percent total body surface burns often develop a reflex paralytic ileus during the latter half of the first 24 h. Unfortunately, vomiting often commences at a time when medical and nursing surveillance has relaxed and the patient is asleep following restoration of fluid volume and administration of sedatives. Thus, pulmonary aspiration of vomitus is not uncommon and is associated with severe morbidity and high mortality. Therefore, prophylactic insertion of a nasogastric tube is strongly recommended in all patients with major burns in order to ensure effective decompression of gastric contents until return of normal gastrointestinal motility is demonstrated.

Frequent inspection of gastric contents removed via the nasogastric tube for frank blood or guaiac-positive material also allows early diagnosis of hemorrhagic gastritis, a complication of severe stress. In addition, hourly installation of antacids through the tube to maintain chemical neutrality of gastric contents has proven effective in preventing the development of superficial erosions of the gastric mucosa.

Transfer of Specialized Centers

Most community hospitals are equipped to provide emergency care for patients with major burns, but few have either the nursing or paramedical manpower to provide sustained specialized care over 2 to 6 months for the occasional admission of severely burned individuals. Because special physical requirements are mandatory for optimum treatment of such patients, most hospitals without specialized units containing designated beds for burned patients arrange patient transfer to specialized facilities as soon as practical.

Previous medical evacuation experience gained during the Korean and Vietnam wars has yielded several guidelines for assuring safe transfer of burned patients. In general, the transfer is best tolerated during the first 24 to 48 h following injury. Intravenous resuscitation with crystalloid should be started prior to transfer. A Foley catheter should be inserted into the bladder of patients with major burns (greater than 20 percent total body surface area), in order that urinary output during the evacuation may be monitored and fluid administration appropriately adjusted. Rapid assessment of pulmonary function is mandatory, and if impending upper airway obstruction or severe smoke inhalation is suspected, endotracheal intubation should be performed prior to transfer. Extensive debridement of the wounds or application of topical chemotherapeutic agents is unnecessary and should be avoided, since such treatment merely delays timely evacuation and later interferes with rapid evaluation of the extent of injury by the receiving hospital. The burn wounds are better treated by the temporary application of sterile dressings to provide maximum comfort during the transfer. Whenever air evacuation (helicopter or fixed-wing aircraft) is utilized, nasogastric tube decompression is mandatory to prevent gastric dilatation at increased altitudes secondary to expansion of intragastric air.

BURN WOUND TREATMENT

Debridement and Excision

Partial-thickness burn injury (second-degree wounds) usually presents as vesicular lesions. In general, the overlying blister should be surgically removed to enable the direct application of topical chemotherapeutic agents to the underlying viable remnants of dermis. The topical chemotherapeutic agents inhibit secondary bacterial infection of deep second-degree burn wounds and in this manner prevent conversion of the partial-thickness injury to full-thickness injury. In most cases, debridement is accomplished without general anesthesia by utilizing careful surgical technique and modest amounts of sedation.

The thermally destroyed skin of third-degree burns is referred to as *eschar*. The eschar is tightly adherent to underlying subcutaneous tissues and, therefore, cannot be sharply debrided without severe hemorrhage. Initially, only loose eschar, which may be debrided without anesthesia or excessive blood loss, is debrided. Bacterial colonization of the remaining eschar is inhibited by the use of topical chemotherapeutic agents. However, it is important to stress that topical chemotherapeutic agents do not prevent bacterial colonization of the third-degree burn eschar, but rather are employed to control the rate of proliferation of bacteria within the burn wound in order to prevent subsequent invasion of underlying subcutaneous tissue and eventual bacteremia. As a result of the slow liberation of bacterial proteases, the third-degree burn eschar eventually separates from the underlying viable tissue between $2^{1}/_{2}$ to 4 weeks following the burn injury. When eschar separation occurs, it must be promptly removed from the body surface, in order to prevent systemic sepsis and localized abscess formation beneath the eschar. Debridement is most easily accomplished by daily hydrotherapy treatments which cleanse the surface of the eschar and allow careful inspection of the wound. The surgeon must unroof the localized abscess pockets and carefully debride all areas of loose eschar.

Immediate, safe surgical debridement of nonviable tissue with immediate wound closure utilizing split-thickness skin grafts would markedly decrease the morbidity associated with major burn injury and significantly shorten hospitalization time. However, immediate total debridement of nonviable eschar has not proved to be a safe procedure in the past because of the associated extensive hemorrhage during the extensive excision of eschar. In addition, limited areas of donor sites in patients with greater than 50 percent total body surface burn has prevented closure of the burn wound. Exposed viable subcutaneous tissue becomes desiccated, forming a secondary eschar which is unsatisfactory for subsequent grafting.

During the past several years, immediate excision of nonviable tissue during the first postburn week has again been attempted by major burn centers with improved results.[14, 15,38,41] In general, two approaches have been utilized to effectively remove nonviable tissue associated with second-degree and third-degree burns. Tangential excision, utilizing either manual or air-driven dermatomes, to sequentially remove layers of eschar in sheets of approximately 0.15 in in thickness has been utilized without excessive hemorrhage. Excision is discontinued when viable tissue is reached, as evidenced by capillary bleeding.

Since the underlying subcutaneous fat is not easily cut at uniform thickness, the procedure may be difficult technically in patients with full-thickness thermal damage. Moreover, the viability of the relatively avascular fat is often difficult to appreciate, and, as a result, nonviable fat may be inadvertently left behind. In addition, the procedure often requires a general anesthetic early in the postburn course when hemodynamic, septic, and metabolic problems may be appreciable. Furthermore, the exposed subcutaneous fat must be immediately covered with either heterograft, homograft, or autograft, in order to preserve its viability. Whenever third-degree burns are relatively limited in size (less than 5 percent), the full-thickness eschar may be primarily excised under anesthesia without excessive hemorrhage. Immediate coverage with autograft may be obtained, allowing decreased hospitalization, postburn morbidity, and often an improved cosmetic appearance. In addition, major burn centers have now taken a more aggressive approach toward the patient with massive burn injury, that is, greater than 70 percent total body surface area burn of which at least 60 percent is third-degree. Primary excision to fascia accomplishes immediate reduction of the burn size to a total body surface area which is more compatible with survival. In general, more aggressive treatment is warranted in patients with advanced age, since survival following the use of conventional techniques is markedly reduced in the aged. Fifty percent mortality is generally observed in patients over the age of 65 with 25 percent total body surface burns when eschar removal is delayed until spontaneous separation occurs. Primary eschar excision of major portions of the body surface should only be attempted in major centers, since this approach is still unproven and requires extraordinary medical, paramedical, and nursing support. If heavy colonization of the burn wound bacteria has already occurred, primary excision is often associated with postoperative systemic sepsis. Therefore, it is mandatory that monitoring of the burn wound with quantitative bacteriological cultures be established shortly after admission to the hospital in order to assure either burn wound sterility or relatively low concentration of bacteria (less than 10^4 organisms per gram of tissue) prior to sharp debridement under anesthesia. When relatively low concentrations of bacteria are present in the burn wound, the preoperative infusion of antibiotics by subeschar clysis provides maximum antibiotic concentration within the relatively avascular eschar and reduces the chances of seeding the bloodstream during the procedure. Both the eschar and the underlying subcutaneous fat are excised, utilizing cold knife excision. The exposed deep fascia is then immediately covered with homograft or, alternatively, autograft if it is available. If immediate physiological coverage of the wound is not accomplished, the fascia rapidly desiccates and becomes secondarily infected. Thus, it is necessary that an unlimited bank of homograft be maintained in those centers in which primary excision is practiced. In addition, massive amounts of both fresh and stored blood must be available to replace the large blood loss associated with the procedure. In the younger age groups, blood loss may be decreased if deliberate hypotensive anesthesia is utilized.

Since patients with electrical injury often have severe damage within the deep muscle compartments of the extremities, early surgical exploration, fasciotomy, and debridement of nonviable muscle must be performed as soon as motor dysfunction or massive edema of the extremity occurs.[12,49] Whenever possible, hemodynamic stability should be obtained via the intravenous administration of lactated Ringer's solution prior to operative exploration.

Another vexing problem occurs when cutaneous thermal burns result from contact with hot tar or asphalt. By the time the patient is brought to the emergency room, the tar has frequently solidified on the burn wound. Removal of the tar is best accomplished by applying generous quantities of Neo-Polycin ointment to the burn wound, after which a large occlusive dressing is applied. The dressing is removed in 18 to 24 h, at which time most of the tar or asphalt will be dissolved and the burn wound can be inspected. A water soluble topical thermotherapeutic agent may then be applied.

Topical Chemotherapy

Modern antibacterial topical therapy was advocated by Monafo and Moyer[42] in the early 1960s. These investigators utilized aqueous silver nitrate (0.5%) solution as a continuous wet soak, in combination with large bulky dressings. Although the agent was effective against most gram-positive organisms, as well as many strains of pseudomonas, silver nitrate is infrequently utilized by specialized burn units today. Whereas the agent often sterilized the surface of the burn wound, it had limited penetration into the depths of the eschar and, therefore, was ineffective when deep bacterial colonization had occurred. In addition, its use was associated with the development of severe electrolyte depletion (primarily sodium and chloride). Furthermore, the necessity for bulky dressings inhibited early active movement of the extremities and often led to less than optimal joint function. Finally, the agent was exceedingly expensive to utilize, since it required increased nursing personnel to effect the multiple dressing changes required. Also, considerable expense was incurred to replace linen, clothes, and equipment as a result of the discoloration caused on contact by precipitation of the silver salts.

In the mid-1960s, Lindberg and Moncrief[34] introduced mafenide acetate (Sulfamylon) as a topical chemotherapeutic agent for the open treatment of burn wounds. This agent proved effective against a wide range of gram-positive and gram-negative organisms, as well as most anaerobes. In addition, it actively diffused through the eschar and therefore provided protection in the depths of the eschar when deep colonization occurred. Since no dressings were required, the treatment did not interfere with intensive physical therapy programs, and its use allowed uninhibited treatment of associated soft tissue injuries. The drug was a potent inhibitor of carbonic anhydrase, and its use led to a decrease in the buffering capacity of the blood as a result of excessive excretion of bicarbonate in the urine. Acidosis frequently developed very rapidly in the presence of pulmonary dysfunction. In addition, the drug was quite painful on application and was associated with cutaneous hypersensitivity reactions in 5 to 7 percent of the population.

Silver sulfadiazine (Silvadene), developed by Fox[26] in the late 1960s, has essentially the same bacterial spectrum as mafenide acetate. However, it does not inhibit carbonate anhydrase activity, and its application is not associated with pain. Betadine, a water soluble-topical antiseptic complex of polyvinyl-pyrrolidone-iodine, may also be used as a topical chemotherapeutic agent. It is effective against a wide range of gram-positive and gram-negative organisms, as well as some fungi. The drug is manufactured both as an ointment and as an aerosol cream. It readily diffuses through the eschar and is absorbed and excreted rapidly. It has a tendency to desiccate the eschar, resulting in interference with progressive active physical therapy programs. In addition, its utilization for partial-thickness burns is often associated with mild to moderate pain.

It has recently been noted that the exclusive use of a single topical chemotherapeutic agent within the environment of an individual burn unit often leads to an increase in incidence of opportunistic infection with relatively resis-

tant gram-negative bacteria. For this reason, many centers utilize several topical chemotherapeutic agents to control the proliferation of bacteria within the eschar, and alter these agents, depending upon in vitro sensitivity to bacteria to the topical agents.

The properties of each of the currently available topical chemotherapeutic agents are summarized in Table 8-2. Newer and even more effective topical agents are currently in clinical trial and may be expected to be marketed in the very near future. The use of topical chemotherapeutic preparations prevents bacterial conversion of deep second-degree burns to full-thickness injury and thus reduces the amount of skin grafting which often is required when the agents are not employed.[45] Furthermore, the application of the agents to third-degree burn wounds has markedly decreased the incidence of invasive burn wound infection, the most frequent cause of death following severe thermal injury prior to the last decade.

Bacteriological Monitoring

Although the utilization of topical chemotherapeutic agents markedly reduced the incidence of systemic sepsis in patients with major burns, their introduction was not associated with improved survival in patients with greater than 60 percent total body surface burns. These patients often exhibited progressive colonization of the burn wound with late invasion of viable tissue and bloodstream dissemination of the bacteria. Therefore, it is still imperative that clinical bacteriological monitoring of the burn would be employed in order to diagnose ineffectiveness of a specific topical agent and provide rapid diagnosis of incipient burn wound sepsis.

Surface cultures from the burn wound have generally proven to be inaccurate with regard to predicting progressive bacterial colonization or incipient burn wound sepsis. There poor qualitative and quantitative correlation

Table 8-2: Properties of Topical Chemotherapeutic Agents

Agent	Antibacterial spectrum	Dressings required	Disadvantages
Sodium mafenide (Sulfamylon)	Gram-positive and gram-negative organisms and most anaerobes	No	Pain on application; skin allergy; carbonic anhydrase inhibition; resistant organisms
Silver nitrate (0.5%)	Most gram-positive organisms and some strains of Pseudomonas	Yes	Hyponatremia; hypochloremia; fails to penetrate eschar; methemoglobinemia
Silver sulfadiazine (Silvadene)	Gram-positive and gram-negative organisms and *Candida albicans*	No	Skin allergy; resistant organisms
Provodine iodine (Betadine)	Gram-positive organisms and fungi; possible less effective vs. some gram-negative organisms	Yes (cream); no (aerosol)	Pain on application; excessively dries eschar

between flora residing on the surface of the burn wound and bacterial colonization of the deep layers of the eschar, where potential invasion of viable tissue will occur. Blood cultures, although helpful if bacterial growth is demonstrated, have not proven particularly useful in the clinical setting, since life-threatening sepsis may occur in the absence of bacteremia, and the presence of bacteria in the bloodstream is a relatively late phenomenon, often just preceding death.[39] Bacterial growth in burn wounds is best monitored by semi-quantitative burn wound biopsy cultures, as advocated by Loebl and his associates.[35,36,37] Serial biopsies are taken from representative areas of the burn wound at 48-h intervals. The tissue is weighed, homogenized, serially diluted, and then inoculated on blood agar and eosin-methylene blue plates. The number of viable organisms per gram of tissue can then be calculated. When greater than 10^5 organisms per gram of tissue, or a 100-fold increase in the concentration of organisms per gram of tissue is observed within a 48-h period, it may be assumed that the organisms have escaped effective control by the topical chemothera-

peutic agent employed. If alternative therapy is not immediately employed, a progressively fatal burn wound sepsis may be anticipated.

Physiological Dressings

Immediately following eschar separation, the wound is seldom ready to accept a cutaneous autograft. During the time interval between eschar separation and definitive cutaneous autograft, the granulation tissue can be temporarily covered with a physiological dressing of either porcine heterograft[13] or homograft (obtained from cadavers.[46] The application of these physiological dressings contributes to the prevention and control of infection, the preservation of healthy granulation tissue, and the maintenance of joint function. In addition, the application of physiological dressings is associated with a decrease in the evaporative water loss from the granulation tissue, and a diminished heat loss secondary to this evaporation. Furthermore, the dressings cover exposed sensory nerves and render the patient more comfortable. Finally, the physiological dressing acts as an excellent test material to determine the optimal time for subsequent autograft. When good adherence of the physiological dressing is observed, the granulation tissue may be assumed ready to accept the application of split-thickness skin grafts (autografts). When autograft is delayed until good adherence of the physiological dressing is observed, the subsequent loss of split-thickness skin graft is minimized.

Physiological dressings may also be utilized to debride untidy wounds immediately after eschar separation. The heterograft or homograft hastens separations of tightly adherent small pieces of eschar left behind after daily local debridement. In such cases, physiological dressings should only be used when more than 95 percent of the eschar has been mechanically removed prior to their application, since, in effect, one is promoting separation of the last tiny pieces of eschar by encouraging bacterial growth.

In addition, both heterograft and homograft have been utilized to immediately cover superficial second-degree burns of less than 20 percent of the total body surface.[19] The principal advantages of such treatment include marked reduction of pain, decreased hospitalization time, early return of joint function, and more rapid reepithelialization of the burn wound. A few important principles, however, must be rigidly followed if heterograft or homograft is to be used in this manner. The wound must be superficial in depth in order that the clinician can be assured that it is, indeed, partial-thickness rather than full-thickness injury. Obviously, the use of physiological dressings over third-degree burn may, in fact, precipitate burn wound sepsis. Also, the homograft or heterograft must be applied within hours after the burn injury, immediately following debridement of the vesicles. The burn wound is then inspected within 24 h to assure continued adherence of the physiological dressings to the dermal remnants. Should the dressing become dislodged, or should fluid accumulate beneath it, the material should be immediately removed and the wound treated in a conventional manner with topical chemotherapeutic agents. However, if the heterograft or homograft remains adherent, it should not be removed, but rather, allowed to separate spontaneously as reepithelialization occurs. Frequent removal and reapplication of adherent physiological dressings applied to second-degree burns results in sequential removal of epithelial cells and may cause conversion to a full-thickness burn wound. Both heterograft and homograft may also be utilized electively over reepithelialized deep second-degree burn wounds, once superficial necrotic debris has been entirely removed by local debridement (usually 8 to 10 days post burn), or following tangential excision of deep second-degree burn wounds. Adherent physiological dressings utilized in this manner promote the rate of reepithelialization and decrease pain associated with the wound.

Split Thickness Skin Grafts

The ultimate objective of all burn wound care is definitive closure of the wounds as soon as possible after injury. When the granulation tissue has been adequately prepared by use of temporary physiological dressings, as described above, it should be promptly covered with the patient's own skin (autograft). The hands, feet, joints, and face should receive priority for coverage with split-thickness skin grafts, in order to preserve function and provide optimum cosmesis. When the wound has been preoperatively prepared by the sequential application of physiological dressings, autografts may be applied as sheets of skin without the need of suture fixation or "pie-crusting" incisions to allow release of plasma. Fixation with bandaging is not required unless accidental dislodgment is likely, e.g., on circumferentially burned limbs, or on burns of patients with uncontrollable motion. Exposure of freshly applied autograft allows early evacuation of any collections of blood or serum that may occur beneath the graft, and provides the physicians and nursing personnel with the opportunity to frequently inspect the graft during the immediate postoperative period. When dressings are utilized, they are usually removed 72 h following application of the graft.

Patients with greater than 40 percent total body surface burns often present with a serious disproportion between the area requiring autografting and available donor sites. In such patients, meshed or expanded grafts may be utilized to cover large areas from limited donor sites.[24,50,51] Mesh grafts are also frequently utilized in elderly individuals in whom the creation of donor sites over considerable portions of the body may be associated with increased morbidity during the postoperative period. The mesh grafts may be expanded up to 6 times the area of the original donor sites. In most cases, the interstices are rapidly closed by epithelialization within 4 to 8 days, resulting in a somewhat thinner but physiologically functional skin cover. When possible, mesh grafts are avoided as skin covers on the face, hands, feet, and flexion creases, since the healed grafts are not only less cosmetically acceptable when compared with sheet autografts, but in addition, they are less able to withstand recurrent localized trauma.

GENERAL THERAPEUTIC CONSIDERATIONS

Metabolism and Nutrition

Major injury is characterized by a hypermetabolic response. Several investigators have shown a direct relationship between the magnitude and duration of the hypermetabolic response and the severity of the sustained trauma. A curvilinear relationship between the resting metabolic expenditure and the magnitude of total body surface burns in human patients has been demonstrated by Wilmore.[56] The resting metabolic rate approached twice normal at the end of the first postburn week in patients with greater than 60 percent total body surface burn. As a result, caloric expenditure exceeds 60 kcal/m² per hour in patients with major thermal injury.[19,56] Total daily energy consumption during the nonresting state in severely burned patients may be approximated by the following formula: 40 kcal/percent burn + 25 kcal/kg body weight.[17] The reader is referred to Chapter 33, "Nutritional Support of the Traumatized Patient," for an in-depth discussion of the pathophysiology associated with posttraumatic hypermetabolism. In addition, the clinical consequences of inadequate nutritional replacement are outlined, and a program for nutritional management of the extensively traumatized patient is suggested.

FUNCTIONAL REHABILITATION

A major complication of severe thermal injury is serious loss of joint function secondary to burn wound contractures. Implementation of a progressive physical therapy program immediately after hospitalization has been associated with the preservation of range of motion of joints. For optimal results, the program must begin on the day of admission and be continued until the burn wounds are healed and normal range of joint motion can be maintained by the patient.[25] Therefore, most major burn centers have found it necessary to employ full-time physical therapists to supervise active physical therapy at the bedside during waking hours. Repetitive exercises are conducted in the direction opposite of that of any anticipated deformity.

Since the patient will assume a "contracture position" spontaneously, proper positioning during bed rest must be monitored, and splints must be manufactured to maintain an "anticontracture position" during sleep.[31,48] Prolonged immobilization is avoided, and early motion following skin grafting should be encouraged. In a retrospective study, Dobbs[25] determined that 85 percent of the joints underlying surface burns should have a normal range of motion at the completion of therapy. Her analysis revealed that the upper extremities were more susceptible to the deleterious effects of prolonged immobilization than were the lower extremities. The ideal position for the lower extremities (knees extended, feet in neutral position) was comfortable for the patient and relatively easy to maintain in either the prone or supine position. However, the shoulders are more difficult to position and splint in patients with extensive burn, and elevation and abduction of the arm at the shoulder joint are often uncomfortable. Therefore, a patient with burns at the shoulder invariably assumes and maintains a position of abduction and extension, if not carefully monitored by nursing personnel and therapists.

Although patient motivation is obviously an important factor in maintaining satisfactory joint function, there is no factor more deleterious to the preservation of motion than delay of treatment. Daily range of motion evaluation and appropriate daily exercises to achieve maximum potential range of motion in joints underlying both second-degree and third-degree surface burns remains of paramount importance. During the early postburn period, the therapist and patient should establish goals which must be rapidly achieved and thereafter maintained. As soon as possible, the patient should be encouraged to pursue these self-care activities. During hospitalization, every effort should be exerted to ensure eventual patient independence. Prior to discharge, the patient should have mastered a home physical therapy program which will ensure maintenance of function with outpatient visits.

The development of hypertrophic scars often occurs following discharge in areas of healed second-degree burn. The resultant scar overgrowth may markedly inhibit function and often is associated with severe disfigurement. Larson and his associates[32,33] have re-ported reduction of hypertrophic scar formation following the application of conforming isoprene splints and/or elastic dressings (Jobst pressure garments) during the convalescent period. By exerting continuous pressure on the hyperactive scar, reduction in local interstitial edema and improved alignment of collagen fibrils is accomplished. Splints and elastic garments must be worn 24 h a day for between 6 and 12 months.

COMPLICATIONS

Smoke Inhalation Syndrome

Smoke inhalation syndrome is defined as acute pulmonary dysfunction related to a lower respiratory tract chemical tracheal bronchitis which occurs within 72 h after exposure to gaseous products of incomplete combustion (primarily aldehydes). The severity of this syndrome is a function of the type of smoke inhaled, the dose of smoke inhaled, and the magnitude of the accompanying thermal injury.[1] Patients with smoke inhalation syndrome frequently exhibit *no* physical signs or symptoms of pulmonary injury during the first 24 h of hospitalization.[23] Severe smoke inhalation should be suspected in patients burned within a closed space, patients injured while under the influence of alcohol or drugs, and in patients who have a history of loss of consciousness. The definitive diagnosis, however, is dependent upon a high index of suspicion and on careful physical and laboratory examination (Table 8-3). Sputum should be obtained from the lower respiratory tract and examined for the presence of carbon. When carbonaceous sputum is noted, the patient should be hospitalized and observed for the development of respiratory dysfunction. Increased concentration of carboxyhemoglobins suggests the inhalation of a significant amount of smoke, and in most cases the patient should be retained in the hospital for observation, since many patients will later develop lower respira-

Table 8-3: Smoke Inhalation Syndrome

Diagnostic tests	Advantages	Disadvantages
Carboxyhemoglobin	Simple; rapid	Nonspecific; rapid disappearance
Fiberoptic bronchoscopy	Simple; rapid; objective	—
^{133}Xenon scan	Objective	Complicated; expensive
A-a Do$_2$ gradient	Simple; rapid; ? objective	Unproven

tory tract pathophysiology following recovery from carbon monoxide poisoning. Following admission to the hospital, fiberoptic bronchoscopy should be performed within 6 to 12 h to assess the lower respiratory tract. The presence of extramucosal carbonaceous material, bronchorrhea, mucosal edema, vesicles, erythema, hemorrhage, or ulceration below the level of the vocal cords are all objective findings associated with the subsequent development of significant pulmonary dysfunction secondary to smoke inhalation.[43] Although the partial pressure of oxygen in arterial blood is relatively insensitive and inaccurate in predicting early smoke inhalation syndrome, a Pa$_{O_2}$ of less than 300 while the patient is breathing 100% oxygen during the first 48 h post burn suggests significant pulmonary dysfunction and often heralds the subsequent development of smoke inhalation syndrome. During the second 24 h, the patient will begin to exhibit progressive bronchial spasm with the development of expiratory wheezes, rales, tachypnea, and progressive respiratory failure. The subsequent development of bronchopneumonia secondary to bacterial superinfection distal to occluding plugs (consisting of inspissated mucus and sloughed bronchial epithelium) within small bronchii is a fairly constant feature. Radiographic changes are usually not apparent until 72 h following exposure to the smoke.

The treatment of smoke inhalation syndrome consists of both nonspecific and specific therapy. Nonspecific therapeutic modalities include rapid fluid resuscitation of burn shock, performance of escharotomies of the chest and the abdomen when indicated, the provision of external dry heat, and frequent monitoring of respiratory function. Restoration of normal intravascular volume prevents exacerbation of central nervous system hypoxia secondary to decreased cerebral blood flow. The provision of an externally warm environment minimizes oxygen demand associated with an increased metabolic rate stimulated by cold stress. Most important, however, is the frequent assessment of respiratory function by repetitive physical examination, serial determinations of Pa$_{O_2}$, and evaluation of the Pa$_{O_2}$/FI$_{O_2}$ ratio, which often decreases prior to a significant fall in the Pa$_{O_2}$.

Specific treatment includes the provision of humidified air and oxygen as required. If respiratory failure is incipient, prompt endotracheal intubation should be performed and the patient supported with mechanical ventilation. Frequently, positive end expiratory pressure (PEEP) must be instituted to obtain adequate arterial oxygenation. Intravenous administration of brochodilators is utilized to alleviate the severe bronchial spasm. In addition, appropriate antibiotics should be administered by a parenteral route when the smoke inhalation syndrome is complicated by pneumonia.

Burn Wound Sepsis

Burn wound sepsis is characterized by the active invasion of microorganisms into viable subeschar tissue, with subsequent bacteremia.[52,53] Because full-thickness burn wounds are essentially avascular, the delivery of antibiotics via systemic routes rarely reaches the eschar in sufficient concentrations to substantially affect microbiological growth (Fig. 8-3). Moreover, host resistance to infection is now known to be markedly diminished in patients with major thermal injury. Complement abnormalities, hypogammaglobulinemia, cellular mediated immunity, decreased neutrophil intracellular bacterial killing, and abnormalities in the inflammatory response within the burn wound have all been described.[2,3,4,5,20,28,44] In addition, a marked decrease in neutrophil and monocyte chemotactic responsiveness has been demonstrated in at least two laboratories.[6,54]

As a result, rapid bacterial colonization of the burn wound results if topical chemotherapeutic agents are not utilized. However, bacterial proliferation may still escape the control of all currently used topical chemotherapeutic agents. When serial quantitative burn wound biopsies suggest incipient burn wound sepsis, the administration of antibiotics by needle clysis beneath the eschar has been employed with success.[8] The antibiotics administered by subeschar clysis should be selected after review of in vitro sensitivity of the offending organisms. The entire daily "systemic" dose of the selected antibiotic is dissolved in a solution of isotonic saline or half-strength saline of sufficient quantity to infuse each 44-cm² area of burn eschar with 25 mL of solution once daily.

Loebl and his associates[36] reported 50 percent survival of children with documented pseudomonas burn wound sepsis accompanied by ecthyma gangrenosum when antibiot-

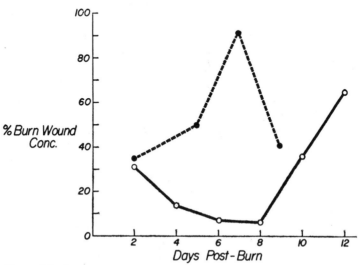

Figure 8-3 Days post burn.

ics were administered by subeschar clysis. Prior to this report, this complication in children was uniformly fatal.

Distant Complications

As a result of decreased host resistance in patients with major thermal injury, distant septic complications are frequently observed. Bronchopneumonia is the most common complicating infection. Microbiological examination of sputum usually reveals the same microorganism which has colonized the burn wound. Bacteria are often aerosolized from the burn wound and inhaled in large doses as the patient is manipulated during the course of daily wound care. About one-third of patients with pneumonia are seeded via the bloodstream (hematogenous pneumonia) as a complication of burn wound sepsis. Conventional treatment with systemic antibiotics and respiratory support is indicated when septic pulmonary infiltrates are diagnosed by physical examination or chest radiography.

The third most frequent septic complication in patients with thermal injury is septic thrombophlebitis. This complication follows prolonged venous cannulation with polyethylene catheters utilized for the delivery of intravenous fluid. Often the patients exhibit no abnormal physical signs, such as calf tenderness and edema, which are associated with bland thrombophlebitis. In fact, most commonly, the patient presents with bacteremia of unknown origin and blood cultures may yield staphylococci. When suspected, prompt surgical exploration should be performed on all peripheral veins which have been cannulated during the hospitalization. The vein is opened and milked in a retrograde manner, and any effluent is observed. If pus is identified, the diagnosis is confirmed. In the absence of liquefied suppurative material within the vein, the suspected vein should be biopsied and subjected to frozen section. Identification of bacterial colonization within the intima of the vein strongly suggests the presence of suppurative thrombophlebitis. The incidence of suppurative thrombophlebitis may be markedly reduced by limiting the duration of any single intravenous catheter to periods of 72 h or less. However, when the complication occurs, the offending vein must be excised in its entirety if fatal bacteremia is to be avoided.

Another common site of distant bacterial infection is thermally injured cartilage. Because the cartilage is relatively avascular, local host resistance to infection is diminished. Since the cartilage of the external ear is covered only by cutaneous tissue, it is frequently injured when full-thickness burns of the ear are sustained. The development of suppurative chondritis may often be prevented in patients with severe burns of the ear by minimizing external pressure upon the surface of the ear. Such patients should sleep without bed pillows and be restrained from assuming a lateral position with the burned ear dependent. Whenever suppurative chondritis occurs, surgical excision of the involved cartilage is indicated to arrest progressive septic destruction.[48]

Gastrointestinal

Gastric and duodenal ulcers (Curling ulcers) were first described in 1842 and have previously been reported to occur in as many as 25 percent of hospitalized burn patients. However, the incidence of Curling's ulcer has been markedly reduced during the past decade, and operative intervention for upper gastrointestinal bleeding following burn injury is only rarely necessary today. In the past, up to 85 percent of upper gastrointestinal hemorrhage was associated with bacteremia. The decreased instance of Curling's ulcers has occurred along with reduced frequency of major septic complications, the prophylactic institution of antacids into the stomach via a gastrointestinal tube (maintenance of neutral pH in gastric aspirate), and the improved provision of nutritional supplements allowing more rapid healing of small, acute mucosal erosions.

SPECIAL PROBLEMS

Long Bone Fractures

Patients incurring long bone fractures with overlying cutaneous burns cannot be treated with closed cylinder casts without a coincidental high risk of burn wound sepsis. The fracture is best immobilized by insertion of Steinman pins or Kirschner wires and institution of balanced skeletal traction. In this manner, the burn wounds remain exposed and topical application of chemotherapeutic agents may be utilized. Daily debridement of separating eschar and careful monitoring of the burn wound by inspection may be readily accomplished.

Bone may be thermally injured by electrical current at sites of entrance and exit. When the underlying bone lies in close approximation to the overlying skin, e.g., scalp, sternum, and anterior leg, debridement of nonviable soft tissue often exposes the bony injury. Such wounds are treated by daily debridement and application of topical chemotherapeutic agents until the soft tissue is covered with granulations. Then definitive closure of the soft tissue defect is accomplished with autograft, and devitalized bone is decorticated in layers until viable bone (as evidenced by bleeding) is encountered.[7] After 10 to 14 days, granulation tissue will develop from the endothelium of intraosseus vessels and eventually cover the remaining viable bone. Split-thickness skin graft may then be applied.

Thermal Injury of Joints

Burn injury may extend to the joint capsule, especially when the overlying skin and soft tissue is relatively thin. Full-thickness burns of the dorsum of the hand and foot are particularly troublesome, in that the interphalangeal joint capsule is often devitalized, leaving the joint open. In such cases, the cartilage within the joint should be surgically removed and a formal arthrodesis performed in order to insure ankylosis in the most optimal position. Interphalangeal joints should be fused in an extended position, or with just a few degrees of flexion. The position may be held with crossed Kirschner wires (which minimize rotational deformity) for a period of 6 to 8 weeks, at which point fusion of adjacent bony surfaces has occurred. When arthrodesis of joints becomes necessary, it is particularly important to maintain full range of motion in adjoining joints if severe long-term disability is to be avoided.

In unusual circumstances, appropriate positioning of extremities cannot be maintained by the application of splints or institution of an aggressive physical therapy program. This problem most frequently arises in infants and young children where not enough finger length exists to allow application of pressure dressings that maintain optimal extremity position within the splint. Temporary insertion of a single, axial Kirschner wire through the interphalangeal joints will often serve to hold the fingers in the desired position. The wires are removed within 2 to 3 weeks, after which active physical therapy is employed to regain joint function.

MORBIDITY AND MORTALITY

Burns of greater than one-third of the body surface area were associated with greater than 95 percent mortality three decades ago. Today, patients regularly survive much greater injury, and mortality rates in most burn centers rarely exceed 10 percent. The poorest results are observed in elderly patients (over the age of 65), in whom only 50 percent survival is observed following 25 percent total body surface burn. Morbidity and mortality in the aged is often related to chronic disease states which interfere with appropriate physiological responses to major injury.

Long-term disability has been markedly reduced during the past 20 years as multidisciplinary burn teams have been developed in burn centers to ensure coordinated attention to all aspects of therapy. At many centers, more than 90 percent of surviving patients return to full-time employment. Self-respect and independence are preserved, and nearly all patients experience a most satisfactory quality of life.

BIBLIOGRAPHY

1 Achauer, B. M., P. A. Allym, D. W. Furnas, and R. H. Bartlett: Pulmonary complications of burns: The major threat to the burn patient, *Ann. Surg.* **177**:311, 1972.
2 Alexander, J. W.: Emerging concepts in the control of surgical infections, *Surgery*, **75**:934, 1974.
3 ———: Host defense mechanisms against infection, *Surg. Clin. North Am.*, **52**:1367, 1972.
4 ———: "Immunologic Considerations and the Role of Vaccination in Burn Injury," in H. C. Polk and H. H. Stone (eds.), *Contemporary Burn Management*, Little, Brown and Company, Boston, 1971, p. 265.
5 ———, R. Dionigi, and J. L. Meakins: Periodic variation in the antibacterial function of human neutrophil and its relationship to sepsis, *Ann. Surg.*, **173**:206, 1971.
6 Altman, L. C., S. J. Klebanoff, and P. W. Curreri: Abnormalities of monocyte chemotaxis following thermal injury, *J. Surg. Res.*, **22**:616, 1977.
7 Asch, M. J., P. W. Curreri, and B. A. Pruitt, Jr.: Thermal injury involving bone: A report of 32 cases, *J. Trauma*, **12**:135, 1972.
8 Baxter, C. R., P. W. Curreri, and J. A. Marvin: The control of burn wound sepsis by the use of quantitative bacteriologic studies and subeschar clysis with antibiotics, *Surg. Clin. North Am.*, **53**:1509, 1973.
9 ———: "Crystalloid Resuscitation of Burn Shock," in H. C. Polk and H. H. Stone (eds.),

Contemporary Burn Management, Little, Brown and Company, Boston, 1971, p. 7.
10 ——— and G. T. Shires: "Early Resuscitation of Patients with Burns," in C. E. Welch (ed.), *Advances in Surgery*, Year Book Medical Publishers, Inc., Chicago, 1970, vol. IV, p. 308.
11 ———, J. A. Marvin, and P. W. Curreri: Fluid and electrolyte therapy of burn shock, *Heart & Lung*, **2**:707, 1973.
12 ———: Present concepts in the management of major electrical injury, *Surg. Clin. North Am.*, **50**:1401, 1970.
13 Bromberg, B. E., I. C. Song, and M. P. Mohn: The use of pig skin as a temporary biological dressing, *Plast. Reconstr. Surg.*, **36**:80, 1965.
14 Burke, J. F., W. C. Quinby, C. C. Bondoc, et al.: Immunosuppression and temporary skin transplantation in the treatment of massive third degree burns, *Ann. Surg.*, **182**:183, 1975.
15 ———, C. C. Bondoc, and W. C. Quinby: Primary burn excision and immediate grafting: A method shortening illness, *J. Trauma*, **14**:389, 1974.
16 Curreri, P. W. and J. A. Marvin: Advances in clinical care of burn patients, *West. J. Med.*, **123**:275, 1975.
17 ———, D. Richmond, J. A. Marvin, and C. R. Baxter: Dietary requirements of patients with major burns, *J. Am. Diet. Assoc.*, **65**:415, 1974.
18 ——— and B. A. Pruitt, Jr.: The evaluation and treatment of the burn patient, *Am. J. Occup. Ther.*, **24**:475, 1970.
19 ———: Metabolic and nutritional aspects of thermal injury, *Burns*, **2**:16, 1975.
20 ———, E. L. Heck, L. Brown, and C. R. Baxter: Stimulated nitroblue tetrazolium test to assess neutrophil antibacterial function: Prediction of wound sepsis in burned patients, *Surgery*, **74**:6, 1973.
21 ———, M. J. Asch, and B. A. Pruitt, Jr.: The treatment of chemical burns: Specialized diagnostic, therapeutic, and prognostic considerations, *J. Trauma*, **10**:634, 1970.
22 DiVincenti, F. C., J. A. Moncrief, and B. A. Pruitt, Jr.: Electrical injuries: A review of 65 cases, *J. Trauma*, **9**:497, 1969.
23 ———, B. A. Pruitt, Jr., and J. M. Reckler: Inhalation injuries, *J. Trauma*, **11**:100, 1971.

24 ———, P. W. Curreri, and B. A. Pruitt, Jr.: Use of mesh skin autografts in the burn patient, *Plast. Reconstr. Surg.*, **44**:464, 1969.

25 Dobbs, E. R. and P. W. Curreri: Burns: Analysis of results of physical therapy in 681 patients, *J. Trauma*, **12**:242, 1972.

26 Fox, C. L., B. W. Roppole, and W. Stanford: Control of *Pseudomonas* infection in burns by silver sulfadiazine, *Surg. Gynecol. Obstetr.*, **128**:1021, 1969.

27 Gruber, R. P., D. R. Laub, and L. M. Bistnes: The effect of hydrotherapy on the clinical course and pH of experimental cutaneous chemical burns, *Plast. Reconstr. Surg.*, **55**:200, 1975.

28 Heck, E. L., L. Browne, P. W. Curreri, and C. R. Baxter: Evaluation of leukocyte function in burned individuals by *in vitro* oxygen consumption, *J. Trauma*, **15**:486, 1975.

29 Hummel, R. P., G. B. MacMillan, and W. A. Altemeier: Topical and systemic antibacterial agents in the treatment of burns, *Ann. Surg.*, **172**:370, 1970.

30 Jelenko, C.: Chemicals that burn, *J. Trauma*, **14**:65, 1974.

31 Larson, D. L., S. Abston, and E. B. Evans: "Splints and Traction," in H. C. Polk and H. H. Stone (eds.), "Contemporary Burn Management," Little, Brown and Company, Boston, 1971, p. 419.

32 ———, ———, ———, et al.: Techniques for decreasing scar formation and contractures in the burn patient, *J. Trauma*, **11**:807, 1971.

33 Linares, H. A., C. W. Kischer, M. Dobrkovsky, and D. L. Larson: On the origin of the hypertrophic scar, *J. Trauma*, **13**:70, 1973.

34 Lindberg, R. B., J. A. Moncrief, and A. D. Mason, Jr.: Control of experimental and clinical burn wound sepsis by topical application of sulfamylon compounds, *Ann. N.Y. Acad. Sci.*, **150**:950, 1968.

35 Loebl, E. C., J. A. Marvin, E. L. Heck, P. W. Curreri, and C. R. Baxter: The method of quantitative burn-wound biopsy cultures and its routine use in the care of the burned patient, *Am. J. Clin. Pathol.*, **61**:20, 1974.

36 ———, ———, ———, ———, and ———: Survival with ecthyma gangrenosium, a previously fatal complication of burns, *J. Trauma*, **14**:370, 1974.

37 ———, ———, ———, ———, and ———: The use of quantitative biopsy cultures in bacteriologic monitoring of burn patients, *J. Surg. Res.*, **16**:1, 1974.

38 MacMillan, B. G.: "Deep Excision and Early Grafting," in H. C. Polk and H. H. Stone (eds.), *Contemporary Burn Management*, Little, Brown and Company, Boston, 1971, p. 357.

39 Marvin, J. A., E. L. Heck, E. C. Loebl, P. W. Curreri, and C. R. Baxter: Usefulness of blood cultures in confirming septic complications in burn patients: Evaluation of a new culture method, *J. Trauma*, **15**:657, 1975.

40 Moncrief, J. A. and B. A. Pruitt, Jr.: Electrical injury, *Postgrad. Med.*, **48**:189, 1970.

41 Monofo, W. W., C. E. Aulenbacher, and E. Pappalardo: Early tangential excision of the eschars of major burns, *Arch. Surg.*, **104**:503, 1972.

42 ——— and C. A. Moyer: Effectiveness of dilute aqueous silver nitrate in the treatment of major burns, *Arch. Surg.*, **91**:200, 1965.

43 Moylan, J. A., K. Adib, and M. Birnbaum: Fiberoptic bronchoscopy following thermal injury, *Surg. Gynecol. Obstetr.*, **140**:541, 1975.

44 Munster, A. M. and C. P. Artz: A neglected aspect of trauma pathophysiology: The immunologic response to injury, *South. Med. J.*, **67**:935, 1974.

45 Pruitt, B. A., Jr. and P. W. Curreri: The burn wound and its care, *Arch. Surg.*, **103**:461, 1971.

46 ——— and ———: "The Use of Homograft and Heterograft Skin," in H. C. Polk and H. H. Stone (eds.), *Contemporary Burn Management*, Little, Brown and Company, Boston, 1971, p. 397.

47 Reckler, J. M., R. J. Flemma, and B. A. Pruitt, Jr.: Costal condritis: An unusual complication in the burned patient, *J. Trauma*, **13**:76, 1973.

48 Salisbury, R. E. and L. Palm: Dynamic splinting for dorsal burns of the hand, *Plast. Reconstr. Surg.*, **51**:226, 1973.

49 ———, J. L. Hunt, G. D. Warden, and B. A. Pruitt, Jr.: Management of electrical burns of the upper extremities, *Plast. Reconstr. Surg.*, **51**:648, 1973.

50 Snyder, W. H., B. M. Bowles, and G. B. Mac-Millan: The use of expansion meshed grafts in the acute and reconstructive management of thermal injury: A clinical evaluation, *J. Trauma*, **10**:740, 1970.

51 Stone, H. H.: "Mesh Grafting," in H. C. Polk and H. H. Stone (eds.), *Contemporary Burn Management*, Little, Brown and Company, Boston, 1971, p. 383.

52 Teplitz, C., D. Davis, A. D. Mason, Jr., and J. A. Moncrief: *Pseudomonas* burn wound sepsis. I. Pathogenesis of experimental *Pseudomonas* burn wound sepsis. *J. Surg. Res.*, 4:200, 1964.

53 ———, ———, H. L. Walker, et al.: *Pseudomonas* burn wound sepsis. II. Hematogenous infection at the junction of the burn wound and the unburned hypodermis, *J. Surg., Res.*, 4:217, 1964.

54 Warden, J. D., A. D. Mason, and B. A. Pruitt, Jr.: Suppression of leukocyte chemotaxis *in vitro* by chemotherapeutic agents used in management of thermal injuries, *Ann. Surg.*, **181**: 363, 1975.

55 Wilmore, D. W., A. D. Mason, Jr., D. W. Johnson, and B. A. Pruitt, Jr.: Affect of ambient temperature on heat production and heat loss in burn patients, *J. Appl. Physiol.*, **38**:593, 1975.

56 ———: Hormonal responses and their effect on metabolism, *Surg. Clin. North Am.*, **56**:999, 1976.

57 Zikria, B. A., G. C. Weston, M. Chodoff, and J. M. Ferrer: Smoke and carbon monoxide poisoning in fire victims, *J. Trauma*, **12**:641, 1972.

Chapter 9

Vascular Injuries

Malcolm O. Perry, M.D.

INTRODUCTION

Over 200 years ago Hallowell successfully repaired a brachial artery by transfixing the edges of the laceration with a steel pin and then looping threads about the pin.[11] By 1900 Carrel and Guthrie had developed suture techniques for repair of arteries and veins, and subsequently described techniques of resection, anastomosis, and graft interposition.[2,5] By 1910 over 100 lateral arterial repairs and 46 end-to-end anastomoses or vein grafts had been clinically performed.[10] These techniques were not widely employed, however, and in World War I and World War II amputation following vascular injuries was common because ligation was utilized as the primary mode of therapy. Hughes reported that from the Korean war the overall amputation rate after ligation was approximately 51 percent,

similar to that obtained during World War II. During the Korean conflict, when arterial repair was undertaken, the subsequent amputation rate was reported to be only 13 percent.[11] It therefore is clear that repair rather than ligation is the treatment of choice for major vascular injuries, and early identification and repair of these injuries are important concepts in the management of vascular trauma.

ETIOLOGY

Aggressive acts of violence are responsible for the majority of vascular injuries encountered in the civilian population. Of over 900 patients undergoing operative exploration for vascular injuries at Parkland Memorial Hospital, gunshot wounds were found to be the cause of injury in 55 percent, edged instruments in 36 percent, and blunt trauma in 9 percent of the cases.[12] The distribution of injuries encountered in this series revealed that the extremity was most often involved, and the femoral, brachial, and carotid arteries were injured more frequently than other vessels. Penetrating wounds of the abdomen are likely to damage the aorta or the renal arteries and are usually associated with major venous injuries (Table 9-1).

It has been clearly demonstrated that associated injuries are often major determinants in the eventual outcome, and Table 9-2 illustrates the incidence of these injuries. It is apparent from these data that in most patients with arterial injury multiple wounds of other systems will be encountered.

PATHOPHYSIOLOGY

Penetrating wounds are the most common causes of arterial injury, and lacerations or transections are usually found. In some cases, mural contusion and severe spasm may produce acute arterial obstruction and ischemia. Multiple, penetrating arterial wounds may be seen as a result of shotgun injuries, and severe arterial and venous disruption may accompany fractures, particularly of long bones. Secondary thrombosis is commonly seen with arterial injuries and may involve the accompanying vein. This is particularly likely to occur when the patient has been hypotensive. In the majority of cases, however, arterial injuries

Table 9-1   Arterial Injuries, Parkland Series

Distribution	Number
Extremity	461
Visceral	24
Aorta	38
Cervical	78

Table 9-2   Associated Injuries

Type	%
Significant vein	34
Major nerve	18
Separate artery	7
Lung, abdominal viscera	39
Shock	36

are not associated with severe distal ischemia and there may be little or no immediate clinical signs of arterial damage.[12]

Arterial injuries as a result of fractures of the long bones may be very difficult to assess because of associated soft tissue swelling and bony deformity.[18] Angulation or compression of the artery may be the cause of initial injury, but this may be complicated by subsequent thrombosis distal to the site of injury. In other cases, kinking of the artery may be associated with contusion, laceration, or even transection, an event most likely to affect the artery where it is relatively fixed by major branches. Supracondylar fractures or dislocation of the humerus or femur are therefore likely to injure or obstruct the adjacent arteries. Less commonly, fractures of the clavicle or of the tibial plateau may produce injuries of the accompanying vessels.

Tolerance of the extremities to ischemia may be difficult to assess because some cells are more susceptible to anoxia than others, presumably as a result of differences in oxygen requirements. There is, for example, a fourfold variation between the respiratory rate of the skin and that of the retina, and it is also believed that the brain is particularly vulnerable to hypoxia because of its relatively large oxygen requirement.[8]

Studies of ischemic skeletal and cardiac muscle suggest that cellular swelling may follow hypoxia and may also play an important role in irreversibility. Volkmann's contracture, for example, has been attributed to obstruction of arterial flow to the extremity, with subsequent fibrosis and contraction of skeletal muscles.[8] Harmen in 1948 produced temporary complete ischemia in the hind legs of rabbits with a tourniquet, and subsequently injected bromphenol blue into the artery to examine the rate of penetration and elimination of this vital dye.[6] He noted that the dye immediately stained normal and mildly ischemic muscle as soon as the tourniquet was released and concluded that the arteries did not remain obstructed. If the ischemia were extended beyond 3 h, however, there was considerable retention of dye within the muscle. If the ischemia lasted as long as 6 h, the dye did not enter the muscle for at least 30 min, findings suggesting that although the circulation was open it was very sluggish. Histological examination of these animals subsequently demonstrated dilated and engorged capillaries, but no thrombi were seen. Generalized swelling of the tissue was documented by demonstration of a gain of weight in the ischemic limb, which increased with the duration of the ischemia.

It is apparent that the susceptibility of different cells to hypoxia varies, and previous studies have indicated that peripheral nerves and muscles have relatively less resistance to ischemia than skin. Many investigators have suggested that irreversible changes in skeletal muscle and peripheral nerves occur after 4 to 6 h of ischemia.[8] This may be demonstrated histologically. Because of these differences in susceptibility to hypoxia, it is clear that the skin and subcutaneous tissue may survive periods of hypoxia which will not be tolerated by skeletal muscles or peripheral nerves.

If the collateral circulation is not well developed, muscle necrosis and irreversible changes often appear within 4 to 6 h. If definitive therapy can be concluded early in the course of ischemia, a successful outcome can be expected; but if revascularization is delayed and 8 to 12 h of ischemia occur, repair is considerably less effective.[11]

CLINICAL MANIFESTATIONS AND DIAGNOSIS

Acute arterial insufficiency usually occurs abruptly and without warning, yet early diagnosis is essential if reconstruction is to be effective. Five cardinal features of arterial insufficiency have been described and are frequently referred to as the "five p's": pain, paralysis, paresthesia, pallor, and pulselessness. In patients with arterial insufficiency, pain occurs acutely in over 75 percent and is well localized in the afflicted extremity. It is usually quite severe, but in patients with good collateral circulation the pain may not be prominent. If there are multiple wounds, it may be difficult for the patient to recognize or describe pain related to ischemia. In some patients the onset of ischemia is sudden and dramatic, and paralysis and anesthesia may occur early, and pain is not a persistent symptom. Paresis and paresthesia are important symptoms in assessing viability of an ischemic extremity; because peripheral nerve endings and skeletal muscle are very sensitive to hypoxia, these symptoms are frequently seen in patients with severe ischemia. It is important to separate perception of light touch from that of pressure, pain, and temperature because the larger fibers serving these latter functions are relatively less susceptible to hypoxia. A patient with ischemia may therefore maintain sensation to pinprick and yet be unable to perceive light touch.

Distal pulses may be absent in patients with an acute arterial injury, but, as alluded to previously, up to 15 percent of patients with proven arterial injuries may have normal distal pulses and pressures.[7,11,12] Despite this, significant disturbances in nutritive flow may occur in these patients, and assessment be-yond the mere evaluation of pulses is impor-tant. Table 9-3 lists the clinical signs which suggest vascular injury. When several of these signs coexist, the likelihood of significant ar-terial injury is very strong, but the absence of these signs does not preclude the presence of a vascular wound (Fig. 9-1).

In some patients detection of distal pulses may be difficult because of swelling of the extremity and associated soft tissue or bony injury. An acutely ischemic extremity is often pale and cool and has empty veins; there may be a definite line of temperature change which is somewhat below the true level of occlusion, usually one joint away from the actual site of occlusion. If the signs of ischemia exist, yet pulses are palpable, further evaluation is re-quired and arteriography is usually needed.

DIAGNOSTIC TESTS

Preoperative arteriography is particularly helpful and offers fairly reliable evidence as to the presence or absence of significant vascular injury. False negative examinations do occur, but with high-grade biplane studies most inju-ries will be detected.[20] Preoperative arteriog-raphy is particularly helpful in assessing frac-tures of the long bones, pelvis, and bones about the thoracic outlet. Because of wide-spread soft tissue and bony damage in these

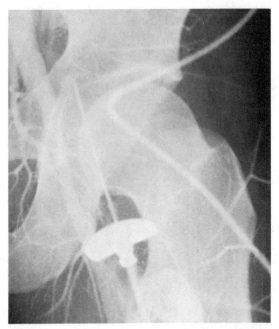

Figure 9-1 Injury of profunda femoris artery. Normal distal pulse and pressure.

patients, accurate evaluation of the severity of the wound and the likelihood of associated arterial or venous injury may be very difficult (Figs. 9-2 and 9-3).

It is difficult to assess the injuries associated with scattered pellet wounds of the leg and forearm incurred as a result of shotgun blasts (Fig. 9-4). In these patients, solid indications for vascular exploration may not exist. How-ever, debridement may be necessary, and one may in the course of such a debridement satisfactorily determine if there is significant arterial injury. However, in some cases de-bridement will be confined to superficial tis-sues, and preoperative arteriography may be of great value in detecting areas of injury and thus avoiding the necessity of an extensive negative vascular exploration.[20]

Arteriography is also of great value in the evaluation of penetrating injuries of the chest and of the neck, especially when the latter is near the base of the skull.[4,12,13,21] Acute false

Table 9-3: Signs and Symptoms Suggesting Arterial Injury

Diminished or absent distal pulse

History of or persistent arterial bleeding

Large or expanding hematoma

Major hemorrhage with hypotension or shock

Bruit at or distal to suspected site of injury

Injury of anatomically related nerves

Anatomical proximity of wound to major artery

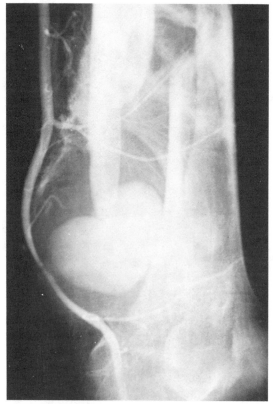

Figure 9-2 Fracture of femur and femoral artery injury. Distal pulse present.

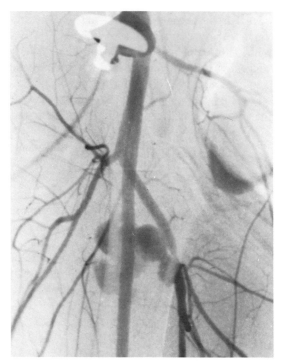

Figure 9-3 Injury of profunda femoris artery.

aneurysms and arterial venous fistulae may be exposed by this technique, and suitable operative preparations may be undertaken prior to encountering the lesion, thus reducing the danger of uncontrollable hemorrhage[16] (Fig. 9-5).

Arteriography is therefore very helpful despite the fact that on rare occasions false negatives may occur. If high-quality films are not obtained or there is a question remaining as to the presence or absence of arterial injury following the initial studies, repeat arteriograms are indicated. It is apparent that when strong indications for surgical exploration exist, delay for arteriography is undesirable. Significant morbidity and mortality may be encountered in patients who have an unstable circulation if they are subjected to prolonged diagnostic procedures and needed surgery is delayed.[12,20]

Other adjunctive methods may occasionally be useful in the detection and management of vascular injuries, and among these the ultrasonic velocity flow detector has been extensively employed. The detection of diminished segmental pressures or obstructed flow signals may be indicative of arterial or venous injuries. These procedures are not entirely reliable because some patients may have normal distal pressures even in the presence of a subsequently proven arterial injury. The Doppler ultrasonic techniques are perhaps of more use in the postoperative period, where the detection of pulses in a swollen extremity may be difficult. In these cases the need for arteriography may be diminished with these tests. Any

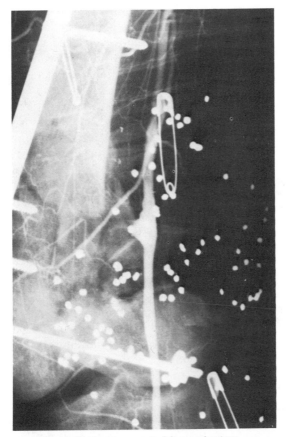

Figure 9-4 Shotgun wound of femoral artery.

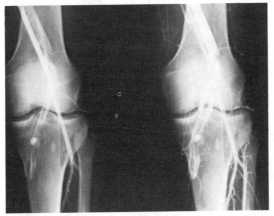

Figure 9-5 Arteriovenous fistula following fracture repair.

discrepancy, however, in pressure measurement or functional evaluation is a clear indication for arteriography.[7,11]

MANAGEMENT

In the management of any trauma patient certain priorities must be established.[4,13] This is particularly true of patients with vascular injuries. As alluded to in the previous section, vascular injuries are commonly associated with serious injuries of other organ systems and are often complicated by marked hypovolemia. An adequate airway must initially be established, and access for the intravenous administration of fluids must be immediately secured. It is important to place large-bore venous catheters into both upper and lower extremities in order to facilitate the treatment of hypovolemia by administration of balanced salt solutions and appropriately matched whole blood. With penetrating injuries of the trunk or chest it is apparent that superior and inferior vena caval injuries may be encountered, and alternate routes for fluid administration must be acquired. In patients who have associated orthopedic injuries stabilization of the extremities should be obtained, thus avoiding continuing damage to the neurovascular bundles. External support is favored in these cases and often can be obtained with a semirigid dressing and splinting.[18] Serious associated injuries of the head, lungs, and viscera are often encountered and must be managed if a successful conclusion is to be obtained. Preparations should be made for arteriography to be accomplished either during or at the completion of contemplated vascular repairs.

The supine position is the most useful in the majority of these patients, and the chest, abdomen, and legs should be prepared appropriately so that access to venous autografts in contralateral extremities is possible. Vertical incisions of the abdomen and the extremities are most useful since they may be readily extended in either direction to allow proximal and distal control of major vascular wounds. Injuries of the neck and thoracic outlet may require thoracotomy for proximal control, and this is usually achieved through an anterior sternal splitting incision or through a thoracotomy to reach the left subclavian artery.[4,7,13] Once exposure of the vessels is obtained, hemorrhage can be controlled by pressure, tapes, vascular clamps, or occasionally balloon catheters. In some cases the remote insertion of a Fogarty balloon catheter may be useful in controlling relatively inaccessible wounds of the arterial tree. This is particularly true in the arch of the aorta and the great vessels, and in the proximal abdominal aorta.[19] Once control of hemorrhage is obtained and exploration is complete, it is wise to pause and complete the resuscitation prior to repair of the damage. In most cases this will require only a few minutes, but this delay for resuscitation is important, and attempts to complete repairs while the patient remains hypovolemic and hypotensive often adversely influence morbidity and mortality.

General Principles

Once control of the injured vessel is obtained, careful evaluation will reveal the type of repair required. When lacerations are encountered in large vessels, lateral repair may be quite satisfactory. This is especially true when minimal debridement is needed. In these cases careful closure is obtained utilizing vascular sutures and assuring intimal coaptation. If this is not possible without undue narrowing of the vessel, patch graft angioplasty may be employed using autogenous material from the saphenous or cephalic vein.

In most instances resection and end-to-end anastomosis is desirable. If the laceration involves more than 50 percent of the vessel lumen, it is preferable to resect the injured area and perform an end-to-end anastomosis in the usual fashion. During mobilization and repair, the vessel should be handled gently because intimal trauma may predispose to the eventual deposition of atheromatous plaques. If, following debridement, suitable end-to-end anastomosis cannot be performed without placing tension on the suture line, interposition of an autogenous graft is preferable, using the saphenous vein, cephalic vein, or autogenous artery. In most injuries of peripheral vessels suitable autogenous grafts are available, but in injuries of the aortoiliac system it may be necessary to interpose plastic prosthesis, although this is particularly undesirable in the presence of associated injuries. In certain cases remote bypasses, such as an axillary-femoral, may be established through clean tissue planes so as to avoid placing plastic prostheses into a contaminated area.

Established vascular techniques are used for the repair of arteries, and the suture material is largely a matter of personal preference. Most vascular surgeons prefer polyester sutures because of their durability and increased tensile strength. Monofilament sutures of prolene are especially useful despite being relatively stiff in comparison with braided Dacron sutures. Careful intimal coaptation and secure repair without undue tension are essential to successful reconstruction. In a large vessel continuous suture techniques are quite satisfactory, but in small vessels or those in which spasm is prominent interrupted techniques are preferable. Careful evaluation of antergrade and retrograde flow should be made prior to completion of the anastomosis, and if clots are encountered during exploration, investigation of the distal bed and removal of clots utilizing Fogarty balloon catheters are advocated. The presence of an intervening collateral bed may produce what appears to be adequate backflow from the distal arterial segment, and yet distal clot occlusion still exists. Irrigation with a dilute heparin solution may be very helpful during the period of arterial occlusion attending repair, and systemic heparin may be utilized in patients where associated injuries do not make its use hazardous. At the termination of the procedure, distal arterial pulses and adequate venous flow must be obtained or operative arteriography is indicated. Many vascular surgeons prefer that each of these procedures be followed by operative arteriography in order to assess the distal circulation, regardless of the physical findings.

Concomitant venous injuries should usually be repaired to prevent late postphlebitic phenomena and also to protect the arterial repair.[14,15] In the extremities there are anatomical provisions for parallel drainage, and ligation of some of these vessels may be acceptable. In most cases where there is disruption of the popliteal, common femoral, portal, or mesenteric veins, repair should be undertaken if at all feasible. The same principles utilized in arterial repair are equally applicable to the repair of veins, but if adequate flow is obtained, operative phlebography is usually not required. Postoperative films are often very helpful and are recommended.

Adjunctive Therapy

Protection of the distal vascular bed is very important and can often be accomplished by local or systemic anticoagulation with intravenous heparin. Administration of other rheologic agents has been advocated, but their usefulness has not been confirmed. Dextran may be of some value in retarding the formation of intravascular thrombosis by increasing the electronegativity of red cells and intima. It may be of particular benefit in enhancing flow through the microcirculation, an effect apart from hemodilution and an increase in circulating volume.

Other rheologic benefits have been claimed for the administration of hypertonic solutions of mannitol. Jameson and others suggest that this agent may be effective in reducing cellular swelling, particularly of perivascular structures, and therefore may prevent the impaired reflow phenomena.[8] In addition, an osmotic diuresis will also follow and may be of value after hypovolemia has been corrected. Mannitol may be of particular benefit in patients who develop myoglobinuria as a result of severe muscle ischemia. In such cases, when the pigment load may further compromise renal failure, establishment of an osmotic diuresis and alkalization of the urine are important therapeutic measures.

It has been demonstrated that potassium may be released as cell membrane integrity is breached and may produce significant cardiac abnormalities. The hyperkalemia may respond to the administration of glucose and insulin and reestablishment of adequate volume and tissue flow. Low flow states of hypovolemia and multiple injuries may induce lactic acidemia, and it has been demonstrated that the increased hydrogen ion concentration may interfere with cardiac function. It is apparent from the studies of Shires, McClelland, and others that the major requirement for correction of such a compositional abnormality is restoration of adequate tissue flow.[12] This is best achieved by repairing volume and improving cardiac output; the judicious administration of sodium bicarbonate may be useful after this stage of treatment.

The management of arterial spasm can be a very difficult problem, but usually responds to gentle, simple, hydraulic, or mechanical dilatation. The administration of drugs such as papaverine, sodium bicarbonate, local anesthetics, and tolazoline has been employed, but these measures have not been consistently effective. Recent experiences in renal transplantation suggest that a 6% solution of magnesium sulfate topically applied may be effective in combatting local areas of severe vasospasm. In most cases, however, simple mechanical dilatation is effective, but care must be taken not to over-distend the vessels as this produces intimal injury which may predispose to thrombosis.

As Patman has demonstrated, adequate early fasciotomy is an important adjunctive procedure in the management of ischemic extremities and may be particularly useful in managing vascular trauma.[11] Even after successful repair, ischemic tissue may swell and, when confined by rigid fascial compartments such as the anterior compartment of the lower extremity, secondary ischemia may result from interference with nutritive flow. Table 9-4 lists the indications most commonly employed for the performance of fasciotomy in relation to vascular injuries. These indications for fasciotomy are relative and, with the exception of swelling of the extremity following repair or ligation, may not be employed as a primary procedure. If the major blood supply to an extremity is impaired or interrupted, however, fasciotomy may be useful from the outset. Many investigators believe that this indication should be extended to include all patients who have combined arterial and venous injuries.

There are numerous techniques employed for fasciotomy, but in most instances fasciotomy through limited skin incisions is satisfactory. The fascia is usually the limiting tissue, and skin may contribute very little to the tamponade. There is little morbidity to the procedure, and often primary closure can be obtained; but if massive swelling of the extremity supervenes, split-thickness skin grafts

Table 9-4:   Indications for Fasciotomy

Combined arterial and venous injury

Massive soft tissue damage

Delay between wounding and definitive repair

Prolonged hypotension

Swelling of extremity

will be required to cover the defects created by the fasciotomy incisions.

In those instances in which tissue swelling has already occurred, wide dermotomy as well as fasciotomy may be required, and then almost always secondary grafting will be necessary to cover these wounds. The anterior compartment of the lower leg is most vulnerable because of its rigid fascial layers, and when fasciotomy is employed this compartment should always be opened. Usually it is also necessary to decompress the deep compartment, and to do this two fascial incisions are needed. In some instances resection of the fibula will be required in order to assure adequate decompression of the compartment, but this is relatively rare. Most failures attributed to fasciotomy are related to delay in use or inadequate decompression, especially of the deep compartment. Superficial infections may occur, but are infrequent if the vascular repair is successful and early cover of the fasciotomy incisions is obtained.

Specific Arterial Injuries

Carotid   Artery   Injuries   In managing wounds of the carotid artery, the neurologic status of the patient may be a critical factor in determining whether repair should be accomplished.[9] Thal and Bradley et al. in recent reports have suggested a plan of management which takes into account several important features   often   encountered   in   these patients.[1,23] The patients are divided into three categories: The first includes patients with carotid artery injuries in whom no neurologic deficit is present; in the second group are those patients who have only a mild deficit; and in the third group are those patients who have a severe neurologic deficit on admission. Data reported by these workers suggest that in those patients in whom no neurologic deficit is present or in whom the deficit is mild and there is uninterrupted flow in the carotid artery, repair is advisable and is safe. In the third group of patients, however, those with severe neurologic deficit, and particularly when associated with altered consciousness, it may be extremely hazardous to repair some of these lesions. The conversion of an anemic to a hemorrhagic infarct is a real threat and is most likely to occur when a completely occluded carotid has been repaired.[9] Therefore, if a residual thrombus is present in the distal carotid, it is probably safer to ligate rather than repair the vessel. When an embolus is present distally in a small artery, it is usually safe to repair the artery. If flow cannot be restored but the collateral circulation is adequate, many patients can be expected to recover.

Arteriography is particularly useful in these patients both preoperatively and at the completion of the procedure.[3] It may be necessary during the course of the operation to perform distal arteriograms in order to determine if the carotid circulation is completely open. The artery is repaired in the usual fashion, utilizing simple suture, resection, or anastomosis and graft interposition as required. In certain instances restoration of flow between the common and internal carotids can be established by utilizing the external carotid as a pedicle graft to bridge the defect created by the vascular wound (Fig. 9-6).

Careful evaluation of the patient's neurologic status in the postoperative period is imperative. Deterioration or change is usually an indication for repeat arteriogram. This is best performed by transfemoral entry, but in certain cases direct puncture of a common carotid low in the neck may be satisfactory. These procedures do not pose a significant threat to the patient at these times, and if emergence of a neurologic deficit is a result of technical inperfections in the repaired area, early arteriography and repair are essential if a successful conclusion is to be obtained.

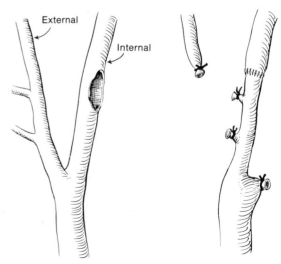

Figure 9-6 See text for explanation.

Although wounds of the innominate and subclavian vessels are usually not accompanied by neurologic deficits, when the complications are present it is reasonable to employ the same considerations which are used to determine the need for and safety of repair in carotid artery injuries.[4,13,20] In most cases special support of the cerebral circulation will not be required, but in some instances temporary inlying shunts may be employed, especially in those patients in whom there is impaired backflow at the time of operation or in whom distal carotid pressures are less than 50 mmHg. Systemic or regional heparinization is a useful adjunct in the management of injuries of extracranial vessels, but associated wounds in the trauma patient may preclude its use. As in the management of other extracranial vessels, arteriography is an important adjunct during the operation and in the immediate postoperative period.

Injuries to the Vessels of the Extremities
Those principles elucidated in the preceding sections are applied to the management of arterial and venous injuries of the extremities.

In certain cases when the multiply injured patient has serious associated wounds, repair of the vessels supplying the extremities may not be feasible. Ligation may be required in order to expedite the procedure. There are specific areas where arterial ligation is associated with less threat of loss of the extremity, and these principles may be applied to the subclavian and axillary arteries in specific instances. It is usually desirable to repair the brachial artery, but ligation may be used distal to the origin of the profunda because of the rich collateral circulation. Viability is usually not threatened, although late functional deficits may occasionally occur.

As a general rule, injuries below the elbow joint are not routinely explored except in specific instances, i.e., when there is a bruit or AV fistula, continuing hemorrhage, extensive soft tissue damage requiring debridement, associated nerve injuries, or evidence of distal ischemia. Distal tissue loss is uncommon except in those cases where there is a combined injury of both radial and ulnar arteries. If exploration is undertaken, ligation may be employed, but it is preferable to repair the arteries.

The femoral artery is the most commonly injured major artery in the lower extremity, and repair can usually be satisfactorily accomplished utilizing the usual techniques. Particular effort should be made to restore the profunda femoral because of the extreme susceptibility of the superficial femoral artery to atherosclerosis. In such cases the profunda will become the primary route of blood supply for the lower extremity.

Injuries of the popliteal artery and vein are particularly prone to produce severe distal ischemia, and early recognition and repair are important.[17] Preoperative and operative arteriography are important adjuncts in the management of these injuries and should be employed if there is any question as to patency of the distal circulation. In cases in which ex-

tended orthopedic manipulations may be necessary, it may be desirable to insert a temporary inlying bypass shunt into the popliteal vessels to restore distal perfusion while such procedures are being completed. At the completion of the procedure, arteriography is recommended to evaluate the distal circulation.

The importance of repair of the popliteal vein has been illustrated by Rich, Richie, and others.[12,15,17] Although the tibial veins are usually paired, as is occasionally the popliteal vein, significant venous outflow blockade in the lower extremity is almost certain to result in early failure of the arterial repair. Previously held opinions that venous repair would lead to an increased incidence of postphlebitic problems and pulmonary embolic phenomena have not been substantiated.[15] In fact the reverse has proven to be true, and there is actually a lower incidence of thromboembolic complications following repair of major veins than following ligation. Although many of these venous repairs will fail in the early postoperative period, subsequent recanalization has been demonstrated to occur in a significant number of cases, and unless the venous repair poses an undue threat to the patient, it should be performed concomitantly with arterial repair (see Table 9-5).

Injuries below the trifurcation of the popliteal, like those injuries distal to the elbow, are not routinely explored unless there are specif-

Table 9-5: Results, Parkland Series

Result	%
Failure of repair	5.2
Bleeding	2.0
Infection	3.1
Amputation	1.8
Mortality	10.4

ic indications. At the completion of repair of combined injuries of the popliteal artery and vein, particularly when associated with severe soft tissue damage or fractures, three-compartment fasciotomy of the lower extremity is an important adjunctive procedure.

Intraabdominal Vascular Injuries Major wounds of the abdominal aorta and its branches are extremely dangerous and are often associated with significant venous and visceral injuries.[21] The infrarenal aorta and iliac vessels are most commonly damaged, and although lateral repair or resection and end-to-end anastomosis may be occasionally successful, it is often necessary to employ plastic prosthesis for the restoration of vascular continuity. If there is associated bacterial contamination, the construction of a remote bypass such as an axillary-femoral through clean tissue planes may be required; then ligation of the injured arteries is performed, and reconstruction is delayed until infection and contamination have been completely controlled.

Special problems are encountered when there are massive pelvic hematomas as a result of blunt trauma. These are not usually explored unless there is evidence of major vascular injury because hemostasis may be extremely difficult to achieve. It is wise not to disturb the tamponade effect of the posterior peritoneum in these patients, but in the event the hematoma is inadvertently entered, direct ligation, suture ligation, and pressure will usually control hemorrhage. Hypogastric artery ligation is usually ineffective in these cases. In contrast are those patients who have penetrating trauma involving the hypogastric plexus. Exploration and repair must be undertaken and in some instances may be extremely difficult. Temporary occlusion of all major vessels proximal and distal to these lesions may be required before hemorrhage can be brought under control. In most instances ligation is the preferred method of treatment, but in patients

who have associated arterial occlusive disease, hypogastric artery repair may be undertaken if it does not pose an undue threat to the patient.

Splanchnic Vessels Injuries of the mesenteric and renal vessels are approached and repaired in the usual fashion. Arteriography may be required for the clear definition of these injuries; this is particularly true in the evaluation of potential renal injuries. The intravenous pyelogram (IVP), although useful, is not a satisfactory screening test, but high-grade arteriography offers valuable evidence as to the presence or absence of a renal injury. In patients who have perinephric hematomas but in whom a normal arterial structure can be demonstrated, exploration is usually not required, unless there are associated injuries to the pelvis or ureter. If temporary interruption of the renal blood supply is necessary, local renal hypothermia may be achieved with simple irrigation with a solution of iced saline.[11] With the renal artery temporarily clamped, significant protective hypothermia of the kidney can be obtained within 3 to 5 min. Ligation of the renal veins is usually tolerated, particularly when performed close to the vena cava; and although a transient rise in the glomerular filtration rate may occur following ligation, significant damage to the kidney is usually not encountered.

Retroperitoneal Hematomas Retroperitoneal hematomas which harbor suspected significant vascular injuries are usually explored, with the exception of the pelvic hematoma associated with blunt trauma.[12] Injuries of the infrarenal vena cava are often encountered, and if tamponade has occurred prior to operation, morbidity and mortality are quite low and repair is relatively simple. If the caval injuries at the time of exploration are still bleeding, there is a significant increase in the mortality. The repairs are effected in the usual fashion, and lateral repair of lacerations is often quite satisfactory. A mortality rate of 13 percent has been reported with repair of infra-renal caval injuries.

Injuries of the inferior vena cava at the level of the renal veins or above the renal veins are quite serious, and the mortality from these wounds is regularly in excess of 50 percent. Exposure and control of injuries of the cava at or above the renal vein can be quite difficult, and exsanguinating hemorrhage may be encountered. Nevertheless, these injuries must be approached and repaired, and the intracaval balloon catheters may be very useful. Techniques of repair are the same as those utilized in other areas. If interposition grafts are required, a section of iliac vein or internal jugular vein may be useful in achieving continuity, especially in the portal system.

Intrahepatic caval injuries are extremely dangerous, and control may never be achieved despite the use of caval shunts inserted through the left atrium. These techniques are very useful in the approach and management of injuries of the hepatic veins and of the intrahepatic cava. Although the injuries are quite serious, some can be successfully managed with early identification and operation.

BIBLIOGRAPHY

1 Bradley, E. L., II: Management of penetrating carotid injuries: An alternative approach, *J. Trauma*, **13**:248–255, March 1973.

2 Carrel, A.:The surgery of blood vessels, *Johns Hopkins Bull.* **18**:18, 1907.

3 Crissey, M. M. and E. F. Bernstein: Delayed presentation of carotid intimal tear following blunt craniocervical trauma, *Surgery*, **75**:543–549, April 1974.

4 Flint, L. M., W. H. Snyder, M. O. Perry, and G. T. Shires: Management of major vascular injuries in the base of the neck: An 11-year experience with 146 cases, *Arch. Surg.*, **106**:407–413, April 1973.

5 Guthrie, G. C.: Heterotransplantation of blood vessels, *Am. J. Physio.*, **19**:482,1907.

6 Harmen, J. W.: The significance of local vascular phenomena in the production of ischemic necrosis in skeletal muscle, *Am. J. Pathol.*, **24**:625–641, 1948.

7 Hewitt, R. L., A. D. Smith, M. L. Becker, E. S. Lindsey, J. B. Dowling, and T. Drapanas: Penetrating vascular injuries of the thoracic outlet, *Surgery*, **76**:715–722, November 1974.

8 Jameson, R. L.: The role of cellular swelling in the pathogenesis of organ ischemia, *West. J. Med.*, **120**:215–218, March 1974.

9 McNamara, J. J., D. K. Brief, W. Beasley and J. K. Wright: Vascular injury in Vietnam combat casualties: Results of treatment at the 24th evacaution hospital 1 July 1967 to 12 August 1969, *Ann. Surg.*, **178**:143–147, August 1973.

10 Nolan, B.: Vascular injuries, *J. R. Coll. Surg.*, **13**:72, 1968.

11 Patman, R. D., E. Poulos, and G. T. Shires: The management of civilian arterial injuries, *Surg. Gynecol. Obstet.*, **118**:725, 1964.

12 Perry, M. O., E. R. Thal, and G. T. Shires: Management of arterial injuries, *Ann. Surg.*, **173**:403–408, March 1971.

13 Reul, G. J., R. C. Beall, G. L. Jordon, and K. L. Mattox: The early operative management of injuries to the great vessels, *Surgery*, **74**:862–873, December 1973.

14 Rich, N. M., J. H. Baugh, and C. W. Hughes: Acute arterial injuries in Vietnam: 1,000 cases, *J. Trauma*, **10**:359–369, 1970.

15 ——, C. W. Hughes, and J. H. Baugh: Management of venous injuries, *Ann. Surg.*, **171**:724–730, May 1970.

16 ——, R. W. Hobson, and G. J. Collins: Traumatic arteriovenous fistulas and false aneurysms: A review of 558 lesions, *Surgery*, in press.

17 Richie, R. E., D. M. Conckle, J. L. Sawyer, and H. W. Scott: Surgical management of injuries of the popliteal artery and associated structures, *Arch. Surg.*, in press.

18 Rosenthal, J. J., M. R. Gaspar, T. C. Gjerbrum, and J. Newman: Vascular injuries associated with fractures of the femur, *Arch. Surg.*, **110**:494–499, May 1975.

19 Smiley, K. and M. O. Perry: Balloon catheter tamponade of major vascular wounds, *Am. J. Surg.*, 326–327, March 1971.

20 Smith, R. F., J. G. Elliott, J. H. Hageman, D. E. Szilagyi, and A. O. Xavier: Acute penetrating arterial injuries of the neck and limbs, *Arch. Surg.*, **109**:198–205, August 1974.

21 Symbas, P. N., E. Kourias, D. H. Tyras, and C. R. Hatcher: Penetrating wounds of great vessels, *Ann. Surg.*, **179**:757–762, May 1974.

22 Thal, E. R., W. H. Snyder, R. J. Hays, and M. O. Perry: Management of carotid artery injuries, *Surgery*, **76**:955–962, December 1974.

23 ———, M. O. Perry, and J. Crighton: Traumatic abdominal aortic occlusion, *South. Med. J.*, **64**:653–655, June 1971.

Chapter 10

Malevolent Inflictions: Bites and Stings

Clifford C. Snyder, M.D.

Gary R. Hunter, M.D.

Earl Z. Browne, Jr., M.D.

HISTORY

When *Homo sapiens* first stepped upon this earth, it was greeted by a barrage of malevolent bites and stings. Preparation to combat these walking, flying, and swimming competitors for life was difficult without protective coverage, instruments, or chemicals, and so wound infections and disease from these inflictions were common. It is interesting to know that fossil bacteria found recently have been predated 300 million years. Reptiles with sharp dorsal spines, insects with barbed stingers, and fish with razorlike teeth were common from Montana to Texas 200 million years ago. Egyptian papyri refer to bites by humans, lions, hippopotamuses, and crocodiles which occurred 2000 B.C., and there is an incident of a scorpion sting recorded in hieroglyphics on a stone.[32] Bites of various sorts are cited over 300 times in the *Greek Herbal of Dioscorides*, written during the first century.[22] Celsus,[6] Galen,[18] and Pliny were aware that human bites were poisonous and were to be considered serious injuries. Although defensive progress against bites and stings has been consistent, current problems tend to be existent.

HUMAN BITES

The oral cavity of the human is recognized as a cache for a variety of microorganisms, among which are the staphylococcus, streptococcus, gonococcus, spirochete, clostridium, pasteurella, Vincent's organism, fusiform bacillus, and even the hepatitis virus and rabies virus.[1,2,4,31,35,51] Because most human bites are inflicted during a period of excitement, the recipient remains for quite some time in a fretful and confused state. The injured fails to recognize the impending infection and delays a visit to the physician. When the wound is first seen by the physician, it is swollen, painful, erythematous, and is manifested by purulent exudate. The local cellulitis is accompanied with lymphangitis, regional lymphadenitis, and hyperpyrexia.[8,12]

Among the least offensive human bites are those of the tongue and buccal mucosa which are accidently self-inflicted during a grand mal seizure or while vigorously chewing gum or eating food. Other causes of mucous membrane bites are ill-fitting dentures and sharp, broken edges of decayed teeth. These bites are usually of little consequence and heal uneventfully in a few days. However, it is not unusual for the bitten area to become abscessed, develop multiple fistulas, burrow into the floor of the mouth, and invade along the fascial planes to the anterior nuchal triangles. The treatment of these bite lesions is to incise and Penrose drain or loosely pack with iodoform gauze. While awaiting the results of a smear test and sensitivity tests, ardent broad-spectrum antibiotic therapy is instituted empirically. Prophylaxis of the bacteria-laden oral vestibule is achieved with mouth washes and gargles of sodium perborate or hydrogen peroxide.

Another source of human bites are the vexatious nail biters who unrelentingly chew the nail into the "quick," which produces paronychial infections one after another. The conventional approach to this lesion is to exploit with the scalpel, but this is a merciless maneuver and terminates with a painful digit for days. A simpler and painless approach to release the incarcerated purulency is to delicately separate the integument from the nail bed with a pointed tissue forceps (Fig. 10-1). Once the purulent loculation is released, a quarter-inch iodoform strip is placed in the

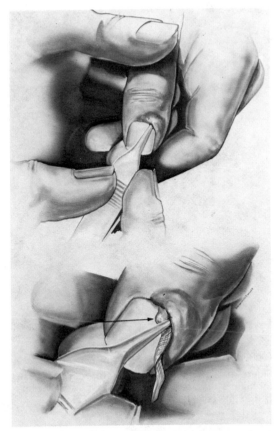

Figure 10-1 Paronychial infections are relieved by subtly separating the skin from the nail with a pointed tissue forceps. The purulent loculation is released (arrow) and an iodoform strip used to assure drainage.

opening. The dressing is changed the following day, and cleanliness is advocated until healed.

The commonest cause of human bites is person-to-person contact ranging from alley encounters (Fig. 10-2) to amorous affairs (Fig. 10-3). When the infuriated or inebriated victim realizes the seriousness of the wound, there is already evidence of spreading infection. All human bites must be regarded as dangerous and need careful management. Because bite wounds are invariably contaminated with anaerobic organisms, they should be irrigated

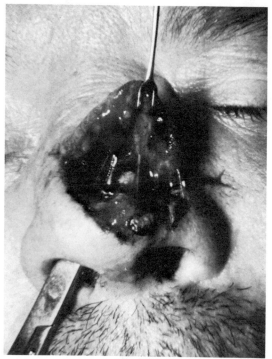

Figure 10-2 Personal quarrels are frequent causes for human bites, and since the nose protrudes invitingly from the face, it is a target for attacking teeth.

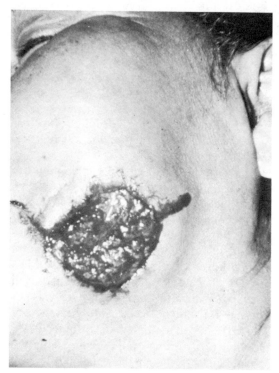

Figure 10-3 During a love affair, the mate was unable to control his tender affections and amorously induced this cheek bite.

with hydrogen peroxide, activated zinc peroxide, or Dakin's solution. Other acceptable irrigants are isotonic saline, Furacin, Betadine, bacitracin, or penicillin. Following thorough flushing, the wound is judiciously debrided. Then the wound may be permitted to remain open, or is loosely packed with gauze. In either case, it should be catheter-irrigated with a continuous drip of organism-specific antibiotic and inspected for impending sequelae daily, or more frequently if necessary. Once it is rendered clean, it may be reasonable to close the wound loosely with sutures or a skin graft or let it heal by second intention. Damaged tendons or nerves are repaired later. Many human bites of a minor nature may be cleansed and closed loosely with a few sutures immediately. The usual precautions are re-

spected and the patient sent home, to return only for suture removal or if infection ensues. Thermal and chemical cautery have no place in human bites.[36] There always remains the possibility of clostridia present in the wound, and therefore tetanus immune globulin or toxoid is indicated.[9] Early extremity bites are loosely dressed and immobilized with the metacarpophalangeal joints placed in flexion while the interphalangeal joints are extended to avoid future contractures. After subsidence of infection, motion exercises are encouraged.

Anesthesia for cleansing, debriding, and dressing the infected human bite wound is usually necessary. Local infiltration anesthesia is not always the approach of choice, but if this method is used, the needle should never penetrate the wound, as the infection may be dispersed. Regional nerve block for bites of the fingers, hand, or arm is preferred; and general anesthesia is used when the patient is hysterical, uncontrollable, or is an apprehensive child. Where it is necessary to explore a bitten hand or tongue, the physician may desire to use a general anesthetic.

MAMMALIAN BITES

Over 2 million humans were bitten by animals in the United States in 1976. With the domestic animal population multiplying as rapidly as it is,[5] and the increase of wild and exotic animals as household pets, physicians must become knowledgeable of the environmental factors associated with these occurrences, ably pursue specific therapy for the conditions, and successfully encounter the sequelae.

It seems to be a perennial problem for parents to purchase rabbits, rats, hamsters, skunks, raccoons, and monkeys for their children, and such is not retributive if a lesson of advice and carefulness accompanies the gift. In fact, the happiness of children having pets and learning to respect living creatures certainly exceeds the hazards incurred from bites by these animals. Regardless, accidents do occur, and physicians must be able to cope with the problems. Until Parrish[38] conducted his study on epidemiology, there were no published data relative to the economic problems of animal bites. He estimated that domestic losses amounted to 1 million dollars annually and medical expenses over 5 million dollars, and he demonstrated the value of controlling bites by animals.

Dog Bites

The animal species responsible for most bites is the dog.[14,20] Nine of every ten humans bitten by an animal have been bitten by a dog.[37,46] Cats are responsible for about 5 percent of mammalian bites, while monkeys, rabbits, rats, bats, foxes, skunks, hamsters, raccoons, horses, camels, and bears are responsible for the remaining 5 percent. Dog breeds answerable for these attacks are mostly German shepherds, collies, spaniels, and terriers. Children are the main recipients of these attacks, predominantly those between the ages of 2 and 15, as parents may become increasingly negligent and children increasingly provocative. It is the child and not the dog who is usually at fault, as children tease and excite the animal. Facial wounds are most common, but lower extremity bites are frequent, as the victims are often running or bicycling. Less frequently, the dog is the aggressor, but in these cases many of the dogs are habitual offenders, especially those taught to be watchdogs. The hapless victims of these canines include postmen, milk carriers, parcel deliverers, and, of course, intruders and trespassers. Occasionally, a veterinarian or an animal caretaker is bitten by a dog unintentionally or as a protective response, but most of these are simple hand wounds which heal without complications.[40]

Established by custom, dog bites are never closed, but left open because of possible bacterial contamination. This method of care is acceptable when skin and fat are avulsed from the host area or when the postbite period is of long duration. In these instances the wound is treated similarly to a human bite of the same nature, that is, with copious irrigation and daily preparation for future coverage. The adage "as clean as a hound's tooth" should be attended with caution, because the dog's oral flora is as abundant with bacteria as is the human's mouth. The bacterium most frequently associated with dog bites is *Pasteurella multocida*.[25] There is a case recorded of osteomyelitis following a dog bite.[29] Yet, there are many such dog bites which should be treated immediately by thorough cleansing with a detergent, debrided of any devitalized tissues, and closed with laxity of the wound margins (Fig. 10-4). The types of wounds which afford this manner of therapy include those involving the face, which may be disfiguring if treated otherwise; those closely related to joints, tendons, nerves, and blood vessels, which may lead to a loss of these vital structures; and those simple lacerations which are superficial and not contaminated. The closure should be achieved without burying sutures and with the wound margins approximated without tension. When indicated, antibiotic therapy and tetanus toxoid or serum are instituted.

Injuries perpetrated by canines can be prevented by proper education of children, by appropriate selection of family pets, and by restraint of watchdogs in the community. The following suggestions are offered:

1 Avoid strange, prowling, or ailing dogs.
2 Use leashes and muzzles on pet dogs in public.
3 Ignore dogs engaged in fighting.
4 Do not pet dogs nursing pups.
5 Do not abruptly awaken a dog.
6 Avoid interruption of a dog that is eating.
7 Instruct children in pet care.

Rabies

Epidemiology The alarming increase in rabid animals continues unabated. The rabies virus and its pathogenesis remain poorly understood, and the disease continues to be a worldwide threat. Nearly half a million people in the world are suspected of being infected by rabid animals every year and are recipients of numerous and sometimes dangerous antirabies treatment.[47] Of the confirmed rabies-infected animals, skunks are involved most, foxes next, and bats are third. The disease is propagated by a multiplicity of animals, but 95 percent of human rabies is caused by dogs. The responsible organism is an ultramicroscopic, filterable, neurotropic virus transmitted to man through bites, skin contact, and inhalation. The incubation period varies from 10 days to a year, but the severity of the disease may lessen this prodromal period remarkably. An early symptom of which the victim complains is pain at the bite site, followed by generalized skin hyperesthesia, photophobia, and objection to loud noises. Soon the pupils become dilated, and the patient begins to perspire profusely. There is then an increase in lacrimation and salivation (hydrophobia). As the patient's status becomes worse, spasms and convulsions ensue, swallowing is difficult, Cheyne-Stokes respiration develops, the body temperature increases, and death is unavoidable.

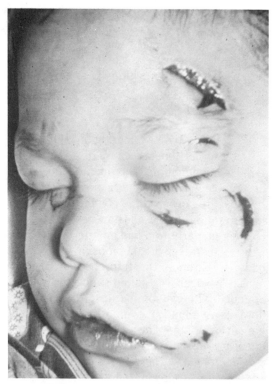

Figure 10-4 Although the conception has been not to close dog bites initially, with antibiotics and careful debridement many facial wounds may be closed early without sequelae.

Diagnosis Confirmation of rabies is possible by various methods, among which are:

1 Direct microscopic examination of brain tissue, which reveals Negri bodies in the motor neurons. These are oval or round bodies seen in the protoplasm or processes of nerve cells and named after Adelchi-Negri, an Italian physician who died in 1912.

2 A chemical test which utilizes a fluorescent antibody response. A smear of brain tissue from the suspected animal is placed upon a glass slide, flooded with rabies antibody, and stained with fluorescein dye. A positive reaction is observed when the virus tags onto the antibody and fluoresces under special light.

3 A biological test based upon the injection of suspected material into the brain of 3-week-old mice, who will succomb in 3 weeks if the material is rabid.

4 The suspected rabid animal is retrieved and kept under surveillance for 10 days, and if it lives without exhibiting suspicion, it is not rabid. If it dies within this period, it is reasonable to suspect infection, and the animal must be studied.

Treatment The possibility of rabies infection should *always* be considered. The incidence of this entity in both wild and domestic animals is high enough to warrant great concern. There is no chemotherapeutic agent or antibiotic which will control this neurotropic virus. Therefore in known cases, immediate local therapy plus active immunization with duck embryo vaccine (DEV) supplemented with human rabies immune globulin (HRIG) may be the difference between life and death. Locally, the bite area is excised even hours after infliction. The open wound is scrubbed briskly with Betadine or Septisol and is not closed. Only 5 percent of infected research animals whose wounds were scrubbed with soap and water developed the disease. In comparison, 90 percent of the controls whose wounds were not cleaned, died of rabies.

Probably the most important decision for an attending physician to make is when to treat and when not to treat.[11] The physician who is not familiar with the disease will merit by consulting public health doctors, who are always cheerful to offer guidance. Although reactions to DEV are uncommon, it is known that these do occur in the form of pain, erythema, pruritis and tenderness at the inoculation site, anaphylaxis, serum sickness, chills, fever, urticaria, intestinal hemorrhages, peripheral neuritis, encephalitis, paralysis, and even death.[28,41] Epinephrine is helpful in most anaphylactic reactions, but cortisone is contraindicated as it decreases the victim's immune reaction and therefore releases the potency of the rabies virus.

Recommendations which may serve as a guide to therapy for rabies is exemplified in Table 10-1.

This table of therapy criteria is merely a guide to help the physician determine which therapy to consider, and must not be used without knowing:

1 The circumstances of the incident at time of the exposure

2 The type of exposure

3 The animal species involved in the exposure

4 The epidemiology of rabies in the area of exposure

5 The vaccination status of the animal

6 The treatment alternatives

The sequence of events involved in a suspected case of rabies and the therapeutic directives may be summarized in the following manner:

1 Was the victim bitten, scratched, or licked by a possibly rabid animal? If the

Table 10-1: Therapy Guide for Rabies

Type of wound	Healthy, domestic, family dog or cat	Unidentified nonvacci- nated domestic animal	Rabid domestic animal	Wild skunk, fox, raccoon
No lesion	No DEV, no HRIG	Observation	DEV, HRIG	Observation
Scratches	No DEV, no HRIG	HRIG	DEV, HRIG	DEV, HRIG
Superficial bite	No DEV, no HRIG	HRIG	DEV, HRIG	DEV, HRIG
Severe attack	HRIG	DEV, HRIG	DEV, HRIG	DEV, HRIG

answer is no, treatment for rabies is not necessary. If the answer is yes, then

2 Is rabies present in the vicinity or suspected in the animal? If the answer is no, do not treat for rabies. If the answer is yes, then

3 Is the animal available? If the answer is no, then

4 Is the animal a dog or cat? If the answer is no, administer DEV and HRIG. If the answer is yes, then

5 Was the person bitten? If the answer is no, give only DEV. If the answer is yes, give DEV and HRIG. If the answer to number 3 above (is the animal available?) is yes, then

6 Is the animal's behavior normal and is it a vaccinated dog or cat? If the answer is yes, then

7 Did the animal become ill during the next 10 days? If the answer is no, no rabies treatment is indicated. If the answer is yes, then

8 Does the laboratory exam of the brain confirm rabies? If the answer is no, forget the treatment. If the answer is yes, then administer DEV and HRIG.

The recommended dose of duck embryo vaccine (DEV) is 40 IU/kg of body weight. Active immunity is achieved in the victim by 14 to 21 daily injections of 1 ml of 10 percent solution, depending upon the severity of the infection. DEV may be doubled daily and the series finished in seven days. Booster injections are given at 10 and 20 days post vaccina-

tion. The vaccine is instituted 24 h after the single dose of HRIG and is given subcutaneously in the abdomen, lower back, and lateral thighs. Vaccination is discontinued if the animal is proven nonrabid or neurological symptoms appear. Passive immunity combined with the vaccine is the best treatment. Passive immunization is accomplished by administering human rabies immune globulin (HRIG) in one intramuscular dose as early as possible following exposure. The usual dose is 40 IU/kg of body weight, but in extensive attacks or bites around the head and neck 50 to 100 IU/kg is used.

A break in the skin is not the only portal through which the rabies virus gains entrance.[10] Eating, drinking, breathing, and handling infected materials may also be cause for rabies infection. It has been shown that contaminated milk has produced rabies through ulcerations in the bowel, and protected, caged animals placed in caves infested with bats died of airborne rabies after only 10 h exposure. It also has been proven that bat urine and guano harbor the rabies virus, and when these excreta are handled, infection may be contracted.

Bites by Other Pets

There is little comparison between cat bites and those inflicted by dogs relative to incidence, but the severity and the complications are comparable. Domestic feline bites account for only 5 percent of all bites inflicted upon humans. Because cats' teeth are needle-sharp and short, the wounds produced are of the puncture type, yet usually are not avulsive in nature. Infective organisms present in the oral cavity of the attacker and those on the victim's skin are driven into the depths of the wound and are difficult to cleanse. Puncture wounds have a tendency to close and serve as an ideal nidus for anaerobic bacteria to multiply. Consequently, these wounds are troublesome to clean with a cloth or brush. Debridement by excision of the wound is the approach to these punctures. If the wound is severe, it should be left open after debridement; if it is a simple wound, it may be debrided and closed.[57] Of course, there are cat and kitten bites which are results of playing without malice or assault intentions, and these need only cleansing without further ado. Scratches by the sharp claws accompanying the cat bite many times create worse problems than the bite. Bites by pet rabbits, rats, hamsters, guinea pigs, and monkeys are treated as those inflicted by cats.

Wild Animal Bites

Any bite by a wild animal which escapes capture necessitates careful attention and observation. The potentiality of rabies infection must be considered, and the incidence of this entity in wild life is high enough to warrant concern. These inflictions are approached therapeutically as those caused by domestic animals, but with more aggression. *Bear* attacks are becoming more frequent because of greater interest in camping and hiking as well as the inviting atmosphere of our national and state forests and parks.[43] Yellowstone National Park has been the source of at least three vicious bear attacks upon humans every year during the summer months. These injuries are devastating because of the large, sharp teeth whose purpose is to pierce and tear into depths of thick and dense objects such as the bark of trees, the scales of fish, and the hard shells of animals. The strong jaws and heavy neck muscles are ideal to avulse masses of tissue from the victim. Bears attack with teeth and claws, and the first bites penetrate the soft tissue deeply (Fig. 10-5). The victim is then helplessly grasped with the bear's long sharp claws and strong forelegs. The teeth engage and avulse large portions of tissue (Figs. 10-6 and 10-7). The treatment for bear bites is instituted immediately (Figs. 10-8 and 10-9). Wound debridement must be thorough, and most of these may be closed at once. When there is a great loss of tissue, reparative surgery is staged using skin grafts and skin flaps (Figs. 10-10 and 10-11). *Zoo animal* bites are of an extensive variety. Camels, zebras, and burros inflict bruising and crushing wounds and many times leave missing sections of tissue (Fig. 10-12). They are very painful and rapidly become infected if care is

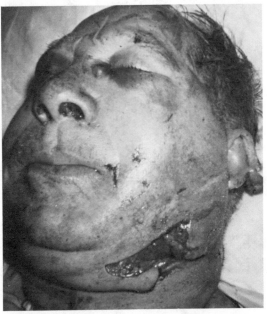

Figure 10-5 The number of bear attacks and the devastating effects are underestimated. Bears are fast runners for 200 yards in the forest.

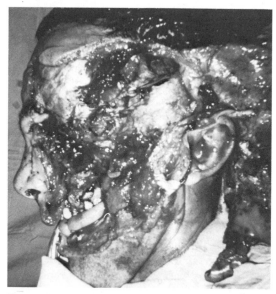

Figure 10-6 Strong jaws and neck muscles enable bears to avulse masses of tissues. Most of this victim's left face, forehead, and eyeball has been torn away.

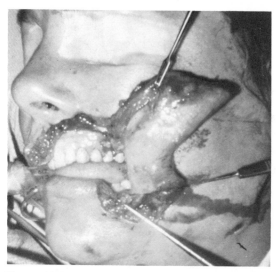

Figure 10-8 This young female victim of bear teeth and claws had most of her upper lip bitten, as well as numerous areas of the scalp, left forehead, neck, upper extremities, chest, and back.

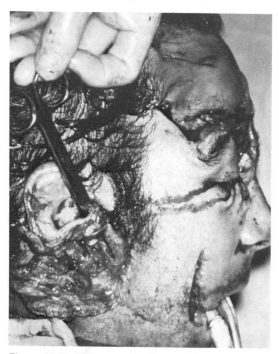

Figure 10-7 The same victim's right forehead, glabella, cheek, ear canal, and ear drum were also areas of deep lacerations and avulsions.

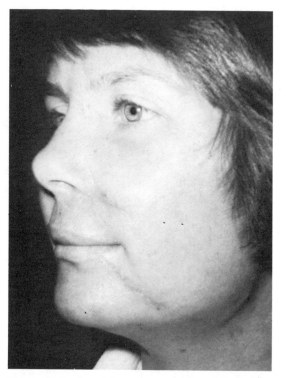

Figure 10-9 Bear bites are treated instantly by thorough debridement and closure if possible. The partial upper lip avulsion and numerous other body wounds healed satisfactorily.

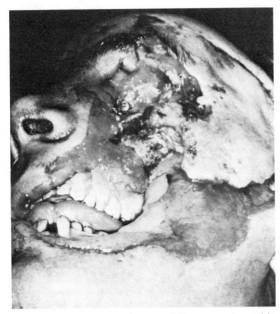

Figure 10-10 Massive losses of tissue, such as this cheek, antrum, and ocular area, are conditioned to repair by soft tissue flaps.

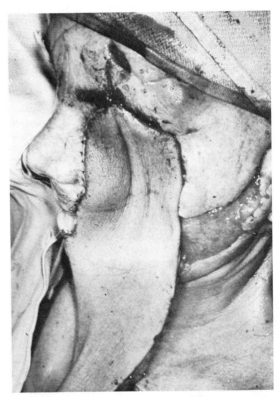

Figure 10-11 A soft tissue flap has been designed as a beginning reparative procedure to symmetrize the facial anatomy.

lacking (Fig. 10-13). For these two important reasons equine bites are cleansed, debrided, and repaired initially. The smaller zoo animals include bobcats, raccoons, weasels, minks, wolverines, and binturongs (Figs. 10-14 and 10-15). Wounds caused by these mammals are debrided and repaired early.

REPTILIAN BITES

Reptiles such as alligators, crocodiles, caimans, and large lizards are endowed with a head which is a mass of nearly solid bone and powerful jaws armed with rows of sharp, conical teeth, which are renewed as fast as they are lost. The alligator, crocodile, and caiman are carnivorous, and the bulk of their food is made up of fish, crustaceans, birds, and mammals. Land animals such as dogs, cattle, and horses can be surprised while drinking from a lake or stream and unknow-ingly pulled beneath the surface of the water and drowned. These reptiles have a highly efficient way of dismembering their prey: their strong tail allows them to revolve in the water, twisting a leg or arm from the victim's body. The chief difference between a crocodile and an alligator is in their behavior; that is, the alligator becomes tame and lazy in captivity, whereas the crocodile retains its vicious nature. The alligator, when enraged, will slowly back away, hissing, opening its mouth, and swinging its tail in warning. The crocodile will often attack by turning toward the enemy, with its body off the ground. The largest of the saurians attain a length of 33 ft, live in the coastal swamps of India and China, and are

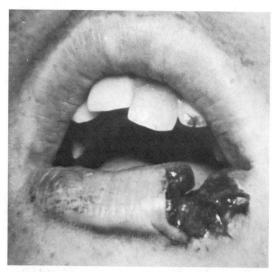

Figure 10-12 This avulsion wound is resultant of a zebra bite, which is representative of horse, camel, and burro, and other equine bites that routinely are bruising and avulsive. They should be debrided and repaired immediately.

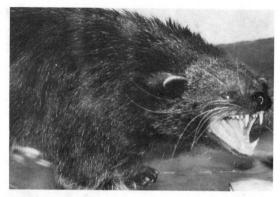

Figure 10-14 The binturong is a small carnivorous animal which is a native of Asia, but popular to the zoo audiences. Its canine teeth are long and very sharp.

rarely dangerous to man. Although a reptile's mouth can be held closed with one human hand, the same hand, regardless of its strength, is unable to pry the mouth open. Alligators and crocodiles have very strong tails and use these to swat their prey into unconsciousness. The bite wounds resultant from these reptiles' attacks are devastating, including leg and arm amputations as well as

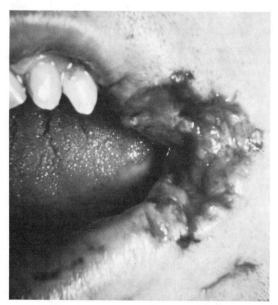

Figure 10-13 Another equine bite (pony) which did not receive early surgical treatment; when seen on the third postbite day, it was complicated with cellulitis and edema and infected with a multitude of various microorganisms.

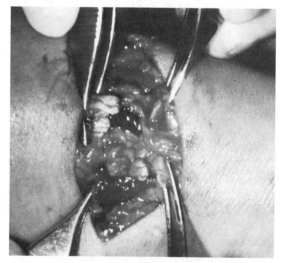

Figure 10-15 This forearm wound with severed tendons and muscles is that of a zoo attendant attacked by the binturong. The tendons were repaired, the wound debrided and closed without complications.

large, gaping body avulsions. Recently a child fell into a reptile pit in a Flordia serpentarium, exciting the crocodile, who raced to the young victim and grasped him in the abdomen. A bystander jumped into the pit and tried desperately to pry the reptile's jaws open, but in vain. The crocodile raised its body and walked to the pool of water, where it slid itself and the victim beneath the water, drowning the child. The boy's death was due to both the crush of the injury and drowning. More recently, a man, while swimming in a Florida river, was attacked and killed by an alligator. Treatment of crocodilian wounds is to control bleeding, irrigate the wound depths profusely, debride devitalized structures, and bring the wound margins loosely into apposition. If the wound is too large to close by suturing, a split-thickness skin graft or an adjacent skin flap will serve the purpose.

There are two species of *lizards* that are venomous, the Gila monster of Arizona and the Mexican beaded lizard. The poison glands are in the maxillary area, and the orifices of the main excretory ducts empty at the base of the teeth, which are grooved. When the lizard becomes angry or apprehensive, there is a profuse drooling of venom, which bathes the teeth. The attack of these lizards is rapid, and the jaws clamp tightly upon the victim. The poisonous venom is comparable to that of some rattlesnakes, and may cause death. The therapeutic approach to the tenacious bite of these lizards is to first release the jaws from the victim and then immediately wash the wound thoroughly to remove as much of the saliva as possible. Any devitalized, hanging skin tabs are superficially debrided to afford a smooth integumental margin for closure. If available, local application of ice to the covered wound relieves the stinging pain in the locale. There is an antivenin,[55] which should be included in the kit of a person contemplating an exploratory or camping outing into Gila monster country and may be purchased from the Poisonous Animals Research Laboratory, Arizona State University, Tempe, Arizona.

Snake Bites

The victim's reaction following a bite from a snake varies from extreme excitement and hysteria to nervous exhaustion, syncope, and shock. These varied reactions and the diversity of symptoms will confuse the physician who is inexperienced with snakebites and will motivate the physician to administer unnecessary therapy to a victim bitten by a poisonous snake.[53]

On April 22, 1977, the Committee on Emergency Medical Services of the National Research Council invited a group of interested individuals to discuss the first aid of snakebite at a meeting in Washington, D.C. There were five who participated, all with varied ideas but a common goal: what to advise those administering the initial care to victims of snake envenomation. Some of the recommendations and procedures will be published in the *Advanced First Aid and Emergency Care,* a textbook published under the auspices of the American National Red Cross.

Incidence   Reliable statistics of snakebite occurrence are wanting, but snakebites take place with greater frequency than is generally realized. Perusal of the literature, unreliable as it is, indicates that there are at least 75,000 human deaths in the world every year from snake envenomation. In the United States there are over 50,000 people bitten by various types of snakes annually, of which about 5000 are by poisonous snakes. Poisonous snakebites in our country seldom terminate fatally, which is reasonable because of the excellent medical care rendered, the educational information afforded the lay public, and the high standard of our nation's living. The morbidity is of greater concern than the mortality. Regional tissue slough usually involves skin, tendons, and bone (Figs. 10-16 and 10-17).

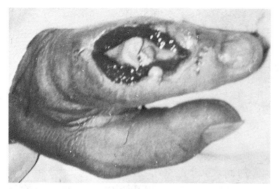

Figure 10-16 This is the site of rattlesnake envenomation which resulted in a loss of skin, tendon, and joint capsule, and a permanent loss of sensation and motility

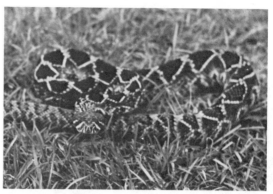

Figure 10-18 The *Crotalus adamanteus* (Eastern diamondback rattlesnake) is a pit viper which is responsible for many of the envenomations in our country.

Permanent paralysis is not unusual in the bite area, and causalgia, atrophy, digital stiffness, limb loss, and even blindness occur. In a great percentage of snakebites the offender remains unidentified because of the victim's fright, the speed of the serpent's escape, and the surrounding occult foliage. In one study, 95 percent of our patients' bites were on the hands, forearms, feet, and legs, and 65 percent of our patients were children under 20 years.[33,52]

The Envenomer Poisonous snakes of North America (Figs. 10-18, 10-19, 10-20, 10-21) stem from the family of Crotalidae (pit vipers) and the family of the Elapidae (represented by the coral snake). The pit vipers consist of three genera, the *Crotalus* (true rattlesnakes), the *Agkistrodon* (including moccasins and copperheads), and the *Sistrurus* (ground rattlers). Pit vipers are so named because of the hole that lies between and below the level of the eye and nostril. The pit is believed to be a sense organ aiding in detecting the proximity of prey or enemies. These poisonous pit vipers may be differentiated from nonpoisonous snakes by their elliptical pupil, fangs, broad head with narrow neck, and single row of scale plates distal to

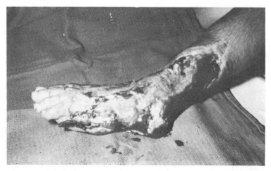

Figure 10-17 A disastrous loss of both soft and osseous tissues, including the fifth digit and calcaneous, as a result of a pigmy rattlesnake bite.

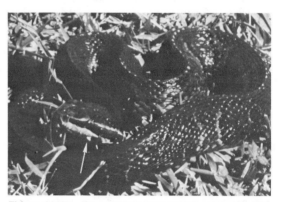

Figure 10-19 The *Agkistrodon piscivorus* is the cottonmouth moccasin which is a large, heavy, dark, swamp snake and is known for its pugnaciousness. The arrow points to the camouflaged head. This snake causes a slough at the site of fang puncture.

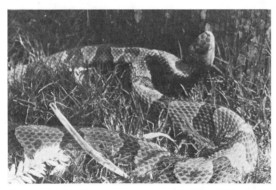

Figure 10-20 The copperhead (*Agkistrodon moka-sen*) is noted for its beautiful red head and hourglass or inverted-Y markings and is extensively distributed in our country.

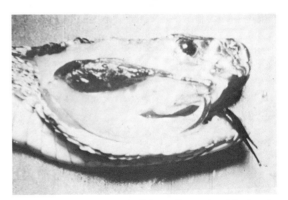

Figure 10-22 A portion of the salivary gland is devoted to venom-producing cells, and the material is propelled through a main duct and specialized teeth (fangs) into the victim or prey.

the anus. Nonpoisonous snakes have round pupils, no fangs, and a double row of plates below the anal orifice. Unfortunately, the coral snake, which is poisonous, has a round pupil and no pit, similar to the harmless snakes. Its fangs are short, erect, fixed to the anterior maxilla, and have either a groove or a canal for guiding the venom.[42]

The venom gland of the snake is analogous to vertebrate salivary glands, and the venom is propelled into the fangs for ejecting (Fig. 10-22). When at rest, the fangs are folded

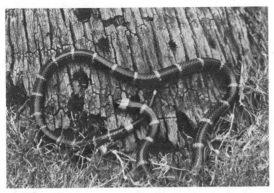

Figure 10-21 The coral snake (*Micrurus fulvius*) is brilliantly colored with rings of red, yellow, and black. It is smooth and glossy, docile and nocturnal, and it injects a very dangerous venom.

against the mouth; when the snake strikes, they are thrust forward for penetration and ejection of venom. The instant that the fangs of a striking snake touch the intended goal, the mouth closes and venom is released. Therefore, when loose clothing and footwear are touched, the snake's mouth is stimulated to close and venom is ejected without piercing the skin of the intended victim. Crotalids bear fangs long enough to penetrate deep into the victim's soft tissue. Hence the depth of bite penetration depends upon covering garments, tissue thickness, fang length, and the angle of penetration. These important factors determine whether the venom is deposited above the muscle fascia or below it, and is decisive in clinical management of the victim.[30] Rattlesnakes can actually control the amount of venom they inoculate, as proven in isotope-tagged venom studies of mice, rabbits, and dogs.[52] This is important to know because many human victims exhibit no symptoms of envenomation (25 percent of bites by poisonous snakes do not result in envenomation), and those treated by bizarre methods (tobacco juice, mystic stone, cackleburr stupes) claim cures which are erroneous. The most toxic venom milligram per milligram of the domestic snakes in this country is that of the coral snake, and the least effective is copperhead venom. Yet rattlesnakes are responsible for more animal deaths than any other snakes because their large venom glands eject more poison into the animal victim, they are more aggressive, and they are awake when most animals are on the move.

The Venom The venom of a poisonous snake is a complexity of several proteins, lipids, enzymes, and other less significant constituents.[4] Several specific toxic enzymatic ingredients have been identified, including proteases, esterases, dipeptidases, hyaluronidase, and phospholipase A, each performing destructive functions to tissues affected. These enzymes and the toxic proteins are the reason that snake envenomation yields a dramatic diversity of symptoms.[7] When a specific snake venom is injected into a laboratory animal, it may cause an embolic phenomenon such as pulmonary embolism; the identical snake venom injected into another similar research animal will cause a hemorrhagic phenomenon such as intestinal hemorrhage. These divergent effects perplex the attending physician and confuse the method of therapy. Such should be known to the doctor so correct therapeusis can be administered. All venoms are composed of so-called neurotoxic and hematoxic components, but are found in different ratios in the various species of envenomers. The neurotoxic elements promote little action at the site of envenomation, but exert their effect on distant tissues. The hemotoxic components are responsible for tissue destruction at the site of infusion. These actions may be exemplified by the following occasions. Elapid (coral snakes, cobras, Russell vipers) venoms may cause little local pain, swelling, or tissue slough, but may result in respiratory and cardiac distress. In comparison, the crotalid (cotton mouth moccasin, rattlesnake) venoms produce immediate local pain, progressive swelling, ecchymosis, and eventually sloughing of tissues.

It is extremely important to differentiate between a poisonous snakebite and a nonpoisonous one, because if the former is not treated, death may ensue, and if the latter is treated with horse serum antivenin, the victim may be allergic to it and irreversible complications, even death, may occur. Today these are liability problems, and legal developments create havoc.

Signs and Symptoms of Envenomation
Cardinal Findings

1 *Fang puncture wounds:* There may be one to six wounds due to more than one attack or because the snake may have one to six fangs (Figs. 10-23, 10-24, and 10-25).
2 *Swelling:* There may be only mild edema and discoloration initially, or the edema may be immediate and progress sufficiently to obliterate superficial venous return (Fig. 10-26).
3 *Pain:* The victim may not experience pain at first, but later the pain becomes excruciating; or the pain may be unbearable immediately and lead to syncope and shock.

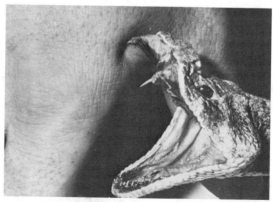

Figure 10-23 There may be one or more fang punctures inflicted during envenomation. This depicts a single fang entrance and therefore one puncture wound.

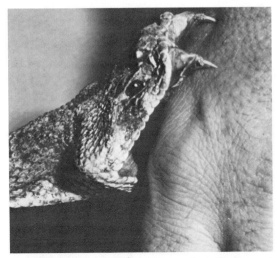

Figure 10-24 This snake was accurate in its aim, and the victim will receive two fang punctures. If it strikes again, there will be more.

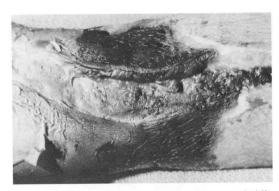

Figure 10-26 Envenomation causes edema and obliteration of venous return, and both are responsible for necrosis. If escharotomy and fasciotomy are contemplated, they should be done early.

Ancillary Findings

1 *Erythema to ecchymosis:* This is usually immediate and progressive.

2 *Bullae:* These may be in the form of clear serum transudate or large blood blisters (Fig. 10-27).

3 *Petechiae:* Venom affects the intima of blood vessels and is also responsible for capillary fragility resulting in minute subcutaneous hemorrhages.

4 *Hyperesthesia to anesthesia:* Venom affects the sensory nerve endings and produces

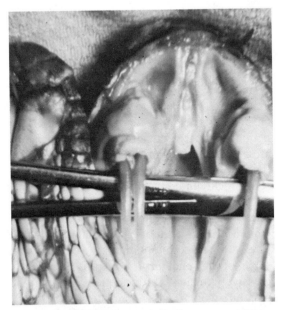

Figure 10-25 Many snakes have three or more fangs, and when they strike, they produce multiple wound punctures. Therefore, the physician must be acquainted with this phenomenon.

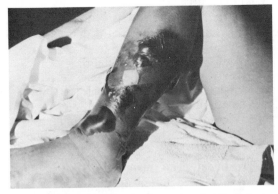

Figure 10-27 Ancillary findings of snakebite poisoning include hemorrhagic transudate, cyanosis, and necrosis, all of which are present in this snakebite victim's leg.

immediate pain, then numbness of the bite area early, which later changes to pain again.

5 *Paresthesia:* This is a later symptom and is in the form of peculiar skin sensations, as formication and tingling, and may terminate with causalgia.

6 *Advancing pitting edema:* This is due to compression of lymph and blood vessels and progresses proximally up a limb.

7 *Cyanosis, necrosis, and tissue slough:* These symptoms are sequential and are a result of compromised blood supply.

8 *Anxiety, nausea, and vomiting:* The central nervous system as well as the gastrointestinal mucosa becomes affected, and this may be accompanied by muscle twitching, convulsions, and paralysis.

9 *Dyspnea, rapid feeble pulse, vertigo, dimmed vision, pinpoint pupils, and general weakness:* These are all prodromal symptoms of shock.

10 *Coma and death.*

Laboratory Findings Moderate to severe envenomation produces evidence of hypothrombinemia, thrombocytopenia, hypofibrinogenemia, and anemia.[27] An x-ray of the chest may reveal pulmonary edema and embolus.

Factors which may influence the severity of symptoms are:

1 Age and size of victim. Children are affected more seriously.[39]
2 Time elapse post snakebite.
3 Location, depth, and number of bites.
4 Species and size of envenomer.
5 Amount of venom injected.
6 Victim's sensitivity to the venom.
7 Efficacy of the initial first-aid treatment.

Treatment The management of persons who have been bitten by poisonous snakes differs because the effects vary in seriousness. Of the more than 200 snakebite patients who have come under our care over the past 33

years, about one-half needed only first-aid therapy, and one-fourth did not even exhibit any signs of envenomation. It is necessary to clarify the differences of opinions regarding snakebites for persons whose occupations place them in snake-infested areas, including those in the armed forces, scout leaders, personnel of the Department of the Interior and the Bureau of Mines, game wardens, and for paramedics, family practice physicians, and the general public who enjoys camping, hiking, hunting, fishing, and other recreations. Therefore, snakebite poisonings need classifying, and an understandable and applicable method is:

1 *Mild:* fang scratch marks, no pain, minimal swelling
2 *Moderate:* fang puncture(s), pain, erythema, local swelling, no systemic symptoms
3 *Severe:* fang puncture(s), immediate or delayed excruciating wound pain (vipers), progressive swelling, ecchymosis, petechiae, bullae, and systemic symptoms of anxiety, hysteria, tingling, nausea, vomiting, fibrillations, vertigo, dyspnea, and syncope

For the *mild* type of bite which is over an hour old, with only fang scratch marks, slight local swelling and no pain, the wound is cleansed with soap and water or alcohol, the patient is not given antivenin, and incisions are not indicated. For the *moderate* snakebite, that is, for the envenomated patient who presents local findings but is without systemic effects, the fang marks are incised with one linear incision through the punctures, the wound is suctioned, but antivenin is withheld. The *severe* snakebite with all the cardinal and some of the ancillary findings is treated aggressively, using a tourniquet, excising the puncture wound area, administering antivenin, and hospitalizing the victim for observation and further therapy. Because some envenomers are more or less poisonous than others, *all* snakebites should not be attended by an "absolute standard" of therapy, but instead the treatment should be tempered to the toxic effects observed. We therefore have divided the modes of therapy into preventive therapy, emergency field therapy, and hospital emergency room therapy.

Preventive Therapy

1 Refrain from hiking or camping in known snake-infested areas, occult foliage, caves, and mines.

2 Be on the alert for snakes sunning on warm days.

3 While walking through forests and deserts, wear protective gear such as snake leggings, boots, long trousers, sleeved shirts, and gloves.

4 Do not reach into ground holes or onto poorly visible mountain ledges.

5 Avoid being alone in the woods; a companion may be a lifesaver.

6 Keep your vehicle near, whether it be 2- or 4-wheeled or 4-legged.

7 Carry a snakebite kit on rural trips, and know how to use it (Fig. 10-28).

8 Do not have poisonous snakes as pets; do not surprise sleeping snakes; do not molest snakes.

9 Inquire in advance about medical aid when traveling in primitive areas.

Emergency Field Therapy

1 Remember there are no absolute rules, only practicable ones.

2 Avoid excitement, exertion, and beverages which may accelerate circulation and rapidly propel the venom throughout the body.

3 Stay and retrieve the offender for identification, but do not exert or endanger yourself.

4 Immediately apply flat tourniquet (belt, bandana, sock, neckerchief) proximal to the extremity bite and only snug enough to permit

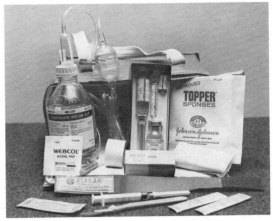

Figure 10-28 Some type of snakebite kit should accompany those who travel in snake-infested areas. Here is the author's kit, which includes antivenim, elastic tourniquet, and other necessities.

introducing one finger beneath it easily. Loosen the tourniquet a little as swelling increases. If swelling is already present, do not apply a tourniquet. Never apply, remove, reapply, and remove a tourniquet intermittently, as this propels the venom into the general system. Release the band completely when antivenin is given intramuscularly or intravenously.

5 Cleanse the bite area, if possible, and cut from one fang mark through the other down to the subcutaneous fat. Do not use cruciate (cross-hatch) incisions as they are harmful, especially on the face and hands.

6 Suction or digitally express fluid (blood and venom) gently from the incised wound without macerating it, but doing this for over 5 min is damaging and useless.

7 Immobilize or rest the bitten limb horizontally at heart level; it should not be above or below heart level because either position will enhance edema and necrosis. Muscular exercise should be inhibited at first as it increases circulation and venom spread.

8 Venom neutralization must be achieved. Wyeth's polyvalent antivenin is the only available therapy to date in the United States, and it has been proven to be lifesaving. The sooner it is administered, the more beneficial it is; yet it has been given 24 h postbite with good results. As it is a horse serum product, the precautions as listed in the package flyer must be heeded.

Emergency Room Treatment

I Identify the venomous injury [fang mark(s), swelling, pain] and the snake if available. Record any history of allergies (drugs, horse serum, novacaine, foods), and note if patient has or had hay fever, asthma, or urticarias.

II If the victim falls into the category of having a severe envenomation, prepare one vial of Wyeth's polyvalent antivenin (Crotalidae) and dilute this 10 mL into 100 mL of sterile normal saline solution and 125 mg of Upjohn's Solu-Medrol (or methylprednisolone equivalent). During this interval, inject into the victim 0.02 mL of a 1:100 dilution in saline of the normal horse serum (included in Wyeth's kit) to raise a small wheal intracutaneously to test for allergy. A control test of normal saline near the horse serum test facilitates interpretation of the findings. A negative reaction shows no local skin changes; a positive response occurs within 5 to 15 min, revealing a white wheal with increasing peripheral erythema, edema, and itching. If the patient has any history of allergies, the antivenin must be tempered to the severity of the snake bite, and a safe starting dose is 0.5 mL of 1:100 dilution. A reaction to this trial dosage is adequate warning not to use the horse serum antivenin. If the person has no allergies and the test response is negative, administer the prepared antivenin intravenously, with epinephrine, corticosteroid, and antihistamine awaiting any untoward reactions. Children and adults are treated alike. It is hoped that our laboratory will have a human antiserum available in the future.

III Local treatment of the snakebitten site is treated as follows:

 A If the envenomation is classed as a *mild* one, do not incise.

 B If the envenomation is of the *moderate* type, a linear incision through the fang punctures to the fascia followed by suction is the course.

 C If the envenomation is *severe*, the fang marks are elliptically excised with an equidistant margin of 1 cm through the fat to the fascia. Bleeding is controlled by an occlusive dressing.

 D Escharotomy is necessary where extreme edema appears to be compromising the blood supply. Fasciotomy is indicated in subfascial envenomation and, when used judiciously can save an extremity.[19]

 E Local remedies such as cautery, acids, alkalies, cruciate incisions, and mystical applications, some of which destroy more tissue than does the venom, are not used.

 F Cryotherapy is advocated by excellent medical serpentologists, but such treatment needs definition. We do not freeze the snakebitten area, but we do cool it. Local hypothermia reduces pain, inhibits venom release, limits edema, and decreases metabolic needs. If not governed carefully however, low-temperature applications will cause bleb formation, necrosis, and gangrene. When used on digits, cold therapy is disastrous in such diseased states as diabetes, arteriosclerosis, cryoproteinemia, scleroderma, Burger's disease, Raynaud's disease, and others. Once the therapeutics of cryotherapy, hypothermia, freezing, and cooling are carefully defined in relation to snakebite, an understanding will lead to better management.

 G Pressure or tight dressings are detrimental.

Tetanus immunization, antibiotics, analgesics, oxygen, calcium, transfusion, tracheotomy, and hemodialysis are all to be utilized when indicated. Hospitalization should be advised for all envenomated snakebite victims because many findings are not distinguishable early. The kin or responsible party should be advised of latent sequelae.

ARTHROPODAL BITES

Arthropods are the most highly developed, specialized, and versatile of the invertebrates. The phylum of joint-footed animals consists of a most important order of membrane winged creatures—the Hymenoptera. Fortunately, of the approximately 800,000 species of arthropods, relatively few are sufficiently venomous or poisonous to be of potential danger to humans. Nevertheless, these animals are implicated in far more poisonings to human beings than all of the other phyla combined. Almost all spiders, approximately 20,000 species, are venomous. Luckily for human beings, only a relative few spiders have fangs long and strong enough to penetrate the human skin. There are some 500 species of scorpions, some of which must be considered lethal. In the order of Hymenoptera (bees, wasps, yellow jackets, and ants) there are numerous genera and species of potential danger to man. Among the ticks, caterpillars, assassin bugs, moths, butterflies, grasshoppers, and other arthropods there are a number of poisonous species. Arthropodal venoms represent some of the most complex and diversified substances known. Many of these animals, such as spiders, use their venom in the gaining of food. Others, such as scorpions, use their venom apparatus chiefly in defense. Still others produce and release a substance from their body surface or special glands that, because of its odor, or irritant, or certain other properties, repels other arthropods and even reptiles and mammals. The massive, hairy tarantula is nothing but a "show-off" and is relatively harmless to man (Fig. 10-29).

The venoms of the various arthropods differ remarkably in their composition and mode of action. Bee venom, a good example of the complexity of an arthropod toxin, contains lipids, peptides, apamines, mellitin, apic acid,

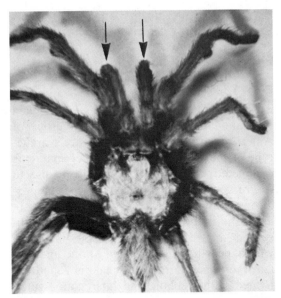

Figure 10-29 Almost all spiders are poisonous, but most are relatively harmless to humans, such as this "showoff" hairy tarantula. Its venom is used in getting food, and it has two fangs (arrows).

sugars, free bases, amino acids, other proteins and enzymes, and a number of unidentified components. There is still considerable question as to which components of bee venom cause sensation, and these may not necessarily be the more toxic ones. Scorpion venoms contain 10 to 15 proteins and at least 6 nonproteins. The lethal and more deleterious components appear to be proteins of low molecular weight. The venom of spiders needs more detailed study. Because of the small yield obtained from each spider, it takes milkings from 1000 spiders to accumulate 1 mg of venom from the smaller species. Ant venoms provide an example of remarkable chemical diversification due to the abundancy of species; some ants sting, some bite, and some spray their venom. More than 3 times as many people in the United States die from arthropod bites and stings than from rattlesnake bites. However, the majority of the arthropod-inflicted deaths can be attributed to anaphylactic response rather than to direct effects of the venoms.[50] Yet deaths from black widow spider bites, brown recluse spider bites, and scorpion stings, as well as from multiple bee and fire ant stings do occur.[15,49]

Black Widow Spider Bites

This creature of arachnology has the justified reputation of being the most dangerous of American arthropods and is nature's archetype of the devouring female. Once mating is completed, the male is of utterly no use to future generations; therefore is it so preposterous that the female often eats her mate after she is through with him? We have observed isolated black widow couples in our lab who appear to have adjusted to one another, and then one morning the male is found entwined with webbing and later gone—eaten alive.

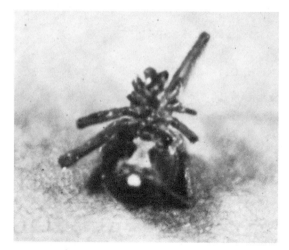

Figure 10-30 The black widow spider is one of the most dangerous of American arthropods and is universally known by its red-orange-yellow abdominal hourglass-shaped figure and, many times, a red taillight.

Habit and Features There are four poisonous species of latrodectus (biting robbers) spiders, and they are found everywhere in the United States from the Bronx to Hawaii, but not in Alaska. One of the largest caches ever was located in the emergency room of a Salt Lake City metropolitan hospital. The female spider's body measures about 15 mm in length and 10 mm across the abdomen, and its slim black legs spread about 50 mm. It is distinguished by a glossy black body, a red-orange hourglass-shaped figure on its abdomen, and often a red taillight (Fig. 10-30). She has two small fangs through which the venom is injected into the victim. The male latrodectus is considerably smaller, not so black, and does not envenomate.

Toxic Manifestations A definite history of spider bite is usually wanting, and it is only after the physician has completed examining the patient and is unable to make a diagnosis that the idea of a possible spider bite is formulated. A careful search then elicits minute red fang marks on the skin. The patient may then recall a sharp pinprick incident which was unperturbing and forgotten (Fig. 10-31).

When a black widow spider bites, there is a moment of sharp pain followed by a dull, numbing ache. If the infliction is severe and on a lower extremity, the pain may progress to the abdomen, where the musculature becomes rigid, simulating an attack of peritoneal irritation. Misdiagnoses of black widow spider envenomation include acute appendicitis, cholecystitis, ruptured peptic ulcer, and ureteral lithiasis. Bites on the upper extremity cause referred pain to the shoulders, back, and chest and sometimes are accompanied by dyspnea, simulating coronary thrombosis or pneumonia. Immediately following the bite there is a minute punctate red mark with a surrounding area of erythema, and mild edema develops. This may disappear and no further signs develop. If the venom spreads through the peripheral nerves to the central nervous system, then other signs and symptoms of varying gradients evolve, such as headache, vertigo, nausea, sweating, salivation, irritability, rest-

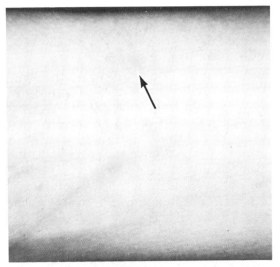

Figure 10-31 Immediately after the black widow spider bites, there appears a minute puncture red mark with surrounding erythema and edema (arrow). This may disappear in 1 to 2 days, or the victim develops constitutional sequelae.

lessness, convulsions, paralysis, eyelid edema with ptosis, shock, and coma. Laboratory findings include leukocytosis, albuminuria, hematuria, and though the spinal fluid pressure may be elevated, the contents are negative. Many of these patients are admitted to the hospital medical service with a pending diagnosis. It is apparent that a number of spider venoms have chemical and pharmacologic properties similar to other venoms, and therefore it is important to encourage the public to bring the offending spider to the appropriate person for identification.

Management Mortality from black widow spider envenomation is around 4 percent. Most of the bites, even in children and the aged, are self-limiting and need only immediate therapy for pain and discomfort.

1 Cold compresses or ice packs reduce local pain.
2 Calcium gluconate, 10 mL of 10% solu-

tion intravenously, repeated at 4-h intervals as necessary for muscle spasms.
3 Diazepam, 10 mg intravenously slowly or by mouth if not nauseated.
4 Methocarbamol, 10 mL intravenously slowly.[26]
5 Add analgesic cautiously; narcotics are generally required.
6 Antihistamines and corticosteroids may be used judiciously.
7 Antivenin is the only specific therapy. The name of the product is Lyovac and it is manufactured by Merck Sharpe & Dohme. It is used only in severe envenomation or in highly susceptible persons. The usual dose is 2.5 mL intramuscularly (not intravenously) and may be repeated. It is a horse serum product, and testing for sensitivity must be conducted as the package flyer indicates.
8 Prompt excision of the bite relieves pain and sequelae, but is not effective if the postbite time is prolonged.

Brown Recluse Spider Bites

This envenomer is a member of the genus *Loxosceles,* and although it is a native of our country, documented cases have only been published since the 1950s. Recluse bites have now been identified in all the southern states from California to Florida, and this is partly due to truck, train, ship, and air freight.

Habitat and Features The average *Loxosceles reclusa* measures about 12 mm long, 6 mm wide, and is light tan to deep brown in color. On its back is a dark brown violin-shaped figure, hence its nickname, the fiddler spider (Fig. 10-32). Another distinguishing characteristic of the fiddler spider is the six eyes positioned on the cephalic end in a semicircle. It prefers the indoors, but lives also in outhouses, in woodpiles, and under leaves. Recently, a housewife in Utah was preparing her flower garden for winter bulb planting, raking the leaves away, and a recluse spider, which she killed and retrieved, bit her

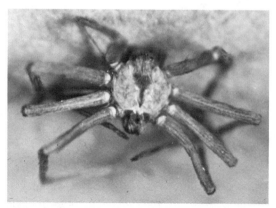

Figure 10-32 *Loxosceles reclusa* (brown recluse) is also known as the fiddler spider because of the violin-shaped figure on its back. It now has been identified in all our southern states and some northern states.

hand. There was no initial pain, and she finished her planting. The next day a bleb was present, but because there was no pain, she did not seek our attention for 2 weeks, by which time an ulcer had developed (Fig. 10-33). A tentative diagnosis of basal cell cancer was made, but upon further questioning and then seeing the spider, the correct diagnosis was confirmed. The wound was closed, and it healed uneventfully.

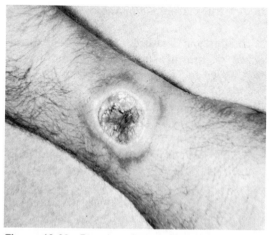

Figure 10-33 Brown recluse spider bite which became ulcerous with an elevated periphery and umbilicated center, resembling a malignancy. It was excised and closed, and it healed uneventfully.

Toxic Manifestations While no symptoms may be apparent initially, in a few hours a small hemorrhagic blister with a white ischemic periphery surrounded by an erythematous halo appears at the site of envenomation. If seen early, this red, white, and blue configuration is nearly pathognomonic of loxosceles poisoning. Lesions caused by the *Loxosceles unicolor, Loxosceles devia,* and *Loxosceles arizona* usually ulcerate and heal without further symptoms, but the *L. reclusa* may cause a large sloughing of tissue and produce systemic manifestations if not treated early.[13] In addition to the cutaneous lesion, generalized findings may include headache, fever, chills, nausea, vomiting, skin rash, and joint pains. Thrombocytopenia, hemolytic anemia, and pulmonary embolism have been responsible for deaths following loxoscelism. Laboratory findings may include leukocytosis, hemoglobinemia, hemoglobinuria, and renal failure.

Management

1 Corticosteroids are effective in early treatment, but must be given in adequate doses, starting with 125 mg Solu-Medrol intravenously immediately and repeated in 12, 24, 36, and 48 h. This should decrease the local necrosis and eliminate the systemic sequelae.[13] Local infiltration of the corticosteroid is as useless as shoes on an insect.

2 In our experience as well as that of others excision of the lesion has been proven clinically to be effective.[16] The earlier this is done, the better the result; but we excise them all and either close them per primamor with a skin graft or flap.[24]

3 Antibiotic is used for secondary infection.

4 Analgesics may be used for pain.

5 Tetanus prophylaxis is given if needed.

6 Antivenin is available in South America, but is not commercially purchasable in the United States. A specific *L. reclusa* antivenin should be manufactured.

7 Peritoneal dialysis and/or hemodialysis

may be indicated in severe arachnidism and renal failure.

In addition to *Latrodectus* and *Loxosceles* genera, at least 50 other species of spiders in the United States have been implicated in biting humans. Bites by most of these species produce some localized pain, swelling, pruritis, and local tissue reaction. These too must be attended according to the degree of envenomation that persists.

Scorpion Stings

It is difficult to realize that such a fragile and delicate creature as the scorpion can be so dangerous to a human. The scorpion has been a resident of this earth nearly 400,000,000 years, and during this time this arachnid has observed animals as large as dinosaurs and mastodons arrive and disappear, yet has undergone little change in habits and life forms itself. There have been nearly 700 species of scorpions identified in the world, and about 40 of these reside in the United States, 20 living in Arizona alone. The most dangerous scorpion of our country and the one responsible for more envenomations than any other is found in the Southwest—*Centruroides sculpturatus.*

   Habitat and Feature   All scorpions are poisonous. Among the species are *Centruroides sculpturatus ewing, Centruroides gertschi stahnke, Hadrurus hirsutus* (hairy desert scorpion), and *Vejovis spinigeris* (stripe-tailed scorpion).[55] Scorpions have a long, thin body and a tail which is segmented and terminates in a conspicuous sharpness. There is a bulbous portion, the ampulla, near the tail tip which contains two poison glands that excrete the venom (Fig. 10-34). When the scorpion stings, the tail tip makes a small wound and the venom is deposited in the wound. As the sharp, pointed tail is withdrawn, the wound also closes to prevent venom escape. Scorpions are nocturnal and search for water and

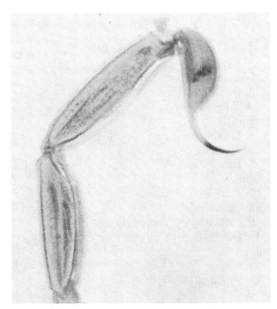

Figure 10-34   All scorpions are poisonous, some relatively harmless, others lethal. The scorpion tail is segmented so it can bend, and near the sharp tip is a bulb (ampulla) containing two poison glands which excrete the venom.

food such as insects, other arachnids, and small rodents. They vary in size from 1.5 to 20 cm in length (Fig. 10-35).

   The Venom   There are two types of scorpion venom: one produces local effects and is relatively harmless, the other contains a neurotoxin which is responsible for fatal reactions and has the following effects:

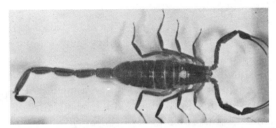

Figure 10-35   There are about 40 species of scorpions in our country, of which 20 are native to Arizona. It is astounding that such a dainty and delicate creature can be so vicious and dangerous to a human.

Signs and Symptoms

1 No local edema or discoloration
2 Sharp pain produced by the venom injection, and then numbness
3 Itching of the nose and mouth
4 Tongue becomes sluggish, with speech impaired
5 Unable to open mouth and difficult to feed; frothing may develop
6 Restlessness, twitchings, muscular spasms
7 Nausea and vomiting
8 Incontinence
9 Convulsions, opisthotonos
10 Death due to circulatory or respiratory failure

Management

I *Relieve pain*
  A Apply household ammonia to sting area immediately or
  B Apply Valisone ointment 0.1% or Disprosone ointment 0.5% (Schering) to infliction.
  C Inject 2 mL 2% Xylocaine (Astra) with epinephrine 1:100,000 into affected area.
II *Inhibit nervousness, hypertension, hypersalivation, muscular fasciculations, convulsions, and shock*
  A Calcium gluconate 10 mL 10% IV and repeat prn.
  B Atropine sulfate 0.6 mg IM.
  C Nembutal (Abbott) 100 mg IV.

Hymenoptera Stings

This order of Arthropoda includes the bees, wasps, hornets, ants, and other membranous-winged insects whose venomers are females. Fortunately, their attacks are more of an aggravation than a disaster, yet some are very envenomous and others kill sensitized persons. About 25 percent of the world's population is sensitive to hymenoptera venoms,[34] and though we have never experienced any disaster, based on other authors' findings at least 25 humans die of insect inflictions yearly in the United States.[17,28] When a fatality occurs, the "literature" average post-sting death time is 10 min! A patrol of soldiers was moving along a jungle path in Vietnam, and one man bumped a bush from which a cloud of angry bees swarmed upon four of the soldiers. A helicopter flew them to the field hospital where, 40 min post sting, they were in shock and suffering from pain, generalized erythema, fast feeble pulse, and periorbital, and labial edema. None had evidence of anaphylaxis. Many living and dead bees were removed from them. From 55 to 76 stingers were removed from each of the four victims. They were bathed, given narcotic analgesics and diphenhydramine for 48 h, and discharged 3 days after hospital admission. Bee specimens were sent to the Pasteur Institute in Saigon, and they were reported to be the Western honeybees (*Apis mellifera linn*). Here is an example of multiple bee stings without critical sequelae and with no anaphylaxis, whereas deaths have been reported from a single sting.

Habitat and Description There is much variation among the species; but all members of the order have two pairs of wings, a head, thorax, abdomen, one pair of antennae, and the females have a tubular ovipositor which has a dual purpose of injecting poison and depositing eggs. Some hymenopteran ovipositors are barbed, and these hook into the victim and tear loose from the insect's body, causing its death; other ovipositors are smooth, and the insect is able to sting repeatedly and fly away for another day.

The Bees
Solitary Bees These live alone, survive for only one season, and include many species, such as the small and large carpenter bees, miner bees, mason bees, and cuckoo bees.
Social Bees These consist of the bumblebees, which are large, noisy, nonaggressive, and the most primitive of the bees; and the

honeybees, which are disciplined workers. The honeybee has a hollow stinging apparatus which is needle-sharp and extrudes when the bee is ready to strike (Fig. 10-36). When injected, this stinging apparatus is avulsed from the bee's body and left in the victim, and the honeybee flies off to die. If the victim is stung on an eyelid, the nonabsorbable stinger remains and may continue to irritate the globe; therefore it must be removed.

The Wasps

Solitary Wasps These have a large thorax and abdomen but a very small waist (Fig. 10-37). These "southern belles" are most useful to man because they destroy large numbers of harmful beetles, caterpillars, spiders, and flies. They build nests from mud (mud daubers) and debris. Because of their narrow waistline, they can only consume liquid food. The stinger is pointed and without barbs, so they can inject multiple victims as many times as their stinger desires.

Social Wasps These number more than 800 different species, and the commoner ones are the *yellow jackets* and *hornets.* They construct nests from wood fragments and leaves, and with their saliva form these particles into a

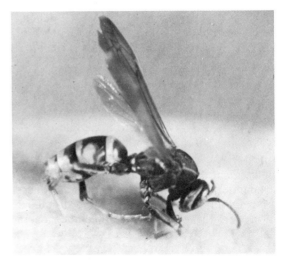

Figure 10-37 There are over 800 species of wasps which bite and sting. Most are aggressive with quick tempers. The stinger is not barbed, so they can inject multiple times and many victims. The hymenoptera kill more people than any venomer in our nation.

paper. It is said the Chinese learned papermaking from these insects. Yellow jackets are very aggressive and have quick tempers. They may first bite and then quickly sting. The hornet, unlike the yellow jacket who paralyzes its prey, butchers the captive alive into small portions to help transport it easily. The stinger or lancet of a wasp is not barbed, so it can be reinserted again and again, and the insect can escape without dying.

The Venom Venoms of the bee, wasp, and hornet contain histamine and phospholipase-A and phospholipase-B. *Bee* venom also consists of serotonin, acetylcholine, melittin, apamin, and a mastocytolytic peptide. *Wasp* venom also contains serotonin, hyaluronidase, and kinin. *Hornet* venom is also made up of serotonin and acetylcholine and produces hypotension and increased vascular permeability. Most of all the components cause pain. The kinins cause vasodilation, increased capillary permeability, diapedesis of cells, and pain.

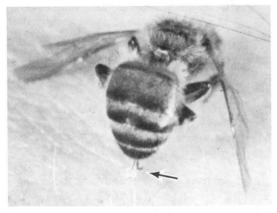

Figure 10-36 This honeybee has a stinger (arrow) which breaks off and remains in the victim as a nonabsorbable foreign body. The stinger should be removed as soon as possible.

Signs and Symptoms These vary depending upon the (1) amount of venom received, (2) degree of patient sensitivity, and (3) site of the sting. A single sting may pass unnoticed, yet it may cause sudden death in a sensitive victim. Effects may be sudden or delayed, and they may last for only an hour or persist for weeks. Reactions are more severe in people over 30 years and are rare in children.[48]

1 *Local:* Sharp pain at sting site, followed by tenderness, itching, swelling, and redness. Usually all symptoms subside and disappear; however, the reaction may become generalized.

2 *Generalized:* Urticaria, anxiety, wheezing, abdominal discomfort, vomiting, and vertigo. These findings may abate or continue.

3 *Critical:* Dyspnea, dysphagia, confusion, collapse, cyanosis, coma, and death.

4 *Delay phenomenon:* After hours or days, redness appears at sting site, followed by urticaria, hemorrhagic bullae, skin necrosis, and anaphylaxis.

5 *Eye stings:* Hazardous with possible penetration of the globe, lens abscess, iris atrophy, and glaucoma. A stinger left in the eyelid may irritate the cornea or sclera for months, causing ulcers, scars, and blindness.

Treatment Hymenoptera kill more people than any venomer in our nation. Therefore, consider a bee sting an acute medical problem deserving emergency attention.[17]

I If the ovipositor is deposited in the skin, it will appear as a black spot and possibly will be covered with a drop of blood. Retrieve it with a No. 11 scalpel blade and without squeezing or pressing it, as the venom sac is attached and venom may be spread further into the wound. Do not use tweezers! Once the ovipositor has been removed, the local sting area is treated the same as an envenomation produced by an unbarbed stinger.

II Local rubor, dolor, and calor is relieved by
  A Valisone ointment 0.1%.
  B Inject 1 mL 1% Xylocaine with epinephrine 1:100,000 into affected area.
  C Ice pack. No heat!
  D Calamine lotion prn.

III Treatment of common toxic effects from venom per se
  A Urticaria, joint pains, nausea, vomiting.

    1 Calcium gluconate, 10 mL 10% IV.
    2 Benadryl 4 mg/kg body weight IV.
    3 Xylocaine 10 mL 1% without epinephrine in 1000 mL normal saline solution given slowly in IV drip.
    4 Corticosteroids.
    5 Tub bath containing a box of Arm and Hammer baking soda.
    6 Intravenous fluids for severe anorexia.

IV Acute generalized allergic reactions need immediate attention
  A Start intravenous normal saline with indwelling catheter.
  B Artificial resuscitation and oxygen.
  C Inject 0.5 mL epinephrine hydrochloride 1:000 subcutaneously, and repeat in 5 min if necessary.
  D Aminophylline 0.25 g in 10 mL IV for bronchospasms.
  E Methamphetamine hydrochloride, 30 mg in 1.5 mL for shock and hypotension.

V Prophylaxis
  A Commercial polyvalent hymenopteran antigens (Center Laboratories, Port Washington, N.Y.) is available.
  B Avoid exposure to infested areas of stinging insects.
  C Avoid preparation with floral or perfume scents when hiking or camping.
  D Wear white clothing and do not go barefoot.

MARINE BITES AND STINGS

There are over 1000 species of marine animals and plants which are capable of inflicting injuries to fishermen, divers, swimmers, bathers, and persons involved in using the waters of the world. The injury mechanisms and their treatment may be divided into groups for simplicity.[56]

Animals that Inflict Trauma

There are a number of marine animals which are potentially dangerous because of their size and ability to inflict injuries. Those most notorious are the shark, barracuda, moray eel, giant sea bass, giant grouper, sea lion, killer whale, and octopus.

Sharks and barracudas are dangerous because their behavior is unpredictable. Although shark repellent is advertised, there is no consistently effective shark repellent proven as such. Observations of shark behavior indicate that they are attracted to sounds resulting from water turbulence and bright objects. Swimmers with red, orange, and yellow bathing suits are like fishing lures to sharks and barracudas. Bathers should be warned not to use plastic floats and surfboards painted with bright colors. Most other marine animals that inflict injury by biting are dangerous only when molested. They may be provoked into attacking when defending their territories, teased by thoughtless divers, or protecting their young.

The most effective measures taken in Natal to reduce shark injuries were preventative.[58] Twenty of twenty-one cases in a recently reported series occurred in areas without protection by elaborate nets along beachfronts. If damage to the protective net is suspected, swimming is banned completely. Bathing in warm water with high optical density in the late afternoon appears to be a contributory factor. Swimming should be curtailed as soon as dirty water invades the protected area. Injuries from sharks cause massive tissue loss and bleeding; therefore emergency medical care to stop the bleeding and treat shock must be instituted immediately. Tourniquet application may be the only feasible method of controlling bleeding from a severed or badly lacerated extremity while or after the victim is

being removed from the water. In the operating room the wound will be found contaminated with beach sand and other debris and will require copious irrigation and estimation of damage. In the common injuries following shark attack by *Carcharodon leucas* (white shark) and related species, excision should be limited to obviously devitalized tissues, as these bites are a combination of incising and avulsing injury, with a minimum of crushing. Careful hemostasis is required, and vascular injuries need primary repair. Covering by soft tissue should be provided for major nerve and tendon injuries, for which secondary suture repair is advised. Primary skin closure is recommended unless there is a large tissue defect for which delayed primary grafting is recommended because there may be considerable oozing from injured muscles. Immediate amputation of an irreparably damaged limb may be required if vascular reanastomosis is not feasible.

Animals that Sting

A group of aquatic animals inflict their injuries by virtue of a stinging apparatus. Jellyfish, the Portuguese man-of-war, sea anemones, hydra, and corals are representative of this class. Toxins are injected by a nematoid apparatus which functions as a microscopic trigger mechanism.[44] Hundreds of thousands of nematocysts reside in the dangling tentacles of jellyfish, and these become imbedded on and in the skin. Swimmers, divers, and lifeguards on beaches come in contact with the tentacles when they are swimming in waters infested by jellyfish. The poison that is discharged onto the skin produces an instantaneous, painful burning which is constant, followed by erythematous streaks wherever the tentacles have touched the skin. The victim becomes very apprehensive and finds that if the lesions are rubbed or scratched, symptoms progress to more pain, itching, and urticaria, which is unbearable. If not treated, headache and mental symptoms appear. In some cases, shock, collapse, and paralysis have occurred within minutes or hours.

The only treatment is emergency:

1 Inactivate the nematocyst by rinsing the involved area with a liquid that has a high alcohol content. If none is available,
2 Pour household ammonia onto the area of skin irritation.
3 Remove the residual tentacles by coalescing them with a drying agent such as flour or baking soda; any mild alkalizing agent will neutralize the acid toxins of the nematocyst.
4 Corticosteroid solutions (fluocinolone acetonide, Syntex) or ointments applied to the affected areas will also achieve relief.

Animals with Spines

A number of marine creatures have body spines, and some of the spines have venom apparatus. These animals are "double trouble," as the venom produces a toxin and the spine produces a traumatic puncture wound that is prone to infection as slime and debris are introduced into the wound. A wide variety of marine animals, including segmental worms, cone shells (five human fatalities), sea urchins, stingrays, catfish, and spiny fish represent this class. Injuries from this group of sea life usually occur on the extremities while the victim is wading or fishing. A common, hand injury occurs when removing a fishing hook from a caught channel catfish. Stepping on a sea urchin or a stingray are everyday casualties in seaboard cities and fishing villages. These marine animals are not aggressive; rather they are docile.

The *catfish* is probably the most prevalent poisonous fish in the United States. There are about 1000 species of catfish, and some of these are endowed with rare characteristics. There is a male catfish which incubates its eggs in its mouth for 2 months; there is the South American astroblepin which climbs cliffs with its mouth; the Amazon catfish that harbors itself in the human urethra; the electric catfish that repels attackers with its electrical plates; and the *Plotosus pincatus,* which is one of the most envenomous fishes known and can cause death. The catfish has dorsal and pectoral fins that erect when the fish desires, and the spines on these fins are dagger-sharp. Some spines have venom glands; others do not, but have mucous cells along the epithelium covering the spine, which are toxic to vascular and neural tissue. The sting of a North American catfish causes an immediate painful and throbbing sensation, which may resolve in a few hours, but can become infected and even be responsible for paralysis (Fig. 10-38). Treatment for deep spine penetrations is to incise the puncture wound and cleanse or debride it thoroughly; or if the puncture is shallow, cleanse to the depths with an applicator soaked in Betadine solution and leave open. A broad-spectrum antibiotic is started, and tetanus prevention is

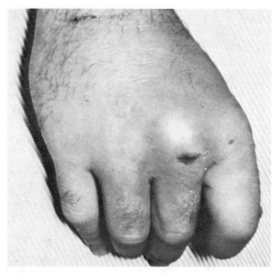

Figure 10-38 Catfish are probably the most prevalent poisonous fish in the United States. This wound was inflicted by the dorsal fin and resulted in a tenosynovitis and infection of the metacarpophalangeal joint. There was also paralysis of the dorsum of the hand and long finger.

instituted. Analgesics usually suffice for the discomfort. The patient must be instructed to return to the emergency room or office the next day or sooner for a recheck.

Stingrays continue to be a menace along the United States coastal waters, being responsible for over 1000 stings annually. There are about 60 species known to be poisonous. This sea animal and its malicious pranks were described circa 100 B.C. by Dioscorides.[22] Stingrays have a furrowed spine on the tail, and it is in this groove where the venom cells and sacs are covered with epitheluim. The venom is released upon penetration of the stinger. Envenomation is evidenced by intense pain, muscle spasms, vomiting, and diarrhea, which may be followed by dyspnea, convulsions, and death. Many treatments have been proposed for stingray envenomation.[23] Therapy for this infliction begins with retrieving the imbedded spine, followed by soaks in less than hot Betadine solution as soon as possible, and continuing with fomentations of the same solution. Other symptomatic therapy such as antibiotics, tetanus prophylaxis, antihistamines, and steroids is instituted as necessary.

BIBLIOGRAPHY

1 Baxter, C. R.: Surgical management of soft tissue infections, *Surg. Clin. North Am.,* **52**:1483, 1972.

2 Bobo, R. A. and E. J. Newton: A previously undescribed gram-negative bacillus causing septicemia and meningitis, *Am. J. Clin. Pathol.,* **65**:564, 1976.

3 Boyes, J. H.: *Bunnel's Surgery of the Hand,* 5th ed., J. B. Lippincott Company, Philadelphia, 1970, p. 616.

4 Bucherl, W., E. E. Buckley, and V. Deulofeu: *Venomous Animals and Their Venoms,* Academic Press, Inc., New York, 1968, vol. 1, p. 168.

5 Carithers, H. A.: Mammalian bites of children, *Am. J. Dis. Child.,* **95**:150, 1958.

6 Celsus: *De Medicina,* translated by W. G. Spencer, Harvard University Press, Cambridge, Mass., 1935–38.

7 Christy, M. P.: Poisoning by venomous animals, *Am. J. Med.,* **42**:107, 1967.

8 Chuinard, R. G. and R. D. D'Ambrosia: Human bite infections of the hand, *J. Bone J. Surg.,* **59-A**:416, 1977.

9 Committee on Trauma, American College of Surgeons: A guide to prophylaxis against tetanus in wound management, *Bull. Am. Coll. Surg.,* **57**:32, 1972.

10 Constantine, D. G.: Rabies transmission by non-bite route, *Public Health Rep.,* **77**:287, 1962.

11 Corey, L. and M. A. W. Hattwick: Treatment of persons exposed to rabies, *J. Am. Med. Assoc.,* **232**:272, 1975.

12 Curtin, J. W. and P. W. Greeley: Human bites of the face, *Plast. Reconstr. Surg.,* **28**:394, 1961.

13 Dillaha, C. J., G. T. Jansen, W. M. Honeycutt, and C. R. Hayden: North American "ell" loxoscelism, *J. Am. Med. Assoc.,* **188**:33, 1964.

14 Douglas, L. G.: Bite wounds, *Am. Fam. Physician,* **11**:93, April 1975.

15 Elgert, K. D., M. A. Ross, B. J. Campbell, and J. T. Barrett: Immunologic studies of brown recluse spider venom, *Infect. Immun.,* **10**:1412, 1974.

16 Fardon, D. W., C. W. Wingo, D. W. Robinson, and F. W. Masters: Treatment of brown spider bite, *Plast. Reconstr. Surg.,* **40**:482, 1967.

17 Frazier, C. A.: Insect sting reactions in children, *Ann. Allergy,* **23**:37, 1965.

18 Galen: *On Medical Experience,* translated by R. Walzer, Oxford University Press, Cambridge, 1975.

19 Glass, T. G.: Snakebite, *Hosp. Med.,* **7**:31, 1975.

20 Goldwyn, R. M.: Man's best friend, *Arch. Surg.,* **111**:221, 1976.

21 Gudger, E. W.: Is the stingray sting poisonous? A historical résumé showing the development of our knowledge that it is poisonous, *Bull. Hist. Med.,* **14**:467, 1943.

22 Gunther, R. T.: *The Greek Herbal of Dioscorides,* illustrated by a Byzantine, A.D. 512, translated by John Goodyear, A.D. 1665, Hafner Publishing Company, Inc., New York, 1968.

23 Halstead, B. W. and U. C. Bunker: Stingray attacks and their treatment, *Am. J. Trop. Med.,* **2**:115, 1953.

24 Hershey, F. B. and C. E. Aulinbacker: Surgical treatment of brown recluse bites, *Ann. Surg.,* **170**:300, 1969.

25 Holloway, W. J., E. G. Scott, and Y. B. Admas: *Pasteurella multocida* infection in man: Report of 21 cases, *Am. J. Clin. Pathol.,* **51**:705, 1969.

26 Horen, W. D.: Arachnidism in the United States, *J. Am. Med. Assoc.,* **185**:839, 1963.

27 Huang, T. T., J. B. Lynch, D. L. Larson, and S. R. Lewis: The use of excisional therapy in the management of snake bite, *Ann. Surg.,* **179**:598, 1974.

28 Jones, R. C. and G. T. Shires: "Bites and Stings of Animals and Insects," in *Schwartz's Principles of Surgery,* McGraw-Hill Book Company, New York, 1974, Chap. 6, p. 207.

29 Lavine, L. S., H. D. Isenberg, W. Rubins, and J. I. Berkman: Unusual osteomyelitis following superficial dog bite, *Clin. Orthop.,* **98**:251, 1975.

30 Lockhart, W. E.: Treatment of snakebite, *J. Am. Med. Assoc.,* **193**:36, August 2, 1965.

31 MacQuarrie, M. B., B. Forghani, and D. A. Wolochow: Hepatitus B transmitted by a human bite, *J. Am. Med. Assoc.,* **230**:723, 1974.

32 Majno, G.: *The Healing Hand,* Harvard University Press, Cambridge, Mass., 1975, p. 86.

33 Minton, S. A.: *Venom Diseases,* Charles C Thomas, Publisher, Springfield, Ill., 1971.

34 Mueller, H. L.: Stinging-insect allergy, *Ped. Ann.,* **3**:43, 1974.

35 Murphy, R., S. Katz, and D. Massaro: Fusobacterium septicemia following a human bite, *Arch. Int. Med.,* **111**:51, 1963.

36 O'Brien, G. R., J. L. Kostecki, and H. Colberg: The human bite, *N.Y. State J. Med.,* **71**:85, 1974.

37 Parks, B. J., L. G. Hawkins, and R. L. Horner: Bites of the hand, *Rocky Mount. Med. J.,* **71**:85, 1974.

38 Parrish, H. M.: Fatalities from venomous animals, *Am. J. Med. Sci.,* **245**:129, 1963.

39 ———, J. C. Goldner, and S. L. Silberg: Comparison between snakebites in children and adults, *Pediatrics,* **46**:251, 1965.

40 Paton, B. C.: Bites: Human, dog, spider and snake, *Surg. Clin. North Am.,* **43**:537, 1963.

41 Pearn, J. H.: Bee stings in operational theatres, *Mil. Med.,* **20**:241, 1972.

42 Ramsey, F. G.: Coral snake bite, *J. Am. Med. Assoc.,* **182**:949, 1962.

43 Randall, P.: Personal communication.

44 Reid, H. A.: Bites and stings in travellers, *Postgrad. Med. J.,* **51**:830, 1975.

45 Riley, H. D.: Brown spider bite with severe hemolytic phenomena, *J. Okla. State Med. Assoc.,* **57**:218, May 1964.

46 Robinson, D.: *Canis familiaris, N. Engl. J. Med.,* **290**:1378, 1974.

47 Robinson, D. A.: Dog bites and rabies: An assessment of risk, *Br. Med. J.,* **1**:1066, 1976.

48 Russell, F. E., J. Wainschel, M. B. Madon, and F. Ennik: Insect and scorpion bites and stings, *J. Am. Med. Assoc.,* **224**:131, 1973.

49 Russell, F. E.: Stingray injuries, *Public Health Rep.,* **74**:855, 1959.

50 Sheffer, A. L.: Therapy of anaphylaxis, *N. Engl. J. Med.,* **275**:1059, 1966.

51 Shields, C., M. J. Patzakis, M. H. Meyers, and J. P. Harvey, Jr.: Hand infections secondary to human bites, *J. Trauma,* **15**:235, 1975.

52 Snyder, C. C.: "Bites and Stings," in *Early Care of the Injured Patient,* American College of Surgeons, W. B. Saunders Company, Philadelphia, 1972, Chap. 7, p. 73.

53 Snyder, C. C., R. Straight, and J. Glenn: The snakebitten hand, *Plast. Reconstr. Surg.,* **49**:275, 1972.

54 Stahnke, H. L.: Arizona's lethal scorpion, *Ariz. Med.,* **24**:490, 1972.

55 Stahnke, H. L., W. A. Heffron, and D. L. Lewis: Bite of the Gila monster, *Rocky Mount. Med. J.,* **67**:25, 1970.

56 Strauss, M. D. and W. L. Orris: Injuries to divers by marine animals: A simplified approach to recognition and management, *Mil. Med.,* **139**:129, 1974.

57 Thomson, H. G. and V. Svitek: Small animal bites: The role of primary closure, *J. Trauma,* **13**:20, 1973.

58 White, J. A. M.: Shark attack in Natal, *Injury,* **6**:187, 1975.

59 Wingert, W. A. and J. Wainschel: Diagnosis and management of envenomation by poisonous snakes, *South. Med. J.,* **68**:1015, 1975.

Chapter 11

Trauma to the Nervous System

W. Kemp Clark, M.D.

The statistical data presented in this chapter are derived from an analysis of the 1086 cases of head injury admitted to the neurosurgical service of The University of Texas Southwestern Medical School–Parkland Memorial Hospital between 1956 and 1965. In the ensuing 10 years, 1965 to 1975, the total experience has enlarged to nearly 2500 cases of the various types of head injury. The incidence and distribution by age has remained essentially constant. The only significant change during this period of time has been the increase in the severe type of closed head trauma. The reason for this apparently lies in more high-speed transportation, with more accidents occurring on the expressways. However, the distribution within the series by type of injury has remained essentially unchanged. The mortality statistics reflect the greater severity of closed head injury by an increased fatality rate in that group. A decrease in mortality in the subdural hematoma group has occurred.

The material presented deals largely with head injuries in the adolescent and adult, who comprise the largest group of patients admitted to a general hospital for treatment of head injuries (Table 11-1). In this chapter, emphasis is placed upon the immediate care of patients who have sustained both serious head and somatic injuries, which occurred in 20 percent of the patients in this series (Table 11-2), and on the surgical treatment of acute head injuries. The distribution of the types of head injuries sustained by the patients in this series is given in Table 11-3.

Brief analysis of this statistical distribution indicates that automotive injuries, falls, and personal violence are the leading etiologic agents. This distribution is similar to that reported in other large head-injury series.

Table 11-1: Age Distribution of 1086 Patients with Head Injuries Admitted to a General Hospital

Age group	Sex M	Sex F	Total number of patients, %
0-1	29	18	4
1-5	121	61	17
5-10	72	19	8
11-20	142	34	16
21-30	150	42	18
31-40	92	40	12
41-50	79	27	10
51-60	76	18	9
61-70	26	15	4
71+	18	7	2
Total	805	281	

Table 11-2: Types of Associated Injuries in 209 of 1086 Patients Who Sustained Both Cranial and Somatic Injuries

Major associated injury	Number of patients
Facial fractures	22
Fracture of extremity	103
Fracture of lower extremity	59
Fracture of upper extremity	39
Fracture of upper and lower extremity	5
Chest injury	29
Pneumothorax	9
Hemothorax	5
Fracture of ribs only	9
Flail chest	5
Intrapulmonary hemorrhage	1
Intraabdominal injuries	41
Urinary tract injury	5
Multiple visceral injuries	36
Vertebral column injuries	14
Fracture of odontoid process	5
Fracture or dislocation of cervical vertebrae	5
Fracture of thoracic vertebrae	2
Fracture of lumbar and sacral vertebrae	2

In the past few years, a decrease in the number of mild closed head injuries has been noted. The reason for this decrease seems to be threefold. First, the decrease in the speed on the highway and streets has effected a reduction in the severity of impact in automobile accidents. Secondly, the increased use of restraining devices in cars has reduced the secondary impact of the person with the car interior. Thirdly, the development of a county-wide ambulance service staffed by experienced, trained emergency medicine technicians and paramedics has reduced the hypoxic injury previously suffered during transportation from the injury site to the hospital. In earlier years, a number of patients were admitted to the emergency room in coma, with partially or completely obstructed airways, adding significantly to their mortality and morbidity.

In recent years, an increased incidence of cervical spine injury has been noted in patients with automotive head trauma. The incidence now is nearly 10 percent in our series. Some of this increased number is related to enhanced methodology. Now all patients with significant head trauma receive at least one x-ray of the cervical spine. If there is any question as to the presence of spine injury, polytomography is done. This method of management has led to increased detection of spine injuries.

In recent years, the number of intracerebral hematomas found in the Parkland Memorial Hospital series has increased significantly. Again, a methodologic change has been largely responsible for this increase. The availability of computerized axial tomography of the head has made the diagnosis of intracerebral hematoma far easier. This noninvasive, accurate technique has resulted in the recognition of an increased number of patients with these lesions. Previously, since the diagnosis required the use of cerebral arteriography, many patients were not studied appropriately, and

Table 11-3:   Types of Head Injuries Sustained in 1086 Patients

Type of injury	Number of patients	% of total	Mortality for this injury	
			Number	%
Closed head injury	758	70	49	7
Compound injuries	182	17	47	26
Penetrating wounds	66	6	32	48
Depressed fractures	116	11	15	13
Intracranial hematomas	146	13	58	40
Epidural	22	2	7	32
Subdural	118	11	47	40
Acute	53	5	38	72
Subacute (3+ days)	21	2	3	14
Chronic (7+ days)	36	3	6	17
Intracerebral	6	1	4	67
	1086	100		

their intracerebral hematomas were not diagnosed.

HEAD INJURIES

Mechanisms of Injury

The effects of compressive blows which produce scalp lacerations, depressed skull fractures, and direct compression and laceration of the brain in compound injuries have been studied extensively by Gurdjian and Webster, using cadavers and dried skulls.[33] With a compressive blow, a concave deformation of the skull occurs at the point of impact. Fracturing of the skull occurs initially at the point of convex deformation, and the fractures spread radially from this convex perimeter of deformation. With higher forces and greater deformation, the entire convex perimeter may fracture and remain in suit or be driven inward, producing a depressed fracture.

However, the widespread brain damage caused by blows producing relatively little damage to the scalp or skull is still inadequately understood because of the difficulty of obtaining a suitable experimental model. Two main theories have been advanced to explain the diffuse and extensive brain damage observed in closed head injuries; the first emphasizes the wave of compression produced by the blow, the second stresses the shearing forces produced by acceleration of the brain. Studies of the effects of a wave of compression produced by a blow have been carried out using transparent models of the skull filled with fluids.[23] High-speed photography and pressure measurements have shown that following the compressive wave which travels outward from the point of impact of a blow, the area through which the wave has passed undergoes decompression, a process similar to the compression and rarefaction produced in a medium when sound waves pass through it. An area of rarefaction may develop cavitation, producing gas bubbles which cause explosive disruption of the fluid medium. The brain, consisting of a semisolid medium separated by dural sheaths and tethered at its base by the cranial nerves and great vessels, has more complex physical characteristics than those of a simple fluid-filled cavity, however. The experiments of Pudenz and Shelden, in which the brain was observed through a lucite calvarium demonstrated that the brain undergoes considerable acceleration and deformation within the skull following a blow.[68] In particular, sliding movements of the lobes and rotation of the brain around various axes were produced by blows to the skull. Denny-Brown and Russell have also shown that blows to the unsupported head of an animal produce greater brain damage than similar blows to a rigidly supported head.[21,65] An analogous situation occurs in boxing, in which the experienced boxer attempts to hold his head rigidly in order to prevent a concussion which would result from a snapping back of the head. Holbourn[37] and Stritch[81] have provided theoretical and neuropathologic evidence that acceleration of the brain caused by a blow produces shearing forces which tear fiber tracts and blood vessels. Lacerations of the white matter of the hemispheres, tearing of veins bridging to the dural sinuses, and contusions of the poles of the brain appear to result from acceleration of the brain within the skull and the concomitant shearing forces developed.

Gurdjian[32] has recently summarized what is known of the biophysics of head injury. He concluded that a variety of effects were possible. These, basically, were impact with compression of the brain secondary to either acceleration or deceleration and impact with direct compression. He pointed out that compression of the closed head produces distortion of the skull with compression of the intracranial contents. The usual acceleration-deceleration type of injury results in a combination of forces within the brain, with both linear and angular acceleration forces. At the time of impact, a variety of compression, tension, and shear forces may be created within the brain. This plus the pressure gradients generated and the movements of the brain relative to the skull are the major factors. It is the vector of these forces that

produces the net extent of damage to the brain.

Pathology of Head Injuries

The most common scalp injury is an irregular linear laceration; less frequent scalp injuries are stellate wounds, wounds with loss of substance, avulsions of the scalp, and subgaleal hematomas.

Of the patients in this series, 39 percent exhibited skull fractures, most commonly of the vault, in the frontal and parietal regions. Fractures of the base of the skull occur most frequently in the floor of the anterior and middle fossae, and the fracture lines tend to run into the foramina of the base of the skull. The most common skull fracture is the simple, linear, nondepressed fracture of the vault, usually occurring without an overlying scalp laceration. Less frequently seen is the complex skull fracture of the vault, usually occurring without an overlying scalp laceration. Even less frequently seen is the complex skull fracture which may be termed a bursting fracture, consisting of radiating fracture lines with comminution of the fragments, and generally associated with overlying scalp lacerations. A variant type of bursting fracture is the circumferential fracture, usually occurring in the horizontal bifrontal plane with elevation of the fractured portion of the calvarium from the base. Bursting fractures result from massive trauma, usually to the frontal area. A second variant of the bursting fracture is the diastatic fracture, with separation of the sagittal suture or a portion of the lambdoidal suture, which results from a severe occipital blow.

Bursting fractures result from compressive forces on the skull, usually when the head is caught between two unyielding surfaces. A variant of the bursting fracture is the diastatic fracture, with separation of the suture. Usually, the diastatic fracture involves the sagittal suture, with the compressive forces anteroposterior; but occasionally the lambdoid suture or the coronal suture may be involved in a diastatic fracture. In any circumstance, the compression force is usually applied parallel to the suture.

The frontal and parietal bones are most often affected by depressed skull fractures. Such fractures are usually caused by a relatively small object striking the head with high velocity. The depth of depression and the size of the bone depressed are a function of the velocity and the mass of the object striking the head. Occasionally, such a large plate of bone may be depressed that it acts as a mass lesion. Usually, depressed skull fractures are associated with scalp lacerations. In fact, one rarely sees adult patients with depressed fractures without an associated scalp laceration. However, in children the reverse seems to be the case. Most depressed fractures in children occur without scalp laceration. The common depressed fracture is comparatively small and generally round or stellate. However, in more severe trauma, depressed fragments of bone may be driven a substantial distance into the brain.

In cases of missile wounds to the brain, the bullet, striking the bone, shatters it, producing secondary missiles of bone. These may be imbedded at a distance from the tract of the missile and produce extensive damage within the brain.

Cerebrospinal fluid (CSF) rhinorrhea or otorrhea is produced by tears in the dura and arachnoid over a fracture at the base of the skull entering one of the air sinuses or the middle ear cavity. This occurred in approximately 5 percent of the patients in this series. It is most frequently associated with fractures around the face and frontal region. The second most common cause is fractures across the petrous ridge. Cerebrospinal fluid rhinorrhea may not be noticed by the patient or the physician if the fluid does not actually run into the nares or external auditory canal. For in-

stance, a fracture through the petrous ridge into the middle ear cavity without a tear of the tympanic membrane may produce a cerebrospinal fluid leak through the eustachian tube into the pharynx, where it may be swallowed. Such leaks can be identified by the presence of fluid in the middle ear cavity.

X-rays of the patient's skull may point to the potential problem of CSF leak. Fractures which enter the frontal sinus, particularly through the posterior rim of the frontal sinus, fractures in or about the ethmoids, and fractures which cross the petrous ridge are likely to produce CSF leak, and it should be sought for.

Patients without an initial CSF leak may develop one later. If the dura is entrapped in the fracture site, the arachnoid may bulge through the tear in the dura and the bone and erode the bone further with the pulsation of the arachnoid fluid. The arachnoid may then rupture, and the patient may develop a delayed cerebrospinal fluid leak.

The brain may sustain either concussion or parenchymatous damage as a result of trauma. Concussion may be defined as a physiologic change due to trauma leading to the loss of consciousness and which may occur without evidence of anatomic disruption of brain tissue. This definition, although imprecise, has clinical usefulness in that it separates the milder forms of head injury from the more severe. The physiologic basis of concussion is still poorly understood. Loss of consciousness in concussion is associated with a rapid pulse rate, shallow respiration, coolness and pallor of the skin, and depression of brainstem reflexes. Although the rapid pulse rate and skin pallor give a superfical clinical impression of hypovolemic shock, the blood pressure is normal or elevated. Studies of the physiologic basis of consciousness by Magoun and co-workers indicate that the thalamic and brainstem reticular formation have a powerful influence in maintaining normal waking cortical activity.[55] It is generally believed that in concussion the electrical activity of the reticular formation is disturbed, and Groat has reported chromatolysis occurring in brainstem neurons after experimental concussion.[31]

Anatomic disruption of brain parenchyma can be either focal or diffuse. Focal injuries are most often caused by high-velocity blows and missiles. Contusions of the summits of cortical gyri are commonly seen under the site of impact and particularly under fractures. *Contrecoup injuries,* which are contusions seen at parts of the brain, particularly at the orbitofrontal, temporal, or occipital poles opposite the site of impact, are commonly found when the injury was caused by deceleration of the moving head, as in a fall.

Injury to the cranial nerves occurred in 6 percent of patients in this series. These injuries were generally associated with fractures of the base of the skull. Most commonly injured are the olfactory and statoacoustic nerves, the nerves to the extraocular muscles, and the facial, optic, and trigeminal nerves, with the frequency of injury being in the order given.

Deep penetrating injuries of the brain are most commonly due to gunshot wounds. In general, in civilian practice, only patients wounded with .22- or .25-caliber pistol bullets survive long enough to come to surgery; .32- or .38-caliber pistols or high-velocity rifles fired at close range usually produce extensive blast effects with secondary missile tracts due to bone and lead fragments, resulting in profound brain steminjury and death, often within a few hours. However, an exception to this pattern of profound destruction is occasionally observed in the transverse frontal, or through-and-through bifrontal wound. Attempts at suicide often result in small-caliber pistol wounds of the temporal area. Frequently, in such cases, the pistol is not held squarely against the head, and the bullet produces only an upward-of-posterior grazing wound or a superficial temporoparietal injury. Assaults with a pistol frequently cause a wound or entry in the frontal area, often through a frontal sinus. The bullet then traverses the skull in an anterior-posterior direction and lodges in the posterior parietal or occipital lobes. Remarkable deflections of bullets can occur within the skull, with intracranial rebounding from dural and skull surfaces. Shotgun blast wounds often produce extensive loss of scalp substance with an underlying depressed fracture, but with penetration of the brain by only a few pellets. The force transmitted by shotgun injury through the intact or partially penetrated skull may be quite high. Thus the fatalities from such injuries tend to be high, largely because of the presence of traumatic cerebral edema secondary to the transmission of such forces.[78]

Approximately 50 percent of patients admitted to the hospital for closed head injuries have blood in the cerebrospinal fluid, arising from tearing of small vessels in the subarachnoid space. In general, the amount of blood present is directly related to the severity of the injury. Focal damage to blood vessels may result in intracranial hemorrhages of a size sufficient to cause compression to adjacent brain tissue and elevation of intracranial pressure. Multiple small petechial hemorrhages may be found scattered throughout the white matter of the hemispheres in closed head injuries, although the temporal lobe is the usual site of large traumatic intracerebral hemorrhages. The other site for the contusional petechial hemorrhages to occur is the orbital surface of the frontal lobes. As rotational and transitional movements of the brain occur inside the skull, the frontal and temporal lobes either slide across the roughened orbital roof or are impacted into the curve of the greater wing of the sphenoid. These movements produce the contusion and petechial hemorrhages in the cortex.

On occasion, these petechial hemorrhages

become confluent, forming an intracerebral hematoma. This type of intracerebral hematoma is a secondary type[20] (Courville). These rarely reach a size requiring surgical intervention, except for a singular circumstance or temporal lobe swelling.

There is a primary type of intracerebral hematoma which is a globular collection of blood, not intermixed with bits of pulped brain tissue. Such hematomas tend to occur centrally in the temporal or frontal lobes, or occasionally in the basal ganglion.[15] These hematomas grow, dependent upon the caliber of the vessel ruptured to produce the hematoma. Occasionally, such hematomas are secondary to anticoagulant therapy in patients who subsequently undergo head injury.

Subdural hematomas occur most frequently over the convexities of the hemispheres, but may be located frontally, under the temporal lobes, or over the cerebellum. Acute subdural hematomas are due to bleeding from cortical vessels following lacerations of the cortex in severe trauma and to tearing of veins which bridge the subdural space from the cortical surface to the dural sinuses. In acute subdural hematomas, the subdural blood tends to clot during the first 24 h following the hemorrhage and then tends to liquefy again during the subacute phase of the injury. Filmy membranes can be seen organizing around subacute subdural collections which are about a week old, and in chronic hematomas these membranes may be thick and firmly attached to the dura and pia-arachnoid. The expansion of subacute and chronic hematomas is probably due to transudation and bleeding into the hematoma from surrounding vessels.[69] The majority of subdural hematomas will probably expand if not surgically removed. However, serial angiographic studies on patients with subdural hematomas that have not been removed surgically show that, in certain instances, spontaneous reabsorption of a subdural hematoma is possible.[28]

Subdural hematomas are not commonly associated with skull fractures, but may be. The outstanding exception to this is subdural hematomas occurring in the posterior fossa. Both epidural and subdural hematomas in the posterior fossa are associated with fractures which cross the transverse sinus and enter the foramin magnum. The presence of this fracture is a warning sign of the potential for posterior fossa clot.

Epidural hematomas are classically associated with tearing of the middle meningeal artery at the pterion. At this point, the artery often runs in a bony canal, making it vulnerable to damage by a fracture crossing the temporal area. However, an epidural hematoma may be produced by any extensive fracture of the skull—such as a bursting fracture, a biparietal fracture that crosses the vertex, or a diastatic fracture—which is associated with massive bleeding from the diplopic space and the small veins passing from the skull to the dural venous sinuses.[80] In the present series of cases, epidural hematomas were more often associated with extensive skull fractures than with discrete tearing of the middle meningeal artery. Epidural hematoma may also occur in the absence of a skull fracture.

Children frequently develop epidural hematomas without evidence of skull fracture because the meningeal arteries are not incorporated into bone.

Certain skull fractures are important prognostic indicators. These skull fractures should be carefully looked for and evaluated. Fractures crossing the middle meningeal groove, or crossing any of the great dural sinuses, may be responsible for the development of an acute epidural or, occasionally, an acute subdural hematoma. Fractures across the dural sinuses may result in the formation of chronic epidural hematomas, particularly occurring at the vertex with blood extruding slowly from the superior sagittal sinus. Patients with such skull fractures should be admitted for observation for at least 24 h after head injury and should be followed closely to be sure they do not develop a more chronic process later in their course.

Similarly, fractures which cross the petrous ridge may be responsible, as described elsewhere, for cerebrospinal fluid otorrhea, which may be hidden. More importantly, such fractures may indicate damage to the hearing apparatus. This damage may include perforation of the tympanic membrane, dislocation of the ossicles of the ear, transection of the facial nerve, damage to the facial nerve with delayed facial palsy, or actual damage to the hearing organ itself. Patients who have such a fracture should be carefully watched for the development of any or all of these complications.

Extensive diffuse parenchymatous brain damage is most often caused by the deceleration accident. In these instances, the moving head strikes an object, as when the patient is thrown from a moving car. Thrombosis of small vessels and small areas of hemorrhage is seen on microscopic examination in cases of acute injury. Changes in neurons similar to those produced by ischemia are seen, with pyknotic neurons exhibiting eosinophilia of their cytoplasm and shrinkage of their nuclei. In addition, chromatolysis and vacuolation in neurons and rapid disintegration of neurons, which appear to be specifically caused by trauma, occur. Multinucleation of nerve cells may also be seen, as described by Rand and Courville.[70]

Swelling of the brain, following head trauma, has been an historic point of interest to the neurosurgeon. As investigations have proceeded, cerebral edema has been recognized to have several etiologic factors. Heavy metal poisoning with triethyl-ten or lead is not applicable to head injury cases. Patients sustaining head injury develop cerebral swelling, or edema, secondary to a variety of mechanisms. The most common mechanism seems to be

that of hypoventilation with resulting hypercapnia and hypoxia. This mechanism is described elsewhere, but will occur in any patient with a disturbed level of consciousness. The additional insult rendered by hypoxia will certainly complicate and add to the other forms of cerebral edema which may be present in patients with head injury.

The other types of edema are pericontusional edema, which is swelling of the brain tissue around areas of blood and pulped brain in a contusion. Second, there is head injury edema which is associated with a loss of autoregulation of cerebral blood flow. There is a loss of resistance to blood flow at the capillary level, so that arterial pressure is transmitted to the passively dilated arterioles directly into the capillary and venous bed, and thus into the tissues. Both pericontusional edema and the type due to the loss of cerebral autoregulation are generally characterized as vasogenic.

Another type of edema is occasionally produced in an iatrogenic way in patients with head injury. Patients with head injury may receive large volumes of hypotonic solutions such as 5% dextrose and water intravenously. If the amount administered is in excess of the capacity of the kidney to excrete the free water load, cerebral swelling will occur. This happens at a rate of about 200 mL/h in an adult.

Both cerebral edema and expanding intracranial hematomas cause herniations of the brain through various dural compartments. Some of these herniations are of little or no consequence; others, however, are extremely important. These herniations are directly responsible for compression of the brainstem, failure of medullary function, and death. Death is usually the result of interference with venous and/or arterial blood supply to the vital centers. Occasionally, such herniation may result in focal neurological deficit. If the medial surface of the temporal lobe herniates through the incisural notch of the tentorium, it may compress the posterior cerebral artery as it comes around the brainstem. This will produce infarction of the occipital lobe, with resulting additional swelling of that lobe. Should the patient survive such an insult, the patient will then have a homonymous hemianopsia, which will be quite severe.

This does not produce any clinical symptomatology, but does produce the radiographic evidence of shift of the anterior cerebral artery across the midline. Occasionally, the temporal lobe will herniate above the wing of the sphenoid. This swelling of the temporal lobe may occur late and be responsible for deterioration of the patient's clinical condition. Such herniation is usually associated with contusions, intracerebral hematomas, and vasogenic edema in the temporal lobe. The cingulate gyrus may herniate under the falx. Temporal lobectomy may be required to salvage the patient.

The most important herniation is herniation of the medial temporal lobe through the incisura of the tentorium. This produces compression of the brainstem and of the third cranial nerve. It is this compression of the cranial nerve which produces the pupillary dilation and loss of the light reflex. It is also responsible for the venous and arterial blood supply to the midbrain with the production of secondary pontine hemorrhages, decerebrate posturing, and death.

Herniation of the cerebellar tonsils through the foramin magnum with compression of the spinomedullary junction is another fatal complication of massive swelling of the cerebellum.

Studies carried on in humans of patients' intracranial pressures have shown that, in cases of herniation, there is a differential of pressure which exists from one dural compartment to another. Kaufmann and Clark measured this differential pressure in transtentorial herniations in humans. This observation gives insight into the intracranial compartmentalization.

Immediate Care of the Unconscious Patient

Initial treatment is directed to ensuring that the patient has an adequate airway and to determining whether the patient's pulmonary ventilation and oxygenation are adequate. The patient's blood pressure, pulse, respiratory rate, and temperature are then obtained, initially at least as often as every 15 min. The signs of hypovolemic shock, low blood pressure, and decreased urinary output are not produced by head injury. Examination of the chest, abdomen, and extremities, with attention paid to the signs of blood loss into these areas, should reveal the sources of hemorrhage leading to shock.[14] Rib fractures, with pneumothorax or hemothorax, may be found on examination of the chest, and, if present, appropriate therapy should be instituted.

Currently, endotracheal tubes are placed in all patients who are unconscious upon arrival in the emergency room at Parkland Memorial Hospital. One must be sure that the tubes are appropriately placed and are not placed down a main-stem bronchus. With the use of paramedic personnel taught to entubate patients, there has been improvement in initial care from site of accident to the hospital.

Usually, the endotracheal tube is connected to a T bar for breathing humidified room air or a 20 to 40% oxygen mixture. Of course, if ventilatory assistance is needed, the patient may be placed on a ventilator, preferably one that is volume-controlled, not pressure-controlled. Suction is easily carried out through the endotracheal tube. The patient can be maintained with endotracheal tube in place for several days without significant complications.

Tracheostomy is now an elective procedure

done in the operating room if the patient remains unconscious for a long period of time. This ensures that the procedure can be properly performed. We have abandoned it as an emergency procedure because of the ease of endotracheal intubation and the tolerance of the endotracheal tube. The complications of the tracheostomy alone merit consideration. Patients with tracheostomy have instance of pulmonary infection. The long-term complications of tracheostomy include stenosis of the trachea in a significant number of patients.

An 18-gauge needle is placed in the forearm vein, which is kept open with isotonic saline or with lactated Ringer's solution. Blood is obtained for laboratory studies, including hemoglobin, hematocrit, white cell count, and typing and cross matching, if shock is present or if surgery is planned. A nasogastric tube is passed to empty the stomach, and an indwelling catheter is inserted into the bladder.

Neurologic Examination

The neurologic examination must be a careful and detailed one and the findings fully recorded, as the course of treatment is determined by the progressive changes found on repeated examinations. The examination is begun with an assessment of the patient's state of consciousness, first by the patient's response to verbal stimuli, and then by the response to vigorous somatic stimulation. In the semicomatose or unconscious patient examination of the head, of the cranial nerves, of motor power, and of the reflexes are the parts of the neurologic examination which yield the most information. Examination of the motor system must be carried out vigorously, and the examiner must determine whether failure to carry out a motor act is due to neurologic damage or to inability of the patient to cooperate. Failure to carry out a vigorous examination may result in severe neurologic damage being overlooked or disregarded. If awake, the patient is questioned about specific areas of pain or tenderness and is asked to point to them. Any repeated complaints of painful areas should be carefully investigated. Often, previously unsuspected fractures or foreign bodies are found in these areas.

The head is palpated and inspected for lacerations, embedded foreign bodies, and depressed fractures. Little information can be gained by immediate palpation in the depths of compound wounds, and it is preferable to apply a sterile dressing and wait until x-rays have been obtained and the scalp is shaved and cleaned before palpating in the wounds with a sterile gloved finger. Ecchymoses over the mastoid prominences and around the orbit, cerebrospinal fluid otorrhea or rhinorrhea, and cranial nerve palsies strongly suggest basilar skull fractures.

Inspection of the fundi, pupils, extraocular movements, and facial movements is the most important step in the examination of the cranial nerves if the patient is comatose and a complete examination cannot be carried out. Early papilledema may be seen only a few hours after a head injury, and this evidence of increased intracranial pressure is indicative of the severity of the injury.

The examination of the motor system provides the greatest amount of information for localizing the sites of brain damage. The essential points are:

1 Whether spontaneous movements are present or whether they have been replaced by reflex posturing, which localizes the rostrocaudal level of damage with respect to the cerebral hemispheres and the brainstem.
2 Whether the motor power is equal in the upper and lower extremities, and on the right and left sides of the body, or whether there is focal weakness, which localizes the damage with respect to parts of the cerebral hemispheres. If the patient makes no spontaneous movement, vigorous sternal pressure is applied and the responses of the upper extremi-

ties noted for any asymmetry of movement. The normal response is a purposeful movement, a flexor response of the arms, which is an attempt to brush away the painful stimulus. Similarly, the normal response to painful stimuli applied to each of the extremities is a flexion withdrawal response. In patients with severe brainstem damage, who often exhibit decerebrate posturing and rigidity, the flexor response to painful sternal stimulation is often replaced by an extensor response of the arms in which the fists are clenched and rotated internally.

The deep tendon and superficial reflexes are then elicited, and, as in the case of motor strength, any asymmetries between the right and left sides of the body are noted.

If possible, a sensory examination is performed, with the particular object in mind of determining whether there is any spinal level of somatic sensory loss, which is indicative of an associated spinal cord or peripheral nerve injury. The cervical spine is carefully palpated for evidence of tenderness and examined for mobility.

A single lateral x-ray of the cervical spine is an essential part of the adequate management of the significantly head-traumatized individual. Approximately 10 percent of head-injured patients will show some abnormality of their cervical spines. Should x-rays disclose any suspicion of abnormality in the cervical spine, the patient should be treated as though there was a cervical spine fracture until proven otherwise. This includes immobilization, preferably with Gardner-Wells skull traction, until one is able to obtain cervical spine films of superior quality. It may be necessary to resort to polytomography to be absolutely certain that no such spinal column injury exists. In the present series, about 2 percent of patients had the triad of head injuries, cervical spine fractures, and cervical cord injuries. A simple outline of important features in any given patient has been developed by the Committee

on Trauma of the American College of Surgeons.

Significance of Signs and Differential Diagnosis in Head Injuries

The essential point in the diagnosis and treatment of head injuries is the recognition of those cases which are to be treated surgically, and their separation from those to be treated medically. Indeed, the earliest known medical text, *The Edwin Smith Papyrus*, gives a number of rules to be used by the surgeon in making this decision.[7] Compound injuries and depressed fractures clearly require surgical treatment. The critical differentiation lies in separating those closed head injuries which have intracranial hematomas of a size sufficient to act as mass lesions and which require surgical evacuation from those closed head injuries in which there is only diffuse parenchymatous damage. It is important to remember in making this decision that only about 13 percent of all acute head injuries develop intracranial hematomas. Therefore, the diagnostic problem may be regarded as one of recognizing this comparatively small subgroup of closed head injuries. It cannot be emphasized too strongly that there is no clinical picture, sign, or pattern of neurologic findings that is pathognomonic of an epidural, subdural, or intracerebral hematoma.[52,53] The classical history of a patient who receives a concussive blow, then regains consciousness (the lucid interval), and subsequently relapses into unconsciousness has been uncommon in our experience. In an industrialized society, the severity of the trauma sustained in accidents frequently produces sufficient parenchymatous brain damage in addition to the hematoma to render the patient comatose at the time of injury and for a prolonged period thereafter. What is highly *suggestive* of the development of a hematoma is the *progression* of neurologic signs pathognomonic of increasing intracranial pressure. These signs are bradycardia, hypertension, bradypnea, headache, vomiting, restlessness, impairment of consciousness, and increasing neurologic deficit. If the increased pressure has been sufficient to cause a unilateral herniation of the uncal gyrus, the neurologic findings typical of this herniation will appear: decerebrate posturing, with an oculomotor nerve paresis ipsilateral to the herniation and a motor hemiparesis contralateral to the herniation. In some cases, the hemiparesis will be ipsilateral to the herniation, however; and in cases in which a dilated pupil and a hemiparesis are found on the same side of the body, the dilated pupil has the greater value in localizing the side of the herniation. Loss of consciousness is a usual, but not necessary, concomitant of uncal herniation. An illustration of this is the case of a patient who observed his right pupil dilate while looking in a mirror and was still conscious, although hemiparetic, 45 min later on arrival at the hospital. A large subacute subdural hematoma with uncal herniation ipsilateral to the dilated pupil was found at surgery. However, the signs of increasing intracranial pressure may be due to increasing cerebral edema rather than to intracerebral hemorrhage. Since the underlying pathology cannot be determined from clinical neurologic examination alone, the signs of progressive, increasing intracranial pressure are investigated by cerebral angiography.

Headache has little pathognomonic value, with the exception of the uncommon case of the conscious patient who has a constant headache well localized to one hemisphere and of a severity far out of proportion to the severity of the lateralizing neurologic signs. A subacute subdural hematoma may be present in this situation.

Diagnostic Tests

Radiographs of the skull are obtained following the neurologic examination. Posterior-anterior, Towne, and right and left lateral views are obtained. Submentovertex views may also be required to reveal basilar fractures, and stereoscopic lateral films are useful for precise localization of small fractures or foreign bodies. The films are examined for fracture lines, and fracture lines which cross major dural vessels are noted. Extensions of fracture lines into air sinuses or the petrous bones are also noted. The characteristic breaks in bone contours and double densities produced by depressed fractures are noted. Figure 11-1 illustrates the importance of obtaining tangential films of any part of the skull in which a depressed fracture is suspected. The surgeon should not assume that a depressed fracture or foreign body seen on x-ray of the skull is necessarily the result of the current injury. In the adult, in particular, any depressed fracture which has smooth contours and which does not have an overlying scalp laceration may be due to previous trauma. Bullets which enter the brain leave a trail of lead fragments which mark the course of the bullet (Fig. 11-2). In some cases, a bullet may only make entrance and exit wounds in the scalp without penetrating the skull. In any severe head injury x-rays of the cervical spine, including odontoid views, are obtained. Chest and abdominal films are also obtained and examined for evidence of pulmonary and visceral damage.

The findings obtained on lumbar puncture have some prognostic value, as the presence of bloody cerebrospinal fluid and high cerebrospinal fluid pressures are positively correlated with serious injuries, as shown by Busch.[9] However, lumbar puncture should not be routinely performed in acute head injuries, as the findings are not pathognomonic for specific pathologic conditions, and may instead be quite misleading. Hematomas, particularly if subacute, can be present without blood being found in the cerebrospinal fluid, and the cerebrospinal fluid pressure can be normal. It should be remembered that the

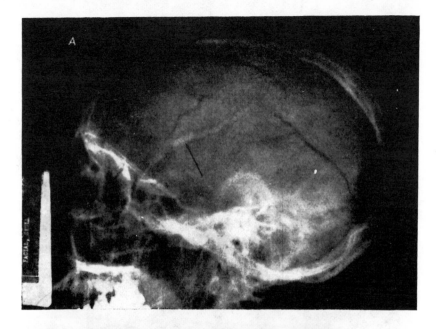

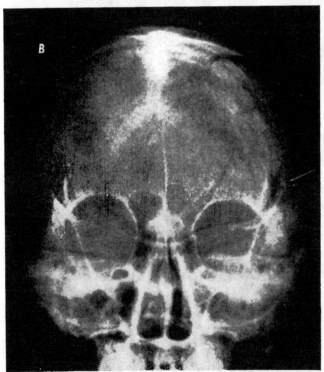

Figure 11-1 Bursting fracture with a depressed fragment. *(A)* Lateral view; area of increased density produced by overlapping of edges of fragment and adjacent bone *(arrow).* (B) Posterioanterior view; the depressed fragment, *(arrow)* was not visualized clearly. *(C)* A view taken tangential to the depression. The site of the depression is visualized *(arrow). (D)* Post-operative lateral view; area of craniectomy required to remove the depressed fragment.

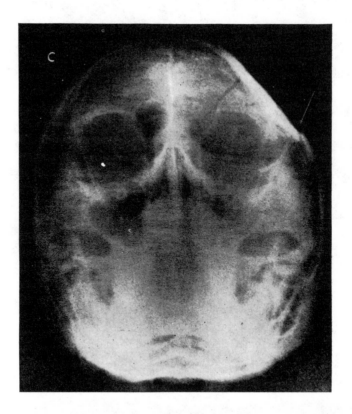

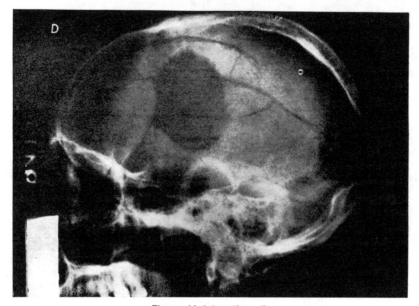

Figure 11-1 (continued)

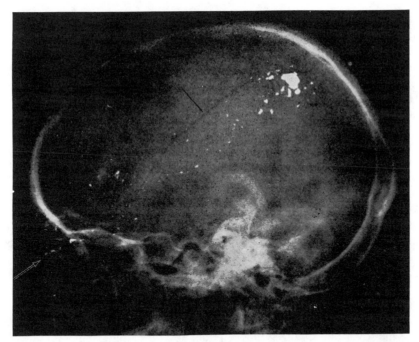

Figure 11-2 Penetrating gunshot wound, small-caliber pistol bullet. Lateral view. Site of entry, left frontal sinus *(arrow)*. Note fragments marking the track of the bullet, and linear skull fracture *(arrow)* due to the bursting effect of the bullet upon entering the skull.

lumbar puncture pressure may not reflect the true intracranial pressure. Significant differential pressure has been demonstrated to be present in man.[44] It has been shown that lumbar puncture in the face of intracranial mass lesion may lead to rapid deterioration and death of the patient. Therefore, lumbar puncture is not a part of the routine care of patients with head trauma.

Intracranial hemorrhages occur following comparatively minor trauma in persons who are receiving anticoagulation therapy or in persons who have disorders of the clotting mechanisms or thrombocytopenia due to blood dyscrasias. If the patient's past medical history suggests such disorders, appropriate studies of the bleeding and clotting mechanisms are carried out and corrective measures taken, if possible, before performing angiography or surgery.

It is generally not practical to obtain an electroencephalographic examination as part of the initial diagnostic studies. However, serial examinations obtained over a period of several days to weeks after an injury can be of diagnostic and prognostic value. As in the case of the neurologic examination, a single electroencephalographic examination is not pathognomonic of the underlying pathology; however, serial electroencephalograms may show progressive changes indicative of the development or resolution of focal brain damage or intracranial hematomas. In coma due to concussion, high voltage and irregular, slow activity in the delta frequency band is seen in tracings taken shortly after the injury. Focal delta activity may also be seen over areas of focal brain damage. The alpha rhythm reappears with progressive return to consciousness. However, asymmetry of the alpha rhythm may be seen, with a lower voltage and a slower frequency over the hemisphere which sustained greater injury. Over epidural or subdural hematomas, either a delta-wave focus or focal reduction in the amplitude of all potentials may be seen.[41]

Ultrasonic echoencephalography is capable of detecting shifts of the midline structures of the brain by means of pulsed ultrasound with an accuracy approaching that of cerebral angiography. Echoencephalography is a useful screening procedure preceding more exact diagnosis of the cause of midline shifts by means of angiography. It is also useful in following the position of the midline after evacuation of mass lesions in patients who are not making a satisfactory recovery and in whom suspicion of recurrence of hematoma exists.[61] Echoencephalography may be misleading if there is significant contusion or swelling of the scalp on one side. Another source of diagnostic error is the presence of matted blood in the hair over one side. Asymmetrically shaped skulls will also give misleading information regarding the midline.

The use of computer axial tomography (CT) has recently entered as a valuable noninvasive diagnostic tool. Because of the precision by which intracranial contents can be surveyed and pathologic processes identified, it is one of the most important tests available to an individual managing patients with serious head trauma. It is possible, by the CT scan, to evaluate serially the progression of cerebral edema and to identify intracranial or intracerebral hematomas. The disadvantages of the test, of course, are its expense and the fact that the restless, uncooperative, obtunded, or combative patient must be put to sleep for a satisfactory CT scan. This means, in essence, that the patient must be managed by anesthesia. Nonetheless, this is an important and significant therapeutic breakthrough.

Cerebral angiography is the test of the greatest value in the diagnosis of intracerebral hematomas in head injuries.[12,38] In view of the problems of differential diagnosis of hemato-

mas, discussed in the preceding section, angiography is done on admission to the hospital in patients with severe focal neurologic deficit. This group of patients is, most commonly, semicomatose or unconscious, with either a hemiparesis or the signs of herniation of the uncal gyrus.

Angiography is usually performed by percutaneous needle techniques. A right retrograde brachial injection is the first procedure. The needle should be introduced into the right brachial artery. Using a pressure injection and a serial x-ray changer, one can demonstrate the posterior fossa and the right cerebral hemisphere. The presence of mass lesions in these areas will be demonstrated. Evidence will be gained pertaining to the left hemisphere, should a shift be demonstrated from left to right. If such be the case, a left percutaneous carotid angiogram should be done. Transfemoral catheter angiography is usually too time-consuming for use in the head-injured patient; however, it is an alternative method.

Serial films should be obtained for study. The presence of shifts in position of intracerebral arteries, veins, and dural venous sinuses are valuable clues to the presence of intracranial hematomas. In bilateral hematomas, or in unilateral chronic subdural hematomas, there may be surprisingly little vascular displacement with little shift of the midline structure; therefore, a unilateral angiogram revealing no shift of vessels cannot be regarded as a definitive study.

In seriously injured patients without lateralizing neurologic signs, the hemisphere contralateral to the side initially injected should be studied by means of either a direct puncture or by the cross-compression technique. Manual compression of the carotid artery contralateral to the carotid already punctured is carried out, and dye is injected. Only an anterior-posterior set of films is taken. The middle and anterior cerebral arteries of both hemispheres are usually filled, via the anterior communicating artery, by this technique, and the positions of these vessels on each side can be compared (Fig. 11-3). In addition to causing a shift of the midline vessels, the acute subdural hematoma of the convexity produces a shift of the middle cerebral vessels away from the hematoma. The angiographic Sylvian point is displaced medially and downward, and the terminal branches of the middle cerebral artery are displaced from their normal position adjacent to the inner table of the skull (Figs. 11-3 and 11-4). The depressed convexity of the hemisphere, which is outlined by the terminal branches of the middle cerebral vessels, retains a normal, convex contour in cases of acute subdural hematoma. The contour becomes concave in cases of chronic hematoma (Fig. 11-4). Epidural hematomas due to bleeding from the middle meningeal vessels produce a shift of the middle cerebral vessels in the Sylvian fissure away from the temporal bone (Fig. 11-5). However, it is not always possible to differentiate between epidural and subdural hematomas by means of angiography.

Figure 11-3 Illustration of cross-compression angiography. Anterioposterior left carotid angiogram performed with manual compression of the contralateral carotid artery, in a patient with an acute subdural hematoma of the right cerebral convexity. On admission the patient exhibited decerebrate posturing without lateralizing signs. Note comparative position of the middle cerebral arteries *(arrow)* with respect to the inner table of the skull *(arrow)* and the shift of the anterior cerebral artery produced by the hematoma *(arrow)*.

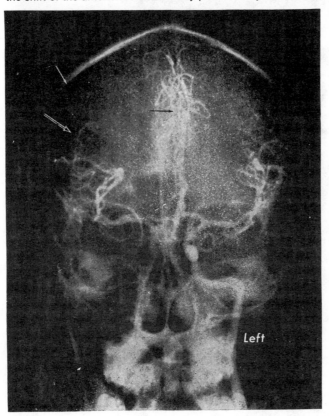

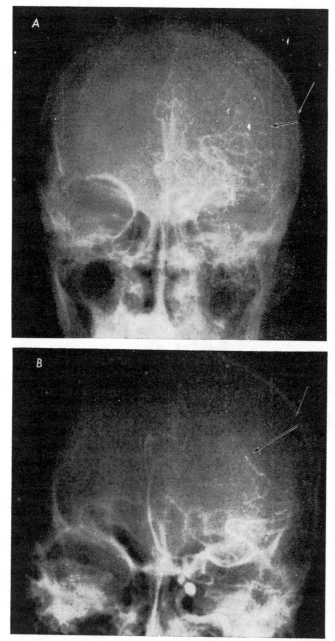

Figure 11-4 Angiographic appearance of acute and chronic subdural hematomas. *(A)* Anterioposterior carotid angiogram in a patient with an acute subdural hematoma. Note convex contour of the depressed cerebral convexity *(arrow)*, which is displaced away from the inner table of the skull *(arrow)*. *(B)* Anterioposterior carotid angiogram in a patient with a chronic subdural hematoma. Note the concave appearance of the depressed hemisphere *(arrow)*.

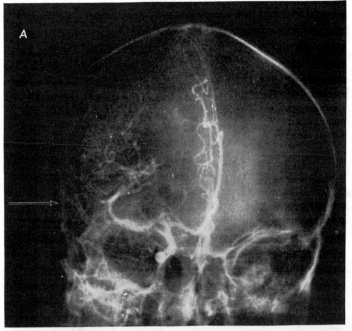

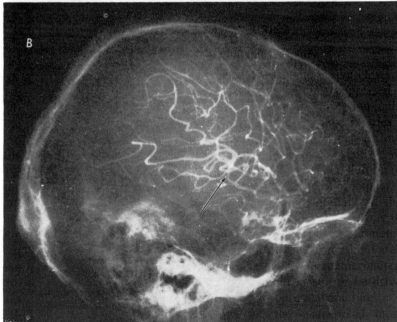

Figure 11-5 Angiographic appearance of an acute epidural hematoma at the pterion. *(A)* Anterioposterior carotid angiogram. Note the medial and upward displacement of the middle cerebral artery away from the temporal bone *(arrow)*. *(B)* Lateral carotid angiogram. Note the upward displacement of the middle cerebral artery *(arrow)*.

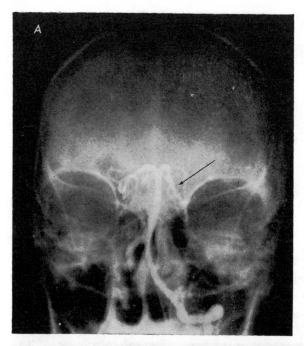

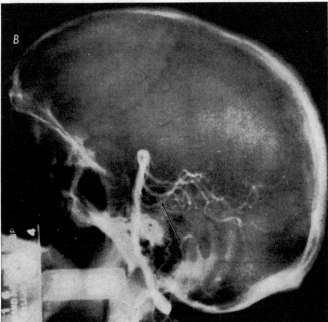

Figure 11-6 Angiographic demonstration of herniation of the uncal gyrus. Vertebral angiograms showing a downward and medial displacement of the posterior cerebral artery *(arrow)* produced by herniation of the uncal gyrus in a patient with an acute subdural hematoma. *(A)* Anterioposterior view. *(B)* Lateral view.

Herniation of the uncal gyrus can be recognized by a downward and medial displacement of the position of the anterior choroidal or posterior cerebral arteries (Fig. 11-6). In some cases of severe head injury, the dye column in the internal carotid artery is arrested at the point where the artery pierces the base of the skull (Fig. 11-7). This stasis appears to result from extremely high intracranial pressure.[59] In our experience, this so-called no-flow syndrome has generally been associated with widespread petechial hemorrhages and massive cerebral edema. Angiography may be repeated after the intravenous administration of hypertonic solutions, which, in some cases, will reduce the intracranial pressure enough to allow arterial filling. No patient demonstrating the no-flow syndrome survived in the Parkland Memorial Hospital experience.

If technical difficulty or the age of the patient prevents the satisfactory performance of cerebral angiography, ventriculography is the procedure of choice. Frontal twist-drill ventriculostomy as described by Kaufmann and Clark is the procedure of choice. Through a small incision in the forehead, a hole is made through the frontal bone and dura by a twist drill. A cannula is passed into the frontal horn of the lateral ventricle. The incision is made 5 cm superior to the nasion and 3 cm lateral to the midline. The twist drill is directed toward the midline at a point 3 cm above the external occipital protuberance. The ventricular needle is then inserted in the same direction. If a soft cannula is used, it may be left in place for measurement, and venting, of the ventricular pressure.[45]

In the case of infants and children up to the age of 1 year, tapping of the subdural space through the fontanelle or a widened coronal

Figure 11-7 Angiographic appearance of non-filling of the intracranial circulation due to increased intracranial pressure. Lateral carotid angiogram. Note arrest of dye column in the carotid artery at the base of the skull *(arrow)* and the filing of the middle meningeal artery *(arrow)* from the external carotid circulation.

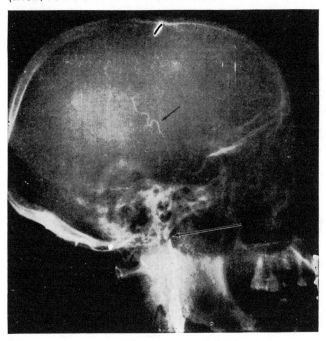

suture should be done. This is performed using a short beveled needle inserted at the lateral edges of the anterior fontanelle tangential to the curve of the skull so that the dura alone is penetrated. Normally, there is no fluid in the subdural space. In the presence of a hematoma lying either in the sub- or epidural spaces, blood will be instantly recovered. All blood which will flow freely from the needle should be removed. The tap should be done bilaterally. Should the taps not find blood, the physician, if still suspicious of increased intracranial pressure, should do a ventricular puncture. Ventricular puncture in very young children and infants is done by inserting a needle at the lateral margin of the anterior fontanelle, aiming in a plane toward that of the pupil of the eye. Normally, the ventricle will be encountered at a depth of approximately 3 to 3 1/2 cm. Ventricular fluid should normally be clear, and not blood-tinged. Venting of the ventricular fluid should result in improvement of the child, if increased intracranial pressure is the problem.

Alternately, if one is concerned about the presence of a mass lesion, an air or positive contrast ventriculogram can be performed. A useful trick is to use 2 mL of Conray mixed with 5 mL of ventricular fluid inserted into the lateral ventricle. A series of anterior-posterior and lateral x-rays are taken, using the angiographic x-ray equipment. This will usually produce adequate films of the entire ventricular system for study.

General Medical Care of the Head-injured Patient

The care of the patient who is in coma or semicoma requires several parameters to be monitored. The first problem is to ensure that no further injury occurs to the already damaged brain. This means that the patient should be carefully watched for evidence of hypoxia or hypercarbia. It also means that the patient should be protected from falling out of bed or

striking the head against a wall or other objects. It requires that the vital signs, intracranial pressure, and neurological status be constantly monitored to be sure that these are not deteriorating. Each of these aspects will be discussed independently, but they are not truly independent of each other. Each will influence the other.

The patient should be protected from injury by the use of mittens. Beds should be equipped with padded side rails. Restraints should be used sparingly. If the patient proves agitated without remedial reason, sedation with chlorpromazine 10 to 25 mg intramuscularly (IM) every 6 h may be used. Paraldehyde, 4 to 8 mL IM every 6 h, is an alternate medication. Restlessness of an increasing nature may represent either air hunger and/or increasing intracranial pressure. Sedation of such a patient is not the correct approach.

Of utmost importance is the maintenance of pulmonary support in the head-injured patient. It has been demonstrated repeatedly that a decreased level of consciousness produces changes in pulmonary ventilation. These changes include both rate and volume. One aspect of these changes is the loss of the voluntary sigh during the respiratory cycle. This loss means that areas of lung will not be aerated and will collapse with microatelectasis and venous shunting. As a result, such a venous admixture produces hypercarbia, initially, and ultimately systemic hypoxia as well. Prevention requires monitoring of the arterial blood gases, with maintenance of the Pa_{O_2} and Pa_{CO_2} and arterial pH within normal ranges. An indwelling arterial line is preferable to repetitive punctures. The radial artery is the most frequent site for sampling.

For correction of respiratory problems, a volume ventilator is best. Appropriate supplemental oxygen via the intratracheal tube is administered in proper concentration. Sighing is done to ensure overinflation of the lung periodically. Such respiratory assistance should be available in all units treating head-injured patients.

Patients who have known or suspected pulmonary dysfunction certainly should be treated in this manner. Patients with emphysema or patients with chronic obstructive bronchopulmonary disease are better managed by controlled-volume regulated respiratory therapy, rather than allowing them to breathe spontaneously on their own.

Certain specific problems arise in the management of patients with head injuries. Among these are the development of seizures. Focal seizures may be the harbinger of an intracranial hematoma. Investigations to rule out a hematoma are necessary.

It is generally considered that generalized seizures are not so frequently associated with intracranial mass lesions. Control of seizures developing post head trauma should initially be by administration of 5 to 10 mg of diazepam intravenously. This can be repeated several times. If seizures continue, phenobarbital, 100 mg intravenously in 1 to 10 min, should be given. Phenobarbital may be repeated to dose levels of 500 to 700 mg in an adult without producing respiratory suppression. It is rarely necessary to use the shorter-acting barbiturates to control seizures and head injury. Diphenylhydantoin should be administered concomitantly with these other drugs. This should be given in doses of 600 to 800 mg per rectum, or in doses of 100 to 300 mg intravenously. Intravenous administration should be slow and carefully monitored by ECG, as arrhythmias and cardiac standstill have occurred during intravenous administration. Intramuscular administration of diphenylhydantoin is contraindicated as it produces a myopathy and an ineffective blood level. Anticonvulsants should be given routinely to all patients with penetrating brain wounds, whether they have had seizures or not. The incidence of posttraumatic seizures in this group of patients[84] is high, and protection

from seizures is indicated. Diphenylhydantoin and phenobarbital should be given parenterally during the period of unconsciousness, and shifted to oral use as the patient clears. It is usually not necessary to give anticonvulsants to patients with closed head injuries. An exception to this rule is an individual with early onset of seizures after a closed head injury.[42]

When there is significant evidence of profound injury to the brain, but without a mass lesion, it is useful to monitor the intracranial pressure (ICP). There are a variety of devices available to do this.

A variety of epidural, subdural, subarachnoid, and intraventricular monitors have been developed in the past few years. This represents the general acknowledgment of the importance of monitoring intracranial pressure in patients who have sustained a significant or serious head injury. Each of these devices has several advantages, and each several disadvantages. The use of an epidural pressure monitor raises the problem of how adequately it reflects the true situation in the intracranial contents, as the dura represents a significant dampening barrier to the transmittal of pressure. All of the devices utilized require a surgical procedure to insert them, and many require a surgical procedure to remove them. They are costly; therefore, it has continued to be our policy for routine measurements of intracranial pressure to use an indwelling ventricular catheter as described elsewhere. The simplest way, however, is to use a catheter placed in the right lateral ventricle through a frontal twist-drill ventriculostomy.[45] This may be connected to a transducer for closed-system pressure recordings, or even to open-fluid-coupled-system for short periods of time.

If a patient develops increased intracranial pressure, several things must be done. An arterial sample for gas determination is drawn, steps to rule out a mass lesion by CT scan or angiogram begun, and a small quantity of ventricular fluid removed, if possible. Any deviation of the blood gases from normal must be corrected.

If this fails to correct the problem and no mass lesion exists, 100 g of mannitol is given intravenously. Furosemide 40 mg may be given as well.

The use of hypertonic solution and diuretics may be continued for several doses or even several days. An electrolyte disturbance may develop, and serial serum electrolyte and urea nitrogen levels should be obtained. If an imbalance occurs, it should be corrected by the usual means. If furosemide is used for a protracted period of time, supplemental potassium, 40 mg/24 h, is indicated.

Corticosteroids have been found to be effective in reducing cerebral edema following ischemic and surgical trauma to the brain.[4,72] The effectiveness of corticosteroids in lowering intracranial pressure in patients with head injuries has not yet been definitely established. However, reduced mortality and morbidity have been reported following the use of corticosteroids, particularly in cases of diffuse brain damage.[79] Corticosteroids are administered parenterally in initial doses of 200 to 300 mg/day for cortisone acetate or hydrocortisone, in doses of 40 mg/day for methylprednisolone, or in doses of 10 to 60 mg/day for dexamethasone. The dosage is then reduced over a period of 5 to 7 days, and then discontinued. Corticosteroids may be beneficial in the treatment of head injury because of the involvement of the hypothalamic pituitary axis in the head injury. The data regarding the effectiveness of corticosteroids in the management of traumatic cerebral edema is confusing.

If these measures fail, the patient should be paralyzed with tubocurarine or decamethonium. Respiration should be by a volume ventilator. Again, constant monitoring of Pa_{CO_2} and Pa_{O_2} should be carried out. An attempt at hyperventilation, reducing the Pa_{CO_2} to 25 torr, should be tried. If there is a mass lesion in an area of the brain, surgical decompression should be undertaken. In the absence of an actual hematoma, the most common circumstance in which this occurs is the bruised, swollen temporal lobe syndrome described by McLaurin. Craniotomy with excision of the pulped, necrotic brain may be the only method of controlling the patient's intracranial pressure.

Bony decompressions in the face of massive cerebral swelling have been tried on a number of occasions. They have usually proven to be failures. However, in desperate situations, a hemicraniectomy has proved lifesaving.

Experience gained at Parkland Memorial Hospital indicates that ICP monitoring is rarely necessary for more than 3 to 4 days post injury. Infections have not been a problem. Less than 1 percent of patients have an infection. No antibiotics are given prophylactically.

The comatose patient should have nothing given by mouth. A nasogastric tube with suction should be used to keep the stomach empty. This will reduce the possibility of aspiration pneumonitis. The endotracheal tube or the tracheostomy tube should be cuffed. This will assist in ventilatory management and in the prevention of aspiration, should vomiting or regurgitation occur. The patient should be turned frequently to prevent the development of pressure sores in bed.

Cerebrospinal fluid rhinorrhea or otorrhea usually stops spontaneously within two to three days. Treatment of patients with this complication should include an upright position in bed. Drainage should not be impeded by the placing of cotton plugs in the nares or the external ear. The patient should be cautioned against coughing, sneezing, straining, or blowing the nose. Daily lumbar puncture may aid in cessation by reducing the pressure. Most importantly, the early, accurate reduction of midface fractures is beneficial. Prompt cessation of cerebrospinal rhinorrhea has occurred in virtually all patients treated on the Parkland Hospital service by this means. Prophylactic antibiotics are not used in patients with spinal fluid leak.

Indwelling bladder catheters should be removed as soon as possible, or replaced with a condom catheter in the male patient. If the bowels are not evacuated regularly without straining, enemas should be given.

The cornea of the comatose patient or of the patient with facial nerve palsy should be observed for drying and inflammation, and methylcellulose eyedrops should be instilled daily.

Intravenous fluid therapy should be directed to replacing daily losses without producing overhydration and intensifying cerebral edema. In most cases, this can be accomplished by the administration of not more than 2500 mL of fluid. In addition, about 75 meq of sodium is also required daily and, after bodily stores are depleted, about 30 meq of potassium. Sodium chloride administered intravenously penetrates the brain slowly, and isotonic salt solution produces less rise in intracranial pressure than does the administration of 5% glucose and water.[25] However, the use of isotonic salt solution to make up the total fluid requirement would lead to hypernatremia. The best compromise between fluid and electrolyte needs is the administration of 500 mL of 5% glucose and water, 500 mL of 5% glucose and isotonic saline, and 500 mL of 5% glucose and water, with each 500 mL being given over an 8-h period.[13,67] Alternately, larger amounts of one-half or one-quarter normal saline can be used in making up the total daily fluid requirements.

The urinary output and specific gravity are measured every 2 h, and serum electrolyte and blood urea nitrogen (BUN) determinations are obtained hourly.

Patients can be maintained on intravenous fluid therapy for about 5 to 7 days, but toward the end of this period, considerable loss of body mass occurs. If the patient has not regained the ability to eat by this time, provision must be made for adequate caloric and protein intake via the alimentary canal. If a nasogastric tube is used, it must be thin and flexible. Complications of the use of nasogastric tubes are gastric reflux and aspiration pneumonia.

Hyperalimentation through a subclavian or superior vena cava indwelling catheter has been used in patients in head-injury coma. This has proved to be superior to the use of feeding enterostomies. Our current practice is to employ this method prior to going to the more complicated feeding-enterostomy procedures. Hyperalimentation can be carried on for several weeks, with adequate installation of calories, amino acids, essential fatty acids, vitamins, and other minerals necessary to improve nutritional state. The use of a hyperalimentation regime carries the risk of producing hyperosmolar coma, unless adequate free water is given concomitantly with the very concentrated hyperalimentation feedings. The other problems encountered with it include those to be expected from having a long-term indwelling venous catheter present. Despite its disadvantages, it is used as an intermediate step between nasogastric feedings and the performance of the feeding enterostomy on the Parkland Memorial Hospital service.

Should any of the laboratory determinations show any abnormality in serum electrolytes or BUN, serum and urinary osmolarities should be obtained. The presence of a rising serum sodium, a rising urinary output, and a rising serum osmolarity with a falling urinary osmolarity indicate the presence of diabetes insipidus. This is secondary to direct damage to the hypothalamus or to the neural hypophysis. Damages to these structures may be anticipated in patients with extensive basilar skull fractures.

When diabetes insipidus occurs, maintenance of adequate water intake is mandatory. Restoration of the serum sodium levels to normal should be accomplished by giving the appropriate determined amount of free water as a 5% dextrose in water IV, or by allowing the patient to drink water freely. If the patient is conscious and rational, with a urinary output less than 10 L/day, the patient can usually manage by oral intake. If it is in excess of this, or if an altered level of consciousness is present, this fluid replacement must be by intravenous route.

Diabetes insipidus follows a number of courses during its natural history. It is not always permanent. It may disappear in a matter of 72 h; however, it may return after a passage of 4 or 5 days. This is the so-called biphasic form. It may remain permanent; or it may simply lessen in degree, so that the individual secretes only 5 to 6 L/day of a rather fixed–specific gravity urine.

The opposing situation, i.e., a rising urinary osmolarity or falling serum sodium, occurs in the syndrome of inappropriate antidiuretic hormone secretion. This is a common complication of head injury, and if looked for, it will be found in a significant number of cases. Usually, it presents no serious problem to the patient, unless the serum sodium falls below 125 meq/L. When this happens, the patient becomes drowsy, somnolent, and confused.

The appropriate treatment is water restriction, with the administration of intravenous electrolyte solutions. If the serum sodium is determined to be extremely low or at dangerous levels, such as 110 meq/L, 3% hypertonic saline intravenously to restore serum sodium levels should be used. One-half of the calculated sodium deficit should be given in the first 12 h. Then, the serum sodium level is measured, and again the serum sodium deficit calculated. One-half of this calculated deficit should then be given over the next 12 h. Water restriction, of course, accompanies the administration of hypertonic saline. The administration of hypertonic saline does not correct the situation, as the sodium is lost in the urine.

Normally, the syndrome of inappropriate ADH secretion reverses itself within a matter of a few days; however, in our series it has persisted for many weeks.

Surgical Treatment

General Principles   Patients with head injuries associated with serious injuries of the chest, abdomen, and extremities require initial treatment of the injury which is most threatening to life. Simultaneous intracranial and visceral or extremity surgery can be performed when required. The presence of a closed head injury with diffuse parenchymatous damage is not a contraindication to performing any required general surgical procedure.[14]

All intracranial surgery for head trauma is carried out under general anesthesia. This ensures more satisfactory control of the patient's airway and behavior on the operation table than is possible by using local anesthesia. Premedication for surgery consists of only the administration of 0.3 to 0.6 mg of atropine. Typing and cross matching for at least 1000 mL of whole blood is performed. Attention should be paid at all times to the amount of blood loss during surgery, as many patients, despite a normal blood pressure, are already hypovolemic from associated injuries. Probably the most common cause of death during the course of intracranial surgery for trauma is sudden blood loss from cranial vessels in a patient already hypovolemic, resulting in shock, anoxia, and cardiac arrest.

Penetrating Wounds   *Indications for Surgery*   Open wounds are debrided and closed primarily as soon as possible after the time of injury. Fractures that are depressed more than 3 mm are elevated. The exceptions to this rule are very small indentations situated over major dural venous sinuses. Although some surgeons have advocated not elevating small, closed, depressed fractures that are not over the motor area,[11] or not elevating closed, depressed fractures as an elective procedure in general, all depressed fractures should be elevated promptly. Delay may result in considerable edema and venous congestion in a brain compressed by bone fragments.

Surgical Techniques Proper positioning of the patient on the operating table aids in the control of venous bleeding. Patients with penetrating wounds near the middle of the skull and sagittal sinus are placed in a semisitting position. The scalp is completely shaved. The operative field, including the scalp lacerations, is scrubbed 10 min, and the wound is copiously irrigated with saline solution. The soiled edges of scalp lacerations and the underlying pericranium are excised. It must then be determined whether to approach the underlying skull and brain damage through the wound or by means of a scalp flap placed to surround the area of injury. In general, if the underlying damage is extensive and the scalp laceration is small, it is preferable to make a scalp flap rather than to extend the laceration. A scalp flap provides wider exposure and better primary healing, and it facilitates cranioplasty. This is important in injuries of the forehead when extension of a laceration may produce a disfiguring scar.

In treating depressed fractures and underlying brain damage, debridement is carried out centripetally, from normal pericranium, bone, dura, and brain into the area of damage. Although large en bloc resection of damaged areas of the skull and brain has been advocated in war injuries to prevent infection,[30] in civilian practice removal of the depressed fragments and necrotic brain will suffice. This produces a smaller skull defect to be covered by subsequent cranioplasty.

The initial step in the elevation of depressed fragments is the placement of a burr hole adjacent to the perimeter of the fracture. The fragments may then be levered into place by an instrument introduced through the burr hole. However, the fragments are usually depressed under the edges of the intact skull and must be removed by ronguering centripetally from the burr hole. Fragments may be removed, cleansed, and repositioned in place as a cranioplasty at the time of the initial procedure. This may be done even though there is gross contamination of the fragments.[58] Surgical judgment regarding replacement of fragments must be exercised, and one should always err on the side of removing a potentially contaminated fragment. In general, all depressed fragments are removed. If the fracture involves a large portion of the orbital rim, however, it is wired back into place rather than removed because of the difficulty of reconstructing the brow area at the time of cranioplasty. If the dura is intact under the depressed area, it is opened and the brain is inspected for bleeding vessels. Fragments driven into the brain over the Sylvian vessels or the dural venous sinuses are not removed until a sufficient area of dura adjacent to them has been exposed. There must be adequate exposure to control massive bleeding from these vessels, which may occur when the bone fragments are removed. Bleeding from major vessels is controlled with silver clips. Bleeding from torn dural sinuses is controlled by inserting the tip of a plug of temporalis muscle into the laceration of the sinus and suturing the muscle down to the adjacent dura.

If the air sinuses of the skull are damaged by depressed fractures, they are unroofed and the depressed fragments removed. The mucous membrane lining the sinus is stripped down and out through the ostium of the sinus. A plug of muscle or Gelfoam is placed in the ostium. This exenteration of the sinus prevents the development of infection or of a mucocele.

Debridement of the injured brain is performed by removing necrotic brain with a No. 7 French suction tip. However, en bloc resection of frontal bone may be done with pulping of the frontal lobe or, in very severe damage to the occipital pole or tip of the temporal lobe. Bullet entry and exit wounds are widely debrided in centripetal manner, as many fragments of lead and bone are scattered around them. The damaged edges of the dura are excised. The bullet tract is then followed into the brain, with the aid of a retractor and suction, and necrotic brain and foreign bodies are removed. When the tract has been debrided to the maximum depth possible, it is inspected for several minutes for bleeding or closing of the tract. A closing tract suggests the presence of an undrained hematoma deeper along the course of the injury, and therefore, the tract should be explored further. It is often impossible to debride a bullet tract to the depth required to remove the missile, as many bullets enter frontally and lodge occipitally. In these cases, the bullet is left in situ if it appears the considerable brain damage will result from attempts to locate and remove it. The position of the bullet is checked by serial radiographs, as it may undergo migration. However, if the bullet lies near the cortical surface, particularly if it is near major vessels, it may have to be removed by a second craniotomy, as there may be intracerebral hematoma formation around it sufficient to lead to the patient's death. Retained small bullet fragments appear to lead to abscess formation only rarely.

The dura is closed in a watertight manner in all penetrating brain injuries in order to prevent infection and the development of brain herniation through the dural opening.[47] The dural defect resulting from the debridement of the lacerated edges of the dura is repaired with a graft of pericranium taken from an adjacent area or with temporalis or occipitalis muscle fascia. It is better to use a pedicled pericranial graft to sew in place to patch the dura. This ensures blood supply to the graft and thus does not contribute to leaving dead and devitalized tissue in the wound. Adequate pericranial tissue or temporalis fascia is usually avail-

able for such flaps. Care should be exercised in initial exposure of such compound wounds to preserve pericranium for this use. If the defect to be covered is larger than the available pericranial or fascial graft, a fascia lata graft is taken from the thigh.

Drainage of the subgaleal and epidural space is done by an implanted Hemovac device. This has proven effective in reducing the amount of hematoma collection in these sites. The device is placed through a stab wound made at a distance from the incisional site. The drains are usually removed about 24 h post surgery.

The scalp flap or the debrided laceration is closed in a single layer with interrupted 32-gauge stainless steel wire, if the wound can be closed with tension. Even though nonabsorbable buried sutures may provide a nidus for infection, it is important to place sutures in the galea if there is any tension in closing the scalp, or healing of the skin edges will be impaired. The minimum number of 3-0 silk sutures necessary to juxtapose the skin edges without tension are placed in the galea, and the skin is then closed with wire. Almost all scalp lacerations can be closed without tension by mobilizing the adjacent scalp by wide undermining between the galea and pericranium and by making the laceration the central segment of a large S-shaped incision and sliding the flaps thus formed. Even with severe loss of scalp substance, the underlying area of damage should always be covered by closing scalp over it. In these cases, the scalp can be mobilized for closure by making large rotational and sliding flaps and then covering the donor sites with skin grafts.

Intracerebral Hematomas *Indications for Surgery* The presence of an intracranial hematoma is an absolute indication for evacuation as soon as is possible.

Surgical Techniques Acute subdural hematomas are those which form within the first 24 h after injury. This mass of blood is usually clotted, and it is impossible to remove this by means of conventional evacuation. There is usually obstruction to venous drainage together with some change in cerebral autoregulation, so massive cerebral edema is usually present under the acute subdural hemorrhage. Evacuation through a burr hole or through small craniectomies usually results in herniation of brain tissue through the cranial openings, with extrusion of edematous and necrotic brain into the operative field or under the galea when the wound is closed. The prognosis of patients treated with burr-hole evacuation of acute subdural hematomas is rather grim. There is between a 70 and 80 percent mortality rate in this group.[57,34] This mortality rate led several investigators to consider a more massive cranial decompression as the treatment for acute subdural hemorrhage.[51, 46,71] The patient who is known or suspected to have an acute subdural hemorrhage is given an osmotic diuretic and furosemide 40 mg intravenously while the operating room is being prepared. With the endotracheal tube in position, the patient is taken to the operating theater, where the head is rapidly prepared to be draped. A linear incision beginning at the nasion and extending back to external occipital protuberance and slightly toward the appropriate mastoid process is made. This is carried down to bone on one layer. This massive, full thickness scalp flap is then reflected, the entire hemicranium is exposed, and a series of perforator holes using the air-driven craniotome are placed. These are usually just to the side of the superior longitudinal sinus and down deep into the temporal fossa. They are connected by the use of the craniotome, and the entire hemicranium is removed. The dura is opened widely and quickly, hinging it along the mesial side at the superior sagittal sinus. The clot is removed, the brain is thoroughly cleansed with irrigating solution, the sphenoid wing is removed using the air-driven drill, and the bone plate is denuded of the pericranium. The dura is then closed, using the entire pericranium flap. The pericranium is sewn to the dura so that a large, floppy pouch is created. The skin is then closed in one layer with nonabsorbable, impervious suture material. The bone flap is saved, placed in triple antibiotic solution, and put in the deep freeze. If the patient survives and has a good functional survival, the bone flap is replaced within 60 to 90 days. In the series quoted,[46,71] the survival has been increased from around 10 percent to 40 to 60 percent by this technique. More importantly, useful survival has been accomplished.

Chronic subdural hematomas are evacuated through three burr holes placed on the side of the hematoma. One burr hole is placed over the contralateral hemisphere if a contralateral hematoma has not been ruled out by bilateral angiography. The patient is positioned in a semisitting position, with the suboccipital area supported by a small headrest to facilitate bilateral trephinations and control of bleeding from veins near the sagittal sinus. The sites of trephination are (1) 3 to 4 cm from the midline anterior to the coronal suture, (2) over the parietal prominence anterior to the lambdoidal suture, and (3) over the pterion. Vertical scalp incisions can be connected to make a scalp flap based on the temporal area, if a parietal bone flap is necessary in order to evacuate a clotted hematoma or to control bleeding.

The majority of subdural hematomas can be removed by passing No. 10 French soft rubber catheters between the burr holes and irrigating with saline solution. If the brain does not re-expand, there may be a retained clot. Conversely, a clot retained subfrontally or beneath the temporal lobe may cause herniation of the brain through the convex burr holes. Other causes of herniation of the brain are associated intracerebral hematomas and cerebral edema due to anoxia and impaired venous damage from the brain.[36] Examination of the position of the endotracheal tube by the anesthetist and hyperventilation using a negative-pressure phase aid in the control of edema due to anoxia and high intrathoracic venous pressure.[35] This facilitates the removal of retained hematomas.

After evacuation of a subdural hematoma, a silver clip is placed on the pia-arachnoid beneath one of the burr holes, and another on the dural edge adjacent to it. Separation of the clips found on postoperative x-rays suggests reaccumulation of the hematoma. Soft rubber drains are placed in two of the burr holes and are removed after 24 h.

Epidural hematomas due to hemorrhage from the middle meningeal artery are evacuated through a subtemporal craniectomy. The middle meningeal artery is identified and cauterized. If the artery is torn in its course along the floor of the middle fossa, it is necessary to occlude it at the foramen spinosum. The middle meningeal artery has an anomalous point of entry in the skull, in some cases at points in the middle fossa other than the foramen spinosum. Epidural hematomas of the convexity, of venous origin, can be evacuated by irrigating through frontal and parietal burr holes. Large epidural hematomas of the convexity which are found to be clotted must be removed through an osteoplastic bone flap made by connecting the frontal and parietal holes with a saw cut and placing additional burr holes as needed.

Extradural hematoma is not nearly so lethal, assuming prompt recognition and surgery. A mortality rate of 15 to 25 percent is usual, but it may go as high as 40 percent.[27,39] This difference occurs if a number of patients are operated on after profound coma or irreversible brainstem signs appear.

Intracerebral hematomas are approached surgically by a small craniotomy or a trephine opening placed over the location of the hematoma. Cerebral angiography is helpful in this localization. The intracerebral hematoma is identified by passing a brain cannula into it through the cortex. A transcortical incision is made, and the hematoma evacuated. The cavity should be thoroughly inspected for bleeding points. The dura is closed, the bone flap replaced, and the wound closed in a routine fashion. Intracerebral hematomas have a mortality of about 25 percent. This is a function of the severity of the injury which produced the hematoma and the time at which the hematoma is detected and removed.[40]

Another mass lesion occurring after head trauma with a rather characteristic pattern is that of swelling of a contused temporal lobe. Typically, the patient has been struck on the occiput or on the side of the head. Skull fracture may or may not be present. Between 48 and 72 h after injury, the patient begins to deteriorate. The level of consciousness begins to slip, and signs of impending uncal herniation, i.e., a progressively stiffer neck, mild ptosis of the ipsilateral eye, and hemiparesis, develop. Angiography discloses elevation of the middle cerebral complex and a shift of the midline structures away from the swollen temporal lobe. Treatment for this condition involves an anterior temporal lobe resection of all the pulped brain. This is usually done through a small temporal craniectomy.[54]

Postoperative Complications Postoperative skull films are routinely taken when the scalp sutures are removed, 3 to 5 days after surgery. The films are studied for evidence of retained bone fragments and foreign bodies, for shifts of normal calcifications and silver clip markers, and for the presence and position of air in the ventricles or over the hemispheres. Abnormal findings may indicate the reaccumulation of intracerebral hematomas or the development of intracranial infections.

Reaccumulation or formation of new intracranial hematomas is the most important surgical complication underlying the failure of a patient to improve postoperatively. Reaccumulation of subdural hematomas is most likely to occur in elderly patients who have had some cortical atrophy prior to the injury.

Cerebrospinal fluid pressures which remain elevated or increase to the level of 350 to 400 mm of cerebrospinal fluid are suggestive of intracranial hematomas. In patients who fail to improve in 3 to 5 days after surgery, or who deteriorate at any time after surgery, cerebral angiography is carried out. Posttraumatic occlusion of intracerebral arteries may also be revealed in this manner.

Early recognition of wound infections and meningitis is made by daily inspection of the wound and by the prompt examination of the cerebrospinal fluid in patients with fever, confusion, and signs of meningeal irritation. It is not uncommon to see meningeal irritation 3 to 5 days after a head injury in which there has been some subarachnoid hemorrhage. The spinal fluid in these cases usually shows an elevated white cell count, with a mixture of polymorphonuclear and mononuclear cells, in addition to many red cells. The glucose content, however, is normal or at the lower limit of the normal range. It may be impossible to differentiate between this type of meningeal reaction and an early stage of meningitis. Daily spinal fluid examinations, including smear and gram stain, culture of the fluid, and neurologic examination, yield the information required for deciding whether antibiotic therapy for meningitis should be started.

The common organisms found in wound infections after surgical debridement of penetrating head wounds are coagulose-positive staphylococcus and gram-negative enterobacilli. Prophylactic use of antibiotics has proven ineffectual in the prevention of these infections. The important aspect is adequate debridement of the wound. If an infection develops, the treatment includes the intravenous administration of methacillin in the dose of 1 g every 4 to 6 h combined with amphicillin in the same dose. If no response occurs prior to the identification of the responsible organism, the addition of chloramphenicol, 2 g every 6 h, is recommended. When the organism is identified, specific therapy is given. It is important to treat meningitis with high doses of antibiotics for at least 7 to 10 days, or longer, depending on the spinal fluid studies.[75]

A brief discussion of all the postoperative complications of head injuries is important. These complications include: posttraumatic epilepsy, osteomyelitis of the skull, leptomeningeal cysts (growing fractures of childhood), porencephalic cysts, ventricular dilation, obstructive hydrocephalus, pneumocephalus, subdural hygroma, traumatic occlusion of the internal carotid artery in the neck (usually at the level of the second cervical vertebra), traumatic occlusion of the middle cerebral artery, aneurysm of the middle meningeal artery, and carotid-cavernous fistula.

Posttraumatic epilepsy occurs in approximately 50 percent of all patients with penetrating wounds of the brain. The use of anticonvulsants has been a subject of investigation and of controversy for some years. It is possible that the only function of the administration of anticonvulsants to such patients is the pretreatment of patients who would otherwise develop posttraumatic epilepsy. Patients with severe closed head injuries are similarly placed at risk of posttraumatic epilepsy. The presence of early seizures in this group of patients is an ominous sign of continuance of their seizure disorder. Patients who have had a seizure in the posttraumatic phase should be considered as having posttraumatic epilepsy, and treated accordingly. Standard doses of anticonvulsants, such as Dilantin 100 mg 3 times a day, and phenobarbital 15 mg 3 to 4 times a day, is adequate in most cases. The patient should not be withdrawn from anticonvulsant medication until at least a 2-year seizure-free period has been obtained. Withdrawal should occur over the next year. The development of a seizure should warn the physician to place the patient on anticonvulsant medication permanently.

Osteomyelitis of the skull following head

injury occurs rarely. It is relatively easily identified by the presence of puffy, tender, fluctuant areas in the region of an old fracture site or penetrating wound. Treatment is surgical incision and debridement, with removal of all infected bone. Cranioplasty, if necessary, should be delayed for at least 1 year.

Leptomeningeal cysts, or growing fractures of childhood, are a complication which leads to underlying brain atrophy and seizures. All children who have sustained a skull fracture should have a second set of skull x-rays done at approximately 3 to 4 months after the injury to see if the fracture is enlarging in size. If so, surgical removal of fracture edges to reach the dural edges, and closure of the defect and primary cranioplasty should be carried out.

Poroencephalic cysts arising from ventricular dilatation in the case of overlying brain atrophy is a complication of head trauma. Surgical therapy is rarely necessary.

Communicating hydrocephalous occurs after head trauma when there have been large amounts of subarachnoid blood as a result of the trauma. Patients with this syndrome complain of increasing headache and become progressively drowsy, confused, and disoriented. A CT scan will make the diagnosis easily. If the patient is symptomatic, a ventriculoperitoneal shunt is the procedure of choice.

Patients after head injury, particularly those with fractures to the base part of the skull, may develop signs and symptoms of a carotid-cavernous sinus fistula. The patient may complain of a noise in the head. Auscultation over the eye will reveal a bruit synchronous with the pulse. The patient may develop chemosis, with injection and redness of the eye, proptosis of the eye, and paralysis of the extra ocular muscles. If truly progressive, the patient's vision is at risk because of the development of closed-angle glaucoma, protrusion of the eye, chemosis, and ulceration of the cornea, leading to perforation, infection, and loss of the eye. Treatment of this condition has proven difficult, but the current methods offer substantial improvement over those of the past. These include embolization of the fistula with a muscle or by occlusion with a Fogarty catheter.

Injury to one or more cranial nerves is not uncommon following head trauma. The olfactory tracts may be avulsed from the cribriform plate at the time of impact. Patients who have sustained this injury complain of the change in the taste of food. Evaluation of the function of the olfactory nerve will disclose the nature of their trouble. Unfortunately, there is no therapy for this injury.

Because of the wide distribution of the visual apparatus through the central nervous system, it is not infrequently damaged. The dangers range from traumatic amaurosis with division of one optic nerve to injuries to the chiasm, to the optic tract, to the optic radiations, and to the occipital cortex itself. Patients who sustain significant head trauma may show forms of homonymous field defects. These usually resolve or improve in time; however, a damaged optic nerve, chiasm, or tract is likely to be permanent.

Injury to the seventh cranial nerve occurs in the fractures of the temporal bone. Injuries to the auditory apparatus may also occur in the temporal bone fracture. These were discussed elsewhere. Damage to the lower cranial nerves is quite rare. Bilateral damage to the ninth nerve occurs in transverse fractures of the clivus.

Prognosis in head injury is a function of many variables. The severity of the trauma, the area of the brain injured, the age of the individual, complications which have arisen in the course of management of the patient, all influence the course and prognosis of a patient with head injury. As a rule of thumb, the longer the period of unconsciousness, the worse the prognosis for recovery of higher intellectual functions. The presence of focal neurologic deficit follows a similar rule: the more dense the deficit and the longer its persistence in the immediate posttrauma phase, the less likely is an eventual complete recovery. The older the individual is, clearly, the worse the prognosis. A child has a better prognosis from a given injury than an adult. A principal point to remember is that, although the patient may appear normal to the examining physician, when placed in conditions of stress or even when attempting to function in a routine environment, the patient may not be able to cope. This may, in time, produce further apparent deterioration. The physician should be extremely cautious in returning individuals after head injury to their normal occupations too soon. This merely produces frustration in patients and their employers. At times, such haste in returning a patient to gainful occupation results in premature termination of employment, whereas a longer period of waiting would have resulted in successful reemployment of the individual.

SPINAL CORD INJURIES

The human spinal cord is well protected. Injury to the spinal cord results from a variety of causes, but the end result is the same: severe neurologic deficit. Injury to the spinal cord occurs most frequently in males, and often during the most productive years. The cost of taking care of a paraplegic patient is high, and many patients may be made unemployable by this injury. Certain select organizations, such as the Veterans Administration, have done a superb job in training the paraplegic for useful lives. However, most patients sustaining a spinal cord injury in civilian life are unable to support themselves.

From Parkland Memorial Hospital, in the original edition, 102 patients were reported as having been treated for acute spinal cord injury. Of this group, 82 were men and 56 were between 20 and 50 years of age. The series of overall mortality was 30 percent.

Two factors markedly influenced the mortality rate: the level of spinal cord injury and the age of the patient. If the cord was totally transected above the fourth cervical level, the mortality was 50 percent within the first 30 days. In contrast, 3 out of 16 patients died within 30 days after an injury at the fifth cervical level, a mortality of 19 percent. The major reason for this disparity is that the major muscles of respiration are paralyzed by injuries above the fifth cervical level.

Age also contributes to the survival of the patient. In the seventh decade, the mortality, regardless of level of injury, was 50 percent; in the eighth decade, 100 percent. There seemed to be little difference between open and closed wounds as to mortality. The rates were 21 and 17 percent, respectively. The slightly higher figure for compound wounds represents the complicating factor of associated injuries occurring with missile wounds.

In the decade that followed the acquisition of those figures, the number of cases (102 patients from 1955 to 1965) had risen to 300 patients. Little change occurred in the distribution of cases between male and female; it remained a disease of young males. The incidence of cervical injuries rose because of the greater use of motorcycles and of higher-speed automobile accidents. This factor tended to increase the mortality slightly overall.

Mechanisms of Injury

The spinal cord may be injured either by direct penetrating wounds or by violent displacement of the component parts of the spinal column. Bullet or missile wounds of the spinal cord may produce injury by directly striking it, producing laceration and contusion of the cord. Alternately, a bullet may strike the bony spine and produce spinal cord injury by transmitted energy. Usually, however, the bullet by striking the vertebra, produces secondary missiles composed of fragments of bone. These splintered bits of the vertebra are driven into the canal and lacerate the spinal cord or nerve roots over a wide area.

Stab wounds may lacerate the cord if the knife has slipped between the lamina into the cord. This injury usually produces a hemisection of the spinal cord with the classic Brown-Séquard neurologic syndrome. Occasionally, a complete transection may occur. A less common injury produced by knife wounds is compression of the cord by a fragment of lamina. The knife may strike the lamina with sufficient force to fracture it. The free fragment of lamina may then be pushed anteriorly and compress the spinal cord.

In closed injuries of the spinal cord, the anatomic structure striking the cord may be vertebral body, lamina, pedicle, intervertebral disk, or ligamentum flavum. The force may be sufficient to produce dislocation of the vertebral column, fractures of the vertebral body, or both. However, occasionally no bony injury can be found by x-ray. The bony fragments and fractures may be too small to be seen on x-ray, or the cord may be compressed by nonradiopaque parts of the vertebral column.

Severe flexion of the spine tends to produce anterior dislocations in which the superior body is displaced forward on the inferior one. Compression fractures of the body or posterior herniations of the intervertebral disk may also occur. If the dislocation is severe, the cord will be caught anteriorly by the lip of the inferior body and posteriorly by the lamina of the anteriorly displaced superior vertebra.[5]

Extension injuries of the spinal cord are produced by sudden, violent, extreme extension of the spine. The likelihood of dislocation of the spine is not great, but the dorsal elements of the column may strike the spinal cord a severe blow. The ligamentum flavum and edges of the laminae may injure the dorsal aspect of the cord, squeezing it between them and the vertebral bodies anteriorly. This type of injury is most likely in the cervical spine and in older persons with spondylotic disease of the neck. It gives a rather characteristic neurologic picture of severe loss in the upper extremities, less severe loss in the lower ones, and more profound loss of sensory function.[76]

Rotary injuries may occur with marked displacement of the spinal column laterally. Usually, such injuries require considerable force, and injury to the spinal cord occurs by direct shearing and tearing as the vertebral column is displaced. Occasionally, rupture of the spinal ligaments allows extrusion of the intervertebral disk, and compression of the cord may occur.

Rarely, direct blows to the spine produce spinal cord injury. Usually, these occur when the patient falls on his or her back with sufficient force to fracture the lamina and pedicles. Spinal cord injury may result from laceration by spicules of bone driven into it or by compression from displaced fragments of lamina or pedicles.

The spinal cord undergoes the same types of pathologic damages in response to trauma as does the brain. It may be concussed, contused, lacerated, and may develop hematomas or edema.

Concussion of the spinal cord is a poorly understood entity. Presumably, it is similar to concussion of the brain, and the cord shows no gross pathologic change. Microscopically, some nonspecific changes have been recorded. These include swelling of the neurons and some loosening of the parenchyma of the cord.

The cord may be contused by missiles or bone. Here, there is bruising of the substance with surrounding edema. This is subpial and extends deep into the cord substance. There may be several areas of contusion which are adjacent but not confluent.

Lacerations of the cord are due to fragments of bone or to missiles which directly strike the cord and cut its substance. There is anatomic disruption of cord tissue. Adjacent to a laceration may be areas of edema and contusion.

Hemorrhage may occur in the substance of the cord or in the meninges around the cord. There are several types of spinal cord hemorrhage. Petechial hemorrhages around blood vessels are called *ring hemorrhages* and are found in many types of injury. Larger nonconfluent areas of hemorrhage are found in contusions and lacerations. These may become large and disrupt cord tissue. *Hematomyelia* is the specific name given to such a large collection of blood.

The spinal cord becomes edematous, as does the brain. The extent of this edema is less than in the brain, as the white matter of the cord is not so extensive. Edema of the cord may produce neurologic deficit, but its true role in spinal cord injuries is obscure. The cord appears swollen grossly and microscopically, and there is loosening of the glial supporting structures.

Signs and Symptoms of Spinal Cord Injury

The spinal cord serves as the main neural connection between the brain and the body; so when it is injured, profound physiologic changes result. Complete interruption of the spinal cord produces total sensory loss and motor paralysis below the level of injury. Associated with these are autonomic dysfunction such as priapism, loss of bowel and bladder control, and loss of sweating and vasomotor tone below the level of the transection.

The autonomic loss causes urinary retention with distention of the bladder. Urinary incontinence is very rare. Males may show priapism. In the Parkland Memorial Hospital series, 20 percent of the male patients had such a symptom. The presence of priapism is generally considered as an ominous prognostic sign. It occurred more commonly in patients with complete spinal cord transection than in those with partial or incomplete lesion.

The interruption of autonomic function causes a loss in vasomotor tone and vasodilation. A rather marked reduction in blood pressure results from this loss of peripheral vascular resistance. This has been termed *neurogenic shock.* This is a poor term, as this condition bears little relationship to surgical shock, if any at all. These patients remain oriented, dry, warm, produce urine, and have full veins. It does produce orthostatic hypotension. The loss of autonomic function also causes loss of sweating below the level of lesion. If the level of cord transection is high, the area for heat loss by evaporation may be reduced considerably. Therefore, the patient may develop hyperpyrexia if left in high ambient temperatures.

The loss of motor function results in paralysis of all muscles below the level of injury. The higher the transection, the greater the area of the body that is paralyzed. If this area involves much of the intercostal muscles, respiration is poor and ineffective and coughing is impaired.

The sudden removal of descending influences from higher centers which modulate spinal segmental activity produces temporary loss of all tendon reflexes. Muscle tone and tendon reflexes are absent, producing a flaccid paralysis. This condition has been termed *spinal shock.* Later in the course of recovery from the injury, return of reflexes occurs. Tendon reflexes are uninhibited by higher control and become hyperactive, resulting in a spastic paralysis. Mass movements of the lower body, the mass reflex, may occur in response to stimuli, and defecation, micturition, and ejaculation may also occur.

Injuries that do not completely transect the spinal cord may produce complex neurologic signs. Classic among the various syndromes of incomplete cord injury is the Brown-Séquard syndrome, resulting from a cord hemisection. The signs are an ipsilateral loss of motor power, light touch, position, and vibration sensory modalities below the level of the injury, and contralateral loss of pain and temperature sensations.

Accident Site and Transportation of Accident Victims

Individuals responsible for the identification, initial care, and transportation of accident victims should be carefully instructed in the management of real or possible spinal cord injuries. The vehicles used to transport such patients should be equipped with proper supports for the spine, particularly for the neck. Individuals responsible for transportation should be instructed to always ask the accident victim to move the arms and legs, to ask about any tingling in arms and legs, and to ask about pain in the back. The presence of any of these are indications for extreme care in moving the patient. In diving accidents, when an individual has struck the head on the bottom of a swimming pool, the patient should be supported in the water until an adequate support for the neck can be obtained. Patients with signs or symptoms of spinal injury should be transported on a spine board. These should be present in all emergency ambulances. The patient should be left on the board during the initial examinations in the emergency room. This includes the x-ray examination.

Treatment in the Emergency Room

The patient with a spinal cord injury should be placed on a flat, hard board without moving the spine. The patient's back should be kept straight. Moving the patient by flexion or extension of the spine may produce increased damage to the spinal cord. When it is necessary to move the patient, four people should be used. Two should exert traction along the spinal axis by pulling at the head and feet of the patient. The other two can then move the patient without bending the spinal column.

Immediate evaluation of the patient should be done—before any attempt to move the patient from the ambulance stretcher is made. The patient should be questioned about pain in the neck or back, any feelings of numbness or tingling in the body, and ability to move the arms and legs. Visual inspection may reveal the presence of the injury and its level. A patient with a spinal cord injury at the sixth cervical level will lie with the arms flexed at the elbows and wrists. This attitude of the upper extremities is characteristic, and should immediately alert the physician to the possibility of cervical spinal cord injury. Priapism is another sign of spinal cord injury.

The neck and back should be palpated by slipping a hand under the recumbent patient. Deformity and points of tenderness should be felt for and noted so that x-ray examination of the appropriate level can be carried out.

The strength and motion of all four extremities should be tested. This is done most easily by asking the patient to flex the elbows (biceps, fifth cervical), grasp and squeeze the fingers of the examiner (finger flexors, eighth cervical), and extend the elbows (triceps, seventh cervical). Next, the pattern of respiration is observed. Paralysis of the intercostal muscles produces paradoxical movement of the chest and abdomen. The patient is asked to cough, then to move the hips, knees, ankles, and toes.

Sensory examination is carried out next. This is done rapidly by using a safety pin and cotton. The patient is instructed to report if the pin feels sharp or dull. No attempt at distinguishing finer qualities of pain perception should be made. Touch is tested by having the patient close his or her eyes and reporting when the examiner touches them with the cotton. The levels of sensory loss, if found, should be marked with a skin pencil or ball point pen. Such marks will make possible accurate comparisons of sensory level upon repeated examinations.

The biceps, radial periosteal, triceps, quadriceps, and achilles reflexes should be tested. Superficial reflexes of the abdominal muscles and cremasterics should then be tested. The plantar response is checked. Usually in acute spinal cord injury, the deep tendon reflexes and the superfical reflexes are lost below the level of the lesion. The plantar response is usually flexor in the acute phase of spinal cord injury.

Careful examination of the vital signs should be made. The presence of true shock in a patient with a spinal cord injury is indicative of some associated injury, as it is rarely seen in spinal cord transection.

Evaluation of the patient's respiratory exchange should be made. If the level of transection is high, so that most of the intercostal muscles are paralyzed, an endotracheal intubation should be done to reduce respiratory effort.

A nasogastric tube should be introduced and connected to suction. Since transection of the spinal cord may produce adynamic ileus, gastric and intestinal distention may occur. This will reduce respiratory exchange and introduce the danger of aspiration.

Since the patient with the spinal cord injury cannot empty the bladder, catheterization should be done. This should be done with care, using aseptic technique and a Foley catheter. The catheter should be taped to the abdomen of the male patient to eliminate the penoscrotal angle, which is a source for infection, periurethral abscess, and urethral fistula formation.

An infusion of Ringer's lactate solution should be begun in an arm vein. The leg veins should not be used in paraplegic patients, as the risk of phlebothrombosis and pulmonary embolism is great in this group of patients. If the spinal cord injury is the sole one suffered by the patient, little need for vigorous fluid therapy exists. However, careful search for other injuries must be made, as the patient may not be able to feel the pain produced by injuries below the level of the cord injury. Associated injuries requiring specific therapy should be treated according to their life-endangering potential, regardless of the spinal cord injury. Abdominal injuries should be explored surgically before attempting definitive treatment of the spinal cord injury. This is particularly important in penetrating wounds of the cord where the missile tract may pass through major vessels or other structures such as bowel or liver. Injuries to these structures should be ruled out before definitive treatment of the spinal cord injury is carried out.

After evaluation of the patient clinically for the level of spinal cord injury and the presence of any associated injury, x-rays of the appropriate spinal segments should be done. Some confusion about the bony level exists; so a few simple rules must be remembered. A neurologic level at the costal margin indicates an injury at the eighth thoracic spinal cord level; the umbilicus, the tenth thoracic; and the inguinal region, the twelfth thoracic. The spinal cord level does not correspond to the vertebral body level, however. The fourth thoracic spinal cord level lies at about the second thoracic body level; the eighth thoracic, at the sixth thoracic body level; the tenth thoracic, at the eighth thoracic body level; the twelfth thoracic, at the ninth thoracic body level; and the lumbar and sacral cord segments, at the level of the eleventh and twelfth vertebral bodies. This difference between bony and cord levels must be kept in mind when ordering x-rays.

Movement of the patient to the x-ray table should be done with care, using the methods described above. X-rays should be made in the anterior-posterior and lateral projections.

They should be of good quality for bony detail. Certain areas of the spine are notoriously difficult to visualize. The cervical thoracic junction is one. All segments of the cervical spine must be seen in the lateral projections to avoid overlooking a fracture or dislocation of the seventh cervical vertebra. Visualization of the seventh cervical and first thoracic vertebra may be improved by pulling down on the patient's arms or by placing one of them overhead and taking the x-rays through the axilla (swimmer's view).

If the patient has a cervical spinal cord injury, some form of skeletal traction should be applied. Crutchfield tongs, or some similar device, should be used. It is crucial that these tongs be applied correctly. The head should be shaved. Crutchfield tongs should be applied at the vertex, parallel to the coronal suture, and directly above the mastoid processes. These bony prominences lie in the plane of the cervical spine and so serve as a useful landmark to ensure proper location of the tongs. The tongs should be centered on the skull, right to left, so that the pull is not eccentric. Similarly, they should be straight across the skull, not more to one side than the other. These tongs are easily inserted through stab wounds through the scalp. The outer table of the skull is drilled, using the Crutchfield drill points. Recently, Gardner has introduced a new device which is easier to apply to the skull. Results are equally satisfactory with the new tongs.[29]

Reduction of a cervical dislocation, if present, within the first few hours after injury should be obtained. Repetitive checks of the position of the dislocation by x-ray are made, and changes in the amount of weight and direction of pull are made.

Surgical Treatment of Spinal Cord Injury

Traditionally, patients with compound injuries of their spinal column and cord have been subjected to decompressive laminectomy. The operation, obviously, should be delayed if any other organs have been injured. For instance, if the patient has suffered a gunshot wound to the abdomen, this must be explored first.

In stab wounds of the spinal cord, or in gunshot wounds of the spinal cord where there is immediate and total transverse injury to the spinal cord, exploration has been used less and less in the Parkland Memorial Hospital series. Review of our statistics indicates that there has not been a significant incidence of infection of the meninges following gunshot or stab wound. The development of a cerebrospinal fistula has occurred in less than 0.5 percent of our cases. Since no patient has been shown to have improved neurologic function after laminectomy for a penetrating wound, its use has been less and less frequent in the past few years.

Injuries to the cervical spine and to the lumbar spine present exceptions. Because of the significant importance of the acquisition of an additional dermatome for a patient with a cervical spinal injury, we have felt that exploration with the removal of an offending fragment of bone, bullet, or disk material from under a nerve root would be beneficial to the patient. Similarly, exploration of the cauda equina should be carried out, as the likelihood of enhanced and more rapid return of function following exploration seems to make the operation warranted. Stab wounds and gunshot wounds to the thoracic cord with complete and total transection rarely require surgical exploration.

Laminectomy for closed injuries of the spinal cord is a more controversial problem. There is some experimental evidence indicating that laminectomy should be done in all cases. Allen,[3] in 1911, did the original experiments, which were confirmed by Freeman and Wright[26] many years later. Clinical experience has been quite varied, however. Wannamaker states that laminectomy is clearly beneficial.[85] Comarr, however, feels that the evidence is unconvincing that laminectomy in humans is of any value.[19]

Clinically useful information to indicate the need for immediate laminectomy and/or anterior cervical fusion is rare. The individual physician is forced to rely on x-ray aids. In the past, routine x-rays were too gross to detect fine fragments driven into the spinal canal. The intervertebral disk is, of course, radiolucent, so no information could be obtained about it. Lumbar puncture and manometrics do not give a clear picture of the spinal canal; and myelography, using Pantopaque, required a great deal of manipulation, and so was hazardous.

The picture has changed with the introduction of air myelography with polytomography. The clear capability of defining the subarachnoid space and its contents in fine detail makes it possible to gain information leading to an appropriate decision regarding surgical decompression.

Similarly, the use of the thoracotomy incision to approach the fractures, thoracic spine, with removal of the vertebral bodies from the anterior, has proven a new advance.

Laminectomy has some clear indications, some relative indications, and some contraindications in the management of closed spinal cord injuries. The positive indications are when there is (1) clear evidence of worsening neurologic deficit, (2) evidence of bony penetration or compression of the spinal canal, and (3) injury of the cauda equina in the lumbar spine. Relative indications include the philosophic concept of ensuring the patient that everything possible is being done, the removal of any loose fragments of bone which may injure the cord during convalescence, and the reduction of secondary scarring about the cord by adequate surgical debridement. Contraindications for exploration of the spinal cord include rapid improvement in neural function; severe associated injuries making surgery hazardous; severe gross bony deformity such as fracture dislocation of the midthoracic spine, which would make it unlikely that the cord is intact; and the presence of a very high, complete cervical cord injury. The patient with severe respiratory paralysis is a very poor surgical risk.[18]

Recently, an anterior approach for the management of cervical spine dislocation has been advocated.[63] This has great usefulness in an acute flexion injury with anterior dislocation of the cervical spine. If an extruded intervertebral disk is present, removal from the anterior is much easier and safer than by laminectomy. Also, since a fusion is also done with this approach, stability of the spine is assured. It should be mentioned that reduction of the dislocation is difficult from this approach. Furthermore, the anterior approach is contraindicated if a tracheostomy is required. The surgical dissection opens the epidural space to the potentially infected tracheostomy site.[17]

Operative care of the patient with spinal cord injury may include open reduction of the dislocation or the performance of a spine fusion for stability. Unilateral dislocations of the cervical vertebrae may be particularly troublesome to reduce, and open reduction should be done early. Unstable fractures of the cervical vertebrae may be stabilized by either anterior fusion or by posterior fusion as advocated by Alexander.[2] Dislocation of the thoracic and lumbar spine may be reduced and stabilized by the Harrington rods. This distraction device greatly facilitates the prompt and accurate realignment of the spine.

The Parkland Hospital series of spinal cord injuries covers 300 patients. The preponderant incidence is in young males. There has been an increase in cervical spine injuries in the decade 1965 to 1975. This is due to the increased use of motorcycles, as well as to more high-speed automobile accidents. However, the basic statistics remain as in the initially reported series of 102 patients. These are divided into four primary groups: closed injury with apparent complete transection of the spinal cord, compound wound with complete transection of the spinal cord, and two groups with incomplete transections. Any patient showing any residual neurologic function in any sphere is included in the incomplete groups. This is an important differential, as the finding of any remnant of function below the level of injury is very important. No patient in our series without such evidence recovered any neural function regardless of the treatment employed and regardless of the type of injury suffered. Therefore, it is very important to make a complete and careful neurologic examination on each patient. The preservation of a single reflex, of a small patch of sensation, or of a flicker of motion is immensely important for the progress of the patient.

The patients with incomplete lesions present another story. In the earlier series of 102 patients, no matter how insignificant the residual function, improvement occurred in 38 out of 47 patients. In 36 of these patients, improvement was judged significant and meaningful to the patient. In the 47 patients with incomplete injuries to their spinal cords, 30 were operated upon. In the operative group, 23 patients were improved neurologically, with 22 of them showing significant improvement. There was one operative death, and one patient was made worse temporarily by operation. In the nonoperative group of 17 patients, 15 showed some improvement in their neurologic findings. Some of these patients showed such prompt improvement in their neurological status that surgical intervention was not contemplated. However, in the patients failing to show such rapid improvement, the amount of function regained was not as good as in the operative group. Again, there was one death in this group, and one patient worsened under nonoperative management.

Long-term survival of patients with spinal cord injury is not good. The average mortality ratio of a patient with paraparesis is little different from the standard population. This rate rises, however, to 216 percent of the normal population for quadriplegia. The most common cause of death after injury and survival of the initial insult was renal failure and cardiovascular disease.[43]

PERIPHERAL NERVE INJURIES

Injuries to peripheral nerves occur with both closed and open wounds of the extremities. Usually, they happen with open wounds such as bullet or fragment wounds, stab wounds, or lacerations. Closed injuries occur with compression, stretching of the extremity, or by entrapment in the healing process.

Usually, manifestations of peripheral nerve injury are present immediately after wounding, but occasionally develop during convalescence. This is particularly true when a long bone is factured near a peripheral nerve. The nerve may be caught in callus formation and be damaged long after convalescence has begun.

In general, some of the same principles of care apply to open, closed, immediate, or delayed injuries to the peripheral nerve. The concept of preventing further injury and observing for signs of return of function are identical. Obviously, there are certain fundamental differences; the appearance of a peripheral nerve lesion after convalescence has begun is an indication of some new problem in the injured area. This usually means a surgical exploration to define and handle it.

Compound wounds present still another significant difference. The anatomic relationship of the peripheral nerve to the arteries, veins, and tendons of an extremity should be borne in mind. Often these lie in immediate proximity to the nerve and may be injured together with it. Such combined neurovascular or neurotendinous injury in an extremity is not uncommon, and exploration must be done immediately to manage the associated injury rather than the peripheral nerve injury. Examination of the patient prior to surgical intervention may disclose the presence of such combined injury. However, too much emphasis should not be placed on the absence of signs of vascular damage. This is emphasized by the reported Parkland Memorial Hospital series of vascular injury. Exploration of the wound throughout its extent is the only way to be sure of finding all structures injured. This is a key principle in the management of wounds of an extremity. A wound which passes near a major neurovascular bundle should be explored promptly to ensure the presence of vascular integrity, regardless of the neurologic deficit present.

Signs of Peripheral Nerve Injury

Each major nerve of the body has certain chief motor and sensory functions. By examining these functions in patients sustaining wounds or injuries of the extremities, the presence of a specific peripheral nerve injury can be identified.

The Upper Extremity   In the upper extremity, there are five major nerves: the circumflex, the musculocutaneous, the median, the ulnar, and the radial. The circumflex nerve supplies sensation to the skin over the deltoid and is the motor nerve to the deltoid muscle. Abduction of the arm at the shoulder is the crucial motor test of this nerve. The musculocutaneous nerve supplies motor function to the biceps and brachioradialis muscles. Flexion of the arm at the elbow is the motor test. The sensory distribution is to the radial side of the forearm. The median nerve innervates most of the flexor muscles of the forearm, particularly the muscles of the thenar eminence. The ability to oppose the thumb to the little finger is the chief motor test. The sensory distribution of the median nerve is extremely important, as this encompasses virtually the entire palmar surface of the thumb, index, and long fingers. The ulnar nerve supplies motor function to the flexor muscles of the ulnar side of the arm and to the intrinsic muscles of the

hand, particularly the interossei and the lumbricals of the third and fourth fingers. Its loss results in inability to abduct and adduct the fingers. Sensation is supplied along the palmar surface of the little finger by the ulnar nerve. The radial nerve has a small sensory distribution, usually over the web space between the thumb and index finger of the dorsal side of the hand. However, the motor function of the radial nerve is quite extensive. Virtually all the extensor muscles of the arm from the triceps down are supplied by the radial nerve. Extension of the wrist and fingers is not possible when this nerve has been injured.

The brachial plexus may be injured. This large, anatomically complex structure, composed of many nerve roots, is the origin of the above-named nerves to the upper extremity. The plexus may be injured by closed trauma, such as occurs during the extreme stretching which occurs during delivery with a shoulder presentation. Open wounds of the brachial plexus may occur with penetrating wounds around the clavicle. Injuries to this complex structure are important for many reasons. Profound neurologic deficit occurs with such injuries, and very perplexing neurologic pictures can be present.

The plexus lies in intimate relationship to the subclavian artery and vein, and these may be injured in open wounds of the plexus. Occasionally, it is assumed that the neurologic deficit of a patient is due to brachial plexus injury. On exploration, a laceration of the subclavian artery is found without any injury to the plexus, the patient's neurologic deficit being purely ischemic in origin.

All open wounds of the brachial plexus demand exploration. The incision should include resection of the medial third of the clavicle, and the insertion of the pectoralis major should be taken down to ensure adequate exploration.

Closed injuries of the plexus are divided into three types: the total, the upper or Erb-Duchenne type, and the lower or Klumpke type. The complete injury implies a loss of function throughout the area supplied by the plexus. In incomplete total injury, the patient may have dissociated loss, so that sensation may be preserved although there is loss of motor function. This occurs because of the greater susceptibility of the large motor fibers to stretch injury. Such patients may be called hysterical; however, the classic findings of dissociated loss should establish the diagnosis. Usually, total injuries are complete, and the patient has a flail, anesthetic arm and hand.

The upper type of brachial plexus injury involves the nerve roots contributing to the most cephalad part of the plexus, the cervical fifth to seventh being involved. The usual mechanism of injury is one of extreme lateral bending of the head away from the side of injury and depression of the ipsilateral shoulder at the same time. Such an injury occurs when a patient lands on the side of the head and point of the shoulder. This injury produces loss of motion at the elbow and shoulder. Loss of flexion of the wrist is less common. Usually function of the hand and wrist is intact. Sensation may be lost in a shield over the deltoid and across the arm and forearm.

Injuries to the lower part of the brachial plexus result from forcible extension of the arm over the head. In this case, the lower nerve roots contributing to the brachial plexus are injured. The patient maintains use of the shoulder and elbow, but has a flail, paralyzed, and anesthetic forearm and hand. Such injuries usually occur when one catches oneself while falling or being thrown from a vehicle.

The Lower Extremity   In the lower extremity, there are three major nerves: the femoral, the obturator, and the sciatic. The sciatic nerve with its two major divisions, the posterior tibial and peroneal, supplies motor and sensory function to much of the entire leg. It supplies the hamstring muscles in the thigh, and its division of the muscles of the leg below

the knee. The tibial nerve supplies the gastrocnemius muscle, the soleus muscle, and the flexors of the toes as well as sensation along the dorsum of the foot. The common peroneal nerve innervates the peroneal and the anterior tibial muscles of the leg and supplies sensation along the lateral aspect of the leg below the knee and on the sole of the foot.

If the major trunk of the sciatic nerve is injured, the site of injury is usually in the buttock or thigh. The patient has an anesthetic foot and has no motion of the foot or toes. If the nerve is injured high in the thigh, loss of hamstring function results in weakness of flexion of the knee. Injury to the tibial branch is usually in the back or calf of the leg or the popliteal space posteriorly. The patient has loss of sensation over the heel and sole of the foot, and cannot plantar flex the foot or toes. The peroneal nerve is usually injured at the level of the fibular head. Such injury produces anesthesia over the lateral aspect of the calf and the foot. Eversion and dorsiflexion of the foot at the ankle are lost.

The femoral nerve supplies motor function to the quadriceps femoris and sensation along the medial side of the foot and leg, extending down as low as the medial malleolus. The femoral nerve is usually injured at the inguinal ligament in the anterior aspect of the thigh. Loss of this nerve produces anesthesia along the medial aspect of the leg and foot and inability to extend the knee.

The obturator nerve supplies the adductor muscles of the thigh, with a small sensory distribution along the medial side of the thigh. This nerve is rarely injured, as it lies deep in the pelvis. Injury to it should be kept in mind when penetrating wounds of the perineum occur. Its loss results in inability to adduct the thigh.

Unlike the brachial plexus, the lumbosacral plexus is rarely injured, except by gunshot wounds. It is well protected from stretch injury by the greater stability of the pelvis and femur as compared with the shoulder girdle and humerus.

Classification of Peripheral Nerve Injuries

Many ways to classify these injuries exist. Each classification requires amplification to describe a given injury. The principal classifications of these injuries are surgical, neurologic, or pathologic. The treatment to be used often depends on the findings leading to a classification of the particular injury.

Surgical classifications define the presence of a closed or an open wound. Usually a compound wound is explored as soon as the patient's general condition warrants it and good operating facilities are available. Closed wounds of the peripheral nerve, however, should be managed by conservative waiting for return of nerve function. Exploration of such injured nerves may be required if this does not occur in a reasonable time. Fortunately, recovery often occurs without surgical intervention.

Neurologic examination of the patient with a peripheral nerve injury defines the clinical status of the patient. From this evaluation, it may be found that a complete lesion of the nerve exists. This means that all functions of the nerve—motor, sensory, and autonomic—have been lost. Or, an incomplete lesion may be found. There may be generally decreased function of the nerve, or a dissociated loss with more motor than sensory loss. With generally decreased function, the damage is usually restricted to a sharply local area of the nerve. However, the larger, more rapidly conducting fibers are more easily damaged by stretching or compression. Since motor nerve fibers are larger than the sensory fibers, the usual finding in dissociated loss is paralysis or paresis without anesthesia or hypalgesia. Occasionally, dissociated sensory loss with loss of light touch and preservation of pain sensation may occur. This is because of the relative size of these nerve fibers, the ones for touch being larger. The classic mechanism producing this type of loss is a stretching of the nerve along its long axis. This produces a long, continuous lesion, often with sparing of some of the function of the nerve. The bizarre patterns produced by such an incomplete lesion may be confusing. The patient may be suspected of malingering or may be thought to be hysterical.

One of the most useful descriptions of the types of peripheral nerve injury was given by Seddon.[77] He categorized the injury as being of three types. The first he named *neurontomesis*. This occurs when both neural and connective tissue elements of the nerve are completely divided. This is complete and total anatomic transection of the nerve. *Axontomesis* implies that only the axon has been cut, leaving the supporting structures intact. Even the Schwann cell tube is left intact in this condition. Finally, he described a condition in which no anatomic interruption of the nerve fiber occurred, but conduction of the neural impulse was blocked. He gave the name of *neuropraxia* to this condition. This classification is useful in understanding the various anatomic and physiologic variables occurring in peripheral nerve injuries.

Management of the Injury

Closed wounds of peripheral nerves are managed by expectant waiting. Recovery should occur in a predictable manner, just as after nerve suture. This recovery time is discussed below.

Exploration of a closed injury should be done if recovery is delayed beyond the predicted time or if the neurologic deficit becomes worse.

Brachial plexus injuries are so crippling as to be a special case. In general, the treatment of closed injuries of the brachial plexus is expectant. The injury to the nerves is diffuse, extends over many centimeters, and exists intraneuronally. Little can be gained from neurolysis or exploration in the usual case. There are two possible exceptions to this rule: (1) If there is clear-cut evidence of worsening of the neurologic deficit after several weeks, exploration is warranted. (2) If the injury producing the plexus injury was a direct blow to the middle third of the clavicle, and a fracture of the clavicle is present, exploration again is probably warranted. In such a case, it is possible that the ends of the fractured clavicle injured the plexus directly.

Some information about the potential for recovery from closed brachial plexus injuries can be gained from the degree of injury and, occasionally, from myelography. If the injury is of the entire plexus and is neurologically complete, the prognosis is poor. In such injuries, if no recovery is present by 2 months, a cervical myelogram should be done. The force of injury may have been so great as to avulse the nerve root from the spinal cord. This produces a characteristic myelographic pattern, with the formation of large diverticula of the arachnoid at the levels of the avulsed nerve roots. Such an injury is irreparable.[62]

Treatment of the patient with a brachial plexus injury should include splinting of the extremity in a functional position with full support of the arm. This will prevent stretching of the deltoid muscle with dislocation of the humeral head.

Repair of Injuries

Timing of Repair Surgical exploration of a peripheral nerve injury can be done at various times. However, exploration of compound wounds of the extremity should be done promptly in order to control hemorrhage, debride dead tissue, define the injury, and repair as much of the damage as possible. During such exploration, a peripheral nerve transection may be the only injury found.

Opinions vary regarding the best way to handle the acute transected nerve. Equally good results can be expected from immediate repair of the nerve or from waiting 6 weeks and performing a delayed repair. There are certain advantages to each course, and each nerve injury should be considered independently. The optimum results will be obtained by careful evaluation of all the factors rather than by following an inflexible course dependent on a hard, fast rule.

Examining the rationale for delayed repair, we can see that there are three major reasons in its favor: ease of defining the extent of the injury, ease of surgical repair after delay, and ability to evaluate the effect of any associated injury on the limb. The extent of injury can be notoriously difficult to define in gunshot wounds where blast injury may be present over a significant area. Certainly, the extent of damage to the nerve may be defined more easily by later exploration, as scarring will be clearly seen throughout the whole injured segment of the nerve. The thickening of the perineurium makes suture technically easier. Another reason for delaying repair is to allow the metabolic demands for axonal regeneration to begin.[22] Finally, other circumstances, such as concomitant injury, may mitigate against immediate repair. For instance, the blood supply to the extremity may be in jeopardy because of arterial or venous injury. The operative repair of an associated injury may be difficult and require long anesthesia, making further prolongation unwise. This may be particularly true if many tendons have to be repaired. Any of these factors indicates that the wisest course is to delay the repair of the peripheral nerve.

If the delay is decided, no attempt to mark or tag the two ends of the nerve should be made. This merely results in additional damage to the nerve. The nerve ends can be found easily by beginning in the normal or uninjured part of the extremity and tracing the nerve into the old area of injury.

Immediate repair in certain cases possesses clear advantages. The patient is spared a second operation. Time is gained in the regenerative process of the peripheral nerve. Usually the problem of defining the extent of damage is not great. Most peripheral nerve injuries seen in civilian practice are due to lacerations, and are usually clean and do not involve widespread tissue injury. The technique of sewing the nerve sheath before the thickening has occurred is not difficult. Using very fine silk and adequate lighting and magnification, good approximation of the nerve ends can be achieved with immediate repair.

One of the more complex problems is that of injury of a peripheral nerve and one or more tendons at the same level in the extremity. The surgeon is faced with the clear-cut requirement of repairing the tendon primarily, and it should take priority. When adequate tendon function has been accomplished, the nerve injury may then be repaired. There are several reasons for this course. The tendon repair may generate considerable scar tissue. The early mobilization required by the tendon repair may jeopardize the nerve suture.

The surgical techniques for repair of the peripheral nerve are standard. However, certain principles are paramount and deserve emphasis. General anesthesia should be used. Local or regional anesthesia may not last long enough and may not produce a large enough area of anesthesia.

Peripheral nerve surgery should not be done under a tourniquet. It is unlikely that adequate exploration and dissection of the peripheral nerve can be carried out in safe tourniquet time. The nerve may be injured in an area in which tourniquet application is very difficult, and the use of the tourniquet may compromise the proximal extent of the incision.

Repair of a peripheral nerve should be carried out through a long incision so as to expose the nerve over a considerable part of its course. The nerve should be identified in a clean area away from the wound, both proximally and distally. It can be traced into the area of the injury. This maneuver ensures correct identification of the nerve and reduces the likelihood of additional damage or trauma to the peripheral nerve. Attempts to find the nerve in the lacerated and distorted area of injury may lead to further damage or to misidentification.

The nerve should be lifted out of its bed and a rubber dam placed around it. This will serve as a handle for the nerve. The nerve should never be squeezed in forceps or handled roughly. To soften them, sponges used in the wound should be moist. The nerve should be kept from drying.

After completing the dissection through the lacerated area, the status of the nerve may be assessed. It will be found to be in continuity, partially severed, or completely transected. If it is in continuity, it should be placed back in the thoroughly debrided wound. The wound should be closed without drainage.

If the nerve is completely severed, the ends should be trimmed to make them square and clean. The nerve ends are placed on a tongue blade and cut with a new razor blade. Pouting of the individual nerve bundles and fascicles indicates that adequate resection has been done. By holding Gelfoam soaked in thrombin lightly against the cut ends of the nerve, bleeding from the nerve ends can be controlled and arrested. All such bleeding must be stopped before attempting repair. This step is vital, as the formation of hematoma between the ends of the nerve will interfere with regeneration of the nerve.

The location of blood vessels on the surface of the nerve and large fascicles of nerve should be used as identifying landmarks to orient the two ends for accurate approximation. The ends of the divided peripheral nerve should lie in approximation without tension or traction before any attempt at suture is made. This requires adequate length to be obtained in the dissected nerve. Three maneuvers are helpful in obtaining this length. Length is gained by dissection along the course of the peripheral nerve, by transposition of the nerve around the joints, and by flexion of the joints crossed by the nerve to shorten its total course. When the ends of the peripheral nerve can be brought into approximation without being held, the suture of the nerve is easy and the repair is not likely to be pulled apart.

Sutures should be placed through the perineurium only. Very fine silk in a swedged needle is used; No. 6-0 or 7-0 silk on an atraumatic eye surgery needle is ideal. Stitches are placed through the perineurium, bringing the two ends into approximation. The perineurium is then closed in a neat, regular fashion using interrupted sutures. There should be no gaps for the growth of nerve fibers out into the surrounding tissue. A technique occasionally useful in peripheral nerve repair is to wrap the repair site with a cuff of some inert material. This is particularly helpful if the peripheral nerve repair takes place in a bed with extensive dissection or destruction of tissue. Here, the surgeon can anticipate an excessive amount of scar tissue. Thin silicone rubber sheet is wrapped around the repair site.[10]

A more difficult surgical problem is presented by partially transected nerves. This situation can present a real dilemma. There are few guidelines as to the best course in such a situation. In general, it is better to do nothing except ensure a good clean bed for the injured nerve and wait and see the amount of recovery after a few months. If the nerve is literally hanging by a shred, then the transection may be completed and repair carried out. The surgeon should remember that a definite decision does not have to be made at the initial operation. He may, and most of the time should, wait and watch for recovery in the incompletely injured nerve.

Either at the time of the initial operation, when an incomplete lesion is found, or at reexploration, when a neuroma incontinuity is present, electrophysiologic efforts may be useful. The use of the stimulating and recording electrodes along the course of the nerve during surgical exploration may give the surgeon significant information about resection of a nerve lesion in continuity. The quality and distances along the distal nerve in which nerve action potentials can be found are important. Similarly, electromyographic recordings with stimulation of the nerve proximal to the site of injury may also give information regarding the nerve lesion in continuity. Before resorting to the radical decision to excise and complete the transection in such cases, it seems prudent to have this type of information available.[64] In case of neuroma incontinuity, internal neurolysis done under magnification can be useful.[8]

After the repair of the peripheral nerve has been accomplished, closure of the wound should be done in anatomic layers. The skin should be closed with fine stainless steel wire, and the extremity placed in a plaster cast. A circumferential cast is used instead of splints or bandages to ensure that the extremity is not forcibly extended. During closure and casting, care must be taken not to extend the extremity or make any movement that might pull the nerve sutures apart. The cast should be left intact for 3 weeks. Following this, if there has been need to flex any joints to gain length in the peripheral nerve, a new cast should be put on, extending this joint about one-third of the way. This cast should be worn a week and then replaced. Again, the joint can be straightened another one-third of the way to neutral. This process is repeated until the joint is completely extended, taking as long as 6 weeks if needed.

Rate of Recovery from Peripheral Nerve Injury

Once a peripheral nerve has been repaired, or in the case of expectant treatment of an incomplete or a closed injury, follow-up is very important. Adequate restoration of function should occur, but it cannot be taken for granted. There are several parameters to consider. The first is the process of degeneration and subsequent regeneration of the damaged axon. At the time of injury, the axon in the proximal end of the nerve degenerates to the nearest node of Ranvier. The axon in the distal segment, being separated from its cell body, degenerates and fragments throughout its entire length. The process occurring in the distal nerve is spoken of as *Wallerian degeneration.* It includes changes in the supporting Schwann cells and the myelin sheath as well as in the axon. The chief events are destruction of the myelin sheath and proliferation of the Schwann cell cytoplasm awaiting the arrival of new axons.

The proximal axon begins to sprout very soon after injury. If these neuron sprouts find an end of a Schwann cell tube in the distal nerve, the successful sprout grows down this axon tube. These new axon sprouts will grow at a rate of roughly 1 in/month. Several factors influence this rate; so it cannot be too rigidly employed. It is influenced by the type of injury, the distance from the central nervous system, the time lapsed since the injury, and the age of the patient. For example, if a nerve is crushed rather than cut, the axon tends to regenerate faster. The closer to the nervous system the axon is injured, the faster its rate of outgrowth. The rate of regeneration tends to slow down as time passes; so the longer the time since injury, the slower the regeneration. Younger persons tend to have a faster rate of regeneration than do older ones.

However, knowing the approximate rate of regeneration and the precise level of the peripheral nerve injury, an approximation of the time required for restoration of function can be made. For instance, if a muscle lies 3 in from the level of transection of its peripheral nerve, restoration of function in this muscle should occur in about 3 months. Voluntary control should return at this time; however, recovery of the previous level of dexterity and strength will require longer. This calculated time of the restoration of function in a muscle just distal to the point of severance of a peripheral nerve is the most reliable sign of adequate repair of an injured peripheral nerve.

There is another sign which is occasionally useful: if a regenerating axon is struck, paresthesias are elicited in the distribution of the peripheral nerve. This is called a *neuroma sign.* If the point at which the paresthesias are elicited advances at a steady rate down the trunk of the peripheral nerve, a Tinel sign is present. This sign is an indicator of the growth of some fibers across the area of injury. It is not a reliable sign of the adequacy of nerve regeneration, but it does indicate that there is some continuity of the nerve trunk.

If signs of recovery do not appear in the predicted time, a reexploration of the peripheral nerve is indicated. Clinically, in calculating the time of expected motor return, the distance from the area of transection to the motor point of the nearest muscle is measured. This distance divided by the predicted rate of regeneration will give the earliest time when recovery may be expected. This time span can be doubled to give the upper limit. Recovery should definitely be present by this later date, and, if not, reexploration is definitely indicated.

Certain exceptions to this rule should be noted. Muscle will not survive beyond 24 months without innervation; so if the calculated time of regeneration approaches 20 months, exploration to ensure continuity of repair may well be indicated in advance of this.

Similar times should be calculated for closed injuries. This is, of course, more difficult, as the precise level of injury in relation to a given muscle is not known. However, a predicted span of time for recovery of the proximal muscle should be estimated. If there is no evidence of regeneration or restoration of function within this predicted period of time, exploration of the closed injured peripheral nerve is indicated.

Results of Peripheral Nerve Surgery

The results of peripheral nerve surgery are dependent on several factors. In general, a nerve containing only one type of fiber, either motor or sensory, will recover more completely than will a nerve containing several types of fibers. Thus, the radial nerve, which is almost a purely motor nerve, recovers much better than the ulnar nerve. The distance the regenerating axon has to travel before reaching its goal is also important. The muscle to be innervated may become fibrotic and disappear before reinnervation occurs. Injuries close to the root of an extremity do not recover as well as those more distal. The primary function of the nerve must be considered. Those which provide innervation for finely skilled muscle control will not have the same quality of return as will those serving more gross motor function. Other factors of importance are the length of resection of nerve trunk required and the delay before repair is accomplished. The longer the length of resection required and/or the longer the delay before repair is done, the worse will be the result. Infection, strangely enough, plays little role in influencing recovery. Finally, there is an order of recovery in the peripheral nerves. This must be considered in the light of the above factors, but certain peripheral nerves seem to recover better than others. The radial, then the median, and finally the ulnar nerve is the order in the upper extremity. In the lower extremity, it is not so clear-cut, but the peroneal nerve is the least likely to recover satisfactorily. Interestingly enough, the complication of causalgia is more likely in either ulnar or peroneal nerve injuries.

Complications of Peripheral Nerve Injury

There are several complications of peripheral nerve injuries. Causalgia is unique to the injury itself. The other complications are secondary to the paralytic or sensory-deprived state of the extremity.

Causalgia may develop at any time following the peripheral nerve injury. It may be present immediately after the injury is sustained, or it may appear several weeks or months later. The pain is quite characteristic, being described as burning and intense, with both hyperesthesia and dysthesia. The extremity may be either cold and clammy or flushed and hot. It may be dry, or it may sweat excessively. It may be blue and discolored. There are always changes in the skin indicating some disturbance of autonomic function. The patient may find that keeping the extremity wrapped or wet is more comfortable. This condition was first described by S. Weir Mitchell in the American Civil War.[60] It is important to recognize causalgia when it develops, as it can become a most intractable and difficult condition to treat. It is more likely to accompany injuries of the median or ulnar nerve in the upper extremity and the peroneal nerve in the lower extremity. Any injury involving the area supplied by these nerves is more likely to be complicated by the development of causalgia.

Initially, the treatment of causalgia is the use of paravertebral sympathetic block with a local anesthetic agent. This block should be performed as soon as the symptoms of causalgia appear, no matter how minor they seem. A few repetitive blocks may relieve the situation permanently. If the relief following sympathetic block is prompt and dramatic, there can be little question as to the diagnosis. After three or four sympathetic blocks, if there is still recurrent pain, a sympathectomy should be performed through an anterior approach, removing the first and second thoracic paravertebral ganglia. For the lower extremities, a retroperitoneal flank incision is usual. The second, third, and fourth lumbar ganglia are removed. Other forms of treatment such as the use of ganglionic blocking agents, local exploration of the nerve, sedatives, and narcotics are not effective, and their use should be restricted to unusual circumstances.

A secondary complication of peripheral

nerve injuries is ulceration of the anesthetic area. Because of the inability of the patient to recognize the damage to the anesthetic skin, the patient may burn or abrade the skin or develop a pressure sore in the area of anesthesia. The patient should be cautioned about this as part of the initial care of the peripheral nerve injury. Any abrasion, superficial or otherwise, occurring in the anesthetic area requires prompt and immediate attention. Care should be taken to be sure that an infection does not develop in this area, as it may become quite severe before systematic symptoms occur. The anesthetic area should be carefully inspected routinely to be sure that no laceration, abrasion, or infection develops. The patient should be warned that infections or lacerations in the anesthetic area may be quite difficult to control and may require amputation.

Another complication is the deformity of joints secondary to the neurogenic muscle imbalance. This imbalance can be corrected by dynamic or static splints to be worn by the patient throughout the period of convalescence. If the problem is discussed with the patient and the importance of preventing deformity stressed, little problem in wearing the splint occurs. It can be pointed out that if peripheral nerve function returns to a deformed and contracted extremity, little has been gained.

BIBLIOGRAPHY

1 Albin, M. S., R. J. White, G. Acosta-Rua, et al.: Study of functional recovery produced by delayed localized cooling after spinal cord injury in primates, *J. Neurosurg.*, **29**:113, July 1968.

2 Alexander, E., Jr., H. F. Forsyth, C. H. Davis, Jr., and B. S. Nashold, Jr.: Dislocation of the atlas on the axis; the value of early fusion of C_1, C_2, and C_3, *J. Neurosurg.*, **15**:353, 1958.

3 Allen, A. R.: Surgery of experimental lesion of spinal cord equivalent to crush injury of fracture dislocation of spinal column: A preliminary report, *J. Am. Med. Assoc.*, **57**:878, 1911.

4 Blinderman, E. E., C. J. Graf, and T. Fitzpatrick: Basic studies in cerebral edema: Its control by a corticosteroid (Solu-Medrol), *J. Neurosurg.*, **19**:319, 1962.

5 Braakman, R. and L. Penning: "Causes of Cord and Root Lesions," in *Injuries of the Cervical Spine*, Excerpta Medica, Amsterdam, 1971, pp. 64–76.

6 Brackett, C. E., J. Overman, and R. Peters: Monitors, ventilators, and the neurosurgeon, *Clin. Neurosurg.*, **18**:166, 1971.

7 Breasted, J. H.: *The Edwin Smith Surgical Papyrus Published in Facsimile and Hieroglyphic Transliteration with Translation and Commentary in Two Volumes,* The University of Chicago Press, Chicago, 1930.

8 Brown, H. A.: Internal neurolysis in the treatment of peripheral nerve injuries, *Clin. Neurosurg.*, **17**:99–107, 1970.

9 Busch, E. A. V.: Brain stem contusions: Differential diagnosis, therapy, and prognosis, *Clin. Neurosurg.*, **9**:18, 1963.

10 Campbell, J. B.: Peripheral nerve repair, *Clin. Neurosurg.*, **17**:77–98, 1970.

11 Carter, N. W., F. C. Rector, and D. W. Seldin: Hyponatremia in cerebral disease resulting from the inappropriate secretion of antidiuretic hormone, *N. Engl. J. Med.,* **264**:67, 1961.

12 Carton, C. A.: *Cerebral Angiography in the Management of Head Trauma,* American Lecture Series, No. 336, Charles C Thomas, Publisher, Springfield, Ill., 1959.

13 Clark, K.: Fluid and electrolyte management in head injury, *Ariz. Med.,* **25**:149–162, February 1968.

14 Clark, K.: Incidence and mechanism of shock in acute head injury, *South. Med. J.,* **55**:513, May 1962.

15 Clark, K.: Intracerebral hematomas, *Arix. Med.,* **25**:200–203, February 1968.

16 Clark, K. and C. C. Watts: "The Multiple Injured Patient," in J. R. Youmans (ed.), *Neurological Surgery,* W. B. Saunders Company, Philadelphia, 1973, vol. 2, p. 865.

17 Clark, K.: "Use of the Anterior Operative Approach: A Treatment of Cervical Spine Injuries," in J. R. Youmans (ed.), *Neurological Surgery,* W. B. Saunders Company, Philadelphia, 1973, vol. 2, pp. 1067–1074.

18 Cloward, R. B.: Treatment of acute fractures

and fracture-dislocations of the cervical spine by vertebral-body fusion: A report of eleven cases, *J. Neurosurg.,* **18**:201, 1961.

19 Comarr, A. E.: The practical urological management of the patient with spinal cord injury, *Br. J. Urol.,* **31**:1, 1959.

20 Courville, C. B.: Traumatic intracerebral hemorrhages with special reference to the mechanics of their production, *Bull. Los Angeles Neurol. Soc.,* **22**:220, 1962.

21 Denny-Brown, D. and W. R. Russell: Experimental cerebral concussion, *Brain,* **64**:93, 1941.

22 Ducker, T. B., L. G. Kempe, and G. J. Hays: Metabolic background for peripheral nerve surgery, *J. Neurosurg.,* **30**:270–280, March 1969.

23 Edberg, S., J. Rieker, and A. Angrist: Study of impact pressure and acceleration in plastic skull models, *Lab. Invest.,* **12**:1305, 1963.

24 Einsbruch, B. C., K. Clark, and F. J. Kuibel: Fluid distribution noted in in vivo and in vitro sections of brain studied by electron microscopy, *Trans. Am. Neurol. Assoc.,* **87**:193, 1962.

25 Fishman, R. A.: Effects of isotonic intravenous solutions on normal and increased intracranial pressure, *Arch. Neurol. Psychiatry,* **70**:1, 1953.

26 Freeman, L. W. and T. W. Wright: Experimental observations of concussion and contusion of the spinal cord, *Ann. Surg.,* **137**:433, 1953.

27 Gallagher, J. T. and E. J. Browder: Extradural hematoma: Experience with 167 patients, *J. Neurosurg.,* **29**:1–12, July 1968.

28 Gannon, W., A. W. Cook, and E. J. Browder: Resolving subdural collections, *J. Neurosurg.,* **19**:865, 1962.

29 Gardner, W. J.: Principle of spring loaded points for cervical traction: Technical report, *J. Neurosurg.,* **39**:543, October 1973.

30 Glaser, M. A. and F. P. Shafer: Depressed fractures of the skull: Their surgery, sequelae, and disability, *J. Neurosurg.,* **2**:140, 1946.

31 Groat, R. A., W. F. Windle, and H. W. Magoun: Functional and structural changes in the monkey's brain during and after concussion, *J. Neurosurg.,* **2**:26, 1945.

32 Gurdjian, E. S.: Certain autobiographical impressions in the life of a neurosurgeon, *Clin. Neurosurg.,* **19**:58–68, 1972.

33 —— and J. E. Webster: *Head Injuries:* Mechanisms, Diagnosis, and Management, Little, Brown and Company, Boston, 1958.

34 —— and L. M. Thomas: Surgical management of the patient with head injury, *Clin. Neurosurg.,* **12**:56–72, 1964.

35 Hayes, G. J. and H. C. Slocum: The achievement of optimal brain relaxation by hyperventilation technics of anesthesia, *J. Neurosurg.,* **19**:65, 1962.

36 Hodash, R. H. and K. Clark: Unpublished observations.

37 Holbourn, A. H. S.: Mechanics of head injuries, *Lancet,* **2**:438, 1943.

38 Huber, P.: *Zerebral Angiographie beim frischen Schadel-Hirn-Trauma,* Georg Thieme Verlag, Stuttgart, 1964.

39 Jamison, K. G. and J. D. N. Yelland: Extradural hematoma: Report of 167 cases, *J. Neurosurg.,* **29**:13–23, July 1968.

40 —— and J. D. N. Yelland: Traumatic intracerebral hematoma: Report of 63 surgically treated cases, *J. Neurosurg.,* **37**:528–532, November 1972.

41 Jasper, H., J. Kershman, and A. Elvidge: Electroencephalography in head injury, in "Trauma of the Central Nervous System," *Res. Publ. Assoc. Res. Nerv. Ment. Dis.,* **24**:388, 1945.

42 Jennett, W. B.: *Epilepsy after Blunt Head Trauma,* Charles C Thomas, Publisher, Springfield, Ill., 1962, pp. 133–134.

43 Jousse, A. T., M. Wynne-Jones, and D. J. Breithaupt: Follow-up study of life expectancy and mortality in traumatic transverse myelitis, *Canadian A.M.J.,* **98**:770–772, April 1968.

44 Kaufmann, G. E. and K. Clark: Continuous monitoring of intraventricular and cervical subarachnoid pressure in neurosurgical patients, *J. Neurosurg.,* **33**:145–150, August 1970.

45 Kaufmann, G. E. and K. Clark: Emergency frontal twist drill ventriculostomy: A new approach, *J. Neurosurg.,* **33**:226–227, August 1970.

46 Kerr, F. W. L.: Radical decompression and dural grafting in severe cerebral trauma, *Proc. Staff Meet. Mayo Clin.,* **43**:853–864, October 1968.

47 Kriss, F. C., J. R. Taren, and B. A. Kahn: Primary repair of compound skull fractures by replacement of bone fragments, *J. Neurosurg.,* **30**:698, June 1969.

48 Larson, S. J., L. Love, and A. Mittelpunkt: Unilateral intracranial hematoma without shift

of the anterior cerebral artery, *Am. J. Roentgenol. Radium Ther. and Nucl. Med.,* **92**:786, 1964.

49 Lundberg, N.: Continuous recording and control of ventricular fluid pressure in neurosurgical practice, *Acta Psychiatr. Scand.* 37: *Suppl.,* **149**:1–193, 1960.

50 ———, H. Troupp, and H. Lorin: Continuous recording of the ventricular-fluid pressure in patients with severe acute traumatic brain injury: A preliminary report, *J. Neurosurg.,* **22**:581, 1965.

51 McLaurin, L. R. and F. T. Tutor: Acute subdural hematoma: Review of 90 cases, *J. Neurosurg.,* **18**:61–67, January 1961.

52 McLaurin, R. D. and F. T. Tutor: Acute subdural hematoma: Review of ninety cases, *J. Neurosurg.,* **18**:61, 1961.

53 McLaurin, R. L. and L. E. Ford: Extradural hematoma: Statistical survey of forty-seven cases, *J. Neurosurg.,* **21**:364, 1964.

54 ——— and F. Helmer: The syndrome of temporal lobe contusion, *J. Neurosurg.,* **21**:296–303, September 1965.

55 Magoun, H. W.: Caudal and cephalic influences of the brain-stem reticular formation, *Physiol. Rev.,* **30**:459, 1950.

56 Marshall, W. J. S., J. L. F. Jackson, and T. W. Langfitt: Brain swelling caused by trauma and arterial hypertension, *Arch. Neurol.,* **21**:533–545, November 1969.

57 Matson, D. D.: *The Treatment of Acute Craniocerebral Injuries Due to Missiles,* American Lecture Series, No. 22, American Lectures in Surgery, Charles C Thomas, Publisher, Springfield, Ill., 1948.

58 Mierowsky, Arnold M. (ed.): *Neurological Surgery of Trauma,* Office of the Surgeon General, Department of the Army, Washington, D.C., 1965.

59 Mitchell, O. C., E. Torre, E. Alexander, and C. H. Davis: The nonfilling phenomenon during angiography in acute intracranial hypertension, *J. Neurosurg.,* **19**:766, 1962.

60 Mitchell, S. W., G. R. Morehouse, and W. W. Keen: *Gunshot Wounds and Other Injuries of Nerves,* J. B. Lippincott Company, Philadelphia, 1864.

61 Muller, H. R.: Zur echoencephalographie; ihre indikation beim schadelhirn-trauma, *Schweiz. Med. Wochenschr.,* **94**:119, 1964.

62 Murphy, F. and J. Kirklin: Myelographic demonstration of avulsing injuries of the nerve roots of the brachial plexus: A method of determining the point of injury and possibility of repair, *Clin. Neurosurg.,* **20**:18, 1972.

63 Norrell, H. and C. B. Wilson: Early anterior fusion for injuries of the cervical portions of the spine, *J. Am. Med. Assoc.,* **214**:525–530, October 1970.

64 Nulsen, F. E. and D. G. Kline: "Acute Injuries of Peripheral Nerves," in J. R. Youmans (ed.), *Neurological Surgery,* W. B. Saunders Company, Philadelphia, 1973, vol. 2, pp. 1089–1140.

65 Ommaya, A. K., S. D. Rockoff, and M. Baldwin: Experimental concussion: A first report, *J. Neurosurg.,* **21**:249, 1964.

66 Osterholm, J. L.: Pathophysiologic response to spinal cord injury: Current status of related research, *J. Neurosurg.,* **40**:5, January 1974.

67 Pitlyk, P. J. and G. S. Moss: Fluid and electrolyte balance in penetrating wounds, *Surgery,* **63**:396–409, March 1968.

68 Pudenz, R. H. and H. C. Shelden: The lucite calvarium: A method for direct observation of the brain. II. Cranial trauma and brain movement, *J. Neurosurg.,* **3**:487, 1946.

69 Putnam, T. J. and H. Cushing: Chronic subdural hematoma: Its pathology, its relation to pachymeningitis hemorrhagica and its surgical treatment, *Arch. Surg. (Chicago),* **11**:392, 1925.

70 Rand, C. W. and C. B. Courville: Histologic studies of the brain in cases of fatal injuries to the head. X. Multinucleation of cortical nerve cells at the margins of traumatic lesions of the human brain, *J. Neuropathol. Exp. Neurol.,* **6**:1, 1947.

71 Ransohoff, J., M. V. Benjamin, E. L. Gage, Jr., and F. Epstein: Hemicraniectomy in the management of acute subdural hematoma, *J. Neurosurg.,* **34**:70–76, January 1971.

72 Rasmussen, T. and D. R. Gulati: Cortisone in the treatment of postoperative cerebral edema, *J. Neurosurg.,* **19**:535, 1962.

73 Reivich, M., W. J. S. Marshall, and N. Kassell: *Loss of Autoregulation Produced by Cerebral Trauma in Cerebral Blood Flow,* Springer-Verlag OHG, Berlin, 1969, pp. 205–208.

74 Roger, L. A. and S. Ousterhout: Pneumonia following tracheostomy, *Am. Surg.,* **37**:39, January 1970.

75 Sanford, J. P.: Pharmocology and modes of action in relation to clinical antimicrobial therapy, *Clin. Neurosurg.,* **14**:178, 1967.

76 Schneider, R. C., G. Cherry, and H. Pantek: The syndrome of acute central cervical cord injury with special reference of mechanisms involved in hyperextension injuries of the cervical spine, *J. Neurosurg.,* **2**:546, September 1954.

77 Seddon, H. J. (ed.): *Peripheral Nerve Injuries,* Medical Research Council, Her Majesty's Stationery Office, London, 1954.

78 Sights, W. P., Jr.: Ballistic analysis of shotgun injuries to the central nervous system, *J. Neurosurg.,* **31**:25, July 1969.

79 Sparacio, R. R., T. Lin, and A. W. Cook: Methylprednisolone sodium succinate in acute craniocerebral trauma, *Surg. Gynecol. Obstet.,* **121**:513, 1965.

80 Stevenson, G. C., H. A. Brown, and W. F. Hoyt: Chronic venous epidural hematoma at the vertex, *J. Neurosurg.,* **21**:887, 1964.

81 Stritch, S. J.: Shearing of nerve fibers as a cause of brain damage due to head injury, *Lancet,* **2**:443, 1961.

82 Tator, C. H. and L. Deeche: Value of normothermic perfusion, hypothermic perfusion, and duratomy in treatment of experimental acute spinal cord fracture, *J. Neurosurg.,* **39**:52, July 1973.

83 Tindall, G. T., G. A. Meyer, and K. Iwata: Current methods for monitoring patients with head injury, *Clin. Neurosurg.,* **19**:98, 1972.

84 Walker, A. E. and S. Jablon: A follow-up study of head-injured men of World War II, *J. Neurosurg.,* **16**:600, 1959.

85 Wannamaker, G. T.: Spinal cord injuries: Review of the early treatment in 300 consecutive cases during the Korean conflict, *J. Neurosurg.,* **11**:517, 1954.

86 Wise, B. L. and N. Chater: The value of hypertonic mannitol solution in decreasing brain mass and lowering cerebrospinal-fluid pressure, *J. Neurosurg.,* **19**:1038, 1962.

Chapter 12

Trauma to the Chest

William A. Gay, Jr., M.D.
John C. McCabe, M.D.

Behind cardiovascular disease and cancer, trauma is the third leading cause of death in the United States. Major injuries of the chest are present in about 50 percent of the deaths due to trauma, and are alone responsible in another 25 percent; therefore chest injury enters into the clinical picture in about 75 percent of fatalities due to trauma.[8] When the thorax alone is injured, the mortality rate is 4 to 8 percent. If another region is involved, the mortality figures rise to about 15 percent, and if two or more additional organ systems are injured, the figure is 30 to 35 percent. Major advances in the rapid transportation of injured patients, including helicopter retrieval, and the use of highly trained and skilled paramedical personnel have resulted in the survival of many seriously injured patients long enough to reach a medical facility. This places extra responsibility upon the accident room staff to act quickly and correctly in handling the seriously injured patient. Delayed or incorrect diagnoses or treatment may be a major factor in the mortality and morbidity in the chest trauma victim.

As can be appreciated from the above statistics, many of the patients with chest injuries also have other serious injuries, and, of course, proper priority must be given to those which may be rapidly fatal. A rapid assessment can be made at the time of the patient's initial evaluation, which would very likely detect the presence of any chest problem requiring immediate treatment (Table 12-1).

Table 12-1: Chest Trauma: Initial Evaluation

Assess adequacy of airway.

Check pulse and blood pressure.

Control any significant external bleeding.

Inspect the totally exposed chest.

Listen to heart sounds.

Listen for bilateral breath sounds.

Palpate upper and lower extremity pulses.

Assurance of a patent and adequate airway is, of course, paramount and can easily be determined by merely placing the examiner's ear close to the patient's nose and mouth and listening to the exchange of air. Sometimes clearing the oropharynx of blood and mucus will improve the exchange of air dramatically. Endotracheal entubation is rarely necessary at this point, and must not be done indiscriminately. Serious and sometimes lethal complications can result from well-intended, but ill-advised, attempts to entubate an awake, frightened, combative patient who may have a cervical spine injury or a ruptured trachea or a full stomach, any of which could lead to disaster. If, however, entubation is necessary under these circumstances, it should be done expeditiously by the most expert person available at the time. If there is any question of cervical spine injury, tracheostomy rather than orotracheal (or nasotracheal) entubation may be preferable. Should there be the possibility of rib fractures on either (or both) sides of the chest, intercostal tubes should be placed (most easily by the trocar technique, using a No. 24 to No. 30 French, and in the fourth to sixth interspace in the anterior axillary line) and connected to water seal units. The reason for this is that should positive pressure ventilation be required, the lung surface may very well be torn by a jagged rib

edge, resulting in a rapidly fatal tension pneumothorax.

Once an adequate airway is assured, *the blood pressure and pulse taken and recorded,* and any significant *externally obvious bleeding controlled,* the *entire chest should be carefully inspected while totally exposed.* In this way any penetrations should be obvious, as would an open sucking wound. Paradoxical motion of a flail segment should be noted, as should the symmetry of motion of the two hemithoraxes. Of course, an open sucking wound should be covered with a petroleum gauze dressing, and an intercostal catheter placed and connected to a water seal system. *The quality of the heart sounds should then be assessed.* Occasionally, relief of tamponade by pericardiocentesis or open thoracotomy can be lifesaving in instances where hypotension, tachycardia, and distant heart sounds occur.[3,4,9] *Breath sounds should then be evaluated bilaterally.* If the patient is ventilating well, no intercostal catheters should be placed, even if breath sounds are absent on one side, until an x-ray can be obtained. For example, absent breath sounds on the left side may be due to the presence of abdominal organs in the chest because of a torn or ruptured diaphragm. *The presence and quality of upper and lower extremity pulses should then be assessed.* If the injury has been a deceleration-type or a severe blunt blow to the anterior chest and the pulses in the lower extremities are diminished or absent, one must think of a traumatic rupture or tear of the aorta and proceed to treat this entity as described later in this chapter. If the pulses, however, are full and equal, if all the other steps in this initial evaluation are completed satisfactorily, and if the immediately life-threatening injuries often associated with major chest trauma have been evaluated and cared for, the other, less urgent injuries may be evaluated and treated.

Since an injury to the chest which appears, at first, to be minor and inconsequential may very rapidly prove to be major and potentially fatal, all persons sustaining significant chest trauma should be admitted to a facility where skilled personnel and adequate monitoring equipment are present (such as a trauma unit or intensive care unit). After the patient has arrived in the trauma unit, appropriate monitoring devices are applied (Table 12-2). These consist of at least a continuous display of the patient's electrocardiogram and arterial blood pressure; other data such as pulmonary arterial (and wedge) pressures as recorded through a flow-guided catheter[45] and frequently determined cardiac outputs using the thermal dilution technique[26] should be available for patients in whom these measurements seem appropriate. A blood gas laboratory which is staffed round-the-clock is a must in caring for seriously injured patients, since important therapeutic decisions are often based on changes in arterial blood gas values. Similarly, facilities for taking, developing, and viewing portable x-rays should be readily available in the area where patients with chest injuries are kept. Although all of these aids to assessing the patient's condition are of great value, there is no substitute for frequent and thorough clinical evaluations by the same observer in order that subtle changes which may occur might be recognized and appropriate therapy begun.

Table 12-2: Chest Trauma: Monitoring

Arterial pressure

Electrocardiogram

Pulmonary artery
  (and wedge) pressure

Cardiac output

Urine output

Arterial blood gases

Protable chest films

BLUNT TRAUMA: NONCARDIOVASCULAR

Rigidly defined, blunt trauma consists of an injury in which there is no communication between the organs of the chest and the outside resulting from the primary impact. The thorax is rather uniquely constructed to serve two functions: provide maximum protection for the organs within and allow movement enough for adequate ventilation to take place (Fig. 12-1). When blunt trauma of the chest is sustained, the extent of injury to the chest wall and the structures within depends upon (1) the magnitude and direction of the force, (2) the area over which the force is applied, and (3) the duration of the force. It has been estimated that the average adult male chest wall can withstand a force of 275 kg for up to a minute, and a force of 500 kg for a fraction of a second. The force of impact of a chest striking a steering post in an automobile collision varies considerably with the weight of the person, the speed of the automobile, and the distance the chest traveled before striking the steering post, but this figure can be over 1300 kg. The thoracic wall and its contents, however, tolerate impacts in this frontal direction much better than in a saggital or longitudinal direction (such as in a fall or jump). It is, therefore, important for the evaluating physician to obtain as much information as possible concerning the mechanism of injury. The great majority of deaths resulting from blunt trauma are due to one of three causes: respiratory failure due to either a ventilatory problem (chest wall injury) or inadequate gas exchange (parenchymal lung damage); hemorrhage due to damage of a major vessel or the heart itself; or injury to other organ systems, usually outside the chest (Table 12-3).

Chest Wall: Ribs, Sternum, Clavicle, and Scapula

Fractures of the bones of the thorax are usually the result of directly applied blunt trauma; however, rib fractures may result

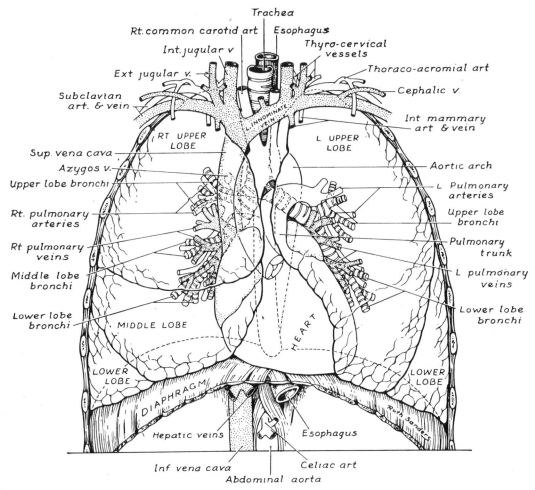

Figure 12-1 Anatomy of the thorax and its contents [*from Shaw, R. R. and Webb W. R. in G. T. Shires (ed). Care of the Trauma Patient, 1/e, McGraw-Hill, New York, 1966.*]

Table 12-3: Blunt Chest Trauma: Causes of Mortality

Respiratory failure
    Ventilatory (chest wall)
    Gas exchange (lung parenchyma)
    Both ventilatory and gas exchange

Exsanguinating hemorrhage

Damage to extrathoracic organs

---

from strenuous coughing in elderly or debilitated patients, or, of course, pathologic fractures may occur in bones affected by malignant disease. Fractures of the clavicle are fairly common in contact sports and are usually reasonably simple to treat with a figure-of-eight bandage which is applied in such a manner as to pull both shoulders backward, reestablishing length and alignment of the clavicle. One should also be wary of the possibility of injury to the underlying subclavian vessels by bone fragments. Although most dislocations involving the clavicle occur at the distal end and involve the acromion, a potentially lethal situation can occur in the setting of a sternoclavicular dislocation with posterior displacement of the clavicular head. In this instance the head of the clavicle rides beneath the sternum and may compress the trachea, resulting in severe embarrassment of respiration, which demands immediate relief. Prompt reduction of the dislocation and relief of tracheal compression may be accomplished by forcefully pulling both shoulders backward, a maneuver which can be lifesaving.

Isolated rib fractures are usually very painful, but rarely serious, injuries. Most often the patient can localize the fracture by pointing to the painful area, and this can be confirmed by careful palpation. The fracture site is exquisitely tender, and, occasionally, movement and/or crepitation can be felt. Chest x-rays should be made in all instances of suspected rib fracture, not only to document the fracture, but also to evaluate the possibility of intrathoracic pathology such as pneumothorax or hemopneumothorax. Rib fractures may not be evident on conventional posteroanterior (PA) and lateral chest films, and overpenetrated, oblique, or "spot" films may be necessary. In the absence of significant intrathoracic injury, the treatment of simple rib fractures is largely symptomatic, consisting of relief of pain and provision for adequate ventilation. In many instances oral or parenteral analgesics (most often narcotic) will suffice. The splinting which occurs in association with the pain of ventilation can cause significant lowering of tidal volume, resulting in hypoxia and hypercardia as well as the risk of subsequent atelectasis and pneumonia. It is gratifying to observe the increase in tidal volume and ability' to clear secretions when the "edge" has been taken off the pain. Care must be taken, however, not to give doses of analgesics which may result in respiratory depression. Intercostal nerve block with long-acting local anesthetics

such as 0.5% bupivacaine (Marcain) can be quite effective as an alternative, or a supplement, to the oral and parenteral analgesics in pain control.[30] These blocks may be repeated as necessary. Strapping or taping of the chest is to be avoided except as a first aid until some other method of pain relief can be obtained. Taping and strapping restrict the motion of the chest and may worsen any ventilatory insufficiency and, if continued for a prolonged period, contribute to the development of atelectasis.

Follow-up chest films should be obtained for several days after the initial injury, because a badly contused lung may appear nearly normal on initial x-rays, progressing to maximum severity in 48 to 72 h.[36] It is worth remembering that the finding of a fracture of the first rib, although rarely seen as an isolated injury, usually denotes that there is serious injury of either nearby or distant (cranial or abdominal) structures.[39] Fractures of the first rib, however, can be iatrogenic, occurring on the opposite side if excessive force is used in removing the upper ribs during a thoracoplasty. Like fractures of the first rib, fractures of the scapula usually mean that massive force has been applied, and intrathoracic injury must be carefully excluded.

Dislocations of the ribs at their anterior cartilaginous joint is a common result of blunt trauma. Like a rib fracture, the primary problem is one of pain. Most often the dislocation reduces itself, and the diagnosis is made by the history of trauma and the finding of tenderness at the affected costochondral joint. Occasionally the painful dislocation persists, and surgical excision of the overriding rib segment is required. Because of the risk of inducing a persistent chondritis in the costal cartilage, the temptation to inject the dislocation site with local anesthetics and/or steroids should be resisted.

Fracture of the sternum is uncommon, but may result from severe blunt trauma to the anterior chest, such as steering wheel injuries. When it occurs, it is often associated with rib fractures or costochondral dislocations. Cardiac contusions may also be seen in patients with sternal fractures.

The diagnosis is usually easily made by combining the history of significant anterior chest trauma with the finding of tenderness and abnormal motion or crepitation over the sternum. If the fracture edges are overriding, the diagnosis is more obvious. Confirmatory oblique films of the chest are warranted, as are standard PA and lateral views. Serial electrocardiograms should be monitored in patients whose clinical cause might suggest the presence of significant myocardial contusion.[35,36]

In most instances symptomatic treatment consisting of relief of pain is all that is required. If the segments override, hyperextension of the chest such as might be accomplished with a dorsocervical back brace may achieve satisfactory alignment. If not, operative fixation using longitudinal pins may be required.

Although somewhat less common than after penetrating trauma, tears or avulsions of the diaphragm resulting in herniation of abdominal contents into the chest can occur following major blunt trauma to the chest and abdomen. This type of injury can be a cause of acute respiratory embarrassment or, on occasion, may be responsible for late complications such as bowel strangulation or intestinal obstruction many years after the initial incident. The left hemidiaphragm is involved in most instances (98 percent), but ruptures of the right side have been reported.[18] The usual site of the tear is in the central portion of diaphragm, but avulsion from the anterior chest wall can occur.[21]

In most reported series of traumatic ruptures of the diaphragm, emphasis is placed upon the frequency with which the diagnosis is missed or delayed, sometimes with serious consequences. The most important factor in making the diagnosis is to think of the possibility of diaphragmatic rupture in patients sustaining major thoracoabdominal trauma. Physical findings may vary, but in those patients who may require urgent surgery there is usually tachycardia, hypotension, and dyspnea which may seem disproportionate to the magnitude of the other injuries. Breath sounds will be diminished or absent on the affected side (nearly always the left). In the acute situation the presence of bowel sounds in the chest is unlikely, because of the paralytic ileus which almost certainly accompanies the injury. The left hemidiaphragm is usually obscure on chest films, and there may be opacification of the lower hemothorax with slight shifting of the mediastinal structures to the opposite side. The temptation to insert an intercostal catheter should be resisted until diaphragmatic rupture has been ruled out. This may be simply done by passing a radiopaque nasogastric tube[31] (Fig. 12-2) or obtaining overpenetrated x-rays, which may reveal typical bowel gas patterns in the chest.

Early operative repair is indicated for diaphragmatic tears. However, the patient's overall condition should be stabilized first if this is possible. It is rare that any significant complication results from a delay of a few hours while other, more urgent, conditions are evaluated and stabilized. In the acute situation the authors recommend that, unless there is other intrathoracic injury which may require attention, exploration and repair be carried out using the abdominal approach. The reason for this is that there are commonly associated intraabdominal injuries which may be more completely evaluated and effectively treated from within the abdomen. When diaphragmatic injury is discovered late after trauma, the transthoracic route is perferable, because there are invariably adhesions between the bowel and the lung which are more satisfactorily handled from within the chest. The defect in the diaphragm may, most often, be

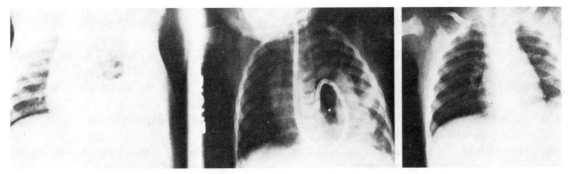

Figure 12-2 Traumatic rupture of the diaphragm with the stomach in the left chest. Radiopaque nasograstric tube documents location of stomach. *(from Melzig. E. P., et al., 1976.)*

repaired by primary suture using nonabsorbable material. If possible, the branches of the phrenic nerve should be avoided in placement of the sutures. Where primary repair without tension is not possible, Marlex mesh has been used effectively.[21]

Major blunt trauma to the chest wall frequently produces multiple rib fractures resulting in flail chest (other names include "stove-in chest," crushed chest, or crushed chest syndrome). Effective ventilation depends upon the presence of stability of the chest wall in order that air may be moved in and out of the lungs as the result of diaphragmatic descent and elastic recoil of the lung. When the chest wall is not intact (Fig. 12-3), ventilatory effectiveness is impaired. Instability results from multiple rib fractures, with the ribs being fractured in more than one place. Steering wheel trauma is a common cause of this type of injury. Flail segments usually occur either anteriorly or laterally because the posterior chest wall is both protected and stabilized by the heavy posterior musculature and the scapula. Therefore, even if multiple posterior fractures occur, instability of the chest wall rarely results.

The physiologic effects of flail chest depend not only upon the results of the flail segment, but also upon the magnitude and type of injury to the lung and the presence of other major intrathoracic injury. The overall effect of the injury, therefore, may be the result of decreased tidal volume from the chest wall injury, increased alveolar-arterial oxygen gradient from the contused lung, and the decreased oxygen-carrying capacity of the contracted blood volume from significant hemorrhage. All of these factors must, therefore, be considered when making decisions regarding ther-

Figure 12-3 An unstable segment of chest wall due to fracture of four ribs, each at two places, with the resulting paradoxical motion during respiration. *(from Ebert, P. A., 1967.)*

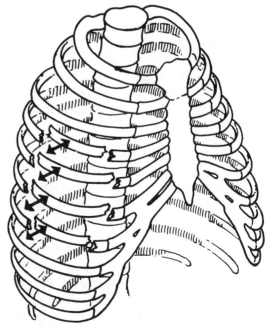

apy. The two important principles to keep in mind as aims of therapy in this type of injury are: (1) full expansion of both lungs and (2) adequate alveolar ventilation.[25] If these criteria can be met, the likelihood of the patient surviving is great, so long as the accompanying injuries are not too serious.

Because of intense spasm of the chest wall musculature overlying the fractures, the flail segment may not be immediately obvious. As the muscles tire along with the overall fatigue experienced by the patient, who is working hard to maintain adequate ventilation, the paradoxical motion of the affected chest wall segment will show itself. If the patient's condition permits, chest x-rays should be taken, not so much to document the number and location of the ribs involved as to ascertain the presence of concomitant injury to the heart or great vessels, to get a baseline view of the status of the lungs, and to detect the presence of pneumothorax or hemopneumothorax. If immediate ventilatory assistance is required before x-rays can be obtained, it is advisable that bilateral chest tubes be placed in order to avoid the possibility of tension pneumothorax due to a lung laceration from inflating the lung forcibly against a jagged rib fracture site. Most patients do not require this and will breathe better after having some of their pain relieved by intercostal nerve block and/or the judicious use of small doses of narcotics.

All patients with multiple rib fractures should be admitted to a trauma unit or intensive care unit (ICU) facility where close, frequent observation is possible. Initial blood laboratory work, in addition to the usual complete blood count (CBC), blood urea nitrogen (BUN), and electrolytes, should include arterial blood gases. In order to facilitate the repetitive drawing of arterial blood for gases and to provide a continuous display of arterial blood pressure, a plastic catheter may be inserted into a radial artery and connected to a pressure transducer and suitable monitoring device. In addition, continuous display of the electrocardiogram is desirable, as is the use of the Swan-Ganz catheter for measurement of pulmonary arterial and capillary wedge pressures as an aid to volume replacement. Some of these flow-guided catheters are fitted with thermistor tips in order to obtain frequent measurements of cardiac output using the thermal dilution technique. Although all the monitoring equipment and frequently determined laboratory values are of considerable value, there is no substitute for frequent personal observations of the patient made by the same examiner. One must remember that the patient with chest trauma of this magnitude is certainly a prime candidate to have significant injuries of other organ systems, which may not have been obvious initially, but which could present at any time. Therefore, the repeated examinations should include an evaluation of the abdomen and extremities and a brief neurologic assessment in addition to determining the status of the already recognized thoracic injury.

There are several effective methods of treating the patient with a flail chest, and the method chosen by individual physicians will depend on such factors as: the age and overall condition of the patient in addition to the severity of the injury, the familiarity of the physician with the methods of treatment and the physician's comfort in utilizing each, and the availability of the equipment and personnel to effectively carry out each method of treatment. For example, the authors agree with Trinkle[49] and his associates, who feel that many of these patients may be effectively managed without mechanical ventilation with improved survival, lessened morbidity, and shortened hospitalization. The selection of this type of treatment, however, places a heavy burden upon the nurses and ICU residents to not only provide intensive pulmonary care but also to make crucial decisions as to when and if to abandon this course of treatment. The use of internal stabilization by endotracheal entubation and mechanical ventilation using a volume-cycled respirator remains the most popular method of treating flail chest injuries[16] and remains the standard against which others must be judged. There is little disagreement that this type of therapy is effective, but there is also little doubt that it is associated with some degree of morbidity and a prolongation of hospitalization in most instances.[49] Operative stabilization[30] of rib fractures using intramedullary pinning of the ribs, sternum, and costal cartilages has proved effective in selected instances. Proponents claim that tracheostomy and mechanical ventilation can often be avoided (or its duration shortened), analgesic requirements can be lessened, and permanent chest wall deformity can be lessened or avoided.

The authors believe the regimen described by Trinkle[49] et al. to be an effective method in managing patients with flail chest injuries (Table 12-4). After the patient has been admitted to the unit, baseline arterial gases are drawn and pain is controlled with small IV doses of narcotics or with intercostal nerve blocks. Fluid administration during resuscitation is

Table 12-4: Blunt Chest Trauma: Management of Flail Chest

Fluid restriction

Diuretics

Steroids

Colloids

Replace blood loss

Intensive pulmonary toilet

Broad-spectrum antibiotics

Control pain

Nasal (mask) oxygen

Entubate and ventilate
  PaO_2 less than 60 mmHg
  $PaCO_2$ greater than 45 mmHg

kept to 100 mL, and then 50 mL/h is given thereafter. Lasix 40 mg IV is given immediately and daily thereafter. Methyl prednisolone 500 mg IV is given immediately and every 6 h for 2 or 3 days. Colloids in the form of plasma or albumin are given daily, and blood loss is replaced with whole blood. Intensive pulmonary therapy with endotracheal suctioning, cupping, posturing, humidification, and incentive spirometry is provided. Intravenously administered broad-spectrum antibiotics are given for a minimum of 5 days. If infection develops, appropriate cultures are taken and specific antibacterial agents used as dictated by sensitivity studies. Control of pain with morphine IV in small doses or intercostal nerve blocks aids the patient in helping him- or herself. Humidified nasal or mask oxygen may be used to maintain Pa_{O_2} at levels of 80 to 100 mmHg. If the Pa_{O_2} falls below 60 mmHg of room air (or less than 80 mmHg with supplemental oxygen) or if the Pa_{CO_2} rises above 45 mmHg, endotracheal entubation and mechanical ventilation with a volume-cycled respirator should be carried out.[49] If entubation—either nasal, oral, or tracheostomy—is necessary, a tube fitted with a high-volume, low-pressure cuff should be used to avoid the possibility of cuff-induced tracheal injuries.[12] Ventilator settings should be made so as to provide for a Pa_{O_2} of 80 to 100 mmHg and a Pa_{CO_2} of 30 to 40 mmHg, with all attempts being made to avoid inspired oxygen concentrations (FI_{O_2}) above 50. Positive end expiratory pressure (PEEP) may be utilized if it does not result in excessive hemodynamic disturbance.

A patient who is being ventilated for flail chest should be on *controlled, not assisted,* ventilation. Since controlled ventilation is desired, if there are no contraindications, the use of paralyzing agents such as curare may be quite helpful not only in preventing the patient from "fighting" the respirator, but also in decreasing the overall body oxygen consumption by blocking neuromuscular activity, resulting in an improvement in Pa_{O_2}. In addition, the use of mild hypothermia (35°C) by using a cooling blanket also decreases oxygen consumption, but shivering must be carefully prevented. Once mechanical ventilation has been instituted, it is probably best to leave the patient on controlled ventilation for at least 4 to 5 days without repeated attempts at weaning the patient from support. However, this must be individualized, as some patients require only a short period of "rest" on the ventilator and are then ready to breathe on their own.

Although the extent of damage to the chest wall is generally obvious within a few hours following injury, the underlying lung may mask its degree of pathology for several days.[36] A badly contused lung may not be clinically evident for 24 to 48 h after the initial injury, at which time it may appear as an area of consolidation on the chest film and may interfere significantly with gas exchange. Lung contusion is generally a self-limited condition which resolves itself and requires only that the patient be supported until resolution occurs. Steroids and antibiotics are always indicated, and mechanical ventilatory support may be used if needed (Table 12-4). Meticulous attention to bronchial toilet will lessen the likelihood of serious complications such as atelectasis and pneumonia.

If blunt trauma to the chest results in a pneumothorax or hemopneumothorax, an intercostal catheter should be inserted at the earliest opportunity in order to achieve full expansion of the lung and complete emptying of the pleural space. In addition, continuing hemorrhage may also be detected by monitoring the drainage from the intercostal tube. If the lung is fully expanded, the pleural space is dry, and the continuing drainage is minimal, the intercostal tube has done its job. If, on the other hand, the lung does not fully reexpand, the pleural space does not empty completely, and/or the chest drainage reaches 1500 mL

total (or continues at 100 mL/h or more for 12 h) early thoracotomy is indicated.[28] At thoracotomy clotted blood should be evacuated, lung lacerations or tears should be loosely sutured, resection of lung tissue should be avoided if at all possible, bleeding chest wall vessels should be ligated, and major cardiac or great vessel injuries should be managed as described later in this chapter. Full expansion of the lung and complete evacuation of the thoracic cavity is the aim of treatment and, when accomplished, will contribute much toward avoiding possible long-term complications.

If there is an unusually large air leak, a significant pneumomediastinum, worsening subcutaneous emphysema, or unexplained failure of a lung to reexpand, injury to the trachea or a major bronchus should be strongly suspected.[7,19,23] Most patients with tears of the trachea or main bronchus also have hemoptysis and dyspnea. The diagnosis is made by bronchoscopy, where precise localization of the tear is the key in planning surgical correction. Tears of the intrathoracic trachea and the right bronchus are best approached from the right side, and the left bronchus is best repaired via a left thoracotomy. The tear should be meticulously repaired, sometimes freshening up the jagged edges a bit, and the suture line covered with a pleural flap or other available autologous material (pericardium, omentum, etc.). Resection of lung tissue is to be avoided. Although tears of the main-stem bronchi may heal and stop leaking spontaneously, the general result is stenosis or occlusion of the bronchus, eventually leading to the destruction of the involved lung.

Of all the important structures within the thorax, the one which is best protected from blunt traumatic injury is the esophagus, but vertical tears may occur. When mediastinal or cervical emphysema is seen, esophagoscopy should be done if bronchoscopy has failed to reveal the etiology. Treatment consists of primary suture repair with wide drainage, as in any esophageal tear.

Traumatic Asphyxia

Traumatic asphyxia (cervicofacial static cyanosis)[42] is an unusual condition which consists of a swollen, violaceous discoloration of the upper chest, neck, arms, and face, along with bulging of the eyes and, sometimes, subconjunctival hemorrhages. These findings are produced by prolonged, severe compression of the lower chest such as might occur during a dirt cave-in or when the victim is pinned beneath a heavy object lying across the chest. The thoracic compression results in obstruction of cardiac venous return, which then causes the massive edema and extravasation of venous blood into the tissues. The edema and reddish purple discoloration of the neck and face make the diagnosis obvious. Occasionally, brain hemorrhages result from the venous stasis, with varying degrees of generalized or focal neurologic sequelae from mild agitation to coma and death. The rather striking cutaneous manifestations of the condition will resolve themselves, and any treatment is directed toward associated injuries and conditions.

BLUNT TRAUMA: CARDIOVASCULAR

Nonpenetrating Cardiac Injuries

Blunt injury to the heart has been sporadically reported for several centuries, but this entity was not clearly documented until 1935, when Bright and Beck collected 175 cases.[11] An increasing awareness of this condition has led to the current estimate that one-fifth of patients sustaining crush injuries of the chest will have cardiac damage. A variety of cardiac lesions may result from blunt trauma, including myocardial contusion and free rupture, ventricular septal defect, injury to valves and their supporting structure, disruption and

thrombosis of coronary arteries, and damage to the pericardium.

High-speed vehicular impact resulting in rapid deceleration accounts for the overwhelming majority of blunt cardiac injuries. Falls from great heights, industrial crush injuries, and blows to the chest are other causes. Injury may result from direct forces compressing the heart between the arterial chest wall and the vertebral column or indirectly from abrupt deceleration of thoracic viscera and from hydraulic force changes which result from abdominal compression. Laceration of the heart can result from fractured ends of the sternum or ribs. Although the bony cage of the thorax provides protection to the intrathoracic viscera, some of the most severe blunt cardiac injuries occur without associated rib or sternal fractures.

Myocardial Contusion Cardiac contusion is the most common injury resulting from nonpenetrating trauma to the heart. It is seen in approximately 20 percent of patients sustaining severe blunt chest trauma, but is rarely fatal.[24] The diagnosis can be easily missed unless an awareness of it exists.

Myocardial damage may vary from edema to necrosis. The surface of the heart may show subepicardial hemorrhage or appear surprisingly normal, as the area of injury can be exclusively intramural or isolated to the interventricular septum. Histological changes mimic those of myocardial infarction, although the transition from normal to abnormal muscle is more abrupt. Myocardial cell necrosis, infiltration of leukocytes, absorption of hemorrhage, and repair by fibrosis are seen. Most often, repair is complete, but with myocardial infarction, muscle necrosis can result in free rupture, ventricular aneurysm, or ventricular septal defect. A diseased heart is more prone to extensive damage from blunt trauma than is a normal one.

Cardiac contusions are among the most

frequently missed or delayed diagnoses because: (1) multiple injuries direct attention elsewhere, (2) there is often little evidence of thoracic injury and, (3) signs of cardiac injury may not be present on initial examination.

The diagnostic features of cardiac contusion are essentially those of acute myocardial infarction. The most accurate method of establishing the diagnosis is by electrocardiography. ST- and T-wave changes similar to those of myocardial ischemia and/or infarction are observed. Serial electrocardiograms (ECG) are necessary, as the initial ECG may be normal. Most injury current changes are apparent by 48 h. These ECG changes are generally reversible, but may take weeks to resolve. Permanent changes do occur and are related to more severe injury with myocardial scarring. Arrhythmias—specifically premature ventricular contractions, varying degrees of heart block, ventricular tachyarrhythmias, and supraventricular arrhythmias—frequently accompany myocardial bruising. Preexisting heart disease may make electrocardiographic diagnosis impossible.

Elevation of serum enzymes (SGOT, LDH, CPK) are usually seen, but are of little value in the presence of multisystem injury. It is possible that the CPK isoenzyme, MB-CPK, will be more specific of myocardial injury. Enzyme determinations take on a greater significance in the absence of associated injuries.

Patients with myocardial contusion frequently complain of anginalike chest pain, but this is difficult to distinguish from pain originating in musculoskeletal injuries of the chest wall. Tachycardia is an important early finding in the absence of other injuries, but is not specific in the severely injured patient. A pericardial friction rub is often heard, but this tends to occur later in the course after inflammation of the pericardium occurs. A collection of blood in the pericardium may result in frank tamponade, but this is uncommon in simple contusion. Severe contusions resulting in depressed myocardial function may produce cardiogenic shock. These extensive lesions may also lead to delayed rupture of the heart or to formation of ventricular aneurysm.

The treatment of uncomplicated myocardial contusion is essentially that of acute myocardial infarction. Complete bed rest and oxygen therapy should be instituted until electrocardiographic changes revert to normal or stabilize, at which time progressive ambulation is begun. Anticoagulation should be avoided because of frequent associated injuries. Cardiac failure and arrhythmias require appropriate drug therapy. Coronary vasodilators have been ineffective in relieving pain, but may be used in an attempt to preserve marginal myocardium. Hypovolemia from associated injuries and, conversely, fluid overload should be avoided, as they may have a cumulative depressant effect on myocardial dysfunction resulting from the contusion. A Swan-Ganz catheter can accurately indicate the optimal filling pressure in this setting. Intraaortic balloon counterpulsation may provide needed support in the rare patient with a low output state from extensive cardiac contusion.

Complications of cardiac contusion such as free rupture, ventricular septal defect (VSD), and aneurysm formation should be managed as those resulting from ischemic heart disease.

Cardiac Rupture Myocardial rupture is the most common cause of fatality in patients autopsied after closed thoracic trauma. Survival longer than a few minutes is rare. The right ventricle is most commonly ruptured, followed by the left ventricle, right atrium, and left atrium in decreasing frequency. As tears are usually rare, the prognosis is worse than with penetrating injury. Survival following repair of atrial tears has been documented, and probably reflects the more tolerable low pressure chamber bleeding. These patients invariably present with the signs of symptoms of cardiac tamponade. Most successful repairs of atrial tears have been done without cardio-pulmonary bypass. It is doubtful that pericar-diocentesis would be effective in this setting, although experience is limited. Rather, imme-diate thoracotomy and digital control should be employed. Atrial tears may be repaired using vascular clamps, and ventricular tears can be sutured beneath a compressing finger. If the location of the tear is such that these maneuvers are impossible, and if time permits, cardiopulmonary bypass should be employed.

Isolated interventricular septal rupture does occur; however it is more often associated with other cardiac injuries. When it is the only defect, the prognosis is related to the size of the defect and the resultant left-to-right shunt. This diagnosis should be considered when a new systolic murmur appears following blunt thoracic trauma. The holosystolic murmur is usually accompanied by a thrill and is heard best at the left third to fourth intercostal space, but it can be confused with murmurs resulting from valvular injury and those of preexisting defects. The diagnosis can be made by sampling blood from the right atrium, right ventricle, and pulmonary artery through the Swan-Ganz catheter as it is inserted and then analyzing it for oxygen concentration. An increased oxygen saturation in the ventricle or pulmonary artery makes the presence of a VSD very likely. If the patient's condition permits, formal cardiac catheterization and ventriculography should be done. Many of these patients will present in pulmonary edema with low output states due to the acute large left-to-right shunt, and these can be managed initially with after-load reduction by counterpulsation. Once the diagnosis is con-firmed, surgical repair should follow urgently in all but the smallest defects.

Repair of traumatic ventricular septal de-fect necessitates cardiopulmonary bypass. The approach to the defect may be determined by associated injuries of the right or left ventricular free wall. If no other cardiac injury is apparent, a fish-mouth incision in the left ventricular apex is most efficacious. Most traumatic septal defects are located low in the septum, making identification and repair diffi-cult from the right ventricular approach.

Damage to Valves Traumatic injury to car-diac valves is relatively rare. When it does occur, it invariably results in significant regur-gitation and cardiac failure. The valves on the left side of the heart, particularly the aortic, are more often involved because of the higher pressures.[14] Previously diseased valves seem to be more susceptible to injury, but damage can occur to a normal valve. Tears of the aortic valve are usually located along the base where the cusp attaches to the annulus or, less often, through the cusp itself. Injuries to the atrioventricular valves more frequently in-volve the papillary muscles and chordi tendini, but cusp tears do occur.

Valvular injury should be suspected when a regurgitant murmur appears after thoracic trauma. The rapidity with which congestive heart failure develops will depend on which valve is involved and the magnitude of the injury. Acute aortic or mitral regurgitation is not well tolerated. Repair of these injuries requires cardiopulmonary bypass and valve replacement. Minor cusp tears and chordal ruptures can sometimes be repaired by valvu-loplasty.

Coronary Artery Injury It is difficult to determine whether coronary artery occlusion occurs as a direct result of blunt cardiac trauma or the trauma merely brings attention to a preexisting lesion. Several instances of left anterior descending coronary artery oc-clusion in very young individuals following nonpenetrating trauma have been documented by coronary angiography.[24,44] These reports suggest that this is a real but rare entity. The diagnosis should be considered in young individuals who demonstrate persistent electrocardiographic changes of acute anterior myocardial infarction. Recovery following conservative management of traumatic coronary artery occlusion has occurred, but selected patients may benefit from coronary arteriography and aortocoronary bypass graft.

Pericardial Injury Virtually all cardiac injuries are accompanied by some degree of pericarditis. It is usually self-limited and without sequelae; however, occasionally recurrent pericarditis with effusion or constriction can develop. Pericardial laceration also occurs from blunt chest trauma. The importance of pericardial tears relates to the integrity of the pericardial barrier. A partial laceration of this barrier may allow the heart to herniate and strangulate or allow exsanguination to occur rather than tamponade. Hemopericardium generally indicates injury to the heart itself rather than to the pericardium. When severe injury to myocardium and pericardium with bleeding coexist, survival is in part dependent on the size of the pericardial rent. Small tears can allow in tamponade, whereas larger ones allow exsanguination into the pleural cavity.

Posttraumatic pericarditis usually responds to conservative measures. Rarely, pericardiotomy or pericardiectomy is indicated for recurrent effusions and constriction.

Tamponade following blunt cardiac injury requires thoracotomy. Pericardiocentesis may be employed in an attempt to gain time. Lacerations of the pericardium should be repaired or widely opened at the time of myocardial repair. Cardiac herniation is most often discovered at autopsy, but if the diagnosis is considered antemortem, immediate thoracotomy and replacement of the heart within the pericardium should follow. The pericardial rent can then be sutured or widely opened.

Nonpenetrating Great Vessel Injuries

Rupture of the Aorta Rupture of the aorta secondary to blunt trauma was described as early as the fifteenth century, but this pathologic entity was not crystalized until 1958, when Parmley and associates reported on 296 cases from the Armed Forces Institute of Pathology.[33] Most patients suffering this injury die immediately of exsanguination; in fact, only 14 percent survived for any period. Associated injuries, particularly cardiac, are common in this group and may be the cause of death. Survival for any period is dependent on containment of hemorrhage by mediastinal structures. This precarious tamponade usually results in delayed fatal hemorrhage from hours to months after the initial injury; however, false aneurysms may develop and persist for years.

The most common cause of aortic disruption is rapid deceleration resulting in extreme forces along a horizontal or vertical plane. These forces affect intrathoracic organs differently, depending on their structure, location, and attachments and the direction of the force. It is thought that the greatest strain produced by these differential forces affects the aortic isthmus, where the relatively mobile thoracic aorta joins the fixed arch, and the ascending aorta, which serves as a pendulum for the mobile heart. Direct compression and a rapid displacement of blood into the thoracic aorta by lower body compression may be additional factors in aortic injury.

The aortic isthmus just beyond the ligamentum arteriosum is by far the most common location for traumatic rupture, followed by the ascending aorta. Tears of the descending thoracic aorta, arch, and abdominal aorta are far less common, but do occur. Rarely, multiple rupture sites are encountered. The actual aortic lesion is usually a rupture in the transverse plane varying from a few millimeters to complete circumferential laceration. Most commonly they are extensive enough to be classified as transections. The injury may be limited to the intima, extend into the media, or, more frequently, involve all three layers of the aorta. Aortic dissection can result from tears limited to the intima and media. The initial hemorrhage may be contained by a remnant of tunica adventitia or by the parietal pleura when the laceration is complete. Delayed free rupture is the rule in this situation, but chronic false aneurysms may result.

Most patients with traumatic aortic rupture have other serious injuries which may dominate the clinical picture. In this setting, the prompt diagnosis of nonpenetrating aortic injury is based on a high index of suspicion following blunt trauma to the chest. The most consistent sign of a ruptured aorta is a widened mediastinum on chest roentgenogram (Fig. 12-4). In a recent review Symbas[48] suggests that a triad of signs is frequently present. The triad consists of (1) increased pulse amplitude and blood pressure in the upper extremities, (2) decreased pulse amplitude and blood pressure in the lower extremities, and (3) roentgenographic evidence of widening of the mediastinum. This acute coarctation syndrome is produced by the mediastinal hematoma compressing the aorta and possibly a ball-valve flap mechanism resulting from the torn intima and media of the distal aortic segment. Other less specific symptoms and signs of aortic rupture include chest pain, dyspnea, hoarseness, paraplegia, systolic murmur, and hemothorax. Ultimately the diagnosis must be confirmed by aortography. This should be obtained on all patients who demonstrate a widened mediastinum or who have a pressure differential between upper and lower extremities as soon as their condition permits. This study will not only establish the diagnosis, but will specifically identify the location and magnitude of the injury. The aortic tear is usually seen as a filling defect created by the elevation of aortic wall by the bloodstream.

Because of the propensity for delayed fatal hemorrhage, surgical repair of acute aortic rupture must be done urgently. The overwhelming majority of patients who survive the initial injury demonstrate tears of the isthmus. The necessity to occlude the aorta to effect repair presents certain problems: specifically, preservation of vital organs distal to the point of occlusion. The spinal cord and kidneys can be vulnerable to even brief periods of ischemia. Various methods have been used to obviate this problem, including (1) short occlusion time, (2) systemic hypothermia, (3) partial left heart bypass, (4) femorofemoral bypass, and (5) the use of shunts.

Surface-induced hypothermia to 30°C was used successfully by DeBakey and Cooley in

Figure 12-4 Transection of the aorta. *(A)* Widened superior mediastinum demonstrated on admission (AP) chest roentgenogram. *(B)* Aortogram reveals complete transection. *(from Blair, E., et al., 1969.)*

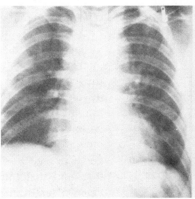 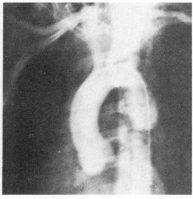

one of the earliest repairs of traumatic aneurysm, but remains of historic interest only.[15] With the advent of perfusion techniques, left atrial–femoral artery bypass and femoral vein–femoral artery bypass using interposed roller pumps and, in the latter case, an oxygenator were popularized. The major disadvantage of these techniques is that they require systemic heparinization, which is undesirable in the multiply injured patient. It also became apparent that ischemic paraplegia can occur despite the use of bypass and lower body perfusion. Because of these factors and a successful experience with aortic occlusion alone, Crawford and coworkers suggest that distal aortic perfusion is unnecessary and hazardous.[14]

An alternative approach that offers many theoretical, if not real, advantages utilizes a temporary heparin-coated shunt. This catheter, pioneered by Gott, precludes the need for systemic heparin and utilizes the left ventricle as the pump. The proximal end can be inserted in the ascending aorta or the left ventricular apex, and the distal end into the descending aorta or common femoral artery. This technique and aortic occlusion without distal perfusion currently enjoy widespread use, but which method is superior must await further experience with each.

Regardless of the technique used to preserve vital organ function, the standard approach is through a left posterolateral thoracotomy, usually the bed of the fourth rib. The aorta is cross-clamped between the left common carotid artery and the left subclavian proximally, and the descending aorta below the apparent hematoma. The aorta or hematoma is then opened, and the tear identified. At this point the occluding clamps may be moved closer to the area of rupture to allow for greater collateral flow and to prevent blood loss from intercostal arteries. Whether an interposition graft or an end-to-end repair is used will depend largely on the magnitude of the aortic wall damage. Most require the use of a woven Dacron graft.

Traumatic rupture of the ascending aorta and the arch requires cardiopulmonary bypass and some method of myocardial protection. The approach is usually through a median sternotomy. Most successful repairs in these areas have involved traumatic aneurysm of a more chronic nature.

Chronic Traumatic Aneurysm Occasionally, acute rupture of the aorta results in a chronic aortic aneurysm. These may be false aneurysms where complete transection has occurred and the pleura serves as the outmost layer, or true aneurysms where some adventitia remain. This distinction is often difficult to make, even at microscopic examination. Circumferential tears usually result in a fusiform shape, whereas limited tears cause saccular- or diverticular-type aneurysms. Both types will frequently calcify with the passage of time.

Most chronic traumatic aneurysms are asymptomatic. When symptoms do occur, they usually result from compression of surrounding structures by progressive enlargement. A widened superior mediastinum or an abnormal aortic contour on chest roentgenogram together with a history of thoracic trauma suggests this diagnosis, but angiographic studies are necessary to confirm it (Fig. 12-5).

The management of an asymptomatic chronic traumatic aneurysm is controversial because the natural history of the lesion is variable. The discovery of seemingly stable aneurysm years after trauma has resulted in the conservative approach, considering only development of symptoms or roentgenographic signs of enlargement as surgical indications. A more aggressive approach for stable chronic aneurysm is advocated by Bennett and Cherry,[6] based on instances of late rupture and instability appearing more than 10 years after injury. There is no question that

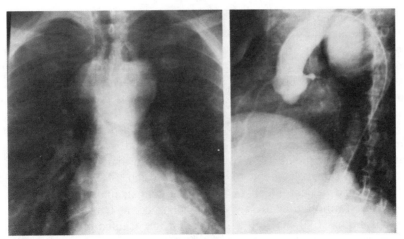

Figure 12-5 Asymptomatic chronic traumatic aortic aneurysm in 34-year-old male noted 10 years after severe deceleration accident. Plain roentgenogram shows widening of the superior mediastinum. Aneurysm distal to left subclavian demonstrated on aortogram.

symptomatic and expanding aneurysm should be resected. The treatment of stable chronic aneurysm should be individualized, depending on location, size, and patient age and condition. Traumatic aneurysms in the usual location and in good-risk patients should undergo repair, as the risk of rupture is always present. The morbidity and mortality of surgical correction in the chronic stage is much lower than immediately after injury.

Rupture of Arch Vessels Avulsion of aortic arch vessels occurs less frequently than aortic rupture. Any or all of the proximal branches can be involved and may be combined with aortic rupture. Survival is rare, but several successful repairs have been reported. The innominate artery is the most frequently involved vessel, and invariably the disruption occurs at its takeoff from the aorta. The same forces involved in aortic injury are encountered; in addition, it has been suggested that hyperextension of the cervical spine can put additional strain on this particular area. The presentation of arch vessel tears is indistinguishable from aortic rupture unless there is compromise to blood flow resulting in diminished pulses or cerebral anoxia. The diagnosis is usually confirmed and is accomplished through a median sternotomy with an oblique extension into the neck on the side of the injured vessel. Cerebral ischemia can be prevented by using a temporary aortocarotid shunt or by establishing flow through a permanent woven Dacron graft from the ascending aorta to the side of the affected carotid artery. Having accomplished this, the injured vessel is excised and its stumps oversewn or repaired directly using a partial occluding clamp on the aorta and a fully occluding clamp on the injured vessel proximal to the shunt. If time does not permit the use of a shunt, repair can be accomplished without one, accepting a slightly higher risk of cerebral complication. Proximal subclavian injuries should be repaired rather than ligated to preclude the possibility of a steal syndrome.

PENETRATING TRAUMA: NONCARDIOVASCULAR

Penetrating wounds of the chest may be conveniently divided into three categories which reflect their severity and, consequently, the urgency with which they must be treated. First is the patient in extremis in whom therapy must be started immediately upon arrival in the emergency room. Second is the responsive but severely injured patient who may be hypotensive and tachypneic but in whom there is adequate time to assess the injury. Third is the patient whose vital signs are normal but whose penetrating chest injury must be totally evaluated to obviate any serious sequelae. For patients in the first of these categories some authorities would recommend pericardiocentesis as an initial procedure for both diagnosis and treatment;[3,9,25] the authors feel that immediate exploration of the chest and pericardium via a left thoracotomy is needed.[4,28,41,43] The patient in extremis with a penetrating injury of the chest should have the chest opened in the accident room with ventilation being provided by the quickest and most readily available method (usually a face mask and an Ambu bag). This incision is easily and quickly made and affords reasonable exposure to the left lung and its hilar structures as well as to the heart and pericardium. Manual cardiac massage may be effectively performed and sites of major bleeding can be identified and controlled so that other resuscitative measures may be instituted. Patients in the second category will most likely require operation, but it can be a planned, definitive procedure done under more sterile and stable conditions.[28] Patients in the third category may require no more than a thorough and comprehensive evaluation with early follow-up examination in order to exclude the possibility of serious intrathoracic injury.

At the time of initial evaluation an accurate history of the injury is desirable. This should include the type of material which penetrated the chest, its approximate trajectory, and an estimate of its speed. This information will give the examiner an idea of the likelihood of intrathoracic injury, the structures possibly involved, and the severity of their injury. For example, although the wound of entrance may be the same for both, a high-velocity missile is more likely to result in severe intrathoracic injuries than one of a lower velocity. If the penetrating object is still protruding through the chest wall at the time of evaluation, such as a knife or sharp metal fragment, it should not be removed until the patient is in the operating room and ready for immediate exploration. Much of what has been learned regarding management of penetrating chest trauma has come from combat experiences, since wartime trauma provides an abundance of this type injury.[40]

These principles are also applicable in treating similar injuries in civilian trauma (Table 12-5) and will result in the fewest possible complications. Complete evacuation of blood from the chest by means of an intercostal tube serves several important functions: it permits full expansion of the lung, it allows the evaluation of the underlying lung for possible injury, and it makes continued bleeding obvious so that operative intervention, when indicated, will not be delayed. Primary closure of obviously contaminated wounds or wounds involving extensive damage to chest wall musculature is never a good practice, as it is an open invitation to potential serious infection.

Table 12-5: Penetrating Chest Trauma: Principles of Management

Early and complete drainage of hemothorax, including early thoracotomy if necessary.

Debridement and secondary closure of external wounds.

Antibiotics.

Avoid resecting lung tissue if possible.

Use physiotherapy liberally.

Avoid prolonged mechanical ventilation.

Instead, this type wound should be debrided thoroughly, the deeper layers approximated to reestablish integrity of the chest wall, and secondary closure of the skin and superficial tissues done at a later date. Antibiotic coverage should include penicillin plus a broad-spectrum agent, and, as in any penetrating wound, tetanus prophylaxis should be given. If thoracotomy is required for any reason, pulmonary tissue should be resected only if it is obviously devitalized, because even the most badly contused lung will likely regain full function. Physiotherapy and meticulous attention to bronchial toilet will prevent many complications and will enable the patient's recovery time to be significantly shortened. If mechanical ventilation is required, its use, unlike in the patient with the crushed or flail chest, should be brief, and attempts to wean the patient from ventilatory support should begin early.

Penetrating Wounds of the Chest Wall

When an open or sucking wound of the chest is present, an airtight dressing is applied and an intercostal tube inserted at another site. If the open area is extensive, such as might be seen in association with a close-range shotgun blast, endotracheal entubation, controlled ventilation, and immediate operation is required.

Less extensive wounds of the chest wall either with or without pleural penetration may require only local treatment and observation of the patient for several days. In the absence of pneumothorax, pleural puncture may be detected by injection of radiographic contrast material into the wound tract just as has been described in penetrating abdominal wounds.[13] If the pleura has not been entered and there are no other serious injuries, the patient may not require hospitalization. On the other hand, if penetration of the pleura has taken place, observation of the patient with repeated x-rays and exams over a 2- to 3-day interval is warranted. Should a pneumothorax or hemopneumothorax develop, it should be managed as described below.

Penetrations of the Lung

When pneumothorax or hemopneumothorax is present, an intercostal tube of reasonably large size (No. 28 to No. 34 French) should be inserted and connected to a water seal drainage and moderate suction (15 cmH$_2$O). The purpose of the tube is to aid in achieving complete expansion of the lung and total evacuation of the pleural space. A properly placed and well-functioning chest tube will also prevent the possibility of tension pneumothorax and will provide an hourly record of any continuing blood loss. Just as in the patient with either bleeding or air leak (or both) due to blunt trauma, frequent chest films and repeated examinations of the patient along with periodic checks of arterial blood gases and hematocrit are necessary. A large air leak with failure to fully expand the lung or the development of subcutaneous emphysema which becomes progressively worse may indicate injury to the trachea or a major bronchus, and bronchoscopy is indicated. If one of these conditions is present, early primary suture repair is required. Should the lung fail to totally expand because of a clotted hemothorax or should active bleeding continue at a rate of 100 mL/h for 15 h or more, surgical exploration of the chest to loosely suture the edges of a lacerated lung or remove a large intrathoracic clot or suture ligate a bleeding chest wall vessel should be done without further delay. Resection of lung tissue should be avoided unless it has been badly fragmented or is the source of uncontrollable bleeding or air leak. Resection of lung tissue leaves a potential space within the pleural cavity, with the ever present possibility of opportunistic infection taking place.

Penetrations of the Diaphragm

Penetrating wounds of the chest and upper abdomen may create a defect in the diaphragm, allowing abdominal organs to herniate into the chest. This occurs almost exclusively (98 percent) on the left side since the liver usually seals perforations of the right hemidiaphragm rapidly. Unless the diaphragmatic defect is large, herniation may not occur right away, and the defect may be missed unless the patient undergoes surgical exploration for other reasons.[27] Therefore, it is always advisable to evaluate the integrity of the diaphragm when exploration of the chest or abdomen is undertaken because of penetration of either of these areas. These hernias may lie dormant for many months or years and present with obstruction and strangulation as a late complication.[18,27] The diagnosis of herniation of abdominal contents into the chest may not be as simple as one may expect. In the acute situation, for example, a paralytic ileus will obscure auscultatory findings, and the chest film resembles a hemothorax. With a penetrating injury anywhere in the vicinity of the diaphragm and the finding of a left hemothorax on chest x-ray, an overpenetrated view is indicated before placing a chest tube. The density in the left chest may be small bowel rather than blood, a finding which would most likely be revealed by overpenetrated films. If the diagnosis is made in the acute stage, surgical repair should be undertaken without delay once the patient's overall condition permits. If the wound of entrance is in the abdomen, a transabdominal route is preferable so as to afford maximum opportunity to search for other intraabdominal pathology. The hernia is reduced from below, and the diaphragmatic defect repaired primarily with nonabsorbable sutures. If the entrance wound is in the chest, a thoracotomy offers a better approach since any attendant lung or cardiac involvement may be easily recognized and treated. A limited exploration of the upper abdomen through the diaphragm may be carried out or, if needed, a separate abdominal incision made. If the wound in the diaphragm is large and the edges ragged, it may be cautiously debrided and the defect closed with Marlex mesh. If the hernia has progressed to chronicity and the diaphragmatic defect discovered months or years after the initial injury, the transthoracic route is preferable since there are usually adhesions between the bowel and the lung which are more easily handled through the chest. The diaphragmatic repair is handled the same way as in the acute situation.

Perforations of the esophagus due to external penetrating trauma occurs rarely, as it is instrumental (iatrogenic) injury which remains the most common source of perforating injuries. Whenever the trajectory of a penetrating object carries to the posterior mediastinum or whenever there is an otherwise unexplained pneumothorax or pneumomediastinum, perforation of the esophagus must be considered. Early recognition and effective treatment is often lifesaving, and delay may cause severe disability or even death.

The diagnosis of instrumental performation is usually obvious, often suspected at the time the procedure is done and confirmed by the presence of mediastinal, cervical, or intrapleural air as a new finding following endoscopy. Cervical tears are usually best treated by simple drainage. Intrathoracic perforations should be repaired by primary suture, with the mediastinum thoroughly drained via the adjacent pleural cavity. Early repair is mandatory because delay usually results in severe mediastinitis or empyema, which, in addition to being a life-threatening event in itself, results in maceration and necrosis of the torn esophagus, making later repair difficult or impossible.

When esophageal perforation is suspected in external penetrating wounds, the diagnosis may be substantiated in several ways. If there is a draining chest catheter, having the patient ingest a little charcoal or even some water soluble food coloring will often stain the drainage enough to make the diagnosis. Also, having the patient swallow some water soluble contrast material such as Gastrografin and watching the material progress to the stomach fluoroscopically will demonstrate any significant leak which might be present. Just as in instrumental perforations, early repair is paramount if good results are to be expected. Primary suture with wide drainage is the procedure of choice. Occasionally, when there has been extensive esophageal destruction from a gunshot wound, or if a simple perforation has been allowed to progress to the stage where extensive necrosis and maceration have taken place, primary repair is not possible. In such instances, what may seem very aggressive therapy is indicated. This consists of exclusion of the esophagus by placing a ligature about the cardia to prevent gastric reflux and diverting the oral secretions by cervical esophagostomy. The treatment also consists of wide drainage of the mediastinum and pleura, construction of a feeding gastrostomy, and vigorous nutritional support by either the parenteral or enteric route (or both). The procedure has been described in detail by Urschel and associates,[50] who recommend reconstruction of the esophagus at a later date after the mediastinum and pleura have had the chance to heal. This seemingly radical approach to treating a group of very ill patients has resulted in decreased mortality and morbidity. The authors feel that this is the method of choice in treating the severely damaged esophagus where primary repair is not possible or has previously failed.

PENETRATING TRAUMA: CARDIOVASCULAR

Penetrating cardiac injuries generally result from gunshot and stab wounds. High-velocity and large-caliber missiles are likely to cause immediate death from exsanguination, as they result in greater damage to the pericardium and myocardium. Low-velocity and small-caliber missiles and stab wounds are more prone to develop pericardial tamponade. Recent years have produced a surge in the number of cardiac wounds produced by guns, to the point that one major trauma center recently reported more cardiac injury from gunshot wounds than stab wounds.[4] The frequency of injury to the various cardiac chambers corresponds to the area of their exposure to the anterior chest wall. The right ventricle is most commonly affected, followed by the left ventricle, right atrium, and left atrium in decreasing frequency. Stab wounds tend to injure single cardiac chambers, whereas bullet wounds frequently result in multiple chamber involvement.

Most patients who survive a penetrating heart wound long enough to reach a hospital do so because of some degree of pericardial tamponade. Usually it coexists with volume depletion due to blood loss into the pleural space. Tamponade results from the accumulation of blood in the tough, fibrous, nondistensible pericardium when the pericardial injury is too small to allow adequate egress of blood or when the injury is sealed by thrombus. The physiologic effects of this increased pressure within the pericardium are manifold. Venous filling of the cardiac chamber is impeded, resulting in elevated central venous pressure, if circulating blood volume is normal. This leads to a reduced cardiac output and, eventually, hypotension. The reduced coronary blood flow results in myocardial ischemia and failure. In the early stages blood pressure is maintained despite a falling cardiac output by peripheral vasoconstriction and tachycardia. Although this process may be lifesaving in that it prevents immediate exsanguination, it invariably proves fatal if allowed to continue. Acute tamponade presents a characteristic clinical picture which includes distant heart sounds, falling blood pressure with narrow pulse pressure, and elevated venous pressure. The degree of shock is out of proportion to the noted blood loss. The facies are typically gray and apprehensive, and the neck veins are distended. A paradoxical pulse may be noted with a blood pressure drop of more than 10 mmHg during inspiration. The central venous pressure will usually be high, unless blood volume is extremely low.

In addition to tamponade, specific intracardiac injury may contribute to cardiac decompensation. Damage to the conduction system may result in various degrees of atrioventricular dissociation and intolerable bradycardia. The production of atrial and ventricular septal defects will produce cardiac failure commensurate with the size of the shunt. Aortic–right ventricular fistulas and direct injury to valves and coronary arteries can also contribute to cardiac decompensation.

The nature of the bleeding from cardiac wounds depends on which chamber has been lacerated. Wounds of the atria bleed continuously because the walls are thin with little contractile power, whereas a laceration of the ventricle may be partially controlled by the thicker muscular wall. In either case hemopericardium is inevitable and is made up of blood and clot formation.

Penetrating wounds of the heart should be suspected in any patient with a penetrating injury of the upper abdomen, neck, or chest, particularly the precordium. A careful search should be made for both entry and exit wounds, as small "ice pick"-type penetrations are often missed. The overriding clinical presentation is usually that of hemothorax and hemorrhagic shock or tamponade. Auscultation of the heart may reveal a precordial crunch (Hamman's sign) if air has entered the pericardium or a murmur produced by a regurgitant valve or septal defect. Electrocardiogram is of little value unless there has been conduction system damage. Chest x-ray may

show a foreign body in or near the heart, but it is of no value in the diagnosis of tamponade, as the pericardium is incapable of distending acutely. The combination of an isolated bullet entry wound of the chest and the absence of a foreign body on chest x-ray should suggest that cardiac penetration and embolization may have occurred. A central venous pressure line is of great diagnostic value in differentiating shock due to cardiac tamponade from shock due to hemorrhage, and should be inserted in any patient with a penetrating chest injury.

The initial management of a penetrating chest wound should include control of the airway and the establishment of centrally located large-bore lines for intravenous infusion. Crystalloid solutions should be used to restore blood volume until specific blood type is available. Autotransfusion may be used if available. Large-bore dependent chest tubes should be placed if hemothorax or pneumothorax is suspected. This should be done prior to obtaining a chest x-ray in unstable patients. When massive bleeding and hypotension do not respond to volume replacement, immediate thoracotomy on the involved side should be done as part of the resuscitative effort. Whether this is done in the emergency ward or the operating room should depend on the rapidity of blood loss and the ability to maintain patient stability. In this setting the existence of cardiac injury is confirmed by direct inspection of the pericardium after thoracotomy.

The diagnosis of cardiac tamponade can be subtle, and its management is far less clearcut. In patients with cardiac tamponade and hemothorax, a marked improvement results from volume expansion, suggesting that the clinical picture is due solely to blood loss. It should be remembered, however, that volume expansion results in an increased filling pressure which will be seen as clinical improvement with tamponade alone or tamponade and hemothorax. This increased filling pressure should be reflected by an elevated central venous pressure and distended neck veins, but an increased venous tone produced by abdominal rigidity and shivering can further confuse the picture. Thus, when the diagnosis of cardiac tamponade is in question, diagnostic pericardiocentesis should be performed.

Pericardiocentesis is performed using a large-bore, thin-walled needle through the left substernal paraxiphoid route. Electrocardiographic control may be helpful in positioning the needle, but it is not essential. The removal of blood from the pericardial space confirms the diagnosis, and may be therapeutic if the source of bleeding has been controlled by thrombus. Because of frequent false-negative and false-positive results with pericardiocentesis, Arom and coworkers have suggested it be replaced by subxiphoid pericardial window.[2] If this procedure reveals tamponade or hemopericardium, it is easily and quickly converted to a median sternotomy and the heart repaired.

For many years, the primary therapeutic approach to heart wounds presenting with tamponade was pericardiocentesis, reserving thoracotomy and cardiorrhaphy for those patients who failed to respond to pericardial aspiration or who had recurrence of tamponade after aspiration.[5] Recently, however, reports from major trauma centers advocate surgery as the treatment of choice for all penetrating heart injuries regardless of presentation, using pericardiocentesis only as a means to provide safe time for surgery.[4,46] This evolution in the treatment of penetrating cardiac injuries has evolved for the following reasons: (1) the duration of an initial favorable response to pericardiocentesis is unpredictable, and rapid deterioration can follow recurrent tamponade; (2) the increasing incidence of gunshot wounds of the heart as compared to stab wounds; (3) the treatment of tamponade by definitive pericardiocentesis requires patient surveillance beyond the capability of

most active trauma units; (4) late sequelae of cardiac injury such as false aneurysm formation and constrictive pericarditis can be avoided; and (5) recent advancements in resuscitation, anesthesia, and cardiac surgery have made surgical intervention relatively safe. In summary, all patients with penetrating cardiac wounds and exsanguinating hemorrhage or unequivocal cardiac tamponade should undergo thoracotomy and cardiorrhaphy; when tamponade is suspected, pericardiocentesis may serve as an interim step in preparation for surgical intervention.

Regardless of the indication, most heart wounds are best approached through an anterolateral left fourth intercostal space incision. The entire chest should be prepared to allow for extension across the sternum or conversion to a median sternotomy–type incision. The costal cartilages on either side of the interspace should be divided to allow for adequate exposure. The pericardium is then opened longitudinally anterior to the phrenic nerve, and the medial pericardium is retracted with heavy clamps to displace the heart toward the left. Hemorrhage may be massive at this point, and the site of bleeding is best identified using suction and copious saline irrigation. Once the heart is exposed, initial control of hemorrhage is by digital compression. Appropriate extensions of the incision can be made at this point if the exposure for repair is inadequate.

Techniques of definitive wound repair and control of hemorrhage depend on the type and location of the penetrating injury (Fig. 12-6). Atrial wounds and laceration of the intrapericardial great vessels can often be temporarily controlled by partial occluding clamps, followed by continuous suture repair. Ventricular wounds are best closed with teflon felt-buttressed horizontal mattress sutures applied beneath the occluding finger. If the wound is in close proximity to a major coronary artery, care must be taken to avoid impingement of

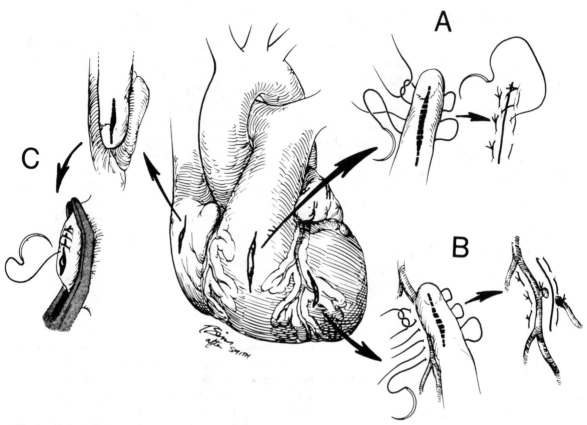

Figure 12-6 Initial control of hemorrhage is obtained by digital compression. *(A)* Ventricular wounds may be repaired beneath the occluding finger with horizontal mattress sutures and reinforced with a continuous suture. *(B)* Wounds in close proximity to coronary vessels are repaired with mattress sutures alone, staying below and away from the vessel. Divided coronary branches and distal vessels are ligated. *(C)* Atrial wounds may be excluded with partial occluding clamps and repaired with continuous sutures. *(from Beall, A. C., Jr., in Resident and Staff Physician, vol. 21, no. 2, 1975.)*

the vessel. Injury to coronary artery branches and laceration of distal major coronary arteries should be ligated to obviate delayed hemorrhage. Division of a proximal coronary artery requires cardiopulmonary bypass, proximal ligation, and distal aorto–coronary artery bypass graft. Wounds of the diaphragmatic surface and posterior aspect of the heart are more difficult to deal with, but must be searched for in every case. Multiple wounds are particularly common with gunshot wounds. Posterior surface injuries can usually

be dealt with by manually luxating the heart until adequate exposure is provided. Occasionally, myocardial irritability or an extensive wound will demand cardiopulmonary bypass for effective repair. Septal defects, fistulas, and valvular injuries are best dealt with at a later time when they can be adequately defined by cardiac catheterization and angiography. Traumatic atrioventricular dissociation may be due to direct conduction system injury or to edema, and should be managed initially by temporary ventricular pacing wires. Permanent transvenous electrodes can be inserted at a later date if necessary.

The type of anesthesia used for thoracotomy and cardiorrhaphy will be dictated by the urgency of the situation and the mental status of the patient. Comatose patients and those in deep shock can be done without anesthesia, but all require endotracheal intubation and positive pressure breathing. Prophylactic broad-spectrum antibiotics are started at the earliest opportunity. The pericardium should be irrigated at the termination of cardiac repair and left open to drain into the pleural space, which is drained by dependent intercostal tube(s).

The prognosis of penetrating injury to the heart depends on both the nature and severity of the injury and on how it is managed. In a recent comparison of various methods of therapy, Symbas reported a 50 percent mortality in those patients who presented with massive or unrelenting hemorrhage.[46] In a group of patients presenting with tamponade and who were treated initially by pericardiocentesis, reserving operation for recurrence or no improvement, the mortality rate was 17.6 percent. This is compared with a mortality rate of 5 percent for that group who had thoracotomy and cardiorrhaphy for tamponade, where pericardiocentesis was used only to provide time to transfer the patient to the operating room. Beall, comparing the same two therapeutic methods, reported a 22 percent mortality for stab wounds and 40 percent mortality for gunshot wounds using definitive pericardiocentesis compared with 13 percent and 31 percent, respectively, using the more aggressive primary thoracotomy. These figures also point out that gunshot wounds are almost twice as lethal as stab wounds despite the method of treatment.

Iatrogenic myocardial perforations may also occur, usually during cardiac catheterization or the insertion of a transvenous pacemaker lead. The increasing use of flow-guided catheters will undoubtedly increase this number. These are usually recognized by an abnormal catheter position or by injecting dye into the pericardial sac. Generally, bleeding is limited and tamponade rarely occurs, but immediate pericardiocentesis and myocardial suture may be necessary in occasional cases.

Penetrating Injuries of the Great Vessels

Penetrating injuries to the thoracic aorta and intrathoracic great vessels carry a poor prognosis, as most result in death by exsanguination. Intrapericardial injuries to great vessels have a better chance of survival because of tamponade than do those which are in direct proximity to the pleural space. Survival in the latter group is possible when intrathoracic bleeding is limited by a tamponading effect of adjacent tissue, or when pleural space is obliterated by an old inflammatory process. Injuries to intrathoracic major veins and the pulmonary arteries are better tolerated because of their comparatively low pressure. Arteriovenous, aortocardiac, and aortopulmonary artery fistulas are occasionally seen after penetrating thoracic injury. Associated major injuries are frequently encountered, usually to lung, heart, and intraabdominal organs. As with cardiac injuries, the wounding agent is usually a knife or gun.

According to Symbas and coworkers, more than 50 percent of penetrating injuries to the great vessels present with massive bleeding.[47] In this case, the diagnosis is made at the time of thoracotomy. In the absence of hemorrhage a careful search should be made for great vessel injury when surface wounds raise the possibility. Wounds of vessels of the thoracic outlet may present as expanding hematomas at the base of the neck or with external bleeding through the entry wound. The pulse distal to the arterial injury may be weak or absent, although a normal pulse does not rule out an arterial injury. Similarly, signs of central nervous system impairment, particularly unilateral, suggest injury to innominate or carotid arteries. Neurological deficits of the upper extremities implicate involvement of the neurovascular bundle to that arm. When a missile has traversed the mediastinum, a widened superior mediastinum roentgenographically suggests injury to the aorta or its proximal branches or their accompanying veins. In addition, the presence of a continuous murmur over the anterior chest suggests great vessel injury and fistula formation. The murmur may be delayed, appearing days or even weeks after surgery, and demands frequent reexamination in these patients. Great vessel laceration can exist without any of the above signs.

When emergency thoracotomy is not indicated for bleeding or tamponade, the suspected diagnosis of great vessel injury should be confirmed and documented by arteriography in order to plan the proper surgical approach.

The initial management of patients with great vessel injury depends on the presentation, but usually includes maintenance of an adequate airway and an attempt at restoration of circulating blood volume. The management of cardiac tamponade is identical to that discussed under cardiac injury, as the source of bleeding is unknown. When profuse and continuous bleeding from chest tubes presents and the site of bleeding has not been identified, the submammary anterolateral thoracotomy affords the best exposure for any eventuality. In addition to the heart and pulmonary hilus, this approach provides access to the descending thoracic aorta and the vessel at the apex of the hemithorax. If exposure is not adequate for repair, bleeding can be stopped temporarily by digital control or sponge-stick pressure until an appropriate extension can be made. For injury to proximal branches of the aorta, this requires conversion to a "trapdoor" or "book" incision by upper median sternotomy and a parallel incision above the ipsilateral

clavicle (Fig. 12-7). Subperiosteal resection of the inner third of the clavicle is required to allow for lateral retraction of the musculoskeletal flap. Although this incision is more time-consuming and associated with greater morbidity than others, it provides access to all cervical and thoracic vessels; an alternative for injury to intrapericardial great vessels would be extension across the sternum to the corresponding opposite intercostal space or conversion to median sternotomy. This latter incision is satisfactory for all wounds of the ascending aorta and its proximal branches as well, but is inadequate for exposure of the descending thoracic aorta and pulmonary hilum and should not be used alone as the primary approach for hemorrhage.[38] Bleeding from the proximal left subclavian artery can usually be repaired through the anterolateral approach, and those of the distal left subclavian and right subclavian arteries can be repaired via a supraclavicular incision after initial control is obtained through thoracotomy.[10] If hemorrhage is found to originate from the descending aorta, the anterolateral incision should be extended as far laterally as possible and inferior ribs should be divided posteriorly to gain added exposure for repair.

When time permits localization of great vessel injury by angiography, the problem of initial surgical exposure is greatly simplified. Midline sternotomy is the incision of choice for injury to intrapericardial major vessels, ascending aorta, arch of the aorta, and innominate and proximal left carotid arteries. Extension of this incision into the neck anterior to the sternocleidomastoid will aid in repairing injury to the innominate and proximal carotid arteries. Extrathoracic injury to the carotid arteries and the jugular veins can be effectively repaired through an oblique incision in the neck. Wounds involving the distal two-thirds of the subclavian arteries, which do not present with massive hemothorax, are best managed through the isolated supraclavicular ap-

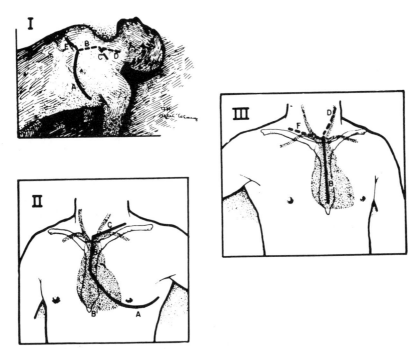

Figure 12-7 Incisions used for the management of penetrating great vessel wounds. Insert II demonstrates the versatile "trapdoor" or "book" incision. Variations of left anterior thoracotomy and midline sternotomy area shown in insert I and III. *(from Symbas, P. N., et al., 1974.)*

proach. Additional distal control can be provided by an incision in the deltopectoral groove or partial subperiosteal resection of the clavicle. Proximal extension requires partial or complete sternotomy. Despite localization of injury, the entire chest and neck should be prepared and draped to provide flexibility of surgical approach should it become necessary.

Regardless of the approach used, the principles of vascular surgery should be applied. When possible, proximal and distal control of a vessel should be accomplished or, alternatively, the defect in the vessel wall should be excluded by a partial occluding clamp. Injuries to innominate and carotid arteries require the use of internal or, more frequently, external temporary shunts to effect repair in most cases. When an injury to the descending thoracic aorta necessitates cross clamping, the principles discussed under blunt injury apply, and a temporary shunt is indicated in all injuries which cannot be repaired expeditiously. The use of internal shunts may be necessary in major laceration of the inferior and superior cavae, when bleeding cannot be controlled by a partial occluding clamp. Total occlusion of either of these structures can result in hypotension and, in the latter case, central venous system injury. However, the introduction of an internal shunt via the atrium can allow exclusion of a caval wound and maintenance of venous return. When irreparably injured, thoracic veins, including the innominate, may be simply ligated.

The type of vascular repair that is used is dictated by the magnitude of the injury. Small lacerations can be controlled by digital pressure or tangential clamping and can be closed by lateral repair beneath the occluding finger or above the clamp with interrupted or continuous vascular sutures. More extensive wounds require resectioned end-to-end repair or interposition grafts, but debridement of a vessel should not go beyond obvious vessel injury. If a graft is required in a medium vessel injury, the saphenous vein serves as the best conduit. Major destruction of the aorta requires the insertion of a prosthetic graft, but carries with it the risk of infection in a potentially contaminated wound.

Certain injuries to the ascending aorta and aortic arch require cardiopulmonary bypass, as do aortocardiac and aortopulmonary fistulas. Although these wounds account for few of the great vessel injuries, accessibility of cardiopulmonary bypass is required should it prove necessary.

Foreign Bodies of the Heart and Great Vessels

Foreign bodies can enter the heart by direct penetration or can embolize within the cardiovascular system from peripheral sites. The most common objects are needles, pins, bullets, shrapnel, and plastic catheters. Sharp objects can enter the bloodstream from the alimentary tract, uterus, bladder, vagina, and bronchial tree, in addition to external surface penetration. Once a foreign body has entered the vascular system, it is subject to the forces of gravity and the force of the bloodstream. Left heart and systemic artery penetration may result in peripheral arterial embolization, whereas entry into the systemic veins and right heart results in embolization to the pulmonary arteries or entrapment in the right side of the heart. Exact location of directly penetrating missiles is often difficult, as they may be within the pericaridium or myocardium, or free in a cardiac chamber.

Foreign bodies which migrate to the heart and pulmonary arteries may be asymptomatic. They are discovered by chest roentgenogram or by the realization that part of an intravenous device is missing. Missiles which penetrate the chest present with the trauma of the initial wound, and if hemorrhage or tamponade is absent, cardiac penetration is suspected by location of a radiopaque object within the heart shadow or by the unexplained absence of the object when there is no exit wound. If peripheral arterial embolization has occurred, signs of ischemia are usually present, particularly with bullets. Significantly, missiles which embolize to the pulmonary arteries from right heart penetration do not result in major pulmonary infarction. However, other complications relating directly to the foreign body do occur.

In a review of intraluminal cardiovascular foreign bodies, predominantly plastic catheters, Hipona emphasizes high morbidity and mortality resulting from unretrieved objects.[22] Among the noted complications are mural thrombosis, venous and arterial occlusion, endocarditis, arrhythmias, myocardial necrosis, abscesses, perforation, and valvular incompetence. Harken, based on an extensive World War II experience, proposed the following reasons for foreign body removal: (1) to prevent embolization of the foreign body or the associated thrombus, (2) to reduce the incidence of bacterial endocarditis, (3) to avoid pericardial effusions, (4) to diminish the danger of myocardial damage with subsequent rupture or myocardial aneurysm.[20] Additional factors which prompt removal are cardiac neurosis and, with iatrogenic foreign bodies, litigation potential. Although Harken successfully removed 13 foreign bodies from the heart, 15 others were not removed because they were asymptomatic and considered to be too small to justify surgical intervention. That some foreign objects in the heart and great vessels remain harmless is documented by many instances of discovery years after initial injury.

Since it is unknown which foreign bodies in the cardiovascular system will cause problems, all must be regarded as a potential threat to life. The risk of removal should then be weighed against the likelihood of complication. The size, location, nature, and length of presence of the foreign body will affect this decision. In most cases, every effort should be made to extract these objects.

There are two methods used to remove a foreign object from the cardiovascular system: (1) a direct surgical approach and (2) an indirect approach using intraluminal transvascular retrieval. The latter technique has gained popularity in recent years because of increasing familiarity with cardiac catheterization techniques, and is particularly useful for the retrieval of embolized plastic catheters. Many devices have been used either percutaneously or by cut-down, including ureteral stone baskets, bronchoscopic forceps, intramyocardial biotomes, and pigtail catheters, but the most effective has been the loop snare.[22] The exact location of the foreign body is verified by angiography and then looped using fluoroscopic guidance. This method has proven effective, safe, and expedient.

When transvascular retrieval is unsuccessful, or when the shape or location of an object does not lend itself to removal by loop snare, thoracotomy and removal under direct vision becomes necessary. The improved techniques of cardiovascular surgery make this a procedure of little risk. The foreign body should be located by palpation prior to cardiotomy if possible, as it can move between cardiac chambers with positioning on the operating table and institution of cardiopulmonary bypass. Objects located in the great veins, atria, and pulmonary arteries can often be removed through a purse-string suture or with partial exclusion without bypass. The timing of removal should be based on the patient's condition, and it is usually not an emergency.

BIBLIOGRAPHY

1 Alberty, R. E. and J. E. Egan: Blunt trauma to the chest, *Am. Surg.*, **42**:511, 1976.
2 Arom, K. V., J. D. Richardson, G. Webb, F. L. Grover, and J. K. Trinkle: Subxiphoid pericardial window in patients with suspected traumatic pericardial tamponade, *Ann. Thorac. Surg.*, **23**: 545, 1977.
3 Beall, A. C., Jr., H. W. Crawford, and M. E. DeBakey: Considerations in the management of acute hemothorax, *J. Thorac. Cardiovasc. Surg.*, **52**:351, 1966.
4 ———, T. A. Patrick, J. E. Okies, D. L. Bricker, and M. E. DeBakey: Penetrating wounds of the heart: Changing patterns of surgical management, *J. Trauma*, **12**:468, 1972.
5 ———, E. B. Diethrich, H. W. Crawford, D. A. Cooley, and M. E. DeBakey: Surgical management of penetrating cardiac injuries, *Am. J. Surg.*, **112**:686, 1966.
6 Bennett, D. E. and J. K. Cherry: The natural history of traumatic aneurysms of the aorta, *Surgery*, **61**:516, 1967.
7 Bertelsen, S. and P. Howitz: Injuries of the trachea and bronchi, *Thorax*, **27**:188, 1972.
8 Blair, E., C. Topuzlu, and R. S. Deane: Major blunt chest trauma, *Curr. Probl. Surg.*, May 1969.
9 Blalock, A. and M. M. Ravitch: A consideration of the nonoperative treatment of cardiac tamponade from wounds of the heart, *Surgery*, **14**:157, 1943.
10 Brawley, R. K., D. G. Murray, C. Crisler, and J. L. Cameron: Management of wounds of the innominate, subclavian, and axillary blood vessels, *Surg. Gynecol. Obstet.*, **131**:1130, 1970.
11 Bright, E. F. and C. S. Beck: Non-penetrating wounds of the heart: Clinical and experimental studies, *Am. Heart J.*, **10**:293, 1935.
12 Cooper, J. D. and H. C. Brillo: The evolution of tracheal injury due to ventilatory assistance through cuffed tubes, *Ann. Surg.*, **160**:334, 1969.
13 Cornell, W. P., P. A. Ebert, and G. D. Zuidema:

x-ray diagnosis of penetrating wounds of the abdomen, *J. Surg. Res.*, **5**:142, 1965.

14 Crawford, E. S. and P. A. Rubio: Reappraisal of adjuncts to avoid ischemia in the treatment of aneurysms of descending thoracic aorta, *J. Thorac. Cardiovasc. Surg.*, **66**:693, 1973.

15 DeBakey, M. E. and D. A. Cooley: Successful resection of aneurysm of distal aortic arch and replacement by graft, *J. Am. Med. Assoc.*, **155**:1398, 1954.

16 Diethelm, A. G. and W. Battle: Management of flail chest injury: A review of 75 cases, *Am. Surg.*, **37**:667, 1971.

17 Ebert, P. A.: Physiologic principles in the management of the crushed-chest syndrome, *Monogr. Surg. Sci.*, **4**:69, 1967.

18 ———, R. A. Gaertner, and G. D. Zuidema: Traumatic diaphragmatic hernia, *Surg. Gynecol. Obstet.*, **125**:59, 1967.

19 Guest, J. C., Jr. and J. N. Anderson: Major airway injury in closed chest trauma, *Chest*, **72**:63, 1977.

20 Harken, D. E.: Foreign bodies in, and in relation to, the thoracic blood vessels and heart, *Surg. Gynecol. Obstet.*, **83**:117, 1946.

21 Hill, L. D.: Injuries of the diaphragm following blunt trauma, *Surg. Clin. North Am.*, **52**:611, 1972.

22 Hipona, F. A., F. D. Sciammas, and U. F. Hublitz: Nonthoracotomy retrieval of intraluminal cardiovascular foreign bodies, *Radiol. Clin. North Am.*, **9**:583, 1971.

23 Hood, R. M. and H. E. Sloan: Injuries of the trachea and major bronchj, *J. Thorac. Cardiovasc. Surg.*, **38**:458, 1959.

24 Jones, J. W., R. L. Hewitt, and T. Drapanas: Cardiac contusion: A capricious syndrome, *Ann. Surg.*, **181**:567, 1975.

25 Kaiser, G. A.: "Emergency Management of Chest Trauma," in J. C. Findeiss (ed.) *Emergency Management of the Critical Patient*, Stratton Co., Stratton, N.Y., 1975, pp. 109–128.

26 Katz, J. D., L. H. Cronau, P. G. Barash, and S. D. Mandel: Pulmonary artery flowguided catheters in the perioperative period, *J. Am. Med. Assoc.*, **237**:2832, 1977.

27 Kessler, E. and A. Stein: Diaphragmatic hernia as a long term complication of stab wounds of the chest, *Am. J. Surg.*, **132**:34, 1976.

28 Kish, G., L. Kozloff, W. L. Joseph, and P. C. Adkins: Indications for early thoracotomy in the management of chest trauma, *Ann. Thorac. Surg.*, **22**:23, 1976.

29 Liedke, A. and W. E. DeMuth: Non-penetrating cardiac injuries: A collective review, *Am. Heart J.*, **86**:687, 1973.

30 McCoy, J. A. and E. Ayim: The management of acute thoracic injuries, *Anesthesia*, **31**:532, 1976.

31 Melzig, E. P., M. Swank, and A. M. Salzberg: Acute blunt traumatic rupture of the diaphragm in children, *Arch. Surg.*, **111**:1009, 1976.

32 Moore, B. P.: Operative stabilization of nonpenetrating chest injuries, *J. Thorac. Cardiovasc. Surg.*, **70**:619, 1975.

33 Parmley, L. F., T. W. Mattingly, W. C. Manion, and E. J. Jahnke: Non-penetrating traumatic injury of the aorta, *Circulation*, **17**:1086, 1958.

34 ———, W. C. Manion, and T. W. Mattingly: Non-penetrating traumatic injury of the heart, *Circulation*, **18**:375, 1958.

35 Pearce, W. and E. Blair: Significance of the electrocardiogram in heart contusion due to blunt trauma, *J. Trauma*, **16**:136, 1976.

36 Pomerantz, M., F. Delagado, and B. Eiseman: Unsuspected depressed cardiac output following chest trauma, *Surgery*, **70**:865, 1971.

37 Powers, S. R.: Management of the flail chest (editorial), *Ann. Thorac. Surg.*, **19**:480, 1975.

38 Reul, G. J., A. C. Beall, G. L. Jordan, and K. L. Mattox: The early operative management of injuries to the great vessels, *Surgery*, **74**:862, 1973.

39 Richardson, J. D., R. B. McElvein, and J. K. Trinkle: First rib fracture: A hallmark of severe trauma, *Ann. Surg.*, **181**:251, 1975.

40 Romanoff, H.: Prevention of infection in war chest injuries, *Ann. Surg.*, **182**:144, 1975.

41 Sanger, P. W.: Discussion of A. C. Beall, Jr. et al., *J. Thorac. Cardiovasc. Surg.*, **52**:359, 1966.

42 Shamblin, J. R. and D. C. McGoon: Acute thoracic compression with traumatic asphyxia, *Arch. Surg.*, **87**:967, 1963.

43 Steichen, F. M.: Penetrating wounds of the chest and the abdomen, *Curr. Probl. Surg.*, August 1967.

44 Stern, T., R. Y. Wolf, B. Reichart, et al.: Coro-

nary artery occlusion resulting from blunt trauma, *J. Am. Med. Assoc.,* **230**:1308, 1974.

45 Swan, H. J. C.: The role of hemodynamic monitoring in the management of the critically ill, *Crit. Care Med.,* **3**:83, 1973.

46 Symbas, P. N., N. Harlaftes, and W. J. Waldo: Penetrating cardiac wounds: A comparison of different therapeutic methods, *Ann. Surg.,* **183**: 377, 1976.

47 ———, E. Kourias, D. H. Tyras, and C. R. Hatcher: Penetrating wounds of great vessels, *Ann. Surg.,* **179**:757, 1974.

48 ———, D. H. Tyras, R. E. Ware, and C. R. Hatcher: Rupture of the aorta: A diagnostic triad, *Ann. Thorac. Surg.,* **5**:405, 1973.

49 Trinkle, J. K., J. D. Richardson, J. L. Franz, F. L. Grover, K. V. Arom, and F. M. G. Holmstrom: Management of flail chest without mechanical ventilation, *Ann. Thorac. Surg.,* **19**: 355, 1975.

50 Urschel, H. C., Jr., M. A. Razzuk, R. E. Wood, N. Galbraith, M. Pockey, and D. C. Paulson: Improved management of esophageal perforation: Exclusion and division in continuity, *Ann. Surg.,* **179**:587, 1974.

Chapter 13

Abdominal Trauma

Erwin R. Thal, M.D.

Robert N. McClelland, M.D.

G. Tom Shires, M.D.

The diagnosis and management of intraabdominal injuries is one of the most challenging areas in clinical medicine. As the incidence of abdominal trauma increases each year, an effective, organized approach coupled with a high index of suspicion and an awareness of the consequences of missed injuries are necessary ingredients in the successful management of these difficult cases. Blunt abdominal trauma generally leads to higher mortality rates than penetrating wounds and presents greater problems in diagnosis. The spleen, liver, kidneys, and bowel are the most frequently injured abdominal viscera.

EVALUATION OF BLUNT TRAUMA

Prompt recognition of intraabdominal injury is the single most important factor affecting ulti-mate morbidity and mortality. Diagnosis is frequently difficult because of associated injuries that tend to mask the presence and severity of abdominal injury. The most frequently associated injuries are those related to the central nervous system, cardiorespiratory system, and musculoskeletal system. Often the patient is unconscious because of alcoholism, shock, or associated head injury. Seemingly minor abdominal trauma and relatively trivial injuries on occasion may cause significant damage, including the rupture of abdominal viscera; hence the index of suspicion must be high if diagnostic errors are to be avoided.

Clinical Manifestations

Evaluation of the patient with blunt abdominal trauma begins with a careful history and physical examination. Knowledge of the mechanism of injury is frequently helpful in discerning the likelihood of abdominal injury. Factors such as rapid deceleration, impaling forces, and seat belt restraints make the abdominal viscera prone to injury. Physical examination in the alert patient is the most reliable predictor of injury, and yet this will be misleading, as either a false-positive or false-negative examination occurs in 10 to 20 percent of patients. The entire patient must be examined as well as the abdomen because of the high incidence of associated trauma. Fitzgerald et al. have reported extraabdominal injuries in 97 percent of patients with abdominal injuries who were dead upon arrival at the hospital and in 70 percent of those admitted alive. When the diagnosis is doubtful, one must often depend on repeated physical examinations alone, done at frequent intervals by the same examiner, to decide whether the patient requires celiotomy. Abdominal pain and tenderness, guarding and rigidity, loss of bowel sounds, and unexplained shock are all parameters that help make the diagnosis of the acute surgical abdomen. Abdominal rigidity, or involuntary guarding, is the most helpful sign, and even when present alone, warrants exploratory celiotomy. Patients with an altered state of consciousness resulting from closed head injuries, alcoholism, or drug abuse frequently do not demonstrate the classic physical findings. Hinton, in 1929, recommended a period of watchful waiting before exploration because of fear of uncontrollable hemorrhage and infection as well as difficulty in performing the necessary surgical procedures under adverse conditions. There is no excuse for this course today, however, and a course of watchful waiting may frequently be disastrous. Clark states that patients with the most severe injuries stand a reasonable chance of recovery only if exploration is performed as soon as possible. Fitzgerald, Crawford, and DeBakey reported no deaths in patients who had an exploratory celiotomy without intraabdominal injury being found. However, in their series three deaths

occurred from intraabdominal hemorrhage because abdominal injury was masked by associated injuries. The negligible mortality for negative abdominal exploration at Parkland Memorial Hospital for cases of suspected abdominal trauma is similar to that quoted above.

In patients with blunt abdominal trauma, determinations of frequent blood pressure are often useful. A valuable sign of continuing intraabdominal hemorrhage is the transient elevation of blood pressure to normotensive levels following the rapid infusion of 500 to 1000 mL of Ringer's lactate solution followed by a return a few minutes later to hypotensive levels. Patients who are hypotensive from minimal blood loss or from neurogenic shock usually do not behave in this manner. The Ringer's lactate solution generally is infused over a period of 15 to 20 min while other measures such as blood typing and cross matching are being carried out. Postural hypotension, when the patient assumes the erect position, is another useful sign of continuing intraabdominal bleeding.

Diagnostic Procedures

Whereas history and physical examination remain the most reliable diagnostic modalities, other diagnostic aids will frequently confirm clinical suspicions. In general, laboratory determinations do not offer much help in the young, previously healthy traumatized patient. Berman et al. state that if the leukocyte count is greater than 15,000 following abdominal trauma, a ruptured solid viscus is likely, especially if other findings are compatible with that diagnosis. Knopp and Harkins, and Williams and Zollinger, however, have not found the leukocyte count to be so helpful. Sudden acute blood loss may not be adequately reflected by early hemograms; hence, a normal hemoglobin and hematocrit shortly after injury may be misleading. Serum glucose and creatinine determinations may be helpful in elderly patients suspected of having diabetes or renal insufficiency. Whereas serum electrolytes are rarely diagnostic, the serum potassium level is extremely important if operation is contemplated. Unrecognized hypokalemia may lead to disastrous consequences. A serum amylase level, when elevated, is a relatively reliable predictor of intraabdominal injury. In addition to being elevated with pancreatic injuries, abnormal amylase levels are also seen in injuries to the duodenum and upper small bowel. Leakage of the amylase-containing fluid is rapidly absorbed into the blood from the peritoneal cavity. Studies of urinary sediment are useful, since hematuria may indicate injury to the genitourinary tract. If the patient with abdominal injury is unable to void, catheterization should be done to obtain urine for examination.

Levin tubes are inserted in all patients sustaining blunt abdominal trauma. The stomach contents are aspirated, and the aspirate is examined for the presence of blood. In addition, a Levin tube provides for decompression of the stomach, prevents gastric dilatation, and prevents aspiration with the induction of anesthesia.

Blood gas determinations should be obtained in all multiply injured patients and, in particular, in those patients with a history of chronic pulmonary disease, chest injuries, or possible aspiration.

Roentgenographic Findings For patients who have sustained severe abdominal injury and in whom other clinical signs obviously point to such injury, roentgenography for diagnosis may dangerously delay surgical intervention. Multiply injured patients should never be left unattended in the x-ray department. However, for about one-third of patients with stable vital signs and questionable diagnosis of intraabdominal injury, x-ray studies may be helpful. Roentgenography is of least aid in injury to solid viscera, notably the liver, spleen, and pancreas.

Patients suspected of having intraabdominal injuries should have upright films of the chest in addition to supine films of the abdomen. Occasionally, additional information can be gained from lateral and left lateral decubitus films. Skeletal parts are checked for fractures or dislocations. Examination of the soft tissues may give information concerning alterations of size, shape, or position of many viscera. Pneumoperitoneum may be diagnosed with the patient in the erect or lateral decubitus position. Indirect evidence of solid viscera rupture with secondary hemorrhage may be presumed by an increase in density in the region, by displacement of neighboring viscera, or by accumulation of fluid between the gas shadows of bowel loops. If a gastric, duodenal, or upper jejunal rupture is suspected, the appearance of pneumoperitoneum may be increased by injecting 750 to 1000 cm^3 of air into the nasogastric tube, after which the patient sits in a semierect position for 10 min before an upright chest film or a left lateral decubitus film of the abdomen is made. Films should also be made prior to air injection for the purpose of comparison, if the patient's condition permits.

Another study which may be useful is examination of the upper gastrointestinal tract by x-ray after ingestion of a water soluble radiopaque medium, which may indicate injury to the stomach, duodenum, or upper small bowel. The use of barium mixtures for this is dangerous, since a severe peritoneal reaction is caused by barium if it leaks through a perforation in the gastrointestinal tract. This is especially true if there is fecal contamination in the peritoneal cavity from a concomitant colon injury.

Intravenous pyelograms should be performed, if feasible, for patients with gross or microscopic hematuria as well as other evidence of genitourinary injury. This will establish the nature and location of the injury, and also determine if both kidneys are functioning prior to surgical intervention in case an injured kidney must be removed. It is important to note that occasional renal injuries are not detected by intravenous pyelography and, if clinically suspected, may be better confirmed by arteriography. If necessary, intravenous pyelograms may be obtained during the surgical procedure to determine the presence of a functional kidney on one side before removing the other kidney.

Cystograms are obtained to determine bladder injury or perforation from blunt abdominal trauma.

Paracentesis Significant intraabdominal hemorrhage due to blunt abdominal trauma can be detected with at least 80 percent accuracy by means of needle paracentesis of the abdominal cavity. This is a useful diagnostic aid only for those cases of abdominal trauma in which, after physical examination, the examiner continues to suspect intraabdominal hemorrhage. The abdominal tap has been particularly useful as a diagnostic adjunct for comatose patients with head injury and in whom adequate physical examination of the abdomen is not possible. A negative tap is not definitive, particularly if other elements of the physical examination indicate other reasons for exploring the abdomen. In female patients with suspected intraabdominal hemorrhage, culdocentesis may be positive for blood when abdominal taps are negative.

The technique is well described by Drapanas and McDonald and is illustrated in Fig. 13-1. The abdomen is surgically cleansed, and an 18-gauge short, beveled spinal needle is attached to a syringe. This is inserted through the abdominal wall after prior infiltration with a local anesthetic agent. Suction is applied to the syringe as the needle is slowly advanced into the abdomen at the site illustrated. Return of a minimum of 0.1 mL of nonclotting blood constitutes a positive tap. Occasionally, an intraabdominal blood vessel may be entered,

but this blood will clot, which differentiates it from blood obtained from the free peritoneal cavity. If the tap is negative in one quadrant, it is repeated at the other sites. Bilateral flank taps are as reliable as four quadrant taps, and may be more reliable if only small amounts of blood are present. Puncture of the rectus abdominis sheath anteriorly should be avoided to prevent rectus abdominis sheath hematoma from injury to the epigastric vessels. This will also diminish the chance of penetration of the bowel, since gas-filled loops of bowel tend to float anteriorly in the abdomen containing fluid or blood. Actually, the danger of penetrating the intestine is slight; several studies have shown that penetration with an 18-gauge needle is harmless, as a hole in the bowel seals off rapidly with no leakage. Other technical considerations include the following:

1 Areas of abdominal scars or other possible points of bowel fixation to the abdominal wall should be avoided.
2 The direction of the needle inside the abdominal cavity should be changed only by withdrawing the point of the needle just superficial to the peritoneum, redirecting the needle, and reintroducing it into the peritoneal cavity.
3 Peritoneal taps should be avoided in the presence of markedly distended bowel, because abnormally elevated intraluminal pressure may cause continued leakage.

Paracentesis is simple and quick, with relatively few complications. Since a positive needle tap is quite accurate, this diagnostic technique is still the initial procedure of choice for detecting intraabdominal hemorrhage. A major drawback is the high percentage of false-negative results.

Peritoneal Lavage Because of the poor reliability of paracentesis, if nonclotting blood is not aspirated, other procedures have been developed to detect intraabdominal injury.

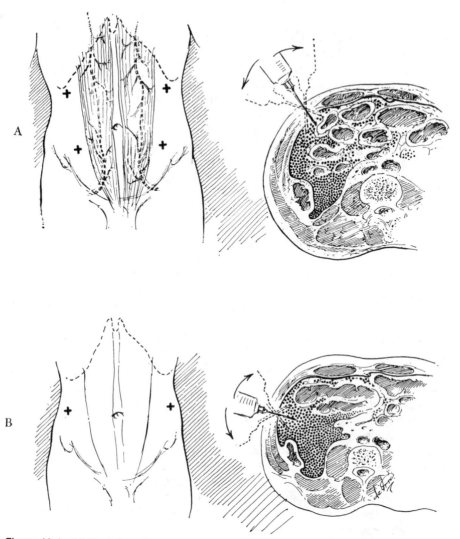

Figure 13-1 (*A*) Technique for four-quadrant peritoneal taps. Preferred location for aspiration of each quadrant is shown. Note that puncture through the rectus sheath is avoided. (*B*) Technique for bilateral flank taps. Aspiration is performed in each flank midway between costal margin and iliac spine. In our experience, bilateral flank taps are equally as reliable and more easily performed than four-quadrant taps in cases of abdominal trauma. (*From Drapanas, T., and McDonald, J.: Peritoneal tap in abdominal trauma, Surgery,* **50**:742, 1961.)

Canizaro et al. described in 1964 the use of intraperitoneal saline infusions in animals. Root et al. described in 1965 the technique of peritoneal lavage in human beings and subsequently reported a series of 304 patients with a 96 percent accuracy. A recent review of this procedure at Parkland Memorial Hospital has proved peritoneal lavage to be a safe and reliable adjunctive procedure for evaluating patients with blunt abdominal trauma. The indications for this technique are closed head injuries, altered consciousness, spinal cord injuries, equivocal abdominal findings, and negative needle paracentesis. It is not recommended for patients with gunshot wounds to the abdomen, stab wounds to the flank or back, multiple abdominal procedures, dilated bowel, pregnancy, or positive needle paracentesis.

The technique used is similar to that described by Perry et al. A point is selected in the lower midline below the umbilicus, approximately one-third of the distance between that and the pubic symphysis. After decompression of the urinary bladder, the skin is cleansed and prepared with an iodinated antiseptic solution. A wheal is raised with 1% lidocaine with epinephrine and the skin incised with a No. 11 scalpel. A standard peritoneal dialysis catheter (McGaw V-4900) is inserted, and the trochar advanced carefully so it just penetrates the peritoneum (Fig. 13-2). An alternative method is to cut the abdominal wall down to the peritoneum and insert the trochar by direct vision. Once the peritoneum is penetrated, the trochar is removed and the dialysis catheter advanced toward the pelvis. A syringe is then attached to the catheter, and the peritoneal cavity aspirated.

Nonclotting blood will often be aspirated

Figure 13-2 Insertion of catheter for peritoneal lavage in the lower midline below the umbilicus. (*From Thal, E. R. and Shires, G. T.: Peritoneal lavage in blunt abdominal trauma, Am. Journal of Surg.* 125:64, 1973.)

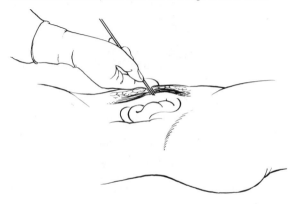

through the large catheter, even with a negative needle paracentesis. If no blood or fluid is aspirated, a liter of balanced salt solution (Ringer's lactate) is rapidly infused into the peritoneal cavity over 5 to 10 min. For children and small adults 10 to 15 mL/kg is used. The patient is then turned from side to side in order to further mix the blood and fluid. If other injuries such as pelvic or long bone fractures are present, this part is eliminated.

The empty intravenous fluid bottle is lowered, and the fluid is siphoned out of the peritoneal cavity. A sample is sent to the laboratory for quantitative analysis. In addition to obtaining red cell and white cell counts, it is important to determine the presence or absence of amylase, bile, or bacteria. Some have recommended colorimetric methods, but these methods do not appear to be as accurate as quantitative analysis of the fluid. The criteria for positive peritoneal lavage include the following: gross blood aspirated prior to infusion of fluid; greater than 100,000 red blood cells per cubic millimeter; greater than 500 white blood cells per cubic millimeter; elevated amylase level; presence of bacteria or bile.

It must be emphasized that the lavage is very inaccurate in indicating retroperitoneal injuries. Unless the posterior peritoneum has been torn or considerable time has elapsed between injury and lavage, most pancreatic injuries are not detected. The same is true for duodenal, urologic, and major vessel injuries which are retroperitoneal. Complications, although uncommon, occur frequently enough that lavage is not recommended for every patient suspected of abdominal injury. However, a negative lavage may spare the patient an exploratory celiotomy.

Arteriography Selective arteriography is another valuable aid in the diagnosis of blunt abdominal trauma. This procedure, advocated by Freeark, and others, employs percutaneous retrograde arteriography by the Seldinger method. Depending upon the skill of the technician, selective catheterization of celiac, mesenteric, or renal vessels may be performed. The arteriogram provides visualization of the arteries supplying the abdominal viscera and pelvis. The film, taken several minutes after injection, can be used as an excretory urogram.

Arteriography is useful in assessing renal artery injury and is routinely employed if a kidney is not promptly visualized with intravenous pyelography. Intimal tears, aortic occlusion, and traumatic aneurysms are often seen in conjunction with seat belt injuries and are occasionally associated with serious lumbosacral trauma.

When continued pelvic bleeding occurs with extension into the retroperitoneal space secondary to pelvic fractures, arteriography may be beneficial in localizing the site of bleeding. Additionally, vasospastic agents may be employed to control hemorrhage. Hemostatic agents as well autologous clot may be embolized to control bleeding.

Benefits of arteriography are directly related to the capabilities of the radiology department. Again, it must be emphasized that time should not be wasted on adjunctive procedures when surgical intervention is indicated.

Scintiscanning   Both liver and splenic scanning have been described in conjunction with blunt abdominal trauma. This technique is primarily limited to those patients whose diagnosis is uncertain and whose conditions remain stable. The radionuclide most frequently used is technetium (^{99m}TC) sulfur colloid. Most series reporting results of this technique are small and emphasize the relative inaccuracy of the examination.

A filling defect representing a parenchymal hematoma is frequently seen with damage to the spleen or liver. In addition, displacement, increased size, and mottled appearance of the spleen may increase suspicion of splenic trauma. Filling defects may also indicate cysts, abscesses, infarction, or tumors.

Other Procedures   Newer, noninvasive modalities, such as sonography and computerized tomography, may have a place in the diagnostic armamentarium, but as yet are unproven. Needleoscopy and laparoscopy provide a less than complete examination and cannot be recommended for the multiply injured patient at this time.

PENETRATING TRAUMA

Stab Wounds

The diagnosis of penetrating injuries of the abdomen does not usually present the difficult problem often posed by blunt abdominal trauma. Three methods of management have evolved: (1) routine exploration of all patients with abdominal stab wounds, (2) selective management, or (3) exploration following demonstration of peritoneal cavity penetration and/or visceral injury.

Before 1960 there was little controversy, since essentially all surgeons agreed that penetrating trauma to the abdomen required exploratory celiotomy to rule out visceral injury. This agreement was first challenged by Shaftan in 1960, who recommended exploratory celiotomy only for patients with physical evidence of injury due to penetrating abdominal trauma and observation in the hospital for those without evidence of visceral injury. The major controversy now revolves around the following issues, which assume paramount importance:

1 How reliable are the various diagnostic criteria for visceral injury?

2 What is the effect of delayed celiotomy on the complication and fatality rate among patients who have no clinical manifestations of visceral injury after penetrating trauma, but

who subsequently develop such manifestations?

3 Does negative celiotomy cause significant morbidity and mortality?

Most clinicians who favor mandatory celiotomy for all patients who have sustained possible abdominal trauma cite the unreliability of physical examination of the abdomen in detecting visceral injury. This point of view is supported by Bull and Mathewson, who found that 23 percent of 78 patients with significant intraabdominal injury confirmed at celiotomy and due to penetrating abdominal wounds had no physical signs preoperatively. In contrast, 18 percent of 100 patients with possible penetrating injuries in whom the peritoneal cavity was not entered did have physical findings suggestive of visceral injury.

In spite of the fact that there is virtually no mortality associated with negative celiotomy, most series report postoperative complications in the range of 10 to 20 percent. A recent review of 175 negative celiotomies performed at Parkland Memorial Hospital revealed a readmission rate of 2 percent for small bowel obstruction. Because of the high incidence of negative celiotomy following routine exploration, most trauma centers have abandoned this approach.

Selective management of abdominal stab wounds is now recommended by many authors. Following clinical assessment, the decision to perform exploratory celiotomy is based on the following factors: (1) physical signs of peritoneal injury; (2) unexplained shock; (3) loss of bowel sounds; (4) evisceration of a viscus; (5) evidence of blood in the stomach, bladder, or rectum; and (6) evidence of visceral injury such as pneumoperitoneum or visceral displacement on x-ray films. Occasionally, other diagnostic studies are employed, including intravenous pyelography, cystography, arteriography, needle paracentesis, or peritoneal lavage. In the absence of any indication of visceral injury, these patients are admitted to the hospital for a 24- to 48-h period of observation. They are reevaluated frequently, preferably by the same observer. If the patient's condition deteriorates, or changes significantly, exploratory celiotomy is performed. Nance reported a reduction in the percentage of negative celiotomies following selective management from 53 percent to 11 percent; 4.8 percent of 210 patients initially observed subsequently required operation when manifestations of visceral injury developed. This delay in surgical treatment caused no mortality or significant morbidity.

An alternative approach other than routine exploration or selective management involves adjunctive methods that help determine whether penetration of the peritoneal cavity has occurred. The decision to operate is based upon confirmation of peritoneal penetration and/or visceral injury. Cornell et al. have described the diagnostic injection of radiopaque contrast material. Following aseptic preparation of the wound site, a small catheter is inserted into the wound and held tightly by a purse-string suture; 50 to 100 mL of contrast media is injected; and anteroposterior, lateral, and oblique films of the abdomen are obtained. Contrast media seen within the peritoneal cavity is an indication of peritoneal penetration. Objections to this technique are the following:

1 Some patients are hypersensitive to the contrast material.
2 Injection of this material may be quite painful, thereby masking further evaluation.
3 The incidence of false-positive and false-negative results is as high as 15 to 25 percent in some series.
4 The technique is impractical for multiple stab wounds.

Local exploration is another modality that may provide useful information. The abdominal wall is prepared with an antiseptic agent. Using local anesthesia, the wound is opened sufficiently to visualize the complete course and depth of the tract. Often with adequate light, instruments, assistance, and exposure, it is obvious that a wound thought to have penetrated the peritoneal cavity is actually superficial and not damaging to the viscera. These patients are managed by simple drainage and outpatient follow-up if other injuries do not require hospitalization. Local wound exploration must involve more than simple instrument-probing to determine penetration. This blind probing may be misleading, since a tortuous wound tract may allow passage of the probe for only a short distance, creating a false impression of nonpenetration. If the end of the tract cannot be visualized or the peritoneum is penetrated, local exploration is considered positive. This technique is equally useful for stab wounds of the back, although the thickness of the paraspinous muscles may prevent visualization of the end of the wound tract. Frequently, innocuous, small stab wounds of the back significantly damage such retroperitoneal structures as the inferior vena cava, ureter, pancreas, or duodenum. A recent review of over 300 abdominal stab wounds at Parkland Hospital indicated that nearly 20 percent of the patients could be discharged from the emergency room without hospital admission based on a negative local exploration that clearly demonstrated the end of the tract.

The abdominal viscera are at risk to injury with stab wounds of the lower chest as well as the abdomen. Figure 13-3 indicates the diaphragmatic excursion with maximal inspiration and expiration and clearly demonstrates elevation of the diaphragm as high as the fourth to fifth intercostal space anteriorly. Wounds at or below this level are therefore evaluated for abdominal injury as well.

If the stab wound to the chest is located below the fifth intercostal space and medial to

the anterior axillary line and there is no obvious indication for operation, peritoneal lavage is performed. If lavage is negative, the patient is admitted to the hospital and observed for 24 to 48 h. If lavage is positive, operation is performed.

Patients with stab wounds of the abdomen located medial to the anterior axillary line are evaluated clinically. If there is no indication for operation, local exploration is performed. If the end of the tract is not visualized or the peritoneum has been penetrated but the abdominal physical findings are considered negative, lavage is similarly performed. Since lavage is unpredictable in determining retroperitoneal injuries, this method of management is limited to lower chest and abdominal wounds that are located between the two anterior axillary lines. Whereas these wounds have previously been treated by routine celiotomy, a recent review of 123 patients treated in this manner successfully reduced the incidence of negative celiotomies from 25.6 percent to 4.1 percent; 70 percent of the patients in this series were spared operative procedures, while 2.3 percent of the 88 patients initially observed were subsequently operated upon, but did not suffer any ill effects from delayed surgical treatment.

Patients with posterior wounds lateral to the anterior axillary line are not lavaged because of this method's unreliability with retroperitoneal injuries. In many centers these wounds are treated according to the criteria for selective management; other institutions recommend operative intervention to rule out visceral injury.

Since lower chest wounds may penetrate the diaphragm, it is important to evacuate air and blood from the pleural space with chest tubes prior to celiotomy. Although a pneumothorax may not be indicated by x-ray or physical examination, prophylactic insertion of an anterior chest tube will decrease the danger of a tension pneumothorax developing

MAXIMUM DIAPHRAGMATIC RESPIRATORY EXCURSION

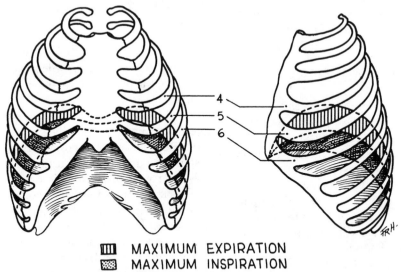

IIIII MAXIMUM EXPIRATION
▦▦▦ MAXIMUM INSPIRATION

Figure 13-3 Diaphragmatic excursion during forced respiration. (*From Shefts, L. M.: The management of thoracoabdominal wounds, Surg. Clin. North Am.,* **38**:1577, 1958.)

during induction of anesthesia and subsequent abdominal exploration.

Gunshot Wounds

The incidence of visceral injury in patients with abdominal gunshot wounds is at least 80 to 90 percent, as compared with 30 to 40 percent in patients with abdominal stab wounds. There is an eight to tenfold difference in mortality rates associated with gunshot wounds when compared with stab wounds.

It is not possible to predict the path of a missile by merely observing the entrance and exit wounds or connecting a line between an entrance wound and the appearance of a bullet on the x-ray film. These missiles may bounce, tumble, ricochet, and embolize.

Extraperitoneal gunshot wounds may produce intraabdominal injury by blast effect. In a report by Edwards and Gaspard, 14 percent of 35 patients sustaining gunshot wounds to the abdomen without penetration of the peritoneal cavity sustained at least one visceral injury.

Any bullet passing in proximity to the peritoneal cavity requires exploratory celiotomy. If the patient's condition permits, anterior, posterior, and lateral films of the abdomen should be made to locate the missile. Selective management, the use of radiopaque material, or local exploration are not recommended.

Once the diagnosis of intraabdominal injury is established and resuscitation instituted, the abdomen is explored. A long midline incision is preferred for the following reasons:

1 It may be made much more rapidly than other incisions, a matter of vital importance when attempting rapid control of exsanguinating hemorrhage.

2 It gives wide access to all parts of the abdomen, which transverse incisions do not.

3 It may be readily extended into either side of the thorax in case of combined thoracoabdominal injury or when better abdominal exposure is required.

4 It may be rapidly closed, which is of great importance in decreasing the anesthesia and operative time in gravely injured patients.

Management of Patients with Exsanguinating Abdominal Hemorrhage

With improvement of prehospital care, more patients are arriving at the hospital in extremis. Frequently this is due to massive intraabdominal hemorrhage that is refractory to standard resuscitative measures. Ledgerwood and associates have recently advocated performing preliminary left thoracotomy and temporary thoracic aortic occlusion prior to opening the abdomen in patients with massive hemoperitoneum, tense abdominal distention, and persistent hypotension. The descending thoracic aorta is quickly and bluntly dissected circumferentially and occluded by a straight vascular clamp just above the diaphragm. Once the abdomen is opened, the aortic clamp can be slowly released following stabilization of the patient and proximal control gained at a lower level. A medium or large Richardson retractor may be used to obtain rapid temporary occlusion of the abdominal aorta just below the diaphragm. The lesser curvature of the stomach is pulled inferiorly, and the flat surface of the retractor blade is compressed firmly against the abdominal aorta, thus occluding it against the vertebra just beneath the diaphragm.

With effective control of massive hemorrhage, resuscitation can be successfully completed, insuring continuous perfusion to the heart and brain and minimizing the possibility of sudden cardiac arrest.

STOMACH INJURIES

Injuries to the stomach from blunt trauma are not common, perhaps because of the relative lack of fixation of the stomach and its protected position. However, penetrating injuries to the stomach from gunshot wounds do occur frequently.

Diagnosis

The diagnosis is generally suspected from the course of the penetrating object, and at times, additional suspicion of gastric injuries arises from the presence of bloody fluid aspirated from the Levin tube. Generally, wounds of the anterior stomach wall are easily seen at celiotomy. Because of the possibility of missing posterior wounds, it is important in all cases of proved or possible gastric injury to open the lesser sac through the gastrocolic omentum. This allows the entire posterior aspect of the stomach to be searched for injury. Points of insertion of the greater and lesser omentum into the greater and lesser curvature of the stomach, respectively, should also be carefully inspected. If a hematoma is noted at the mesenteric attachment, it should be evacuated and the stomach wall at that site carefully inspected for injury.

Treatment

Gastric wounds are repaired by first placing a continuous, locked No. 2-0 absorbable suture through all layers of the gastric wall; a pursestring suture does not give adequate hemostasis. A hemostatic stitch is very important to control extensive bleeding which may occur from the rich submucosal network of blood vessels in the stomach. Following the first layer of closure, an outer inverting row of interrupted nonabsorbable mattress sutures of the Lembert or Halsted type is placed. The outer row of sutures provides adequate serosal approximation of the stomach wall, seals off readily, and prevents leaks. These sutures of the outer layer should not be through-and-through, as is the first row of sutures, but should extend through the seromuscular coat to the submucosal layer of the stomach. Wounds of the stomach are not drained, since they are unlikely to break down and leak, as duodenal wounds sometimes do. However, it is very important to suction the peritoneal cavity, with particular attention to the subhepatic and subphrenic spaces as well as the lesser sac, so that all food particles and gastric juice spilled into these areas are removed.

After operation for a gastric wound, Levin tube suction should be maintained for several days until active peristalsis has resumed and the danger of postoperative gastric dilatation has passed. The gastric aspirate should be observed for inordinate bleeding, which may occur if the hemostatic suture line is inadequate. If bleeding is brisk or persists, the patient should be immediately reexplored for control of the gastric bleeding point. After peristalsis resumes, gastric aspiration is discontinued, and the patient is started on clear liquids in the usual fashion and advanced to a normal diet.

Complications

Complications which may develop following stomach wounds are hemorrhage from, or leakage of, the suture line and development of subhepatic, subphrenic, or lesser sac abscesses secondary to spilling of contaminated gastric contents. The development of such abscesses is suspected following gastric wounds in patients who fail to do well postoperatively and who persist with unexplainable fever for more than a few days. If contamination seems heavy, the skin should be left open until the wound appears clean.

DUODENAL INJURIES

Mortality rates for duodenal injuries have steadily decreased and are directly proportional to the number and severity of associated injuries as well as the time interval between injury and treatment. Lucas reported a mortality rate of 40 percent in those patients who were not operated upon in the first 24 h after injury, as contrasted to a mortality rate of only

11 percent among the patients operated upon within less than 24 h. The average overall mortality rate is about 20 percent. The mortality rate for simple stab wounds involving only the duodenum should be significantly less than 5 percent, while the mortality rate for severe blunt trauma or shotgun wounds to the duodenum ranges from about 35 percent to more than 50 percent, especially when combined with serious pancreatic injuries.

Diagnosis

The diagnosis of blunt trauma to the duodenum and the small bowel is considerably more difficult than that of penetrating trauma to these organs. With duodenal or small bowel trauma, all the characteristic signs of trauma to the abdominal viscera may be minimal or absent, particularly in the early period following injury, for several reasons:

1 The injury of the duodenum following blunt trauma is frequently retroperitoneal, so that duodenal contents leak into the retroperitoneal area rather than into the free peritoneal cavity.

2 Duodenal and small bowel fluid is generally sterile and does not lead to early signs of bacterial peritonitis, as occurs following colon injury.

3 The pH of the small bowel contents is frequently near neutral and, thus, produces only slight chemical irritation of the peritoneum. This is not true of injuries to the duodenum in which duodenal fluid freely flows into the peritoneal cavity. The highly alkaline pH of this fluid causes immediate chemical irritation of the peritoneum and physical signs of such irritation.

One should be suspicious of injury to the duodenum or upper small bowel in patients who have received a blow to the upper abdomen or lower chest, such as from a steering wheel. Testicular pain should raise suspicion of a retroperitoneal duodenal rupture. Also, pain referred to the shoulders, chest, and back is associated with perforation of the duodenum and small intestine.

Several diagnostic aids may be helpful in determining rupture of the duodenum or small bowel. Needle paracentesis of the abdomen, particularly in the right gutter region or in the upper quadrants, may be helpful if blood, bile, or small bowel contents are aspirated. Peritoneal lavage may likewise be beneficial, but it must be reemphasized that lavage is not accurate with retroperitoneal injuries.

Roentgenograms are helpful and may be diagnostic, but the absence of free intraperitoneal air does not rule out bowel perforation. Retroperitoneal rupture of the duodenum is not often diagnosed by x-ray. However, it may be made based on the finding of a large accumulation of air around the right kidney. It is also important to inspect the psoas muscle margins on the plain film of the abdomen for the presence of air, indicating retroperitoneal rupture of a viscus. When the diagnosis is delayed for more than 24 h, the retroperitoneal dissection of air becomes obvious, as it extends massively down the right gutter and into both sides of the pelvis, up into the mediastinum, and occasionally above the right hemidiaphragm. After initial films are obtained, it may be helpful to inject air into the Levin tube. This may confirm a suspicious injury not demonstrated on previous films. Additionally, water soluble radiopaque dye can be given in an attempt to detect a duodenal injury. This contrast material washes out so fast it is not reliable in detecting small bowel leaks. Such diagnostic procedures are unnecessary if other clinical signs indicate the need for exploratory celiotomy.

Treatment

When celiotomy is done for suspected intraabdominal injury, duodenal lesions are often missed, especially retroperitoneal lesions of the third and fourth portion. This is due to superficial observation, inadequate exposure, and lack of persistence on the part of the surgeon. To avoid overlooking a duodenal injury, which contributes to the high mortality from these wounds, it is important to inspect the entire duodenum during abdominal exploration. This is particularly true when a retroperitoneal hematoma is noted near the duodenum or if there is crepitation or bile-stained fluid along the lateral margins of the duodenum retroperitoneally. As Cohn et al. state, the following signs, in addition to those mentioned, indicate careful exploration of the duodenum in the retroperitoneal area: elevation of the posterior peritoneum with a glassy edema; petechiae or fat necrosis over the ascending and transverse colon or mesocolon; retroperitoneal phlegmon; hematoma over the head of the pancreas extending into the base of the mesocolon; fat necrosis of the retroperitoneal tissues; and/or discoloration of retroperitoneal tissues—dark from hemorrhage, grayish from suppuration, or yellowish from bile. If these signs are noted or if the duodenum is contused, the duodenum should be widely mobilized by the Kocher maneuver, incising the peritoneum along its lateral margins, so that it is completely mobilized along with the head of the pancreas. Thus, small areas of perforation in the retroperitoneal aspect of the duodenum may be seen.

A report from the Lahey Clinic describes a technique for wide exposure of the third and fourth portions of the duodenum. This involves mobilizing the cecum, right colon, hepatic flexure of the colon, and mesenteries of these organs up to and including the ligament of Treitz, carrying the dissection of the mesocolon along the attachment to the root of the small bowel mesentery, as shown in Fig. 13-4.

Often retroperitoneal wounds of the duodenum which have been missed are not recognized until several days later, when bile-stained fluid drains from the abdominal wound of a patient who has continued to do poorly postoperatively.

The local treatment of the duodenal perfo-

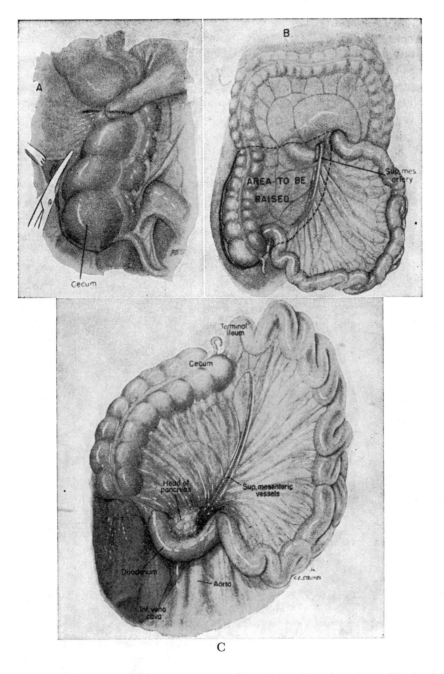

Figure 13-4 A technique for the exposure of the third and fourth portions of the duodenum. (*A, B*) Initial dissection for mobilization of the right side of the colon, small intestine, and mesentery. (*C*) Exposure obtained of the third and fourth portions of the duodenum. (*From Cattell, R. B., and Braasch, J. W.: A technique for the exposure of the third and fourth portions of the duodenum, Surg., Gynecol. Obstet., 111:379, 1960. By permission of Surgery, Gynecology & Obstetrics.*)

ration itself will depend more on the size of the perforation than on any other single factor. Generally, an attempt is made to close a duodenal perforation, if this can be done without decreasing the lumen of the duodenum. This closure is performed with a continuous locking No. 3-0 absorbable suture through all layers of the duodenal wall, followed by an outer layer of nonabsorbable interrupted mattress sutures in the seromuscular layer. After this, the duodenum should be carefully palpated to exclude stenosis. If the perforation is so large that closure will cause a stricture of the duodenum, consideration should be given to (1) complete division of the duodenum and an end-to-end anastomosis or (2) division of the duodenum, closure of both ends, and a gastroenterosotomy.

Kobold and Thal have reported another method of handling large duodenal defects which previously might have necessitated one of the above techniques of duodenal division. This consists of bringing up a retrocolic loop of proximal jejunum and suturing it over the large defect in the duodenum, with an inner row of absorbable sutures taken between the torn edge of the duodenum and the seromuscular layer of the jejunum and an outer layer of nonabsorbable mattress sutures taken between the seromuscular coats of the duodenum and the jejunum. Animal studies, as well as clinical usage, have demonstrated the feasibility of this "patching" technique in managing large duodenal defects (Fig. 13-5). This technique may also be applicable for less severe duodenal injuries that cannot be securely closed. Buttressing of a tenuous closure by either a jejunal patch technique or reinforcement with an omental patch may improve the repair.

When there is sufficient loss of duodenal tissue to obviate suture repair, the duodenal defect may be closed, if the medial duodenal wall and ampulla are intact, by performing a side-to-side or end-to-side duodenojejunos-

tomy. This is done by constructing a defunctionalized Roux-Y jejunal limb approximately 35 to 40 cm in length. The end of the jejunal limb is closed and brought up in a retrocolic position so it lies lateral to the large duodenal injury. The defect in the duodenum is then closed simply by performing a side-to-side anastomosis between the duodenum and the defunctionalized jejunal limb. The side-to-side anastomosis is preferred to the end-to-side anastomosis since it permits a longer duodenal defect to be covered by the jejunum, the suture line is under less tension, and the anastomosis has a better blood supply.

Berne et al. have described a duodenal "diverticulization" procedure for combined extensive injury of the duodenum and pancreas or severe injury of the duodenum alone. The essential components of the operation consist of suture closure of the duodenal injury, gastric antrectomy with end-to-side gastrojejunostomy, tube duodenostomy, and generous drainage (Fig. 13-6). The bypassed duodenum with its associated biliary and pancreatic ductal system becomes a very low pressure diverticulum. Duodenal diverticulization is an approach to combined injury to the duodenum and pancreas that may avoid both the potential undesirable sequelae of simple closure of the duodenum and the magnitude of pancreaticoduodenectomy. For combined duodenal and pancreatic injury or severe duodenal injury so treated, Berne reports a mortality of 16 percent, which is extremely low for these types of injuries.

The common bile duct should be identified, with insertion of a T tube, if the region of the ampulla is involved. Reimplantation of the common bile duct sometimes may be necessary. Approximately 75 to 80 percent of all duodenal injuries may be closed by debridement of the wound edges and simple suture. For the other 20 to 25 percent, one of the repair procedures described above or recommended by Cleveland and Waddell is used

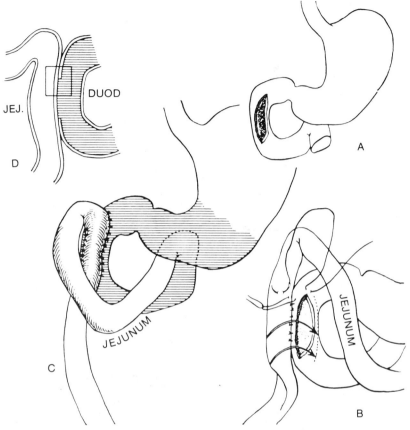

Figure 13-5 (*A*) Area of excision of duodenal wall. (*B*) Technique of placement of intact jejunum over the wound to form a patch. (*C*) The completed closure. (*D*) Cross section of the completed closure showing the relationship of the intact jejunum to the duodenal perforation. The area enclosed within the box is the site from which tissue was subsequently removed for study. (*From Kobold, E. E., and Thal, A. P.: A simple method for the management of experimental wounds of the duodenum, Surg., Gynecol. Obstet., **116:**340, 1963. By permission of Surgery, Gynecology & Obstetrics.*)

(Fig. 13-7). Rarely, even a pancreaticoduodenectomy may be necessary to manage large defects of the duodenum and periampullary region.

It is important after repair of duodenal injuries to establish adequate drainage. This is accomplished by the use of Penrose and sump drains. Care is taken to place the drains near the injury but not on the suture lines, since placement directly on the sutures might cause leakage of the repair. It is even more important to institute drainage if there appears to be

an associated pancreatic injury, as often occurs.

Fistulas

Duodenal fistulas develop in about 5 to 10 percent of patients sustaining duodenal trauma. Fistula formation following duodenal injury occurs because of poor blood supply, infection, excessive tension on suture lines, or distal obstruction, and may lead to a mortality rate approaching 50 percent. The occurrence may be related to a lack of serosal surface in

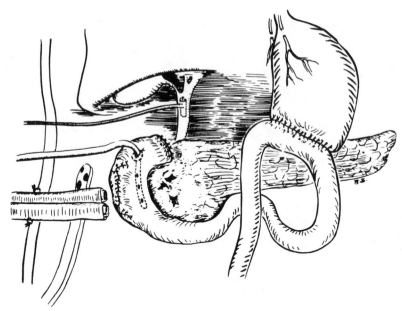

Figure 13-6 The essential components of duodenal diverticulization, including gastric antrectomy, tube duodenostomy, gastrojejunostomy, and drainage. Vagotomy and drainage of the biliary tract may be advisable. (*From Beane, C. J., Donovan, A. J., White, E. J., and Yellin, A. E.: Duodenal diverticulization for duodenal and pancreatic injury, Am. Journal of Surg.* **127**:503, 1974.)

Figure 13-7 Diagrammatic representation of various operative procedures in present series of cases. (I) Simple closure. (II) End-to-end duodenoduodenostomy. (III, IV) Closure of both ends of duodenum and gastroenterostomy. (V) Closure of distal duodenum and duodenoje-junostomy. (VI) Duodenojejunostomy and gastroduodenostomy. (VII) Resection of fourth part of duodenum and duodenojejunostomy. (*From Cleveland, H. C., and Waddell, W. R.: Retroperitoneal rupture of the duodenum due to nonpenetrating trauma, Surg. Clin. North Am.,* **43**:413, 1963.)

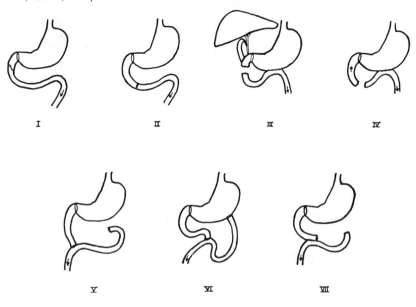

I II III IV

V VI VII

which to sew the retroperitoneal portion of the duodenum, so that an insecure closure is obtained. Fistulas may be prevented by prolonged decompression of the duodenum following closure of the wound. This is especially indicated in more severe injuries of the duodenum and is accomplished by several means:

1 A Levin tube may be threaded through the entire course of the duodenum with sufficient holes in the tube to allow simultaneous decompression of the duodenum and stomach. The tube may be brought through the anterior wall as a gastrostomy tube and placed on suction, or it may be inserted through the nasopharynx.

2 A tube may be inserted through a Witzel (serosal-lined) tunnel and threaded in a retrograde direction so that its tip lies within the duodenum just below the fistula. Suction is applied to this tube, which is brought out as a jejunostomy and greatly reduces the volume of drainage, thereby promoting closure of the fistula.

3 A No. 10 Foley catheter may be placed through a small stab wound in the duodenum, adjacent to the area of duodenal injury to serve as a vent. The tube is maintained under suction until active bowel sounds return. At this time, suction is discontinued, and the tube is attached to a glass Y tube fixed to a stand at the level of the duodenum. This arrangement does not allow siphonage of duodenal contents, as does gravity drainage, but does provide a decompressive vent if the pressure rises in the duodenum. After 9 or 10 days, at which time a fibrinous tract has formed about the small Foley catheter, the bag, which contains only 2 mL of water, is deflated. The Foley tube is again placed on gentle suction and is pulled just outside the duodenum, where it remains on suction for an additional 24 h. At the end of the 24-h period, the Foley catheter is removed if drainage is minimal. It is reemphasized that a small No. 10 Foley is used since a tube of this size provides very adequate decompression without causing a fistula when it is removed.

Postoperative Care

Postoperative care of these patients may be extremely difficult. Extracellular fluid volume deficits may be large, particularly if fistulas, retroperitoneal inflammation, or pancreatitis occur. It is very important to maintain the extracellular fluid volume with adequate infusions of balanced salt solution. In addition, these patients should be maintained on adequate doses of broad-spectrum antibiotics administered intravenously. Gastric and duodenal decompression should be continued for long periods of time in order to protect the suture lines. The average period of gastroduodenal decompression for duodenal wounds is about 5 to 7 days following exploration. If a fistula forms, gastroduodenal decompression should be continued for longer periods and a sump drain should be inserted into the drain site for continuous active suction of the fistulous tract. This is instituted to prevent the collection of duodenal fluid with possible spread throughout the abdominal cavity, to promote collapse and healing of the fistulous tract, to prevent digestion of the skin by duodenal fluid draining onto the skin, and to aid calculation and replacement of fluid and electrolyte losses.

When a duodenal fistula develops, the patient should be placed on central intravenous hyperalimentation according to the principles of Dudrick and associates. This regimen maintains excellent nutrition and may reduce the volume of gastrointestinal secretions.

With central intravenous hyperalimentation, it is now frequently unnecessary to perform feeding jejunostomies to provide nutritional support for patients with duodenal fistulas. If for some reason central intravenous feeding is not possible, a feeding jejunostomy may become necessary. Standard jejunostomy feedings are given as tolerated by the patient. Duodenal fluid recovered from the fistulas may be refed through the jejunostomy tube.

If, after 5 to 7 days of Levin tube or gastrostomy decompression of the duodenum, the patient is doing well, shows no evidence of duodenal leak, and has adequate bowel activity, the patient is given 1 oz of water orally every hour for approximately 12 h, after the Levin tube is removed or the gastrostomy tube clamped. If water is tolerated, diet is increased in the usual fashion. Also, after feeding has been instituted for 1 to 2 days and there has been little or no drainage, the Penrose drains are advanced and removed over 3 days unless further drainage ensues. In the face of continued drainage, the drain should be left for at least 2 or 3 weeks, or as long as any significant drainage continues. After about 3 weeks, if drainage persists, the Penrose drains may be removed; the only drainage tube which should remain is the sump drain, which is removed when drainage has dropped to a minimum.

Occasionally, the duodenal fistula does not close despite adequate nonoperative treatment as described above. In such cases, when a reasonable trial of conservative treatment has been made and the patient is in optimal condition for reoperation, the abdomen is opened and completely explored to rule out distal bowel obstruction, which may be causing the fistula to persist. The fistula is exposed and a Roux-Y defunctionalized limb of proximal jejunum is brought up and anastomosed to it. This procedure permanently diverts the fistulous drainage internally and has been very effective in treating persistent duodenal fistulas.

Intramural Hematoma

Another interesting but infrequently reported lesion of the duodenum secondary to trauma is intramural hematoma of the duodenum. This lesion is generally caused by blunt abdominal trauma which causes rupture of the intramural duodenal blood vessels with formation of a dark sausage-shaped mass in the submucosal layer. The hematoma causes partial or complete duodenal obstruction. Patients show signs of high small bowel obstruction with nausea and vomiting associated with abdominal tenderness and sometimes a suggestion of a right upper quadrant mass. If there is any suspicion of a traumatic perforation, however, the upper gastrointestinal (GI) series should be done with water soluble contrast media. If this shows no evidence of perforation, barium is then given to provide the sharp detail necessary for demonstration of the so-called "coiled-spring sign" or "stacked-coin sign" in the second and third portions of the duodenum. The serum amylase level may be elevated. This lesion may occur spontaneously in patients on anticoagulants.

Treatment generally consists of celiotomy, evacuation of the duodenal hematoma, and closure of the defect in the seromuscular coat of the duodenum with interrupted nonabsorbable sutures after control of any bleeding points. Fullen has recently recommended conservative treatment of this injury. Eleven patients treated with restriction of oral intake, nasogastric suction, and intravenous fluids and electrolytes all survived without complication. Nonoperative treatment is only considered after satisfactorily excluding the possibility of duodenal perforation or other associated injuries requiring celiotomy.

SMALL BOWEL INJURIES

Injuries to the small bowel are more frequent than injuries to the duodenum or colon. The usual mechanism of small bowel injury from blunt trauma is the crushing of the small bowel against the vertebral column. Rupture of the small bowel is also caused by shearing and tearing forces applied to the abdomen, but rarely by sudden elevation of intraluminal pressure unless a closed loop of bowel is present.

Penetrating trauma to the small bowel from

a gunshot wound or stab wound is frequent, although, surprisingly, it has been noted that in patients who have stab wounds to the abdomen, the small bowel has been spared. This is probably because the great mobility of the small bowel allows it to slide away from the knife, a much less likely occurrence with gunshot wounds than with stab wounds.

In exploring the abdomen for injuries to the small bowel, it is important to inspect completely the circumference of the small bowel and its attached mesentery from the ligament of Treitz to the ileocecal valve. The bowel may be completely transected in one or more places by blunt trauma with or without severe injury to the mesentery and its blood supply; at times, the mesentery may be torn from a segment of bowel, thereby depriving the bowel of its blood supply.

Treatment

Small, single perforations of the small bowel may be closed safely with a single layer of interrupted nonabsorbable mattress sutures which include and invert the seromuscular and submucosal coats of the bowel. A hemostatic stitch as required for stomach wounds is not necessary for small bowel wounds because the small bowel does not tend to continue bleeding from the submucosal plexus as does the stomach. Individual bleeders, however, should be ligated with fine suture material. An advantage of a single layer closure is its rapidity of performance, which is important to patients in precarious condition following multiple trauma.

Two small perforations of the bowel which are close together may often be repaired by converting the wounds into one and closing the resulting defect as a single linear wound. This type of repair does not constrict the lumen of the bowel as much as two separate lines of suture placed close together and is more secure. Multiple perforations of the small bowel may occur following injury from

shotgun pellets. Each one of these injuries should be carefully sought out and closed with interrupted rows of nonabsorbable mattress sutures.

Long linear lacerations of the lumen should also be closed with a single row of nonabsorbable sutures after ligating any persistent bleeders with small nonabsorbable sutures. Longitudinal lacerations may be closed in a longitudinal direction or transversely according to the Heineke-Mikulicz principle.

Injuries produced by high-velocity missiles may cause severe contusion of the tissue surrounding the actual perforation. Because the contusion is a site of potential tissue necrosis and bowel leakage caused by thrombosis of vessels in the area of blast injury, it should be debrided. The debridement should extend back to the viable bowel where active bleeding is obtained.

If the wound is large or long and longitudinal, the damaged segment should be resected to avoid compromise of the lumen. Also, if there are multiple wounds in a short segment of bowel, it is much safer and easier to resect the injured segment than attempt to suture each of the closely spaced wounds. Perforations and lacerations at the mesenteric border, unless they are quite small, are difficult to repair and are frequently associated with vascular impairment. They also should be managed by resection of the involved segment when adequate closure cannot be obtained without interference of the blood supply. Bowel transections should be reanastomosed after debriding the contused and damaged bowel on either side of the wound back to normal bowel with good blood supply. Careful attention should be given to ensuring uninjured mesentery adjacent to the suture line of the anastomosis. Extensive segments of bowel may be avulsed from the mesentery with resultant loss of blood supply. All necrotic or potentially necrotic bowel and injured mesentery must be resected, and an end-to-end anastomosis made between uninjured bowel attached to uninjured mesentery.

Contusion of the small bowel should be assumed to be larger than is apparent. Such injuries are dangerous since they may lead to necrosis and perforation. Contusions up to 1 cm in diameter may be turned in with a row of fine, nonabsorbable mattress sutures. Larger contusions should be resected.

Postoperative care of patients with wounds of the small bowel should include maintenance on nasogastric suction and no oral intake until adequate bowel activity has returned. Also, these patients are maintained on antibiotics which are begun preoperatively. Usually, the antibiotic is discontinued about the time the nasogastric tube is removed unless there is some indication to continue treatment. Leakage from suture lines and intestinal obstruction are rarely seen if the wounds are properly managed. In a report by Giddings and McDaniel concerning wounds of the jejunum and ileum during World War II, leakage from suture lines occurred in only 1 percent and intestinal obstruction in 1.7 percent in a series of 1168 patients with small bowel injuries, most of whom had multiple visceral injuries. Again, extracellular fluid volume deficits should be replaced in patients with small bowel injury with adequate amounts of balanced salt solutions.

COLON INJURIES

The morbidity and mortality from acute injuries to the colon have been significantly reduced by an aggressive surgical approach. This has been largely influenced by the experiences of military surgeons beginning in World War II. This improvement was due to several factors, including improved methods of triage and transportation, effective replacement of blood and fluid, and early surgical intervention combined with the ancillary use of antibiotics. The mortality rate for wounds of the colon of 37 percent in World War II was reduced to approximately 15 percent during the Korean conflict, and in most recent civilian series is reported to be between 3 and 9 percent. The majority of military surgeons treating acute injuries of the colon tended to exteriorize the wound as an artificial anus to prevent further soilage of the peritoneal cavity. This approach to these particular wounds was duly carried over into civilian practice and reflected in the subsequent reduction in mortality and morbidity. In the later phase of the Korean conflict, however, some modification of this aggressiveness was noted in that small primary wounds, treated early, were handled by primary closure without exteriorization.

Acute wounds of the colon which occur in a civilian environment exhibit features that may modify indications for exteriorization of the wound. Types of injuries noted in a military situation resulted from either high-velocity missiles or fragmentation missiles in which there was massive destruction of tissue and usually gross soilage of the peritoneal cavity. In the civilian environment, the wounds are more often caused by a low-velocity missile and usually are unassociated with massive destruction of surrounding organs and tissues. The time from wounding to initial treatment in the civilian situation is generally somewhat less than that noted during military conflict. Similarly, associated injuries occurring in civilian accidents do not tend to be so numerous nor so massive as those in military environment, and this has had a definite influence on morbidity and mortality.

Etiology and Diagnosis

Acute injuries of the colon may be divided into penetrating wounds and wounds resulting from blunt trauma. In the former group, colon injuries may be the result of industrial accidents involving explosions resulting in impalement, penetrating injuries from flying objects, or blast injuries. These injuries may be either the direct result of explosives or accidents involving sources of compressed air. External acts of violence constitute an important source of injuries to the colon. These are generally penetrating injuries caused by guns or knives or, on rarer occasions, blunt abdominal trauma.

A systematic, diagnostic approach to problems of abdominal trauma is necessary, but specific examination of the colon may be necessary to delineate an injury. This is particularly pertinent in instances in which instrumentation is the cause of suspected perforation. Rectal examination and sigmoidoscopy should occupy a prominent place in the examination of these patients. Diagnostic abdominal x-ray studies are employed to determine if there is a perforation of the colon with leakage of air into the peritoneal cavity. Anteriorposterior and lateral decubitis views are particularly helpful in these instances. Contrast studies of the colon should be employed rarely and cautiously in view of the morbidity and mortality associated with leakage of barium and feces into the free peritoneal cavity. Water soluble opaque contrast media is preferable when penetration of the colon is suspected, if these studies are deemed necessary.

Treatment

The treatment of colon injuries continues to be controversial. Some surgeons contend that more complications, chiefly intraabdominal abscesses, develop if primary suture repair or resection are employed to treat colon injuries, in contrast to others who argue that there are fewer complications following primary repair. Fortunately neither group advocates exclusive use of their methods, and they agree that each patient should be selectively managed.

Anatomic location of the colonic wound is an important factor in determining the choice of repair. Small perforations of the cecum and ascending colon in good-risk patients with minimal fecal spill lend themselves to primary repair. This is accomplished with a two-layer closure employing No. 3-0 absorbable suture as an inner layer and No. 3-0 nonreactive nonabsorbable suture as an outer layer. When injury to the cecum or right colon is more extensive, the decompression of a primary repair may be accomplished by the use of a cecostomy. If the injury is near the appendix, operative trauma may cause obliteration of the appendiceal lumen, which may lead to postoperative appendicitis. Decompression in these cases can be accomplished by removing the appendix (which is not routinely done with abdominal trauma patients) and inserting an appendicostomy tube for decompression. Seromuscular sutures are placed about the base of the appendix and secured to the lateral peritoneum in order to prevent intraperitoneal leakage about the area of tube insertion. When the appendicostomy tube is removed, barring distal obstruction, the appendicostomy site will close spontaneously.

Serious injury to the right colon involving loss of extensive tissue may require a primary resection. Because of the low bacterial population in the right colon, in most instances it is safe to perform a primary ileo–right transverse colostomy. In gravely ill patients, it may be necessary to construct a temporary ileostomy and mucous fistula of the distal colon.

Injuries located in the transverse or left colon are managed somewhat differently. Primary repair is considered only for minor, clean perforations with no fecal spill. Specifically, primary repair should be avoided if there is: (1) gross fecal material in the peritoneal cavity at a distance of more than 5 cm from the site of perforation, (2) shock, (3) significant associated injuries, or (4) considerable time between injury and repair.

Injuries that are considered too extensive for primary repair are exteriorized as a loop or diverting double-barrel colostomy if located in the transverse or sigmoid colon. If it is not possible to mobilize enough bowel for exteriorization, then the perforation is primarily closed and a proximal diverting colostomy performed in the right transverse colon. The right transverse colostomy is preferable to a left transverse colostomy because of greater mobility and ease of closure. In cases of multiple injury, the distal wounds are closed primarily and the proximal wound exteriorized as a colostomy or, if it does not lend itself to a colostomy, is likewise closed and a right transverse colostomy performed. If excessive colon is blasted away, it may be necessary to resect the injured segment and form a proximal colostomy and distal mucus fistula or oversew the distal end and return it to the peritoneal cavity for reconstruction at a later time. There is virtually no place for a resection and primary anastomosis in the treatment of transverse and left colon injuries.

A compromise between immediate colostomy and primary closure has been advocated by Beall and associates. These authors advocate exteriorization of a loop containing the primarily repaired injury. Following 10 to 14 days of observation, the segment is returned to the peritoneal cavity under local anesthesia. Hunt and his associates emphasized that the ideal milieu for colonic healing is the peritoneal cavity; exclusion of anastomosis of the peritoneal cavity increases the incidence of disruption. Exteriorized colon suture lines are infected since serositis inevitably develops in a few days, and leakage from such exteriorized closure does not mean the same result would have occurred intraperitoneally. Either primary closure alone or establishment of a colostomy as the initial procedure is preferable to exteriorization of sutured perforations.

Postoperative management of the patient with a colostomy is facilitated by good enterostomal therapy. Many hospitals now employ the use of enterostomal therapists who assist patients in the management of their appliances and stomal-related problems.

Early closure of the colostomy is indicated in patients who have completely recovered and have no distal colon injury. It is desirable to close the simple colostomy in 7 to 10 days if a single injury has been exteriorized. Frequently this will not be possible, and the timing of the colostomy closure will be dependent upon complete recovery from associated injuries. Prior to closure, both wounds should be visualized radiographically to assure that no lesion persists.

RECTAL INJURIES

Rectal injuries present challenging problems not associated with injuries to other parts of the large bowel. These injuries are difficult to visualize, hard to repair, and are often associated with massive soft tissue infection. The mortality has steadily decreased with improvement of surgical technique and is generally reported to be between 10 and 20 percent. A majority of these injuries occur as a result of some act of violence; occasionally, however, they may occur with instrumentation, administration of enemas, or foreign body perforation.

Diagnosis may be difficult, but all patients suspected of having rectal trauma should have a careful anorectal examination including preoperative sigmoidoscopy. Less obvious injuries may be detected by the presence of guaiac-positive stool.

Aggressive management of extraperitoneal rectal injuries is essential if serious septic complications and increased mortality is to be avoided. Experience from military injuries has provided the guidelines for sound surgical principles.

It is emphasized that about 25 to 35 percent of rectal injuries are associated with some injury to the distal urinary tract. The possibility of such associated injuries must always be considered, and appropriate diagnostic studies, including an intravenous pyelogram and a cystourethrogram, should be obtained.

Treatment

Fecal diversion and presacral drainage are the two essential elements necessary for proper management of rectal injuries. Regardless of how minor the injury may seem, it is necessary to divert the fecal stream by means of a sigmoid diverting colostomy. It is not necessary to repair the injury unless it is easily accessible. Attempts to visualize and close a distal rectal wound may lead to troublesome bleeding deep within the pelvis.

Drainage of the retrorectal area is extremely important. This can be established by making a curvilinear incision in the posterior perianal area, incising the anococcygeal ligament and bluntly dissecting into the presacral space (Fig. 13-8). Two Penrose drains will usually suffice, but with extensive injuries it may be necessary to utilize sump drainage for a few days.

Lavenson and Cohen, based on their experience from the Vietnam conflict, strongly recommend removal of all feces from the distal rectum. This is accomplished by irrigating copious amounts of saline solution through the defunctionalized segment until the return is clear. They report a significant decrease in mortality and complication rates when utilizing this technique. Military injuries are generally associated with high-velocity missiles and cause more fecal contamination and blast injury to surrounding pelvic tissue. In civilian injuries, distal irrigation may not be as important, as evidenced by Trunkey and associates, who report a lower morbidity and mortality rate in their series, in which distal irrigation was not employed.

Serious perineal injuries are treated in a similar manner. Even in the absence of rectal

Figure 13-8 A curvilinear incision is made over the posterior anal area. By blunt dissection the retrorectal area is entered and Penrose drains are inserted. (*From Trunkey, D., Hays, R. J., and Shires, G. T.: Management of rectal trauma, Journal of Trauma,* **13**:411, 1973.)

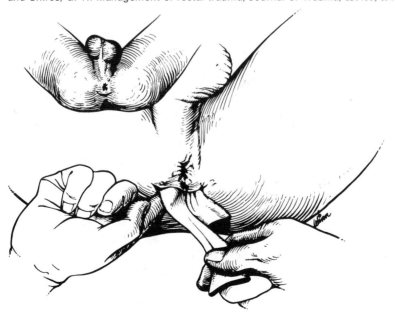

injury, sepsis can be avoided by early fecal diversion. Failure to recognize this potential problem may lead to extensive soft tissue infections extending from the knee to the axilla with potential involvement of the anterior and posterior abdominal wall.

LIVER INJURIES

Injury to the liver is suspected in all patients with penetrating or blunt trauma that involves the lower chest and upper abdomen. Among patients with penetrating abdominal trauma, the liver is second only to the small bowel as the structure most commonly injured; among those with blunt trauma, the liver is second only to the spleen as the most commonly injured organ. About 80 percent of liver injuries occur as a result of penetrating trauma from stab wounds or gunshot wounds, whereas only 15 to 20 percent occur with blunt trauma. In the past decade, the incidence of stab wounds has diminished while the incidence of gunshot wounds, especially those caused by high-velocity and large-caliber missiles, and blunt trauma has increased. These changes in the types of liver injuries, the more rapid transport of patients with hepatic trauma to treatment facilities, and better resuscitation methods have caused an increase in severity of liver injuries that are likely to confront the surgeon.

Early exploration, prompt replacement of blood and use of balanced electrolyte solution, use of antibiotics, proper choice of surgical treatment, plus adequate drainage are all factors that have led to increased survival rates. The average overall mortality rate of patients with hepatic trauma is about 13 to 15 percent. However, this rate is directly related to the severity of the liver injury and injuries to other intraabdominal organs. The mortality rate of stab wounds to the liver without associated organ injury is only about 1 percent. When significant liver trauma is associated

with injuries of more than five other intraabdominal organs, or major hepatic resection is required to control bleeding, the mortality rate rises to about 45 to 50 percent.

Treatment

After initial resuscitation and diagnostic maneuvers, patients with suspected hepatic injuries are rapidly moved to the operating room. The entire abdomen and chest are prepped and draped, and a long upper midline incision is made. Sources of bleeding from the liver and the abdomen are quickly appraised, and temporary control of the bleeding is achieved by manual compression of packs placed over the bleeding sites and by temporary occlusion of appropriate major vessels. Digital compression of the hepatic artery and portal vein to temporarily occlude the blood flow to the liver (the Pringle maneuver) may control or slow hepatic hemorrhage in some patients, but more often it is necessary to combine the Pringle maneuver with compression packs placed over the liver injury to effectively control hemorrhage. There is general agreement that, in the normothermic liver, complete occlusion of blood flow to the liver can be safely sustained for about 15 min without causing any hepatocellular damage. If it is necessary to occlude the hepatic blood supply for more than 15 min, the vascular occlusion can be briefly interrupted every 10 or 15 min to allow short periods of uninterrupted hepatic blood flow.

Definitive treatment may be accomplished by drainage alone, suture or hemostatic maneuvers and drainage, or variations of hepatic resection.

Drainage Alone Hepatic hemorrhage will have ceased spontaneously by the time the abdomen is opened or stops soon after compression of the bleeding site in about 50 to 70 percent of patients with liver injuries. In such patients, the only treatment necessary is adequate drainage of the injury. Suturing of non-bleeding liver injuries is unnecessary. This is emphasized by Lucas and Ledgerwood, who reported no rebleeding among 284 patients with liver injuries that stopped bleeding spontaneously or soon after temporary pack compression. Suturing of nonbleeding liver wounds may cause bleeding and needlessly traumatize hepatic tissue.

All liver injuries should be drained with large, 1-in-wide Penrose drains, and several drains should be used in patients with larger injuries. The drains are brought out postero-laterally, as dependently as possible, through an abdominal wall stab wound in order to achieve the best drainage by gravity. This greatly reduces the formation of infected collections of bile, blood, and tissue fluid in the subphrenic and subhepatic spaces. Also, dependent gravity drainage is more reliable than nondependent suction drainage. In most patients with liver injury it is unnecessary to resect the twelfth rib to achieve dependent drainage. Usually the drains can be brought through the stab wound at the tip of, or just below, the twelfth rib. However, in large patients with more extensive liver wounds, it may be preferable to resect the lateral half or two-thirds of the right twelfth rib, as described by Coln, to achieve more effective drainage (Fig. 13-9). An adequate opening, easily admitting two fingers, must be made in the abdominal wall to be certain these injuries are effectively drained. The drains are left in place 5 to 10 days thereafter, being slowly removed over a 3-day period. Not until the end of this time is a firm, fibrinous tract formed about the drains, which insures adequate external drainage of any material that accumulates in the abdomen after the drain is removed.

Suture, Hemostatic Techniques, and Drainage Bleeding persists despite temporary compression packing of the injury site in 30 to 50 percent of patients with liver injuries. De-finitive hemostasis of persistent bleeding liver injuries usually can be achieved by liver sutures. Simple interrupted sutures are placed 2 cm from the wound margins, using No. 2-0 or No. 1-0 chromic suture swaged onto a 2-in blunt-tipped "liver needle." This will allow gentle but firm approximation, thereby stopping most bleeding which originates from the outer 2 cm of the liver parenchyma immediately beneath the capsule of the liver. Larger wounds may require placement of figure-of-eight liver sutures to prevent cutting through the liver capsule. Passage of the liver suture through buttressing materials such as Surgicel, Gelfoam, or omentum is seldom needed if the sutures are placed 2 cm from the margin of the injury and tied gently. However, if a bolster is needed, it is preferable to use a vascularized pedicle of omentum instead of foreign material. Trunkey, Shires, and McClelland have abandoned the technique, previously described, using interlocking mattress sutures for hemostasis. These authors now recommend direct suture ligation of the bleeding vessel as an attempt to reduce the chance of strangulation and subsequent necrosis.

Recently, microcrystalline collagen powder (Avitene) has been reported to be successful in controlling bleeding from liver wounds. Unlike other material such as Gelfoam, Avitene can be left in liver wounds without inciting significant foreign body reaction. The use of other hemostatic agents as well as gauze packs to tamponade hemorrhage is not recommended.

The use of liver sutures to obtain hemostasis from both the entrance and the exit sites of long gunshot tracts in the liver is controversial. However, Lucas and Ledgerwood state that this technique was successfully used in several of their patients who otherwise would have required extensive surgery. Placement of the liver sutures at both ends of the bullet tract stops bleeding arising from the subcapsular area, which is the usual source. During their

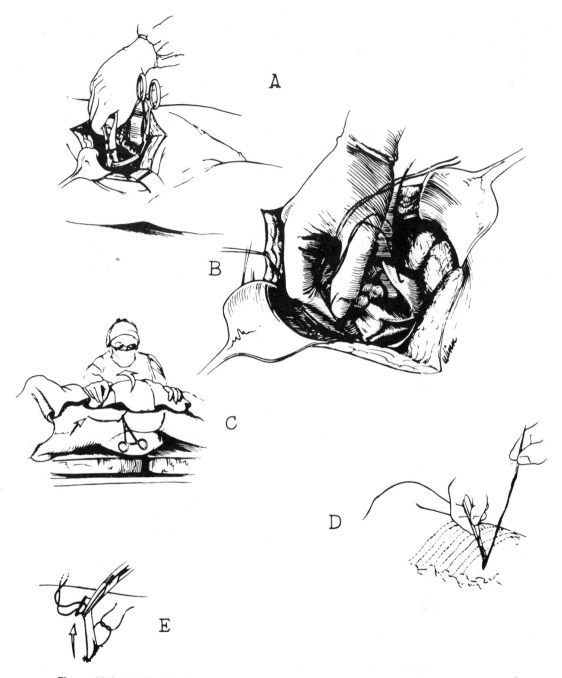

Figure 13-9 (*A*) Twelfth rib removed. (*B*) Threaded needle passed through rib bed. (*C*) Needle located and suture pulled through. (*D*) Incision made along course of wire. (*E*) Drain located, pulled through, and anchored. (*From Coln, Dale: A Technique for drainage through the bed of the twelfth rib, Surg. Gynecol. Obstet. 141:608, 1975.*)

5-year prospective review, Lucas and Ledgerwood found that only one patient developed an intrahepatic abscess following this technique and no patients developed hemobilia after closure of both ends of a long gunshot tract. Continued bleeding, which persists after closure of both ends of the tract, is usually identified at the initial operation by blood oozing between the liver sutures or by an increase in the size of the liver within 10 min after placement of the sutures. If the persistently bleeding tract is short and close to an accessible surface of the liver, hemostasis can be achieved by limited wedge resection or by resectional debridement, incorporating the tract as part of the debridement. Persistent active bleeding from deep bilobar tracts that do not lend themselves to resectional debridement is best controlled either by ligation of an appropriate branch of the hepatic artery or by tractotomy and ligation of the intraparechymal bleeding vessels. However, tractotomy may cause further bleeding, and for this reason, ligation of one of the main hepatic artery branches is preferable since it usually stops arterial bleeding from deep tracts and is likely to cause less morbidity than tractotomy.

Ligation of an appropriate major branch of the hepatic artery (i.e., the right or left branch) is a safe and effective means for controlling liver bleeding in patients with active arterial bleeding from wounds that do not permit suture ligature or wedge resection and in whom bleeding stops with temporary hepatic artery occlusion. Mays reported achieving liver hemostasis in 15 of 16 patients who underwent ligation of hepatic artery branches. Lucas and Ledgerwood did not find ligation of major branches of the hepatic artery as effective in arresting hemorrhage as did Mays, possibly because some of their patients were bleeding from major venous injuries. It is suggested that the right or left hepatic artery should not be ligated if a simple temporary compression pack or suturing of a bleeding liver injury controls the hemorrhage. However, if compression or suturing does not control bleeding and temporary occlusion of the hepatic artery branch supplying the injured area of the liver does stop hemorrhage, then the appropriate major hepatic artery branch should be ligated, especially if the alternative treatment is a hepatic resection.

Resection Resectional debridement or limited wedge resection is recommended for control of bleeding from the ragged liver injuries that may be caused by shotgun wounds, high-velocity rifle wounds, and severe blunt injuries. Limited resectional debridement of shattered liver tissue usually achieves hemostasis from such injuries effectively and safely. The margins of resectional debridement should be 2 or 3 cm byond the point of injury, and bleeding during debridement is controlled by digital parenchymal constriction and/or temporary occlusion of the inflow of blood to the liver at the porta hepatis. The liver parenchyma is separated bluntly by finger fracture, a suction tip, or a scalpel handle. Vessels and bile ducts are secured by individual suture ligation or metal clips as they are encountered. It is not necessary to oppose the margins of resection with interrupted liver sutures if bleeding from the resected surface is controlled. This suture technique may be undesirable, since it may create a potentially infected closed space within the liver.

Anatomic hepatic lobectomy for control of bleeding, especially from the right lobe, is best reserved for patients in whom: (1) hepatic suturing is unsuccessful, (2) resectional debridement or hepatotomy with intraparenchymal hemostasis is precluded by the anatomic location of the injury, or (3) occlusion of the hepatic artery is ineffective in controlling hemorrhage. Although resectional debridement or sublobar hepatic resection may be required in about 4 or 5 percent of all patients with liver injuries, no more than 2 or 3 percent require anatomic lobar resection to control hemorrhage. Most of the few patients with liver injuries who require major hepatic lobectomies to control bleeding have massive shattering injuries of the liver, injuries of the retrohepatic vena cava, or injuries to the major hepatic vein (Fig. 13-10). If it becomes apparent that major lobar resection is necessary, the hepatic bleeding is temporarily controlled by manual compression packing and a Pringle maneuver while the midline abdominal incision is extended by performing a median sternotomy.

A median sternotomy is much more quickly and easily made and closed than a right thoracoabdominal incision, causes considerably less diaphragmatic injury, provides much easier access to the vena cava and hepatic veins, permits easier insertion of a retrohepatic vena caval shunt, if this is required, and causes less postoperative pain and pulmonary morbidity than a right thoracoabdominal incision.

After wide exposure is obtained by the median sternotomy extension of the midline abdominal incision, Rumel tourniquets are placed about the vena cava superior and inferior to the liver. The superior tape is placed about the vena cava superior to the central tendon of the diaphragm after this portion of the vena cava is exposed by opening the pericardium. These tapes permit temporary occlusion of the vena cava for insertion of a retrohepatic intracaval shunt if vascular isolation of the liver is required during hepatic lobectomy because of major retrohepatic vena cava or major hepatic vein injury. The hepatic artery, portal vein, and bile ducts supplying the lobe to be resected are then suture ligated and divided (Fig. 13-11). After this, hepatic resection can be carried out by dividing Glisson's capsule with a cautery along the line appropriate for the lobe being removed (Fig. 13-12). The lobe is removed by fracturing through the liver substance along the line of resection with the thumb and forefinger or with the tip of an abdominal suction tube from

Figure 13-10   Typical liver injury requiring hepatic resection. (*From McClelland, R., Shires, T., and Poulos, E.: Hepatic resection for massive trauma, J. Trauma, 4:282, 1964.*)

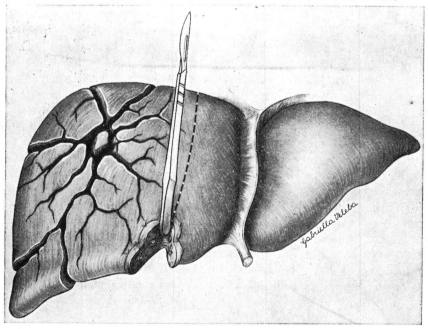

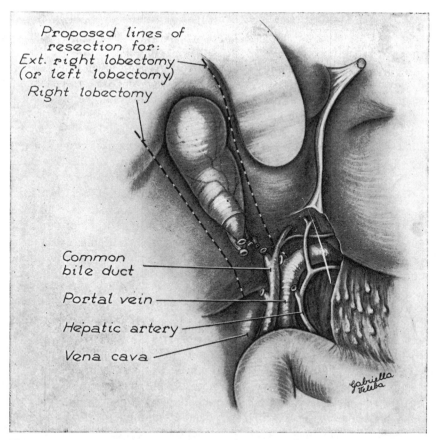

Figure 13-11   The individual vessels and hepatic duct going to the lobe are dissected out and individually ligated as in elective hepatic resection. (*From McClelland, R., Shires, G.T., and Poulos, E.: Hepatic resection for massive trauma, J. Trauma,* **4**:282, 1964.)

Figure 13-12   Healey's newer anatomic concepts of the distribution of the hepatic vessels with the lines of lobar resection superimposed over the vascular distribution. (*After Healey, from Braasch, J. W.: The surgical anatomy of the liver and pancreas. Surg. Clin. North Am.,* June, 1958.)

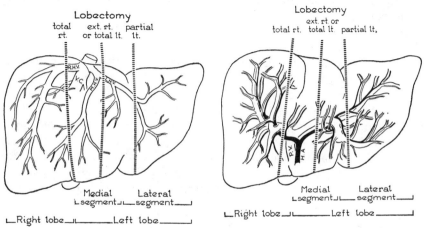

which the guard has been removed. The back of a scalpel handle may also be used to fracture through the liver parenchyma. As the blood vessels and bile ducts are encountered within the liver, they are isolated by passing a right angle clamp around them and are sharply divided after the larger vessels and ducts are suture ligated and the smaller ones are secured with tantalum (Weck) clips. No attempt is made to secure the hepatic veins at their junction with the retrohepatic vena cava before beginning the resection; instead, it is much easier and safer to isolate and suture ligate or oversew the appropriate major hepatic veins as they are encountered posteriorly during the liver resection. The resection begins anteriorly and progresses posteriorly toward the right or left side of the vena cava, keeping to the right or left of the middle hepatic vein (depending upon whether a right or left lobectomy is being done). The middle hepatic vein demarcates the right from the left lobe of the liver and passes in a line from the middle of the gallbladder bed posteriorly to the midportion of the retrohepatic vena cava. The hepatic veins and other large vascular structures must be oversewn since simple ligatures on these large structures often slip off and cause catastrophic bleeding.

The recently described Lin liver clamp may be helpful in performing resections. There is considerable reduction in blood loss and operating time with the use of this clamp, but its availability should not cause a broadening of the indications for liver resection. The clamp can be used only for resecting the liver when it has been severely shattered and devitalized without injury to the retrohepatic vena cava or the major hepatic veins near the junction with the vena cava (Fig. 13-13).

Although Merendino et al., Longmire and Marable, and Perry and LaFave suggest that T-tube drainage of the common bile duct should be carried out after hepatic resections, reports by Lucas and by Pinkerton et al.

suggest that septic complications and bleeding from gastroduodenal stress ulcers are significantly increased by this. Although T-tube drainage may not lower pressures in the common bile duct and therefore probably does not prevent bile leakage from the liver and bile collections in the operative site, the T tube does help identify the right and left hepatic ducts with certainty during liver resections and thus aids in preventing operative injury to the remaining major bile duct. Also, the T tube does provide a useful port through which such postoperative complications as hematobilia and biliary fistula formation can be recognized and the type of drainage can be observed. Cholangiography may also be done through the tube postoperatively, and this may be very useful in determining the cause of prolonged jaundice after hepatic resections. Lucas and Walt, in a well-controlled prospective study, support the position that effective biliary decompression is not achieved by the T tube and drainage of the common duct may, indeed, increase the incidence of complications in patients with hepatic trauma, especially complications due to infection and bile duct obstruction (i.e., jaundice, cholangitis, and bile duct stricture). The increased likelihood of bleeding from gastroduodenal stress ulcers caused by T-tube drainage of the common bile duct after hepatic resection may be offset by frequently lavaging the stomach with antacid solution through the Levin tube to maintain a high gastric pH for several days postoperatively, as suggested by Curtis and associates.

Vascular Isolation Vascular isolation may be required in a highly selected group of patients with liver injuries. This technique allows the surgeon to control bleeding from and to repair retrohepatic vena caval or major hepatic venous injuries. Vascular isolation of the liver is attained by using one of two techniques. The first technique was initially described and reported by Heaney in 1966;

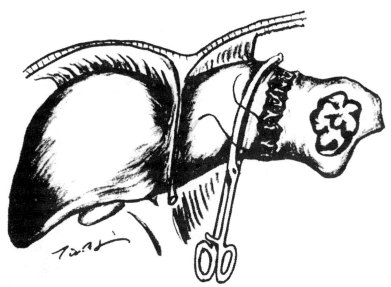

Figure 13-13 T. Y. Lin's liver resection instrument. (*A*) Hepatic clamp. (*B*) Hepatic crush clamp. (*C*) Scissors. The hepatic clamp in place, the liver parenchyma is crushed with the crush clamp through the incision on the superior surface of Glisson's capsule. On release of the crush clamp, the vascular and ductal structures remain as whitish cords bridging the two parts of the liver. (*From Lin, Tien-Yu, A Simplified technique for hepatic resection, Annals of Surgery,* **180**:285, 1974.)

when this method of vascular isolation is used, occlusive vascular clamps are placed across the aorta just below the diaphragm, the porta hepatis, and the inferior vena cava above and below the liver. This technique may be associated with cardiac dysrhythmias and renal insufficiency. The second technique for obtaining vascular isolation of the liver was first described and reported by Shrock and associates from the University of California in San Francisco in 1968. When this technique is used, retrohepatic vena caval and hepatic venous isolation is attained by inserting an intracaval shunt via the right atrial appendage of the heart, and control of vascular inflow to the liver is obtained by placing a Rumel tourniquet or vascular clamp on the porta hepatis (Fig. 13-14). Defore and associates reported survival of 7 of 15 patients with major vena cava or hepatic vein injuries following vascular isolation and the introduction of intracaval shunts. The introduction of the intracaval

shunt via the right atrial appendage is most expeditiously done via a median sternotomy. It is suggested that three equidistant "guy" sutures be placed in the right atrial wall somewhat outside the atrial purse-string suture before making the atrial opening in the center of the purse-string suture to insert the shunt. These "guy" sutures are then split apart and held up by assistants as the atrium is opened, which greatly facilitates the insertion of the shunt as the atrial wall is stabilized.

Another method for controlling hemorrhage from the retrohepatic vena cava or major hepatic veins has been described by Fullen and associates and Yellin and his colleagues. If the major venous laceration is in such a position in the suprahepatic vena cava or the extrahepatic portion of the hepatic veins, a Foley catheter may be quickly inserted into the exposed laceration. The balloon of the Foley catheter is then inflated and pulled up against the wall of the vena cava or hepatic

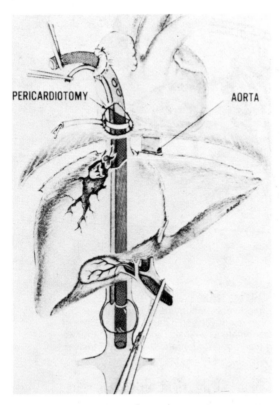

Figure 13-14 Vascular isolation of avulsion of right hepatic vein by use of internal vena caval shunt inserted through right atrium. (*From Yellin, A. E., Chaffee, C. B., Donovan, A. J.: Vascular isolation in treatment of juxtahepatic venous injury, Archives of Surg.* **102**:566, 1971.)

vein to occlude the laceration, arrest the hemorrhage, and thus permit repair of the venous laceration with relatively good exposure and little blood loss.

It is reemphasized that these methods should not be used unless there is a skillful and experienced surgeon in whose judgment exsanguination will occur unless vascular isolation is carried out.

Subcapsular Hematoma

The treatment of subcapsular hematomas is somewhat controversial. Left alone, these may: (1) resolve spontaneously; (2) expand and burst with delayed intraperitoneal bleeding; (3) cause development of hepatic abscess; or (4) decompress into the biliary tree and cause hemobilia. The risk of inducing massive hemorrhage, at times uncontrollable, accompanies attempts at incision and evacuation.

Richie and Fonkalsrud report a series of patients treated nonoperatively. They emphasized that severe bleeding may result in some patients in whom hematomas of the liver are unroofed, and they further note that since some hematomas are centrally located within the liver, they often do not lend themselves to resection or control by hepatic artery ligation. These authors recommend performing an emergency liver scan on patients with probable blunt hepatic trauma who do not have evidence of persistent hemorrhage or shock and who do not have other indications for immediate celiotomy, such as positive needle paracentesis of the abdomen or positive peritoneal lavage. If the patient's condition remains stable and a subcapsular hematoma is seen on liver scan, they recommend close observation of the patient in the hospital by means of frequent physical examinations, serial hematocrits, and performance of liver function studies. The status of the hematoma is appraised by serial liver scans to be certain it is resolving and not increasing in size.

Emergency hepatic arteriography in stable patients with probable intrahepatic hematomas due to blunt trauma is probably preferable to emergency scanning. Arteriography more definitely delineates the size and location of a subcapsular or intrahepatic hematoma, indicates whether there is persistent intrahepatic or extrahepatic hemorrhage, and may show the source and severity of the bleeding.

Another notable advantage of hepatic arteriography in some stable patients with intrahepatic hematomas is that this technique may be used therapeutically as well as diagnostically. If a site of arterial hemorrhage is visualized arteriographically, the hemorrhage may be stopped nonoperatively and atraumatically by embolizing several 2-mm^2 pieces of Gelfoam through the hepatic catheter. These emboli obstruct the bleeding site and thus prevent further bleeding.

Hemobilia

Hemobilia is caused by arterial hemorrhage into the biliary tract after liver trauma and classically presents with a triad of findings consisting of upper or lower gastrointestinal hemorrhage, obstructive jaundice, and colicky abdominal pain. In the past the standard treatment for this condition has consisted of hepatic resection or hepatotomy with direct exposure and suture ligation of the bleeding artery. Such treatment is often associated with considerable blood loss and a high operative mortality and morbidity rate. There are now several reports of successful management of traumatic hemobilia by ligation of the hepatic arteries supplying the involved lobe of the liver. Recent experience with hepatic artery ligation in the management of hepatic trauma and hepatic tumors has proven this to be a safe technique.

Complications

Major nonfatal complications occur in approximately 20 percent of patients with liver injuries. Since the thorax is involved in a large number of hepatic injuries, there is a high incidence of pulmonary complications. A large number of patients develop intraabdominal abscesses, and approximately 50 percent of these are associated with injuries to the colon.

Patients with major lobar resections may be expected to have some degree of postoperative bilirubin elevation, secondary probably to transient biliary obstruction by blood clots and temporary hepatic insufficiency (due to shock, loss of hepatic mass, operative trauma,

and, on occasion, perhaps secondary to postoperative sepsis). Such hyperbilirubinemia usually disappears in about 3 weeks, with no further surgical treatment for the relief of jaundice required. Liver function studies generally demonstrate hepatic impairment, but usually return to normal after several weeks. Glucose metabolism is altered following resection, and in the early postoperative period it may be necessary to supplement the patient with glucose solutions. Studies indicate that survival is possible with only 20 percent of the normal hepatic mass and that within 1 to 2 years most of the resected hepatic tissue is replaced as a result of hepatic regeneration.

GALLBLADDER INJURIES

Although perforations of the gallbladder due to blunt trauma are very unusual, penetrating abdominal trauma frequently causes gallbladder injury. Penetrating or avulsion injuries of the gallbladder are best managed by cholecystectomy, but in unstable patients with other severe injuries when, in the surgeon's judgment, cholecystectomy is inadvisable, a tube cholecystostomy should be done with placement of Penrose drains around the gallbladder in the subhepatic space. In general, simple suture of a gallbladder perforation is not recommended because of the probability of bile leakage. After about 4 weeks, if a patient who has had a tube cholecystostomy is doing well, a cholangiogram is performed through the cholecystostomy tube, and if this shows that the gallbladder and biliary ducts are normal with free flow of contrast material into the duodenum, the cholecystostomy tube can be removed. Routine cholecystectomy after removal of the cholecystostomy tube in patients who have sustained gallbladder trauma is unnecessary, but it is probably advisable to perform an oral cholecystogram several months after injury to determine the status of the gallbladder.

EXTRAHEPATIC BILE DUCT INJURIES

Penetrating Injuries

The diagnosis of penetrating injuries of the extrahepatic biliary tree generally presents no problem as compared with the diagnosis of blunt trauma of the biliary tree, which may be difficult unless intraabdominal hemorrhage occurs. When the hepatic artery and portal vein are involved, the mortality is inordinately high because of massive hemorrhage which may be virtually impossible to control before irreversible hypoxic damage occurs to the brain and myocardium. Most patients with injuries to the extrahepatic biliary tree do not survive when injured with large-caliber, high-velocity missiles.

On opening the abdomen, blood and bile seen in the area of the subhepatic space indicate possible injury to the biliary tree. At times, the amount of bile, blood, or contusion may be minimal. If so, the gallbladder, cystic duct, and hepatoduodenal structures must be carefully inspected to evaluate the significance of any subserosal hematoma or bile staining. Many times in obtaining exposure of the hepatoduodenal ligament structures, clots which have formed and caused tamponade of the major bleeding sites may be dislodged, with recurrence of vigorous bleeding from the portal vein, hepatic artery, or their branches, which are frequently injured when the bile ducts are injured.

Generally, hemorrhage may be immediately arrested by placing the fingers in the foramen of Winslow and compressing the hepatoduodenal ligament. Following this, after removing the free blood and obtaining good exposure while maintaining the finger tamponade as above, more definitive control of the hemorrhage may be obtained by placing vascular clamps or rubber-shod clamps across all struc-

tures in the hepatoduodenal ligament. One clamp should be placed as far distal as possible on the hepatoduodenal ligament. This maneuver is facilitated by performing a Kocher maneuver and mobilizing the duodenum and head of the pancreas mediad. Another clamp is then placed on the hepatoduodenal ligament through the foramen of Winslow as near the liver hilus as possible.

After hemorrhage is controlled, the serosa of the hepatoduodenal ligament at the point of the hematoma formation is incised, and the disruption of the portal vein or hepatic artery is visualized by rapidly dissecting out these structures. When the defects in the major vessels are located, repair is performed with No. 5-0 vascular suture using the general principles and techniques of vascular surgery. The vascular repair should be done only after careful exposure of the defect, but also with dispatch, since the safe occlusion period of hepatic vascular inflow is only 15 to 20 min unless the patient is under hypothermia.

After repair of any vascular injuries, the biliary tract is carefully dissected out along the course of the penetrating wound. Knife wounds of the bile ducts may be closed with interrupted No. 4-0 Prolene sutures. The common duct should be decompressed with a T tube inserted through a separate incision in the ductal system a short distance above or below the injury, so that one arm of the T tube serves as a stent for the wounded portion. For injuries caused by bullets or other large penetrating objects which may produce destruction or avulsion of a segment of the biliary ductal system, the wound should be carefully debrided and all devitalized tissue removed. This may require completing a partial transection of the bile duct, so that an end-to-end anastomosis may be made between the viable portions. This anastomosis is again made with interrupted simple sutures of No. 4-0 Prolene, and the repair is stented with a rubber T tube placed through a separate incision in the duct, above or below the injury. Medial reflection of the duodenum, by the Kocher maneuver, relaxes tension and allows the ends of the divided ducts to come together more readily.

If the loss of biliary ductal tissue is extensive, end-to-end repair of the duct may not be possible, and a bypass procedure is necessary. This is done by bringing up a 30- to 40-cm Roux-Y limb of jejunum made by transecting the jejunum about 30 cm below the ligament of Treitz. The end of the defunctionalized limb of jejunum is closed with two layers of suture. Following this, the distal end of the common duct is doubly ligated with heavy nonabsorbable suture material, and the choledochojejunostomy is performed in the following manner: A small incision is made in the side of the defunctionalized limb of jejunum about 2 cm from the closed end, at the site where the free limb of jejunum comfortably opposes the divided proximal bile duct. The anastomosis is performed by placing a posterior row of No. 4-0 Prolene sutures between the seromuscular coat of the jejunum and the common duct. Usually, it is possible to place only two or three sutures in the posterior row.

The inner row of the anastomosis is made with No. 4-0 absorbable sutures, placing the sutures so that the knots are tied within the lumen. These catgut sutures are continued around from the posterior to the anterior row, and, again, it is usually possible with a small duct to place only four of these sutures. Following this, the anterior row of Prolene sutures is placed in the same manner as described above for the posterior row. It is best to perform this anastomosis over a T-tube stent to help prevent stenosis of the anastomosis and to reduce bile leakage from the anastomosis in the immediate postoperative period. The T tube should be placed in the bile duct, just above the anastomosis to the jejunum, so that one limb of the tube goes across the suture line. If the anastomosis is made so

high in the hilus of the liver that it is impossible to place a T tube above it, then the T tube may be placed through a stab wound in the wall of the jejunal limb and one limb led through the anastomosis into the biliary ductal system. A purse-string suture should be placed in the jejunum about the T tube to secure it in position.

The abdomen should be closed with extensive drainage of the biliary-jejunal anastomosis. The T tube should be left in place for 3 or 4 weeks, following which cholangiography is performed to assure adequate healing and a patent anastomosis. If the cholangiogram shows no leakage or obstruction of the duct, the T tube may be safely removed. The drains are left in until all biliary drainage has ceased, or until a firm drainage tract has formed, which occurs about 3 weeks postoperatively.

If the gallbladder and cystic duct are intact, the bypass may also be done between the gallbladder and jejunum with ligation of the distal and proximal limbs of the damaged common duct. Also, it may be more expedient at times to use a simple loop of jejunum instead of a Roux-Y limb to perform the bypass procedure.

If the patient is in poor condition and cannot tolerate a prolonged procedure for definitive repair, then the defects in the biliary ductal structures may be repaired by simple bridging with a T tube fixed in place with a suture at either end of the ductal defect; secondary repair may be done later as soon as the patient can tolerate it. If possible, however, definitive repair should be done, since recurring strictures are more likely to occur following the more difficult secondary repair of the bile duct.

Blunt Trauma

Blunt trauma to the biliary tree deserves separate discussion, not because the surgical management differs, but because of its relative rarity and difficulty of diagnosis. According to

Rydell, complete division of the common duct by blunt trauma was reported in 25 cases up to the year 1970. The usual mechanism of closed injury to the extrahepatic biliary tree is a shearing force applied to the common duct or impingement of the bile duct between the vetebral column with a crushing force applied to the abdominal wall. The common bile duct and extrahepatic bile ducts are more likely to be injured by blunt trauma than the gallbladder, hepatic artery, or portal vein. There are two hypotheses that may explain this relatively large number of bile duct injuries. First, a widely patent cystic duct permits rapid emptying of the gallbladder when pressure due to blunt trauma is applied to the gallbladder, and while this emptying prevents rupture of the gallbladder, it fills the common bile duct with bile, thus making this tubular structure rigid and more susceptible to injury by a shearing force. Second, the extrahepatic bile ducts are relatively more fixed at the superior edge of the pancreas and at the liver hilus than at the portal vein or hepatic artery, and this greater fixation makes the extrahepatic bile ducts more subject to avulsion injury than the vascular structures in the hepatoduodenal ligament.

When blunt trauma to the biliary tree is severe enough to result in a free flow of bile, the characteristic picture of bile peritonitis occurs. These patients usually present with severe pain and, occasionally, hypotension. The hypotension is usually of relatively short duration, seldom more than a few hours. Generally during this period, the diagnosis of probable intraabdominal injury may be established by signs of peritoneal irritation, such as abdominal rigidity and guarding. Bile or non-clotting blood may be found on peritoneal tap or lavage. Shock is usually secondary to the marked outpouring of extracellular fluid into the peritoneal cavity due to the chemical irritation of the peritoneum by bile. The initial chemical peritonitis caused by bile may be

followed shortly by bacterial peritonitis. If biliary leakage is minimal, shock may be of relatively short duration or absent, and abdominal signs may be slight initially. This may be followed by the recovery and well-being of the patient, which lasts for periods of up to 5 or 10 days. However, the onset of jaundice on about the third day is a fairly constant sign. The appearance of clay-colored stools and the presence of bile in the urine may be noticed from about the second to the fifth day after injury.

A considerable gradual increase in abdominal size occurs during the first 10 days, but may be unattended by the usual signs of peritonitis. This condition is accompanied by progressive signs of extracellular fluid volume deficit and by evidence of infection, such as rising temperature and elevated white cell count. Intravenous cholangiography and visceral angiography may help establish the diagnosis of trauma to the extrahepatic bile ducts. If other studies are inconclusive, a "skinny-needle" percutaneous cholangiogram performed with a Chiba needle may detect the lacerated bile duct.

In the reported cases of complete transection of the common duct, the site of transection was uniformly in the retroduodenal area, thus again indicating the importance of extensive medial reflection of the duodenum by the Kocher maneuver to explore the retroperitoneal duodenum as well as the distal common duct and pancreas.

When blunt trauma to the extrahepatic biliary tract is diagnosed, the repair is generally the same as in the previous discussion of penetrating trauma. End-to-end repair of the ducts over a T tube should be done, if possible, or a bypass procedure between the ducts and the jejunum should be done by bringing up a Roux-Y limb or loop of jejunum to perform an anastomosis between the biliary tract and the jejunum as described in the discussion of penetrating trauma. The ducts should not be implanted in the duodenum, since anastomotic leaks occur more often with this than with the anastomosis to a defunctionalized limb of jejunum. Leak of a choledochoduodenal anastomosis produces not only a biliary fistula but a duodenal fistula as well, with all the grave consequences of such a fistula. If a biliary-jejunal anastomosis leaks, only a bile leak occurs, which is easier to manage generally and has a better prognosis than a biliary duodenal fistula.

Primary repair of small, thin-walled bile ducts may be associated with an inordinately high incidence of subsequent anastomotic stricture. Therefore, it is probably preferable to ligate the distal and proximal ends of very small extrahepatic bile ducts that have been severed and to reestablish biliary-enteric continuity by performing a widely patent cholecystojejunostomy.

The postoperative therapy of biliary tract injuries, in which bile peritonitis is an important complicating feature, should include adequate replacement of extracellular fluid volume deficits, which may require several liters of balanced salt solutions in 24 h. Broad-spectrum antibiotics should be given prior to the surgical procedure and continued throughout the procedure and for several days after, until the chances of sepsis and infection have diminished.

Mortality from biliary tract injuries should be less than 5 to 10 percent if they are discovered early and treated appropriately.

PORTAL VEIN INJURY

Approximately 90 percent of portal vein injuries occur as a result of penetrating trauma. They are frequently associated with other visceral injuries, most commonly injuries to the inferior vena cava, liver, pancreas, and stomach. Mattox and associates recently reported a survival rate of 50 percent in their series of 22 patients.

Lateral venorrhaphy, if possible, is the preferred method of treatment. Mattox suggests performing a portacaval or mesocaval shunt as an alternate treatment of portal vein injury if suture repair is impossible and the patient's general condition is stable. Fish, on the other hand, reported that four of five patients who had portacaval shunts for portal vein reconstruction after trauma developed hepatic decompensation or encephalopathy, whereas these complications were not observed in patients undergoing portal vein ligation.

The insertion of an autogenous vein graft to bridge the defect in the portal vein (using the left common iliac vein, left renal vein, or a paneled saphenous vein graft) may be preferable to a portacaval shunt if the patient's condition is stable and the proximal and distal ends of the injured vein are suitable for the insertion of a graft. This procedure should prevent portal hypertension or hepatic deterioration that may occur if the vein is ligated. If, however, associated injuries are severe, then ligation of the portal vein may permit salvage of the patient. Even though portal vein ligation may cause portal hypertension, interruption of the vein is compatible with the patient's survival in about 80 percent of the cases. It should, of course, be emphasized that in those associated hepatic arterial injuries, a good repair of the hepatic artery must be achieved before accepting treatment of portal vein injuries by ligation.

PANCREATIC INJURIES

Travers described the first reported pancreatic injury found in an intoxicated woman struck by a stagecoach wheel in England in 1827. Although about two-thirds of pancreatic injuries are caused by penetrating trauma, recently there has been an increase in the incidence of blunt pancreatic trauma, most of which is caused by steering wheel injuries. Northrup and Simmons recently reviewed 734 cases of pancreatic trauma in the English literature. They describe three basic mechanicisms of blunt pancreatic trauma. First, when the blunt forces are concentrated to the right of the vertebral bodies, the head of the pancreas may be crushed and, in addition, there may often be hepatic lacerations, avulsions of the common bile duct, and rupture of the duodenum. Second, when the blunt abdominal trauma is concentrated in the midline, where the pancreas normally crosses the vertebral bodies, the classic pancreatic transection injury is often produced, frequently without associated injuries. Third, if the impact forces are directed to the left of the vertebra, distal pancreatic contusions and lacerations with associated splenic lacerations may occur.

Diagnosis

Diagnosis of pancreatic injuries is based upon a complete history (including the mechanism of injury), thorough physical examination, serum amylase level, and adequate visualization of the pancreas at surgical exploration. The history of trauma may be the only clue to the diagnosis of pancreatic injury. Signs and symptoms may initially be absent. In fact, in patients with isolated blunt pancreatic trauma, clinical manifestations of the injury typically appear slowly. Symptoms have been reported to be absent for as long as 5 days, even after a complete pancreatic transection, and for up to 92 h after avulsion of the pancreatic and biliary ductal systems from the duodenum. Moreover, symptoms following isolated blunt pancreatic trauma may even be delayed until a pseudocyst develops weeks, months, or years later. The delay in appearance of symptoms in patients with isolated pancreatic injuries may be caused either by an initial secretory inhibition of the pancreas after injury or by failure of pancreatic enzymes to be activated in the absence of other visceral injuries.

Not only are symptoms of isolated blunt pancreatic trauma often mild and delayed, but physical signs may also be absent or minimal. Usually, however, there is at least mild upper abdominal tenderness, but in the absence of a history of significant trauma or severe symptoms this sign may be overlooked. Injuries to retroperitoneal organs such as the pancreas may not produce clinical findings of loss of bowel sounds, tenderness, guarding, or spasm for several hours.

Serum Amylase Determination Over 25 years ago Matthewson and Halter advocated routine serum amylase determinations in patients sustaining blunt trauma and emphasized that pancreatic injury was more common than had been previously appreciated. Serum amylase elevation alone has not been considered an indication for exploratory celiotomy. If signs of peritonitis are present, such as spasm, tenderness, and absent bowel sounds, then a celiotomy is performed. Unrecognized severe pancreatic injury can be a fatal lesion, particularly when it is accompanied by disruption of pancreatic tissue and leakage of pancreatic juice.

Many patients have been found to have an elevated serum amylase level but negative abdominal findings. These patients are closely observed for evidence of peritonitis or until the amylase level returns to normal. An amylase determination is performed on peritoneal lavage fluid, but the elevation is more often due to small bowel injury than to pancreatic injury.

Recent studies by Olsen, Moretz and associates, and White and Benfield, have indicated that improper interpretation of elevated amylase determinations may be misleading. Olsen stated that 33 percent of patients with hyperamylasemia had no significant intraabdominal trauma, and in his series no patient with hyperamylasemia had significant intraabdominal injury without other evidence of such trauma. He reemphasized the fact that hyperamylasemia alone, without any other evidence of visceral injury, is not an indication for exploratory celiotomy. White and Benfield found that only 26 percent of the patients in their series who had significant blunt or penetrating pancreatic trauma had preoperative hyperamylasemia.

While these various reports show that it is unwise to perform exploratory celiotomy on the basis of elevated amylase levels alone, nevertheless, the detection of hyperamylasemia in asymptomatic patients who have sustained abdominal trauma cannot simply be dismissed. These patients are admitted to the hospital and are closely observed. Plain abdominal x-ray films may show evidence of retroperitoneal trauma. This is suspected when there is obliteration of the psoas margin, retroperitoneal air along a psoas margin or around the upper pole of the right kidney, or displacement of the stomach. Upper gastrointestinal studies with water soluble media may show leakage of contrast media from the retroperitoneal duodenal area. Serial sonographic studies of the upper abdomen, when strongly positive, may also indicate pancreatic or other retroperitoneal injuries and thus give sufficient reason for performing exploratory celiotomy in patients with blunt abdominal trauma who have asymptomatic hyperamylasemia.

Visceral arteriography may be helpful in these diagnostically challenging patients. It may clearly show vascular injuries in the region of the pancreas that definitely indicate the wisdom of exploratory celiotomy. As more experience is gained with endoscopic retrograde pancreatography, it is quite possible that this technique may have a role in the diagnosis of pancreatic injury.

Surgical Exploration When preoperative diagnostic studies indicate a probability of pancreatic injury, it is very important to visualize the entire pancreas. The head of the pancreas and the duodenum are completely mobilized to the midline by performing a Kocher maneuver. The gastrocolic omentum is also divided in order to enter the lesser sac and view the entire body of the pancreas. The tail of the gland is mobilized by freeing the spleen and retracting it medially along with the tail of the pancreas, thus allowing direct visualization and palpation of both sides of the distal part of the gland. Cattell and Braasch described a technique that provides easy access to the third and fourth portion of the duodenum, the head and part of the uncinate process of the pancreas, and the superior mesenteric vessels where they cross the duodenum. This technique entails mobilization of the right colon and its mesentery along with the small bowel and its mesentery from the retroperitoneal attachments (Fig. 13-4).

Any retroperitoneal hematoma in the upper abdomen or any peripancreatic hematoma should be considered presumptive evidence of pancreatic injury and should be explored.

Associated Injuries

Isolated pancreatic injury is rare and occurs in less than 10 percent of all patients with pancreatic trauma. Associated injuries are usually more obvious indications for surgical exploration than is suspected pancreatic injury. Death and serious complications are frequent in pancreatic trauma, but are only rarely caused by the pancreatic injury. Massive hemorrhage from associated vascular, hepatic, or splenic injury is the main cause of death.

Although the pancreas is a vascular organ, it is not often responsible for uncontrollable hemorrhage. When profuse bleeding occurs from the pancreatic area, the pancreas is mobilized and the superior mesenteric vessels, splenic vessels, aorta, and vena cava are inspected, since they are often the source of severe hemorrhage. Because of the location of the pancreas, injuries to the liver and the stomach are frequent. In a series of 175 pancreatic injuries reported by Jones and Shires,

58 percent had an associated retroperitoneal injury in addition to the pancreatic injury.

Management of Pancreatic Injuries

It is essential to control all bleeding at the time of initial exploration of pancreatic injuries. Bleeding vessels in the pancreas are exposed by carefully debriding surrounding devitalized tissue sufficiently to gain secure hemostasis by precise placement of shallow mattress sutures of fine nonabsorbable material. Complete mobilization of the injured pancreas permits temporary control of bleeding by anterior and posterior digital compression of the bleeding site with the fingers of one hand while hemostatic stitches are placed with the other hand. Nonabsorbable sutures must be used since absorbable material is quickly digested away by the proteolytic enzymes from the pancreas. Suturing of the bleeding points should be done without preliminary application of hemostatic clamps, since such clamps cause more damage to the viable pancreas and often cause tearing and further bleeding from the fragile pancreatic vessels. Control of bleeding from the pancreas should not be attempted by blind clamping, by mass ligatures, or by deep sutures, since these may injure or obstruct major pancreatic or biliary ducts or major mesenteric blood vessels and thus cause further serious complications.

After bleeding from the pancreas or from adjacent major blood vessels is controlled, the extent of the pancreatic injury is determined. In general, pancreatic injuries may be classified as follows: (1) simple pancreatic contusion without rupture of the pancreatic capsule or significant hemorrhage; (2) more severe contusion and disruption of the pancreatic parenchyma with rupture of the capsule but without major ductal injury; (3) severe pancreatic injury with major ductal disruption; and (4) combined pancreatic and duodenal injury.

Simple Contusions without Capsular or Ductal Disruption   Simple pancreatic contusions without capsular or ductal disruption and without persistent hemorrhage require no suturing or debridement. These injuries should be drained with a sump drain and several large Penrose drains placed directly at the site of the pancreatic contusion and brought out along a short, direct tract. A properly functioning sump drain allows air to enter the tract, preventing the occurrence of a vacuum. It also allows measurement of the amount of pancreatic juice being lost and helps prevent skin digestion. These drains should exit through a stab wound in the upper flank, which is placed as dependently as possible and made sufficiently large to easily admit two fingers. The drains are left in place for 10 days to 2 weeks since moderate drainage may not occur during the first week following injury. Drainage from the pancreas might not be expected with a simple contusion and an apparently intact pancreatic capsule; however, minor capsular disruptions might be easily missed during exploration of the pancreas. Lack of drainage to such areas of unrecognized capsular injury may lead to complications associated with intraabdominal collections of pancreatic secretions such as pseudocysts, pancreatic abscesses, lesser sac abscesses, and subphrenic abscesses.

Capsular Laceration without Ductal Injury   Most surgeons agree that simple pancreatic penetration or lacerations with capsular disruptions without loss of tissue or major ductal injury are best treated by simple suture of the capsule with nonabsorbable material and extensive drainage. Such injuries with significant loss of pancreatic tissue that precludes suture repair to the capsule obviously can be treated only by direct suture of any bleeding points and by extensive drainage. Extensive drainage to control leakage from a pancreatic injury is more important than attempting to prevent a fistula by capsular repair.

Injury with Ductal Disruption Disruption of the main pancreatic duct is a much more serious injury than capsular disruption and requires especially careful management. Major ductal injury almost always causes a pseudocyst or abscess if not recognized and drained. If treated by drainage alone, these injuries usually produce a troublesome and persistent fistula.

Distal Pancreatectomy An effective method of treatment for pancreatic injuries with disruption of the pancreatic duct in the body or tail of the gland is distal pancreatectomy. This is performed at the point where the main duct is injured and allows removal of the traumatized and devitalized tissue.

When performing a distal pancreatectomy, suture-stick ties are placed in the superior and inferior borders of the pancreas approximately 1.5 to 2 cm from the edge. This, along with isolation of the splenic vessels during distal pancreatectomy, prevents unnecessary blood loss and provides better visualization. In resecting the distal pancreas, the cut edge is beveled in a fish-mouth fashion. This enables a better closure of the proximal end of the pancreas. The transected duct of the Wirsung in the remaining proximal gland is ligated with a transfixion suture of fine monofilament nonabsorbable material such as Prolene to discourage fistula formation. The cut surface of the transected proximal pancreas is oversewn with interrupted, interlocking mattress sutures, which facilitate hemostasis. The stump of the pancreas is extensively drained with a sump drain and large Penrose drains.

Yellin and associates reported excellent results with distal pancreatectomy in 60 patients. In eight of their patients, the injury was located considerably to the right of the superior mesenteric vessels, and as much as 13 to 15

cm of distal pancreas was resected. (The average normal pancreas has a length of 15 cm, is 3 cm thick, and weighs 60 to 125 g.) Only one patient (1.6 percent) developed diabetes mellitus after distal pancreatectomy. Jones, in reviewing 300 pancreatic injuries from Parkland Hospital, reported 8 patients who had a greater than 80 percent resection. Three of the 8 patients developed diabetes, a fourth had a slightly elevated FBS, and a fifth a slightly abnormal glucose tolerance test. It seems, therefore, that greater than 80 percent of the pancreas (> 11.5 cm) must be resected. These patients must be followed closely for the development of diabetes.

Distal Pancreatectomy with Roux-Y Anastomosis This technique has been utilized in patients undergoing primary distal pancreatectomy for trauma when there is much contusion and edema of the remaining pancreatic head. In these cases the surgeon may anticipate that there will be significant obstruction in the proximal ductal system, leading to persistent leakage of pancreatic secretions from the end of the transected pancreas if the pancreatic duct and stump are simply oversewn and drained instead of being implanted in a defunctionalized Roux-Y limb of jejunum. This procedure is time-consuming and is not recommended in patients whose condition is often tenuous because of hemorrhage and severe injuries to structures adjacent to the pancreas.

Roux-Y Pancreaticojejunostomy Several methods of treating pancreatic transection have been described. For the completely transected pancreas over the superior mesenteric vessels and to the right of these vessels, a Roux-Y anastomosis suturing both ends of the pancreas to the defunctionalized limb has proved satisfactory (Fig. 13-15). This treatment has been recommended by Jones and Shires for treatment of injuries which require removal of 75 percent or more of the pancre-

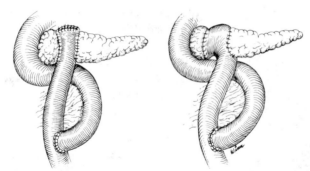

Figure 13-15 Techniques of Roux-Y anastomosis of both ends of transected pancreas. (*From Jones, R. C., Shires, G. T.: Pancreatic trauma, Archives of Surgery,* **102**:424, 1971.)

as. Transections of less magnitude are treated by simple distal pancreatectomy. A Roux-Y anastomosis to both ends of the severed pancreas has eliminated the need to find a severed duct or to reanastomose it. This method leaves all functioning pancreatic tissue, thereby avoiding the possibility of pancreatic insufficiency or diabetes. The risk of injury to the underlying superior mesenteric vessels seems less with this mode of treatment than with resection. The possibility of fistula and pseudocyst formation is also minimized.

The easiest method of accomplishing the Roux-Y anastomosis to both ends of the severed pancreas is an end-to-end anastomosis of pancreas to jejunum and end of pancreas to side of jejunum. This is accomplished using permanent sutures placed approximately 1 cm apart in a single-layer anastomosis. Once this anastomosis is accomplished, drainage with Penrose and sump drains is placed to the pancreatic injury.

Jordan and associates advocate complete transection of the pancreas with a Roux-Y anastomosis to the pancreatic fragment with oversewing of the proximal pancreas. The Roux-Y limb should be at least 30 cm in length and is usually passed through the transverse mesocolon to the site of injury. As long as the duodenum is intact and viable, there is little justification for a pancreaticoduodenectomy for this type of injury.

Unless the completely severed pancreatic duct is managed with definitive surgery, a pseudocyst or fistula will almost always result. A Roux-Y anastomosis to one fragment of the severed pancreas is little more time-consuming than resection of the distal fragment, which requires a splenectomy.

If location of the pancreatic injury suggests the possibility of injury to the intrapancreatic portion of the common bile duct, the common bile duct is opened in its supraduodenal position and a cholangiogram obtained. If a partial tear of the distal common duct has occurred but some ductal continuity remains, a T tube is inserted for decompression.

Repair and Stent of Pancreatic Duct It is difficult to locate the pancreatic duct when there is considerable bleeding and hematoma, and it is even more difficult to suture it after it is found. Nevertheless, several reports have appeared in which the pancreatic duct has been identified, found to be completely transected in the region of the neck of the pancreas, and successfully repaired by stenting and suture repair. The stent may be inserted into the duct at the area of injury and threaded through the ampulla into the duodenum. The second method by which this has been accomplished is by duodenotomy and catheter cannulation of the pancreatic duct through the ampulla, with or without a sphincterotomy, with passage into the distal pancreatic duct past the point of transection. The pancreatic duct is then reapproximated with No. 6-0 or No. 7-0 nonabsorbable suture. This is not a preferred, but an alternate, method, which might be of some benefit in selected cases in which the injury would require radical resection of the pancreas in the critically ill patient. Although either fistula, late stricture formation at the site of injury, or recurrent pancreatitis secondary to partial obstruction of the pancreatic duct is possible, these complications have not been reported.

Anterior Roux-Y Pancreaticojejunostomy A Roux-Y pancreaticojejunostomy may be placed to the anterior surface of the pancreas over the injury in selected cases. This method of treatment has been satisfactory only if the posterior pancreatic capsule is intact. If the posterior pancreatic capsule is torn, drainage will continue into the retroperitoneal space rather than into the Roux-Y limb, and result in abscess, pseudocyst, or fistula formation.

The most severe form of pancreatic injury is extensive laceration and shattering of the head of the pancreas, which leaves virtually none of the proximal pancreas or its main ductal system intact. Extensive injuries of the pancreatic head not involving the duodenum are preferably treated by either a Child 95 percent pancreatectomy or a Jones-Shires double pancreaticojejunostomy. Only rarely should pancreaticoduodenectomy be done for injuries of the pancreatic head alone.

Combined Duodenum and Pancreatic Injuries Northrup and Simmons reported an overall mortality of duodenal injuries alone of 20 percent, which is equal to the overall mortality of pancreatic injuries alone. Combined pancreatic and duodenal injuries, however, increase the mortality rate to an average of 44 percent, with some reports exceeding 60 to 70 percent; 30 percent of duodenal injuries are associated with pancreatic trauma, and approximately 20 percent of pancreatic injuries are associated with duodenal trauma. The high mortality among patients with combined injuries is related to the intensity and severity of forces that cause injury not only to the pancreas and duodenum but also frequently involve the adjacent major blood vessels, with resultant immediate or early death from hemorrhage. A large amount of devitalized tissue and complicated pancreaticoduodenal fistulas also contribute to the high mortality rate.

Combined injuries of the pancreas and duodenum are treated by either a Berne duodenal "diverticulization" procedure (Fig. 13-6), as previously described under duodenal procedures, for relatively less severe combined injuries or a Whipple procedure for very severe combined pancreaticoduodenal injuries.

Pancreaticoduodenectomy Prior to performing a pancreaticoduodenectomy, the presence of a pancreatic ductal injury should be verified. This may be accomplished by duodenotomy, cannulation of the pancreatic duct, and pancreatogram. The common duct is identified and proved to be intact by operative cholangiogram. An alternate method of determining ductal injury is by mobilizing the tail of the pancreas and performing a pancreatogram through the distal pancreatic duct. Hemostatic sutures are placed 1.5 to 2 cm into the superior and inferior portion of the pancreas prior to incising the tail. If the common bile duct and major duct system are intact and the duodenal injury can be closed, then a pancreaticoduodenectomy is usually not indicated.

Indications for pancreaticoduodenectomy include rupture of the duodenum and head of the pancreas, avulsion of the common duct from the duodenum with an avascular duodenal wall, and stellate fracture with bleeding from a crushing injury of the head of the pancreas. This procedure is also indicated for combined injuries to the head of the pancreas and duodenum, with destruction of both, to control hemorrhage, remove devitalized tissue, and restore ductal continuity. The overall condition of the patient and associated injuries must be considered prior to submitting the patient to several more hours of surgery. There are times when this procedure is necessary, but they are rare, particularly if the duodenum is intact. Complications following pancreaticoduodenectomy are common. Thus, mortality of this procedure must be low to justify its use.

In addition to fistula formation and abscesses, marginal ulceration with upper gastrointestinal bleeding has occurred following pancreaticoduodenectomy in which a vagotomy or subtotal gastric resection was not performed. Symptoms of dumping, diabetes, and weight loss with diarrhea and semiformed bowel movements have occurred following pancreaticoduodenectomy for trauma. Foley and associates have reported a postoperative complication following pancreaticoduodenectomy with bleeding into the intestinal tract from the site of the pancreaticojejunostomy, which was demonstrated by arteriographic studies and required reoperation to achieve hemostasis.

The average mortality for patients treated with the Whipple procedure continues to be about 35 percent, with some series reporting as high as 50 to 60 percent. This high mortality rate is frequently due to associated injuries, and it is probable that some of these patients would have died if a pancreaticoduodenectomy had not been done. Despite a very justifiable concern about the inappropriate use of the Whipple procedure in the treatment of less serious pancreatic and duodenal injuries, Yellin and Rosoff conclude that pancreaticoduodenectomy is an effective procedure for removing severely devitalized pancreas and duodenum when these organs are irreparably injured.

Complications

Complications following pancreatic trauma include fistula, pancreatic abscesses, vascular necrosis with hemorrhage from the drain site, pseudocyst formation, and duodenal fistula secondary to suture line breakdown from pancreatic juice activation.

Pancreatic enzymes liberated in an inactive form do not digest living tissue. In extensive injuries, duodenal and biliary enzymes are often released and the proteolytic pancreatic enzymes activated. Trypsinogen activated by enterokinase and hydrolyzed to trypsin breaks down protein. Mixtures of bile, gastric, and pancreatic juices are capable of digesting soft tissues with which they come in contact. As a result of digestion of surrounding tissues, any attempt at delayed definitive operation in this area becomes hazardous.

Fistula Jordan et al. have reported the occurrence of pancreatic fistula as the most common complication following operative therapy, occurring in 35 percent of the cases and usually following blunt trauma. Most pancreatic fistulas are minor and close within a period of 1 month. Major pancreatic fistulas have been arbitrarily defined as those which drain longer than 1 month. The serum amylase is frequently elevated while the fistula is present, probably because of transperitoneal absorption.

Almost all pancreatic fistulas will eventually close spontaneously; therefore treatment is mainly conservative. Attention must be given to preventing autodigestion of the surrounding skin. Dressings should never be applied to any fistula since skin irritation will result from the fistula fluid in the dressings, even in the presence of relatively bland pancreatic juice.

The use of Stomahesive provides an excellent method for managing the drainage from pancreatic or other types of gastrointestinal fistulas. An opening is made in the Stomahesive sheet just large enough to permit drains from the fistula tract to pass through. Stomahesive securely adheres to the skin for several days before it must be replaced and is virtually nonreactive and nonallergic. A gas-sterilized polyethylene bag with adherent backing and a "drainable stoma" at the bottom is applied so that it adheres to the Stomahesive sheet rather than to the patient's skin. The Penrose drains, if these are still in place, are completely contained within the bag and the suction catheter in the fistula tract exits through the "drainable stoma" in the bag. Leakage is prevented by placing rubber bands around the suction catheter and the polyethylene bag in order to make a tight seal where the catheter passes through the stoma. This method protects the skin, isolates the drains from outside infection, and permits accurate measurement of fluid loss from the fistula.

Vigorous fluid replacement with balanced salt solution to prevent volume deficit is indicated: the volume may be equal to that lost through the fistula. In order to minimize fluid and electrolyte losses, the pancreatic fluid from a fistula may be returned to the alimentary tract by way of a nasogastric tube, a gastrostomy tube, or a jejunostomy. However, except with very large volume fistulas, refeeding of this fluid usually is unnecessary.

Many patients with pancreatic fistulas can continue oral intake of food, especially if the fistula drains less than 500 to 600 mL each day and the volume does not increase significantly when the patient eats. In the presence of large-volume pancreatic fistulas, it is preferable to institute intravenous hyperalimentation. Intravenous hyperalimentation has two beneficial effects on such patients: (1) it maintains excellent nutrition and nitrogen balance without stimulating the pancreas as do oral feedings, and (2) intravenous hyperalimentation can significantly reduce the volume of pancreatic exocrine secretion by one-half or more.

Baker and associates have advocated the use of atropine or other anticholinergics to reduce pancreatic secretion and decrease fistula drainage. These agents may cause discomfort to the patient by inducing dryness of the mouth, blurring of vision, urinary reten-tion, and inspissation of pulmonary secretions.

With good supportive care of the patients who develop pancreatic fistulas following pancreatic trauma, surgical repair should be necessary in less than 5 percent. Although there are no rigid criteria indicating when conservative treatment should be abandoned, Baker and associates suggest that closure should probably be carried out in most patients who have fistulas that have persisted for more than 60 days and continue draining more than 1000 mL/day. Internal drainage of these fistulas via a Roux-Y defunctionalized limb of jejunum is a very satisfactory method of management.

Pseudocyst A pancreatic pseudocyst is a cyst whose wall of inflammatory fibrous tissue does not contain epithelium, but is made of those structures surrounding the region of the pancreas in the retroperitoneum. The most frequent symptoms associated with a pancreatic pseudocyst are an abdominal mass, pain, nausea, and vomiting. The serum amylase level is usually elevated for a prolonged period of time during this illness. The pseudocyst rarely resolves spontaneously. Pancreatic pseudocyst is now a rare complication following pancreatic trauma if the pancreas has been explored and managed appropriately, including adequate drainage with a sump and numerous drains. The preferred method of draining pancreatic pseudocysts is internally by either cyst gastrostomy or Roux-Y cyst jejunostomy.

Sepsis Intraabdominal abscess is a common complication following multiple abdominal trauma. Although pancreatic fistulas rarely cause death, they occasionally give rise to pseudocyst formation and lesser sac abscesses requiring reoperation for drainage. A lesser sac abscess may contribute to either sepsis or retroperitoneal bleeding and death. Cultures of the abscess grow a predominance of mixed gram-negative organisms; however, staphylococcus and enterococcus may often be present. Serum amylase is not consistently elevated in patients with a pancreatic or lesser sac abscess.

The method of management of pancreatic abscesses consists of adequate debridement and drainage plus insertion of gastrostomy and feeding jejunostomy tubes. Complications are often associated with a duodenal fistula. If this is present, a Roux-Y jejunostomy is placed over the duodenal fistula wall when possible. Antibiotics are instituted in all cases.

Mortality

The mortality rate caused by pancreatic injury is quite variable and is chiefly related to hemorrhage from adjacent major blood vessels. Northrup and Simmons in a review of 734 patients found that the wounding agent was directly related to the mortality rate as follows: stab wounds, 8 percent; gunshot wounds, 25 percent; steering wheel injuries and other severe blunt trauma, up to 50 percent; and shotgun wounds, 60 percent. Whatever the wounding agent, the average mortality rate of pancreatic head injuries was 28 percent in contrast to the mortality rate of 16 percent from all types of injuries to the body or tail.

Early surgical intervention in both blunt and penetrating abdominal trauma, meticulous abdominal examination of all organs, and an aggressive approach to pancreatic injuries including resection when indicated are essential if mortality is to be lowered. Jones and Shires reported a decrease in mortality due to blunt trauma to the pancreas from 37 percent in 1965 to an overall 16 percent in 1970. The mortality for isolated pancreatic injury was less than 5 percent.

SPLENIC INJURIES

The spleen is the abdominal organ most frequently injured by blunt trauma, representing approximately one-quarter of all blunt injuries of the abdominal viscera. The spleen is also often injured by penetrating abdominal trauma and is frequently associated with blunt and penetrating thoracoabdominal injuries.

Diagnosis

The diagnosis of splenic injury is usually easily made with penetrating trauma, but is often more difficult in patients sustaining blunt trauma. The clinical manifestations are the systemic symptoms and signs of hemorrhage and local evidence of peritoneal irritation in the region of the spleen. Only about 30 to 40 percent of patients with splenic injury present with a systolic blood pressure below 100 mmHg. However, many patients with splenic trauma may develop hypotension and tachycardia when assuming the sitting position. A tender abdomen with guarding and distention is apparent in only about 50 to 60 percent of those patients with splenic rupture.

A history of injury, which may be seemingly slight, followed by abdominal pain, predominantly in the left upper quadrant, left shoulder pain, and syncope is very significant. Often the left shoulder pain, or Kehr's sign, occurs only when the patient is in a supine or head-down position. This is caused by irritation of the inferior surface of the left diaphragm by free blood or blood clots. Elevation of the foot of the bed or pressure in the left subcostal region may occasionally reproduce pain at the top of the left shoulder. Ballance's sign, which refers to fixed dullness to percussion in the left flank and dullness in the right flank that disappears on change of position of the patient, thus indicating large quantities of clot in the perisplenic region and free blood in the remainder of the peritoneal cavity, may be helpful in establishing the diagnosis. Whereas a decreased or falling hematocrit, leukocytosis of more than 15,000, x-ray findings such as fractures of the left lower ribs, gastric displacement, loss of splenic outline, and splinting or elevation of the left diaphragm are useful diagnostic findings, they are frequently absent. Abdominal paracentesis and diagnostic peritoneal lavage are extremely helpful in establishing the diagnosis in doubtful cases, particularly in patients who are obtunded by other injuries. In patients with splenic trauma the incidence of false-negative diagnostic peritoneal lavage is reported in repeated series to be less than 1 percent.

Delayed rupture of the spleen was first described by Baudet in 1902, and the asymptomatic interval between abdominal injury and rupture of the spleen is known as the latent period of Baudet. It was postulated that bleeding appeared several days after injury because: (1) a subcapsular splenic hematoma gradually increased in size until it caused a delayed rupture of the splenic capsule and intraperitoneal hemorrhage, or (2) there was initial bleeding from a splenic laceration which ceased spontaneously but began again in several days or weeks when the perisplenic hematoma became dislodged. This concept has recently been challenged by Olsen and Polley and Benjamin and associates. These authors report a delayed rupture of the spleen of less than 1 percent in over 600 patients. They suggest that splenic rupture is an unusual occurrence and that the 15 percent incidence reported in older papers actually represents a delay in diagnosis rather than a delayed rupture in those patients.

Treatment

Splenectomy remains the only acceptable treatment for splenic injury. Even a slight nonbleeding tear of the splenic capsule may lead to recurrent fatal bleeding. Also, it is likely that a splenic hematoma will increase in size secondary to increasing osmotic pressure of the hematoma and imbibition of fluid, even though no further hemorrhage occurs. The splenic hematoma eventually reaches such size that the spleen ruptures, either spontane-

ously or following slight trauma, causing massive bleeding which may be rapidly fatal.

Nonoperative treatment was recognized very early to carry a high mortality rate; when no operation is performed, the mortality rate is 90 to 95 percent. If an attempt is made to suture the spleen to stop bleeding or to tamponade it with omentum or other hemostatic agents, the estimated mortality rate ranges from 25 to 50 percent because of the high incidence of rebleeding.

Controversy surrounds the proper treatment of a minor nonbleeding splenic injury in the pediatric age group. Singer reported an incidence of fatal sepsis in children that was 58 times greater than that in the general population following splenectomies for trauma. Increasing experimental data and clinical evidence indicate that an intact spleen is required to produce important opsonic antibodies which are necessary for optimal function of the macrophage system in production of immunoglobulins.

Sepsis is a rather frequent occurrence following splenectomy for certain hematologic disorders, many of which have a diffuse reticuloendothelial abnormality. Many of these patients however, receive various forms of therapy that alter immunity and response to infection.

There is no large series of carefully evaluated patients having had splenectomy for trauma in which overwhelming infection has developed. Without more proof that splenectomy in a patient with a normal reticuloendothelial system predisposes to infection, it is difficult to justify conservative management or partial splenectomy for splenic trauma, even in infants.

Another area of controversy is the issue of prophylactic antibiotics in the postsplenectomized patient, particularly in the pediatric age group. Most authors advocate prophylactic penicillin therapy until at least age 5; but it has been recommended that protection be extend-

-ed into the teen-age years, and isolated reports suggest indefinite protection. The use of long-term antibiotics is not without untoward effects such as drug sensitivity, bacterial resistance, and suppression of natural immunologic defenses.

Operative Technique Splenectomy is best performed through a long, upper midline abdominal incision. The advantages of this incision are:

1 It can be made very quickly.
2 It offers easy access not only to the spleen but to other intraabdominal organs that may be injured.
3 It can be closed quickly and heals securely if closed with nonabsorbable, interrupted sutures of appropriate strength.

Good exposure can be obtained by downward retraction of the splenic flexure of the colon and the body of the stomach and by firm retraction on the left upper portion of the midline incision. The operator's right hand is then placed below and posterior to the spleen, and the spleen is grasped and delivered into the wound, either directly or after freeing the peritoneal reflection, which often attaches the lateral surface of the spleen to the diaphragm. Warm, moist sponges are packed into the splenic bed to aid in controlling bleeding from the bluntly divided ligaments and diaphragm and to maintain exposure of the spleen. Occasionally it is necessary to divide the splenorenal ligament by sharp dissection to obtain complete rotation of the spleen and optimum delivery through the incision. If there is considerable splenic hemorrhage, bleeding may be temporarily controlled by compressing the pedicle of the spleen between the index and middle fingers of the left hand or, if necessary, by placing a nontraumatic clamp such as a DeBakey vascular clamp or a Glassman clamp across the pedicle.

In some patients in whom the splenic pedi-cle cannot be quickly mobilized and compressed in order to control hemorrhage, the lesser sac can be rapidly entered by pulling the stomach inferiorly, opening the gastrohepatic omentum above the lesser curvature of the stomach, and then grasping and occluding the splenic artery and vein at the superior margin of the tail of the pancreas with the fingers of the left hand. This then permits rapid mobilization of the spleen and its pedicle by blunt dissection with the right hand, with much less blood loss during the mobilization.

Rotation of the spleen anteriorly and medially out through the midline abdominal incision in order to visualize the posterior aspect of the splenic pedicle is very important. This is necessary to avoid injury to the pancreas and to permit individual ligation of the hilar vessels of the spleen under direct vision. Whitesell, in performing 50 anatomic dissections, found that the tail of the pancreas was either intimately applied to the spleen or within 1 cm of it in half of the dissections, and in another 15 percent the tail approached to within 1.5 cm of the splenic hilus.

When the spleen is delivered, the pedicle is divided between long chest Pean clamps and ligated with heavy nonabsorbable suture. Suture ligatures should be used to control the portions of the pedicle containing the splenic artery and vein.

When delivering the spleen through the midline incision, care must be taken to avoid tearing the gastrosplenic vessels. These must be carefully ligated in order to avoid injuring the wall of the stomach by including it in a mass ligature. Such injuries may cause necrosis of the stomach at this point and subsequent formation of a gastric fistula. After the spleen has been removed, the proximal greater curvature of the stomach should be carefully inspected, and if there is any question about the integrity or viability, the questionable area should be buttressed by imbricating the fundus on itself with several interrupted Lembert sutures.

Although drainage of the splenic bed following elective splenectomy is controversial, there is little question that drainage should be employed when splenectomy is performed under emergency conditions. The incidence of drain-tract infections and subphrenic abscesses has been reported to be as high as 25 to 50 percent when drains were used, in contrast to 5 to 12 percent when drains were not employed. Many of these infections, however, were related to the presence of associated injuries, usually in the GI tract, or to the immunologic defects often present in patients requiring splenectomies for conditions other than trauma and not to the drains per se. The routine use of drains following splenectomy for trauma is supported by the series from Parkland Hospital reported by Naylor and associates. These authors reported the incidence of subphrenic abscess to be only 3.4 percent in 408 patients undergoing splenectomy for trauma. Among the 72 patients who had splenectomy for trauma involving the spleen alone, there were no subphrenic abscesses and an incidence of drain-tract infection of only 1.3 percent.

Thus, while it cannot be proved that drainage of the splenic bed after splenectomy for trauma reduces the incidence of subphrenic collections, it is most probable that drainage in such cases does not increase the incidence of subphrenic abscess. Also in those instances of splenic injury in which there is any question of associated pancreatic or gastric trauma, drainage of the splenic bed may prevent complications that could arise if such unrecognized injuries were not drained. Even those authors who incriminate the usage of splenic bed drains report no higher incidences of subphrenic abscess or other infections if the drains are removed before the sixth postsplenectomy day.

Mortality

Factors contributing to mortality following splenic injury include (1) associated injury, (2) mechanism of injury, (3) presence of shock on admission, and (4) advanced age. Naylor and associates reported an overall mortality rate of 11.2 percent in their series of 408 patients, which compares favorably to other reports.

RETROPERITONEAL HEMATOMA

The management of traumatic retroperitoneal hematoma is a controversial subject. The most common cause of retroperitoneal hemorrhage according to Baylis et al. and according to the experience at Parkland Memorial Hospital is pelvic fracture, which accounts for about 60 percent of all traumatic retroperitoneal hematomas. The diagnosis of retroperitoneal hematoma is most difficult following blunt, nonpenetrating trauma to the abdomen, and should be suspected in any patient following trauma who has signs and symptoms of hemorrhagic shock but no obvious source of hemorrhage. Hemorrhage within the retroperitoneal area may be massive and may exceed 2000 mL of blood. Experimental data have shown that as much as 4000 mL of fluid can extravasate into the retroperitoneal space under pressure equal to that in the pelvic vessels.

Diagnosis

Abdominal pain occurs in approximately 60 percent of patients, and back pain in about 25 percent. The abdominal pain is usually vague and generalized, but is occasionally localized over the hematoma. Local or generalized tenderness is present in about two-thirds of the patients, and shock occurs in approximately 40 percent. Occasionally, a tender mass is palpable through the abdomen or in the flanks, and in some cases, rectal examination will reveal a boggy mass anterior or posterior to the rectum. Dullness to percussion over the flanks or the abdomen, which does not vary with changing positions of the patient, has been recorded in some instances. At times, discoloration of the flanks from retroperitoneal hemorrhage has been noted after the lapse of a few hours (Grey Turner's sign). Progressive decrease in the hemoglobin and hematocrit is a consistent finding, and hematuria is found in 80 percent of patients. Hematuria may represent the first clue to the development of a retroperitoneal hematoma.

Somewhat more than half the patients produce free, nonclotting blood on diagnostic paracentesis or lavage of the abdomen, which is generally related to the presence of both retroperitoneal and intraabdominal hemorrhage. However, if the retroperitoneal hematoma which occurs without intraperitoneal hemorrhage is large enough to yield a so-called "false-positive" peritoneal tap or lavage from retroperitoneal hemorrhage alone, then the hematoma itself may require abdominal exploration to search for the persistent source of the retroperitoneal bleeding.

Roentgenography, according to Baylis et al., has been valuable in several respects: close to two-thirds of the patients with retroperitoneal hematoma have had fractures of the pelvis, and other x-ray findings have included obliteration of the psoas shadow in 30 percent, abdominal mass in 5 percent, and paralytic ileus in 8 percent. Also, displaced bowel gas shadows and fractured vertebrae have been noted. Baylis et al. also noted that in one patient a pelvic phlebolith was displaced by an expanding retroperitoneal hematoma. Intravenous pyelograms and/or retrograde cystograms are routinely obtained in all patients with suspected retroperitoneal hematomas, if the patient's condition is stable enough to have these studies performed. Arteriography has also been helpful in establishing the diagnosis of retroperitoneal injury. In the deteriorating patient, however, immediate exploration is performed without obtaining such studies in order to attempt rapid control of progressive bleeding. Most retroperitoneal hematomas from pelvic fractures will tamponade themselves within a short time; and the patient's condition will remain stable and the

hematocrit normal, perhaps after transfusion of several units of blood.

Treatment

It has been recommended by some that retroperitoneal hematomas not be explored at the time of operation. This nonexploration is considered poor practice, an opinion, based on experience, which indicates that nonoperative treatment of retroperitoneal hematomas, with the exception of retroperitoneal hematoma secondary to pelvic fracture, has led to an excessive mortality from continued or recurrent hemorrhage from injured retroperitoneal vessels such as the vena cava, aorta, lumbar veins, or renal veins. In addition, it is felt that nonexploration of retroperitoneal hematomas adjacent to partially extraperitoneal bowel is dangerous because of the possibility of missing a perforation in the bowel's extraperitoneal portion (e.g., duodenum). Consequently, it is recommended to explore all retroperitoneal hematomas discovered during celiotomy for the source of bleeding, as well as for associated injuries to the bowel, kidney, ureter, bladder, etc. This is done regardless of the size of the hematoma or whether it is increasing in size or not at the time of exploration. This policy has not been associated with any complications arising solely from such exploration.

Warnings have been made that if a small hematoma which is not enlarging is disturbed, uncontrollable bleeding may occur. However, it is felt that if such bleeding is to occur, it is best for it to take place at the time of the surgical procedure rather than postoperatively. If major vessels are not explored at the time that hematomas occur near them, major and sometimes fatal postoperative bleeding may occur. Present day vascular surgical techniques obviate the fear of incurring massive hemorrhage as a contraindication to exploring retroperitoneal hematomas. This is with the sole exception of the treatment of large retroperitoneal hematomas due to pelvic fracture.

In massive retroperitoneal hematomas following pelvic fractures, it is often impossible to adequately control multiple small bleeding points. Consequently, it is advisable not to explore this type of massive pelvic hematoma for fear of causing bleeding which may be very difficult to control unless the hemorrhage from the fracture site fails spontaneously to tamponade itself and exsanguination threatens. However, spontaneous tamponade usually occurs. It is important to be certain that there is no injury to the distal aorta, common iliac, or external iliac vessels when not exploring these hematomas.

Seavers et al. advise that the ligation in continuity of one or both hypogastric arteries may, at times, control persistent bleeding in the pelvic retroperitoneal space from pelvic fractures which cannot be controlled by any other means. This will often control the venous bleeding from this source, also. Certainly it is preferable to locate a single vessel which is bleeding and either ligate or repair it, rather than blindly ligating the hypogastric arteries. Recent studies now indicate that infusion of vasospastic drugs or the embolization of autologous clots or hemostatic agents may be beneficial in controlling this type of hemorrhage. On rare occasion it may be necessary to pack the pelvis with large lap packs for 24 to 48 h in order to achieve hemostasis.

FEMALE REPRODUCTIVE ORGANS

Injuries of the female reproductive organs are infrequently seen following either blunt or penetrating trauma to the abdomen. A series reported by Quast and Jordan revealed only 27 patients with gynecologic injuries in a 16-year period at their hospital. Two of those injuries resulted from blunt trauma with rupture of the uterus in patients who were in the immediate postpartum period. These are apparently the only cases recorded of rupture of the non-pregnant uterus. The remaining injuries were penetrating wounds. An enlarged uterus was present in 10 of their patients. Six patients were pregnant, two had large uterine myomas, and two were in the postpartum period. No cases of rupture of an unenlarged uterus by blunt trauma have been recorded, however. Rupture of the pregnant uterus as a result of blunt trauma is rare, but has occurred in a number of instances. Of blunt and penetrating wounds to the female reproductive tract, 90 percent involve the uterine corpus, and 10 percent involve the remaining adnexa.

Treatment

The signs and symptoms from a ruptured pregnant uterus are those of abrupt and massive intraperitoneal hemorrhage. Associated with these findings are generalized abdominal pain and tenderness, abdominal distention, ileus, and the absence of fetal heart sounds and movements. If the patient arrives at the hospital alive (which is not often the case), immediate blood volume and extracellular fluid replacement must be instituted through several large-bore intravenous catheters, preferably placed in the upper extremities since there may be an interference with venous return from lower extremities of these patients. Urgent celiotomy is necessary to control hemorrhage, even though the patient may still be in shock at the time, since the only means of controlling the shock is to stop the hemorrhage. Probably the only anesthesia which will be required is assisted ventilation with 100% oxygen administered through an endotracheal tube. Other agents may be added if and when shock abates. The treatment of choice is evacuation of the uterus, closure of the disruption with large chromic catgut sutures, and thorough peritoneal toilet with removal of all blood and foreign tissue.

Wounds of the uterus and adnexa are repaired by figure-of-eight chromic catgut sutures without drainage in most instances, although in occasional patients hysterectomy is indicated, as in injury of the lower uterine segment and major uterine vessels caused by high-velocity missiles. In these instances, hysterectomy is preferable to an attempted suture repair, since repair may cause stenosis of the cervical canal with resultant hematometra and dystocia. Also, hysterectomy for lower uterine segment injuries is indicated to obtain proper control of bleeding vessels and to help rule out urethral injury at the point where the ureter and uterine artery are in juxtaposition.

It is best to leave the vaginal cuff partially open following hysterectomy for trauma, because of the likelihood of vaginal cuff or cul-de-sac abscess formation, especially if there is appreciable blast injury or concomitant colon injury. If abscesses occur and the vaginal cuff has been left open, it is usually a relatively simple matter to drain the abscess with a finger inserted through the vagina into the open cuff. If gross fecal contamination is present from colon injury, the cuff should be left open and a Penrose drain led out of the vagina from the cul-de-sac. This drain may be secured to the vaginal cuff by a single small chromic catgut suture.

If massive uncontrollable or recurrent bleeding occurs following trauma to the female pelvic organs, it may be rapidly and adequately controlled by bilateral incontinuity ligation of the hypogastric arteries with nonabsorbable suture material. This will not often be required, but should be borne in mind as a very helpful and possibly lifesaving procedure.

Following injury to the pregnant uterus, the loss of the fetus is quite high. Quast and Jordan reported a salvage of only 1 of 10 pregnancies. One patient who was pregnant at the time of a tangential knife injury of the uterus had a uterine repair for penetrating trauma and subsequently delivered the child uneventfully per vagina.

Other instances have been reported in which penetrating uterine injury during pregnancy has been repaired with ensuing normal delivery. Quast and Jordan found that 81 percent of their patients with uterine injuries during pregnancy delivered subsequently per vagina with no difficulty. The cesarean section rate was 19 percent. Of the patients they followed after uterine injury, all who were in the childbearing age subsequently were able to conceive children. In this group, the abortion rate for these latter pregnancies was 16 percent with no apparent cause found.

By far the majority of pregnant patients with uterine injuries will abort shortly after the injury, frequently requiring curettage to control bleeding after spontaneous abortion. Others will require elective emptying of the uterine contents at the time of celiotomy in order to secure adequate hemostasis and uterine repair. Intravenous oxytocin should be given in such instances to aid in uterine contraction and hemostasis after hysterotomy.

ABDOMINAL WALL

Injury to the abdominal wall without peritoneal injury is often difficult to diagnose. Muscular guarding and rigidity are frequently present, and it may be impossible to rule out intraabdominal injury from a hematoma of the abdominal wall. Such hematomas are usually due to rupture of the rectus abdominis or the epigastric artery by direct trauma or severe muscular exertion. The epigastric artery may be injured also by penetrating trauma, so that a hemoperitoneum results. The patient may become hypotensive from such an injury because of the severe intraperitoneal bleeding which sometimes occurs.

The mass from the rectus abdominis hematoma is below the umbilicus in over 80 percent of the cases. To distinguish this mass from intraperitoneal masses, the patient should be requested to raise his or her head against resistance; the mass should disappear if it is intraperitoneal and remain the same if it is in the abdominal wall (Bouchacourt's sign). This sign is not completely reliable, and if adjunctive diagnostic aids such as paracentesis and lavage are equivocal, then abdominal celiotomy should be performed.

BIBLIOGRAPHY

1 Ahmad, Waheed and Hiram C. Polk, Jr.: Blunt abdominal trauma: A prospective study with selective peritoneal lavage, *Arch. Surg.*, **111**:489–492, 1976.

2 Anane-Sefah, John, Lawrence W. Norton, and Ben Eiseman: Operative choice and technique following pancreatic injury, *Arch. Surg.*, **110**:161–166, 1975.

3 Anderson, Charles B., John P. Connors, Duvan C. Mejia, and Leslie Wise: Drainage methods in the treatment of pancreatic injuries, *Surg. Gynecol. Obstet.*, **138**:587–590, 1974.

4 Awe, William C. and Larry Eidemiller: Selective angiography in splenic trauma, *Am. J. Surg.*, **126**:171–175, 1973.

5 Backwinkel, K.: Rupture of the rectus abdominis muscle, *Arch. Surg.*, **90**:35, 1965.

6 Baker, R. J., R. T. Bass, R. Zajitchuk, and E. L. Strohl: External pancreatic fistula following abdominal injury, *Arch. Surg.*, **95**:556, 1967.

7 Baker, R. L., W. F. Dippel, R. J. Freeark, and E. L. Strohl: The surgical significance of trauma to the pancreas, *Arch. Surg.*, **86**:180, 1963.

8 Barnes, J. P. and J. S. Diamonon: Traumatic rupture of the gallbladder due to nonpenetrating injury, *Tex. State J. Med.*, **59**:785, 1963.

9 Bartizal, John F., David R. Boyd, Frank A. Folk, Durand Smith, Theodore C. Lescher, and Robert J. Freeark: A critical review of management of 392 colonic and rectal injuries, *Dis. Colon Rectum*, **17**(3):313–318, 1974.

10 Bass, E. M. and J. H. Crosier: Percutaneous control of post-traumatic hepatic hemorrhage by Gelfoam embolization, *J. Trauma*, **17**(1):61–63, 1977.

11 Baudet, quoted by J. H. Terry, M. M. Self, and J. M. Howard: A discussion of injuries of the spleen, *Surgery*, **40**:615, 1956.

12 Baylis, S. M., E. H. Lansing, and W. W. Glas: Traumatic retroperitoneal hematoma, *Am. J. Surg.*, **103**:477, 1962.

13 Beall, Arthur C., Donald L. Bricker, Francis J. Alessi, Hartwell H. Whisennand, and Michael E. DeBakey: Surgical considerations in the management of civilian colon injuries, *Ann. Surg.*, **173**:971–978, 1971.

14 Benjamin, Charles I., Loren H. Engrav, and John F. Perry, Jr.: Delayed rupture or delayed diagnosis of rupture of the spleen, *Surg. Gynecol. Obstet.*, **142**:171–172, 1976.

15 Berman, J. K., E. D. Habeller, D. C. Fields, and W. L. Kilmer: Blood studies as an aid in differential diagnosis of abdominal trauma, *J. Am. Med. Assoc.*, **165**:1537, 1957.

16 Berne, Clarence J., Arthur J. Donovan, Edward J. White, and Albert E. Yellin: Duodenal 'diverculization' for duodenal and pancreatic injury, *Am. J. Surg.*, **127**:503–507, 1974.

17 Biggs, T. M., A. C. Beall, Jr., W. B. Gordon, G. C. Morris, and M. E. DeBakey: Surgical management of civilian colon injuries, *J. Trauma*, **3**:484, 1963.

18 Bollinger, J. A., C. F. Fowler: Traumatic rupture of the spleen with special reference to delayed splenic rupture, *Am. J. Surg.*, **91**:952, 1956.

19 Bracey, D. W.: Complete rupture of the pancreas, *Br. J. Surg.*, **48**:575, 1961.

20 Brawley, R. K., J. L. Cameron, and G. D. Zuidema: Severe upper abdominal injuries treated by pancreaticoduodenectomy, *Surg. Gynecol. Obstet.*, **126**:516, 1968.

21 Bull, J. C., Jr. and C. Mathewson, Jr.: Exploratory laparotomy in patients with penetrating wounds of the abdomen, *Am. J. Surg.*, **116**:223, 1968.

22 Burrington, John D.: Surgical repair of a ruptured spleen in children: Report of eight cases, *Arch. Surg.*, **112**:417–419, 1977.

23 Burrus, G. R., J. F. Howell, and G. L. Jordan: Traumatic duodenal injuries: An analysis of 86 cases, *J. Trauma*, **1**:96, 1969.

24 Buscaglia, L. C., W. Blaisdell, and R. C. Lim: Penetrating abdominal vascular injuries, *Arch. Surg.*, **99**:764, 1969.

25 Butler, E., E. Carlson: Pain in testicle: Symptoms of retroperitoneal traumatic rupture of duodenum, *Am. J. Surg.*, **11**:118, 1931.

26 Canizaro, P. C., C. T. Fitts, and R. B. Sawyer: Diagnostic abdominal paracentesis: A proposed adjunctive measure, *U.S. Army Surg. Res. Unit Ann. Rep.,* June 1964.

27 Cattell, R. B. and J. W. Braasch: A technique for the exposure of the third and fourth portions of the duodenum, *Surg. Gynecol. Obstet.,* 111:379, 1960.

28 Cerise, Elmo J. and James H. Scully, Jr.: Blunt trauma to the small intestine, *J. Trauma,* 10(1):46–50, 1970.

29 Clark, K.: The incidence of mechanisms of shock in head injury, *South. Med. J.,* 55:513, 1962.

30 Cleveland, H. C. and W. R. Waddell: Retroperitoneal rupture of the duodenum due to nonpenetrating trauma, *Surg. Clin. North Am.,* 43:413, 1963.

31 Cohn, I., Jr., H. R. Hawthorne, and A. S. Frabese: Retroperitoneal rupture of the duodenum in nonpenetrating abdominal trauma, *Am. J. Surg.,* 84:293, 1952.

32 Coln, Dale: A technique for drainage through the bed of the twelfth rib, *Surg. Gynecol. Obstet.,* 141:608, 1975.

33 Cornell, W. P., P. A. Ebert, L. J. Greenfield, and G. D. Zuidema: A new nonoperative technique for the diagnosis of penetrating injuries to the abdomen, *J. Trauma,* 7:307, 1967.

34 Counseller, V. S. and C. J. McCormack: Subcutaneous perforation of jejunum, *Ann. Surg.,* 102:365, 1935.

35 Crosthwait, R. W., J. E. Allen, F. Murga, A. Beall, and M. E. DeBakey: The surgical management of 640 consecutive liver injuries in civilian practice, *Surg. Gynecol. Obstet.,* 114: 640, 1962.

36 Curtis, L. E., S. Simonian, L. A. Buerk, E. F. Hirsch, and H. S. Soroff: Evaluation of the effectiveness of controlled pH in management of massive upper gastrointestinal bleeding, *Am. J. Surg.,* 125:474, 1973.

37 Defore, W. Wilson, Jr., Kenneth L. Mattox, George L. Jordan, Jr., and Arthur C. Beall, Jr.: Management of 1,590 consecutive cases of liver trauma, *Arch. Surg.,* 111:493–497, 1976.

38 Dickerman, Joseph D.: Bacterial infection and the asplenic host: A review, *J. Trauma,* 16(8):662–668, 1976.

39 Drapanas, T. and J. McDonald: Peritoneal tap in abdominal trauma, *Surgery,* 100:22, 1960.

40 Dudrick, Stanley J., Douglas W. Wilmore, Ezra Steiger, Julius A. Mackie, and William T. Fitts: Spontaneous closure of traumatic pancreatoduodenal fistulas with total intravenous nutrition, *J. Trauma,* 10(7):542–553, 1970.

41 Edwards, James and Donald J. Gaspard: Visceral injury due to extraperitoneal gunshot wounds, *Arch. Surg.,* 108:865–866, 1974.

42 Felson, B. and E. J. Levin: Intramural hematoma of the duodenum: Diagnostic roentgen sign, *Radiology,* 63:828, 1954.

43 Fish, J. C.: Reconstruction of the portal vein: Case reports and literature review, *Am. Surg.,* 32:472, 1966.

44 Fitzgerald, J. B., E. Crawford, and M. E. DeBakey: Surgical considerations of abdominal injuries: Analysis of 200 cases, *Am. J. Surg.,* 100:22, 1960.

45 Fogelman, M. F. and L. J. Robison: Wounds of the pancreas, *Am. J. Surg.,* 101:698, 1961.

46 Foley, W. J., R. D. Gaines, and W. J. Fry: Pancreaticoduodenectomy for severe trauma to the head of the pancreas and the associated structures: Report of three cases, *Ann. Surg.,* 170:759, 1969.

47 Forde, Kenneth A. and A. P. Ganepola: Is mandatory exploration for penetrating abdominal trauma extinct? The morbidity and mortality of negative exploration in a large municipal hospital, *J. Trauma,* 14(9):764–766, 1974.

48 Freeark, R. J.: Role of angiography in the management of multiple injuries, *Surg. Gynecol. Obstet.,* 128:761, 1969.

49 Fullen, W. D., J. G. Selle, D. H. Whitely, L. W. Martin, and W. A. Altemeier: Intramural duodenal hematoma, *Ann. Surg.,* 179:549–556, 1974.

50 ——, J. J. McDonough, M. J. Popp, and W. A. Altemeier: Sternal splitting approach for major hepatic or retrohepatic vena cava injury, *J. Trauma,* 14(11):903–911, 1974.

51 Giddings, W. P. and L. H. Wolff: Penetrating wounds of the stomach, duodenum, and small intestine, *Surg. Clin. North Am.,* 38:1605, 1958.

52 —— and J. R. McDaniel: "Wounds of the Jejunum and Ileum," in *Surgery of World War*

II, Office of the Surgeon General, Washington, 1955, Chap. 19.

53 Graham, A. X.: Penetrating wounds of the colon, *Surg. Clin.*, 1960, p. 1639.

54 Griswold, R. A. and H. S. Collier: Blunt abdominal trauma, *Surg. Gynecol. Obstet.*, **112**: 309, 1961.

55 Haddad, G. H., W. F. Pizzi, E. P. Fleishmann, and J. M. Moynahan: Abdominal signs and sinograms as dependable criteria for the selective management of stabwounds of the abdomen, *Ann. Surg.*, **172**:61, 1970.

56 Hinshaw, D. B., G. R. Turner, and R. Carter: Transection of the common bile duct caused by nonpenetrating trauma, *Am. J. Surg.*, **104**: 104, 1962.

57 Hinton, J. W.: Injuries to abdominal viscera: Their relative frequency and their management, *Ann. Surg.*, **90**:351, 1929.

58 Jones, R. C.: Management of pancreatic trauma: *Annals of Surgery*, **187**:555, 1978.

59 Jones, R. C., R. N. McClelland, W. H. Zedlitz, and G. T. Shires: Difficult closures of the duodenal stump, *Arch. Surg.*, **94**:696, 1967.

60 —— and G. T. Shires: The management of pancreatic injuries, *Arch. Surg.*, **90**:502, 1965.

61 —— and G. T. Shires: Pancreatic trauma, *Arch. Surg.*, **102**:424, 1971.

62 Jordan, G. L., G. R. Burns, and J. F. Howell: Surgical management of pancreatic injuries, *Am. J. Trauma*, **1**:32, 1940.

63 King, J. C.: Trauma to the abdominal and retroperitoneal viscera as it concerns the radiologist, *South. Med. J.*, **49**:109, 1956.

64 Knopp, L. M. and H. N. Harkins: Traumatic rupture of the normal spleen, *Surgery*, **35**:493, 1954.

65 Kobold, E. E. and A. P. Thal: A simple method for the management of experimental wounds of the duodenum, *Surg. Gynecol. Obstet.*, **116**: 340, 1963.

66 Lauritzen, G. K.: Subcutaneous retroperitoneal duodenal rupture, *Acta Chir. Scand.*, **96**:97, 1947.

67 Lavenson, George S. and Arthur Cohen: Management of rectal injuries, *Am. J. Surg.*, **122**:226–230, 1971.

68 Ledgerwood, Anna M., Maris Kazmers, and Charles E. Lucas: The role of thoracic aortic

occlusion for massive hemoperitoneum, *J. Trauma*, **16**(8):610–615, 1976.

69 Letton, A. H. and J. P. Wilson: Traumatic severance of pancreas treated by Roux-Y anastomosis, *Surg. Gynecol. Obstet.*, **109**:473, 1959.

70 Lim, Robert C., Morton G. Glickman, and Thomas K. Hunt: Angiography in patients with blunt trauma to the chest and abdomen, *Surg. Clin. North Am.*, **52**(3):551–565, 1972.

71 Lin, Tien-Yu: A simplified technique for hepatic resection, *Annals of Surgery*, **180**:285, 1974.

72 LoCicero, Joseph, III, Tomoo Tajima, and Theodore Drapanas: A half century of experience in the management of colon injuries: Changing concepts, *J. Trauma*, **15**(7):575–579, 1975.

73 Longmire, W. P. and S. A. Marable: Clinical experiences with major hepatic resections, *Ann. Surg.*, **154**:460, 1961.

74 Lucas, Charles E.: What is the role of biliary drainage in liver trauma?, *Am J. Surg.*, **120**:509, 1970.

75 —— and Alexander J. Walt: Analysis of randomized biliary drainage for liver trauma in 189 patients, *J. Trauma*, **12**(11):925–930, 1972.

76 —— and A. J. Walt: Critical decisions in liver trauma, *Arch. Surg.*, **101**:277–283, 1970.

77 —— and Anna M. Ledgerwood: Factors influencing outcome after blunt duodenal injury, *J. Trauma*, **15**(10):839–846, 1975.

78 —— and Anna M. Ledgerwood: Prospective evaluation of hemostatic techniques for liver injuries, *J. Trauma*, **16**(6):442–451, 1976.

79 McClelland, R. N., G. T. Shires, and E. Poulos: Hepatic resection for massive trauma, *J. Trauma*, **4**:282, 1964.

80 —— and G. T. Shires: Management of liver trauma in 259 consecutive patients, *Ann. Surg.*, **161**:248, 1965.

81 ——, P. C. Canizaro, and G. T. Shires: "Repair of Hepatic Venous, Intrahepatic Vena Caval, and Portal Venous Injuries," in G. F. Madding and P. A. Kennedy, *Trauma to the Liver*, 2d ed., W. B. Saunders Company, Philadelphia, 1971, Chap. 10, pp. 146–153.

82 ——, R. C. Jones, G. T. Shires, and M. O.

Perry: "Trauma to the Abdomen," in G. T. Shires (ed.), *Care of the Trauma Patient*, McGraw-Hill Book Company, New York, 1966, Chap. 18.

83 McInnis, W. D., J. B. Aust, A. B. Cruz, and H. D. Root: Traumatic injuries of the duodenum: A comparison of 1° closure and the jejunal patch, *J. Trauma*, 15(10):847–853, 1975.

84 Madding, G. F., K. B. Lawrence, and P. A. Kennedy: War wounds of the liver, *Tex. State J. Med.*, 42:267, 1946.

85 Matthewson, C., Jr. and B. L. Halter: Traumatic pancreatitis with and without associated injuries, *Am. J. Surg.*, 83:409, 1952.

86 Mattox, Kenneth L., Rafael Espada, and Arthur C. Beall, Jr.: Traumatic injury to the portal vein, *Ann. Surg.*, 181:519–522, 1975.

87 Maynard, A. L., and G. Oropeza: Mandatory operation for penetrating wounds of the abdomen, *Am. J. Surg.*, 115:307, 1968.

88 Mays, E. Truman: Lobar dearterialization for exsanguinating wounds of the liver, *J. Trauma*, 12(5):397–407, 1972.

89 Merendino, K. A., D. H. Dillard, and E. E. Cammock: The concept of surgical biliary decompression in the management of liver trauma, *Surg. Gynecol. Obstet.*, 117:285, 1963.

90 Miller, D. R.: Median sternotomy extension of abdominal incision for hepatic lobectomy, *Ann. Surg.*, 175:193, 1972.

91 Moore, S. W. and M. E. Erlandson: Intramural hematoma of the duodenum, *Ann. Surg.*, 157:798, 1963.

92 Moretz, J. Alfred, III, David P. Campbell, Donald E. Parker, and G. Rainey Williams: Significance of serum amylase level in evaluating pancreatic trauma, *Am. J. Surg.*, 130:739–741, 1975.

93 Morgenstern, Leon: Microcrystalline collagen used in experimental splenic injury: A new surface hemostatic agent, *Arch. Surg.*, 109:44–47, 1974.

94 Morton, Jeremy R. and George L. Jordan: Traumatic duodenal injuries: Review of 131 cases, *J. Trauma*, 8(2):127–139, 1968.

95 Naffziger, H. C. and H. J. McCorkel: Recognition and management of acute trauma to pancreas with particular reference to use of serum amylase test, *Ann. Surg.*, 118:594, 1943.

96 Nance, Francis, C., Martin H. Wennar, Lester W. Johnson, James C. Ingram, and Isidore Cohn, Jr.: Surgical judgment in the management of penetrating wounds of the abdomen: Experience with 2212 patients, *Ann. Surg.*, 179:639–646, 1974.

97 ——— and I. Cohn, Jr.: Surgical judgment in the management of stab wounds of the abdomen: A retrospective and prospective analysis based on a study of 600 stabbed patients, *Ann. Surg.*, 170:569, 1969.

98 Naylor, Rebekah, Dale Coln, and G. Tom Shires: Morbidity and mortality from injuries to the spleen, *J. Trauma*, 14(9):773–778, 1974.

99 Northrup, William F., III, and Richard L. Simmons: Pancreatic trauma: A review, *Surgery*, 71(1):27–43, 1972.

100 Olsen, William R. and Theodore Z. Polley, Jr.: A second look at delayed splenic rupture, *Arch. Surg.*, 112:422–425, 1977.

101 ———: The serum amylase in blunt abdominal trauma, *J. Trauma*, 13(3):200–204, 1973.

102 ———, H. C. Redman, and D. H. Hildreth: Quantitative peritoneal lavage in blunt abdominal trauma, *Arch. Surg.*, 104:536–543, 1972.

103 O'Mara, R. E., R. C. Hall, and D. L. Dombroski: Scintiscanning in the diagnosis of rupture of the spleen, *Surg. Gynecol. Obstet.*, 131:1077, 1970.

104 Parvin, S., D. E. Smith, W. M. Asher, and R. W. Virgilio: Effectiveness of peritoneal lavage in blunt abdominal trauma, *Ann. Surg.*, 181:255–261, 1975.

105 Pellegrini, J. N. and I. J. Stein: Complete severance of the pancreas and its treatment with repair of the main pancreatic duct of Wirsung, *Am. J. Surg.*, 101:707, 1961.

106 Penberthy, G. C. and C. R. Reiners: Visceral injury resulting from nonpenetrating abdominal trauma, *J. Mich. State Med. Soc.*, 54:1057, 1955.

107 Perry, J. F., Jr. and J. W. LaFave: Biliary decompression without other external drainage in treatment of liver injuries, *Surgery*, 55:351, 1964.

108 ———, J. E. DeMeules, and H. D. Root: Diagnostic peritoneal lavage in blunt abdominal trauma, *Surg. Gynecol. Obstet.*, 131:742–743, 1970.

109 Pinkerton, J. A., J. L. Sawyers, and J. H. Foster: A study of the postoperative course after hepatic lobectomy, *Ann. Surg.*, **173**:800, 1971.

110 Pringle, J. H.: Notes on the arrest of hepatic hemorrhage due to trauma, *Ann. Surg.*, **48**:541, 1908.

111 Printen, K. J., R. J. Freeark, and W. C. Shoemaker: Conservative management of penetrating abdominal wounds, *Arch. Surg.*, **96**:899–901, 1968.

112 Quast, D. C. and G. L. Jordan: Traumatic wounds of the female reproductive organs, *J. Trauma*, **4**:839, 1964.

113 Quattlebaum, J. K. and J. K. Quattlebaum, Jr.: Technique of hepatic lobectomy, *Ann. Surg.*, **149**:648, 1959.

114 Reich, W. J. and M. J. Nechtow: Ligation of the internal iliac (hypogastric arteries): A lifesaving procedure for uncontrollable gynecologic and obstetric hemorrhage, *J. Int. Coll. Surg.*, **36**:167, 1961.

115 Reinhardt, George F. and Charles A. Hubay: Surgical management of traumatic hemobilia, *Am. J. Surg.*, **121**:328–333, 1971.

116 Roof, W. R., G. C. Morris, and M. E. DeBakey: Management of perforating injuries to the colon in civilian practice, *Am. J. Surg.*, **99**:641, 1960.

117 Root, H. D., C. W. Hauser, C. R. McKinley, J. W. LaFave, and R. P. Mendiola, Jr.: Diagnostic peritoneal lavage, *Surgery*, **57**:633–637, 1965.

118 Rosoff, Leonard, J. Louis Cohen, Nancy Telfer, and Mordecai Halpern: Injuries of the spleen, *Surg. Clin. North Am.*, **52**(3):667–685, June 1972.

119 Rydell, W. B., Jr.: Complete transection of the common bile duct due to blunt abdominal trauma, *Arch. Surg.*, **100**:724, 1970.

120 Ryzoff, R. I., G. W. Shaftan, and H. Herbsman: Selective conservatism in abdominal trauma, *Surgery*, **59**:650, 1966.

121 Salyer, K. and R. N. McClelland: Pancreaticoduodenectomy for trauma, *Arch. Surg.*, **95**:636, 1967.

122 Schrock, T., F. W. Blaisdell, and C. Mathewson: Management of blunt trauma to the liver and hepatic veins, *Arch. Surg.*, **96**:698, 1968.

123 ——— and Norman Christensen: Management of perforating injuries of the colon, *Surg. Gynecol. Obstet.*, **135**:65–68, 1972.

124 Seavers, R., J. Lynch, R. Ballard, S. Jernigan, and J. Johnson: Hypogastric artery ligation for uncontrollable hemorrhage in acute pelvic trauma, *Surgery*, **55**:516, 1964.

125 Shaftan, G. W.: Indications for operation in abdominal trauma, *Amer. J. Surg.*, **99**:657, 1960.

126 Sheldon, G. F., L. Cohn, and W. Blaisdell: Surgical treatment of pancreatic trauma, *J. Trauma*, **10**:795, 1970.

127 Shires, G. T., D. Jackson, and J. Williams: Temporary duodenal decompression as an adjunct to gastric resection for duodenal ulcer, *Am. Surg.*, **28**:709, 1962.

128 Singer, D. B.: "Postsplenectomy Sepsis," in H. S. Rosenberg and R. P. Bolande (eds.), *Perspectives in Pediatric Pathology*, Year Book Medical Publishers, Inc., Chicago, 1973, vol. 1, pp. 285–311.

129 Smith, A. D., Jr., W. C. Woolverton, R. F. Weichert, and T. Drapanas: Operative management of pancreatic and duodenal injuries, *J. Trauma*, **11**:570, 1971.

130 Smithwick, W., III, H. R. Gertner, Jr., and G. D. Zuidema: Injection of Hypaque (sodium diatrizoate) in the management of abdominal stab wounds, *Surg. Gynecol. Obstet.*, **127**:1215, 1968.

131 Sparkman, R. S.: Massive hemobilia following traumatic rupture of the liver, *Ann. Surg.*, **138**:899, 1953.

132 Sperling, L. and L. G. Rigler: Traumatic retroperitoneal rupture of duodenum: Description of valuable roentgen observation in its recognition, *Radiology*, **29**:521, 1937.

133 Sturmer, F. C. and K. E. Wilt: Complete division of the common duct from external blunt trauma, *Am. J. Surg.*, **105**:781, 1963.

134 Thal, E. R.: Evaluation of peritoneal lavage and local exploration in lower chest and abdominal stabwounds, *J. Trauma*, **17**(8):642–648, 1977.

135 ——— and N. Saretsky: Negative laparotomy, morbidity, mortality and rationale. In preparation.

136 ——— and G. T. Shires: Peritoneal lavage in

blunt abdominal trauma, *Am. J. Surg.*, **125**:64, 1973.

137 Travers, B.: Rupture of pancreas, *Lancet,* **12**: 384, 1827.

138 Trunkey, Donald, G. Tom Shires, and R. N. McClelland: Management of liver trauma in 811 consecutive patients, *Ann. Surg.*, **179**(5):522–528, 1974.

139 ———, Robert J. Hays, and G. Tom Shires: Management of rectal trauma, *J. Trauma,* **13**(5):411–415, 1973.

140 Vannix, R. S., R. Carter, D. B. Hinshaw, and E. J. Joergensen: Surgical management of colon trauma in civilian practice, *Am. J. Surg.,* **106**: 364, 1963.

141 Weckerson, E. C. and T. C. Putman: Perforating injuries of the rectum and sigmoid colon, *J. Trauma,* **2**:474, 1962.

142 Weichert, R. F., III, R. L. Hewitt, and T. Drapanas: Blunt injuries to intrahepatic vena cava and hepatic veins with survival, *Am. J. Surg.,* **121**:322–325, 1971.

143 Werschky. L. R. and G. L. Jordan: Surgical management of traumatic injuries to the pancreas, *Am. J. Surg.,* **116**:768, 1968.

144 White, P. H. and J. R. Benfield: Amylase in the management of pancreatic trauma, *Arch. Surg.,* **105**:158–163, 1972.

145 Whitesell, F. B.: A clinical and surgical anatomic study of rupture of the spleen due to blunt trauma, *Surg. Gynecol. Obstet.,* **110**:750, 1960.

146 Wilder, J. R., M. W. Lotfi, and P. Jurani: Comparative study of mandatory and selective surgical intervention in stab wounds of the abdomen, *Surgery,* **69**:546–549, 1971.

147 ———, E. T. Habermann, and S. J. Schachner: Selective surgical intervention for stab wounds of the abdomen, *Surgery,* **61**:231–235, 1967.

148 Williams, R. D. and R. M. Zollinger: Diagnostic and prognostic factors in abdominal trauma, *Am. J. Surg.,* **97**:575, 1959.

149 ——— and F. T. Sargent: The mechanism of intestinal injury in trauma, *J. Trauma,* **3**:288, 1963.

150 Witek, J. T., R. P. Spencer, H. A. Pearson, and R. J. Touloukian: Diagnostic spleen scans in occult splenic injury, *J. Trauma,* **14**:197–199, 1974.

151 Yajko, R. D., F. Seydel, and C. Trimble: Rupture of the stomach from blunt abdominal trauma, *J. Trauma,* **15**(3):177–183, 1975.

152 Yellin, A. E., T. R. Vecchione, and A. J. Donovan: Distal pancreatectomy for pancreatic trauma, *Am. J. Surg.,* **124**:135–142, 1972.

153 ——— and L. Rosoff, Sr.: Pancreatoduodenectomy for combined pancreatoduodenal injuries, *Arch. Surg.,* **110**:1177–1183, 1975.

154 ———, C. B. Chaffee, and A. J. Donovan: Vascular isolation in treatment of juxtahepatic venous injuries, *Arch. Surg.,* **102**:566–573, 1971.

Chapter 14

Trauma to the Genitourinary System

Paul C. Peters, M.D.
Thomas C. Bright, III, M.D.

GENERAL CONSIDERATIONS

The urologist's role in the management of the multiple injury patient is most often that of consultant. The urologist is usually called to the emergency room after hematuria or evidence of pelvic injury has been discovered. Attention is initially given to the nature of the injury, and the patient is examined. Fracture sites, particularly involving the eleventh and twelfth ribs posteriorly, should be sought. Inspection should be made to ascertain the presence of hematoma in the flank, which may be an indication of retroperitoneal hemorrhage. Severe tenderness to palpation in the hypogastrium should alert one to the possibili-

ty of bladder rupture. The presence or absence of pelvic fracture should be noted. In 543 patients with a pelvic fracture seen from 1956 to 1971 at Parkland Memorial Hospital, 5 percent were found to have simultaneous bladder rupture. Examination of the genitalia and perineum for sites of hemorrhage may give a clue to urethral rupture. Inspection of the meatus for blood, indicating urethral trauma, is of importance prior to instrumentation. Careful rectal palpation is mandatory. Lacerations of the urethra superior to the urogenital diaphragm may be detected by the inability to palpate the prostate in its normal position. At this point, a urologic trauma work-up is carried out; this consists, first, of careful examination of the urine sediment, if available, to confirm the presence of hematuria and to determine the possibility of preexisting renal disease. Next, integrity of the lower urinary tract is ascertained by retrograde injection of the urethra with a contrast agent or by the passage of a soft catheter when there is no history of potential urethral trauma, e.g., a straddle injury. After catheterization, 300 to 400 mL of contrast material is instilled by gravity into the urinary bladder. A film is made of the full bladder, which is then drained and another film taken. The second exposure will occasionally show minute extravasation which was obscured by the distended bladder. After cystography, an excretory urogram is performed to determine the integrity of the upper urinary tract or the presence of any abnormality. This is done by injecting 1 mL/lb of iodine-containing contrast material into the venous system and making films at appropriate intervals. The first exposure is taken 1 min after the injection to evaluate the nephrogram appearance; a second picture is made 5 min later to ascertain the integrity of the collecting system. In most patients, a nephrogram may be expected within 30 sec after completion of the injection of the contrast material; 10 to 15 min is required for proper opacification of the ureters. Therefore, the usual trauma series consists of a cystogram and urethrogram done initially, followed by an intravenous pyelogram with films at appropriate intervals, usually 1, 5, 15, and 30 min. This is usually possible in the patient who has suffered blunt trauma, but there is not always time for this in the patient with penetrating injury to the genitourinary tract.

Genitourinary trauma is most common in young adults. Motor vehicle accidents and penetrating missile injuries constitute the most common etiologic agents of genitourinary insult. A history of a deceleration-type injury is important in the initial evaluation.

RENAL TRAUMA

Renal injuries are most commonly due to motor vehicle accidents and gunshot wounds. In the Parkland Memorial Hospital series, 80 percent were caused by these etiologies. In addition, renal injuries are most commonly associated with trauma to other organs (80 percent in our series). Simultaneous bilateral renal injuries are rare, occurring in 4 of 150 renal injuries at Parkland Memorial Hospital. Renal injuries are significant because: (1) shock or death from blood loss may follow; (2) sepsis may occur from an unrecognized or untreated urinary extravasation; (3) renal failure may occur secondary to hypotension and diminished renal perfusion; (4) renal parenchymal loss may result, particularly in patients with solitary kidney; and (5) renal loss may occur by failure to recognize or suspect renal artery thrombosis in deceleration injuries.

Diagnosis

Renal injury must be suspected initially from the history of penetrating missile to the abdomen in the region of the kidney. Evidence of fall or motor vehicle accident with subsequent deceleration injury should also be investigated. Renal injury should be sought in the conscious, traumatized patient with costovertebral angle pain and tenderness. Also suspect are patients with gross hematuria, a bruise over the posterior aspect of the eleventh or twelfth rib, or a bruise and discoloration of the flank. Persistent flank pain may be a clue to renal artery thrombosis secondary to a deceleration injury; this is of current paramount importance because angiographic support is available to establish the diagnosis promptly and minimize renal loss. The normal kidney is difficult to feel, even in a relaxed patient during routine physical examination. Palpation of a large flank mass should make one suspicious of an abnormal kidney, e.g., renal trauma with hemorrhage and extravasation or preexisting disease. The presence of casts or protein should suggest previous renal disease. The amount of hematuria does not correlate well with the magnitude of renal injury. Four mL of blood will make a liter of urine appear grossly red, and the urine may be, therefore, grossly bloody even with mininal renal injury. Conversely, severe renal injury may be present with little or no hematuria. At Parkland Memorial Hospital, 20 percent of patients subsequently proved to have a renal injury had no hematuria on admission. Preexisting renal disease, such as renal neoplasm, glomerulonephritis, hydronephrosis, or congenital variations of the urinary tract, should be suspected when hematuria is out of porportion to the severity of the injury.[7] Of importance, also, is the fact that a deceleration injury with subsequent renal artery thrombosis may be present with no evidence of microscopic hematuria.

When renal injury is suspected because of the presence of physical signs or blood in the urine, excretory urography and cystourethrography are immediately indicated. A plain film of the abdomen is taken initially and examined for the presence of rib or vertebral fractures (particularly transverse process displacement), displacement of bowel shadows, abnormal calcifications, and visceral organ enlargement. Calcifications may be noted to be curvilinear, laminated, or mottled. Attention should also be given to the presence of gas outside the confines of the bowel, which may indicate injury to a hollow viscus, i.e., the colon.

After careful inspection of the plain film of the abdomen and a cystogram has been made, contrast material is injected as an intravenous bolus. A dose of 1 mL/lb of body weight is injected over a 1-min interval. A volume of 150 mL of 29% iodine-containing material is commonly used; e.g., meglumine diatrizoate and sodium diatrizoate (Renografin-60). Exposures are made at 1, 5, 15, and 30 min after completion of injection.

A sensitivity to contrast material is difficult to anticipate. The patient should be questioned as to the occurrence and nature of reactions at the time of previous intravenous injection of contrast agents. Prior to the bolus injection of the contrast material, the conscious patient with a history of allergy to seafood, such as shrimp and lobster, should be given an initial test dose of 1 to 2 mL by slow intravenous injection and be observed for hypotension, urticaria, nausea, and vomiting.

Disparity in renal size may be a clue to preexisting renal disease. Delay in visualization may indicate renal injury or previous renal disease. The presence of renal fractures or urinary extravasation should be sought.

Of current paramount importance is the recognition of the significance of the nonvisualizing kidney by excretory urography. When found, these patients need prompt investigation by retrograde femoral arteriography and selective renal arteriography. This is done in order to diagnose intimal tears occurring from deceleration injury of the renal artery, so that prompt exploration and vascular repair may result in salvage of these kidneys. Historically, the conservative observation of the patient with a nonvisualizing kidney is based in the hope that subsequent films, a week to 10 days later, may show return of function. This management has led to the loss of renal units. Cystoscopic examination and retrograde pyelography has been advocated as a sequential step in the diagnosis of the patient with the nonvisualizing kidney. When this is done, the absence of urine production has suggested to the operator the presence of a vascular injury. Current diagnostic procedure at our institution is to bypass this step and proceed directly to angiography, which is diagnostic of an arterial intimal tear with renal artery thrombosis. Venous injuries, even main renal vein lacerations, do not result in a completely nonvisualizing kidney.

The mechanism of the deceleration injury deserves special consideration (Fig. 14-1). In this situation, usually secondary to a fall from a height or a motor vehicle accident, the kidney is suddenly stretched on its pedicle when the moving body comes to an abrupt halt. The media and adventitia are quite elastic and stretch readily. The intima lacks the elastic properties of the media and adventitia and is often torn in the process. When the kidney returns to its resting position, the torn intima is present and thrombosis quickly follows at this site. The lesion may be suspected clinically if the patient complains of severe back pain on one side, which is persistent. Microscopic hematuria is not a necessary concomitant. An exemplary case is illustrated in Fig. 14-2. Intimal thrombosis following deceleration injury is not often suspected initially, and delay in diagnosis greatly reduces the chances for successful revascularization and renal salvage.

The role of angiography has been an increasing one in recent years. Selective angiography techniques are in common usage in radiology departments today and are readily available in most hospitals caring for the renal trauma patient. Renal arteriography most clearly defines the extent and nature of a renal injury. It does not dictate the need for surgery. This decision should be made on the nature of the injury (all penetrating renal injuries are explored) and the condition of the patient. Judicious sequential diagnostic steps may be required in the blunt trauma patient. The renal scan and sonogram may be of benefit in evaluating renal trauma, though not as accurately as arteriography does. The two former techniques, being noninvasive, are of particular use in postoperative follow-up and in monitoring the nonoperated blunt trauma patient. The renal scan is useful in predicting the recovery of function of renal parenchyma or loss thereof, and sonography is of special value in delineating fluid collections about the kidney and in estimating their progression or regression in size when compared with plain films and excretory urograms. Therefore, it is the excretory urogram and the selective angiogram that provide the radiographic support to the trauma surgeon evaluating the acutely injured patient.

Classification and Treatment

Classification of renal injury is helpful in subsequent management. Major renal injuries consist of: (1) lacerations of the parenchyma through the collecting system with subsequent hematoma and extravasation; (2) pedicle injuries with major artery thrombosis or avulsion of a major artery or vein; (3) massive perirenal expanding hematoma; and (4) total renal fracture. Minor renal injuries are considered to be: (1) contusion, (2) laceration through the capsule and into the parenchyma, and (3) small subcapsular hematomas (Fig. 14-3).

Penetrating renal injuries, regardless of their extent, should be explored. This is primarily because of the high association of other visceral organ injuries, rather than fear for the life of the patient or complications from the renal injury. A patient suffering minor injuries to the kidney, sequential to blunt trauma, will usually have a normal excretory urogram showing, at most, a slight delay in function with either microscopic or no hematuria. Such a patient, after careful physical examination, is usually dismissed from the hospital and followed as an outpatient until hematuria has cleared. Patients with presumed minor renal trauma and gross hematuria are admitted to the hospital for further examination and treatment. In the follow-up of these patients, it is imperative that they be examined closely. Periodic monitoring of the hemoglobin, hemat-

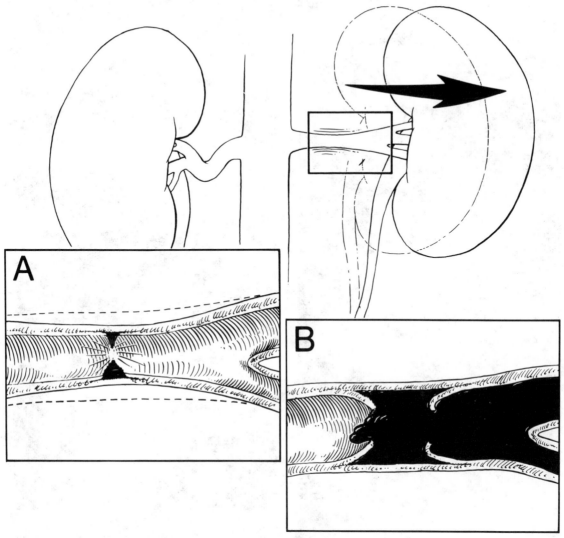

Figure 14-1 Mechanism of renal artery thrombosis in blunt traumatic injury. The kidney remains in motion in reference to the more stationary aorta. (*A*) The media and adventitia, because of their elasticity, stretch readily. The intima, being not so elastic, tears. (*B*) The intimal flap initiates the clotting mechanism and the thrombus is quickly propagated distally.

ocrit, and urine output is mandatory. Aliquots of the urine may be taped to the foot of the bed to ascertain whether the degree of hematuria is increasing or decreasing. Repeated palpation of the flanks by the same examiner is necessary to detect enlarging flank masses.

Appropriate markings may be made on the skin of the patient's abdomen to ascertain a change in size of a flank mass. Sonography and repeat excretory urography are of value in following extravasations of blood or urine. Historically, these patients do quite well on

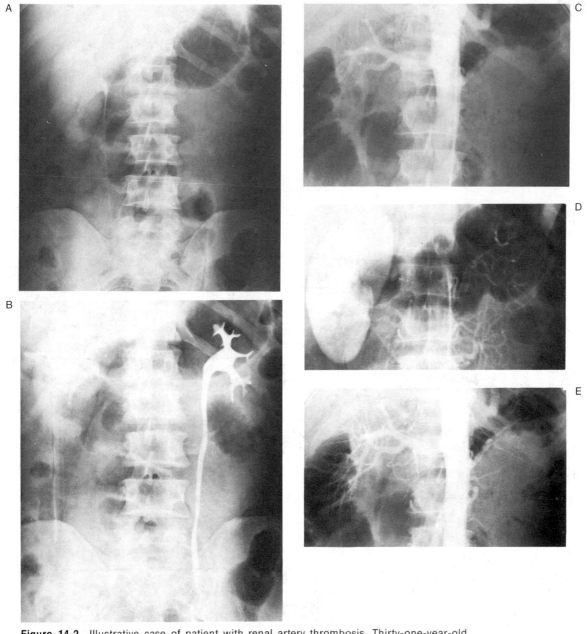

Figure 14-2 Illustrative case of patient with renal artery thrombosis. Thirty-one-year-old white male, PMH #569734, admitted 12:00 midnight 4/23/74 involved in motor vehicle accident (motorcycle), estimated speed 40 mi/h. Chief complaint: severe left back pain on admission. Poor quality plain abdominal film interpreted as negative. Urine microscopically clear. Peritoneal lavage was negative. Twenty-four hours later, severe left back pain persisted; BP 130/70; greater than 40 red blood cells per high-power microscopic field; repeat KUB; fracture of transverse process of L-1 on the left; excretory urogram performed. (*A*) Nonvisualizing left kidney. (*B*) Retrograde pyelogram interpreted as showing structurally normal collecting system. (*C, D*) Immediate angiography followed retrograde; thrombosis found in main left renal artery; immediate exploration and repair of vascular injury completed. (*E*) Follow-up arteriography showed incomplete visualization of the vasculature.

Minor renal trauma

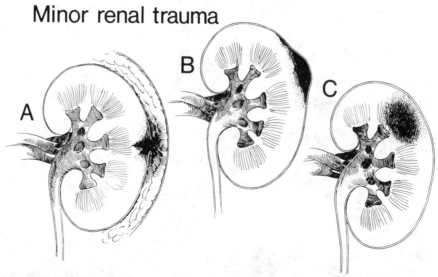

Figure 14-3 *Minor renal injuries:* (*A*) Simple laceration. (*B*) Subcapsular hematoma. (*C*) Renal contusion. *Major renal injuries:* (*A*) Renal rupture. (*B*) Laceration of renal artery and vein. (*C*) Perirenal hematoma. (*D*) Laceration through collecting system.

bed rest; less than 5 percent usually demand subsequent exploration. The patient is allowed to ambulate when gross hematuria disappears. The patient is usually discharged if he or she remains afebrile after ambulation and the urine shows less than 500 red blood cells per high-power field (gross hematuria). Rarely, indications for surgery develop in the patient suffering minor trauma who is at bed rest. These are: (1) the development of sepsis; (2) failure to sustain the hemoglobin and hematocrit with fluid and blood administration; (3) an expanding perirenal mass which is associated with a fall in hemoglobin and hematocrit; and (4) failure to sustain adequate blood pressure with supportive care.

Major renal injuries, for example, major pedicle injury, rupture of the kidney (polar or total), or large expanding perirenal hematomas, usually require surgery. In our original series, this was 91 patients of 182 patients hospitalized for renal trauma. Immediate exploration and surgical repair of the lesions of major trauma result in increased renal salvage

and diminished long-term morbidity in complications for the patient.

Operative Techniques

Operations for the management of renal trauma should be performed with the patient in the supine position with endotracheal anesthesia and nasogastric suction in place. The abdomen is opened through a midline xiphoid-to-pubis incision. The parietal peritoneum is exposed posteriorly by moving the colon superiorly and laterally and the small bowel to the side opposite the affected lesion. Medial to the inferior mesenteric artery, an incision is made in the parietal peritoneum overlying the aorta, and the renal artery on the appropriate side is located. The renal pedicle is mobilized by a combination of blunt and sharp dissection. The artery is secured with a vascular clamp, the colon is reflected, and Gerota's fascia is incised. Hemorrhage from the transected parenchyma or a renal vessel is thus controlled by the initial maneuvers to secure the renal pedicle (Fig. 14-4).

Major renal trauma

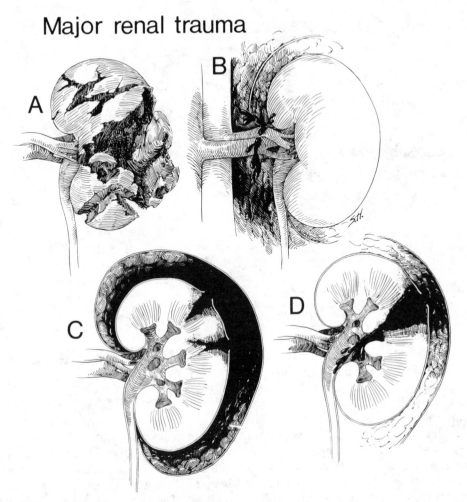

Figure 14-3B   Continued

Management of Individual Renal Parenchymal Lesions   Simple parenchymal lacerations that are not bleeding may be simply closed with through-and-through No. 3-0 chromic gut sutures which are tied over a piece of fat to prevent tearing the capsule by the suture material. One or two Penrose drains are brought out of a stab wound in the flank. Major lacerations, partial amputations, and polar ruptures involving both the parenchyma and collecting system are best treated by guillotine amputation of the affected part (Fig. 14-5). After the capsule has been reflected, the ne-

crotic or devascularized parenchyma is sharply cut away. Next, individual arcuate artery ligation is performed with No. 4-0 chromic gut figure-of-eight sutures, and the calyx is closed with running, inverting No. 4-0 chromic gut sutures. Finally, the denuded portion of the kidney is covered with capsule, adjacent perirenal fat, or live omentum. The omentum may be obtained by making a small incision in the adjacent peritoneum if one desires a vascularized pedicle flap to cover the raw area of the kidney. Collecting system repairs, such as major lacerations of the renal pelvis, should

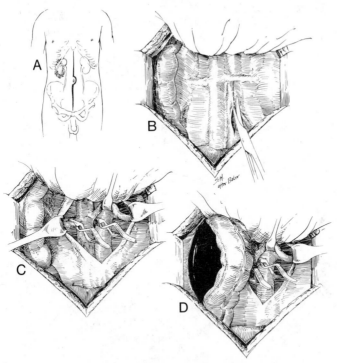

Figure 14-4 Operative approach to renal pedicle. (*A*) Midline xiphoid-to-pubis incision. (*B*) Incision of posterior parietal peritoneum over aorta medial-to-inferior mesenteric vein. (*C*) Vascular clamps on renal artery and vein. (*D*) Reflection of colon to explore Gerota's fascia and enclosed hematoma.

be repaired with No. 4-0 absorbable sutures with care taken to exclude it from the lumen of the urinary tract, lest it provide a nidus for stone formation. Attention must be given to the two fundamental principles in ureteropelvic junction repair, i.e., the creation of a funneled outlet and a dependent ureteropelvic junction to ensure most efficient emptying and to avoid an abrupt transition in lumen. If a large pelvic injury exists, a flap of renal capsule may be dissected to cover the defect.[26]

Repair of Renovascular Injuries Intrarenal venous connections are profuse. When there is a major renal venous injury, one may simply treat the vessel by ligating it unless it is the only renal vein. In this case it must be re-

paired, preferably by using No. 6-0 nonabsorbable sutures such as Prolene. The left kidney may drain adequately from the left adrenal and left gonadal vein, so that the left renal vein may be ligated if absolutely necessary. If the renal vein is avulsed and its continuity with the inferior vena cava cannot be reestablished, one must either consider autotransplantation or anastomosis of the right renal vein to the portal vein. Every effort should be made to restore its continuity to the inferior vena cava.

Renal arteries, in contrast, are end arteries, and the vessel must either be repaired or the parenchyma supplied by a given vessel amputated. One may elect to ligate a polar artery, particularly if it supplies the upper pole of the

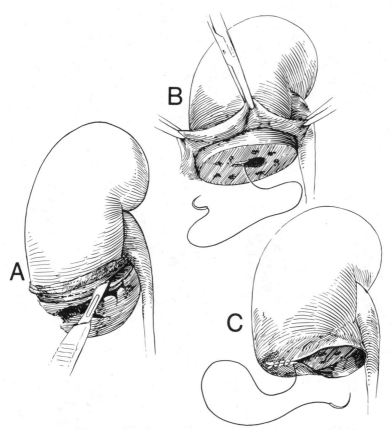

Figure 14-5   Repair of polar rupture. (*A*) Guillotine amputation of macerated or devitalized renal parenchyma. (*B*) Suture of collecting system with continuous interlocking suture and individual arcuate artery ligation. (*C*) Closure of renal capsule over operative defect.

kidney. More care should be observed in ligating a lower pole accessory renal artery, particularly if the kidney has been previously mobilized, as these vessels supply not only the parenchyma, but also a major portion of the lower calyx and renal pelvis. Their interruption may cause subsequent mucosal slough with urinary extravasation. If a polar vessel is ligated, there is a risk of subsequent hypertension. Most renal trauma series have reported an incidence of hypertension of less than 5 percent, though Boeminghaus and Gotzen[4] reported an incidence of 19 percent in the follow-up of patients who had elective ligation of an accessory renal artery at the time of

ureteropelvic junction repair. When arterial repair is indicated, a variety of techniques are available to the experienced operator. Thrombectomy with excision or fixation of an intimal flap, with or without patch graft angioplasty, may be performed. Arterial resection and reanastomosis may be feasible for lesions of short extent (< 2 cm). Dacron interposition to the aorta may be considered as a less reasonable alternative. Hypogastric artery segments may be used adequately to replace renal artery segments. There are reports of aneurysmal formation of the saphenous vein when it is substituted for renal artery. Ovarian vein, although readily accessible, is entirely unsatisfactory, as it appears too weak to support arterial pressure.[25] Nonabsorbable sutures, such as No. 6-0 Prolene or No. 6-0 Ethiflex, should be used for arterial repair. An interrupted suture line is generally preferred to a continuous one, particularly if a child's kidney is involved or if subsequent growth is anticipated. This lessens the chance of stenosis and development of hypertension.

Complications of Management of Renal Trauma

Immediate complications, such as sepsis and hematoma formation, are best prevented by meticulous attention to hemostasis at the time of surgery, adequate debridement of injured tissue, and appropriate drainage for predicted extravasation of urine. It is difficult to achieve watertight closures of the collecting system, particularly in the partially devitalized renal tissue, and urinary leakage should be anticipated. This often resolves spontaneously following the law of fistula within 9 to 20 days after the operative procedure. Urinary leakage persisting longer than 6 weeks after surgery usually indicates that the natural pathway for elimination of urine is obstructed. Efforts should then be made to diagnose and repair structural alterations in the collecting system to permit the normal flow of urine to the bladder. It is seldom necessary to resort to operative closure of a urinary fistula. When a fistula does persist, antegrade and retrograde pyelography will assist in localizing the site of the urinary obstruction which is usually responsible for the fistula. Retained foreign bodies, such as suture material and drains, must always be considered when urinary fistula persists.

Polar or accessory artery ligation may result in necrosis or partial sloughing of the collecting system; this may be responsible for delayed infection or extravasation of urine. Following initial exploration, necrotic parenchyma may result from infection, operative

vascular damage, or the "blast effect" of a high-velocity missile. Selective arteriography may be useful in delineating this infarcted tissue prior to the reexploration. Provision of adequate drainage for the urine is mandatory when operating on the victims of high-velocity missile injuries.

Hypertension as a complication of renal trauma occurs in 2 to 5 percent of the patients postoperatively. It is most commonly seen in those patients who required renal arterial repair at the time of the injury or in those patients who had a large subcapsular or perirenal hematoma. The long-term constrictive effect of an organizing perirenal hematoma compressing the renal parenchyma and resulting in persistent diastolic blood pressure elevation has been amply described by Page[19] in his experimental surgical approach in wrapping the kidney with cellophane. Several clinical examples of hypertension produced by an organizing perirenal hematoma have been reported. It is recommended that patients who have had a massive perirenal hematoma or who have had ligation of a segmental artery be followed for a minimum of 5 years postsurgery to ascertain that renal hypertension will not supervene.

Abscess formation in the kidney is rare if adequate initial debridement and hemostasis is achieved and drainage of the wound is provided. Patients who have fragments of foreign body, such as gunshot wadding or bits of clothing in the region of the kidney, are particularly suspect. Patients are explored transperitoneally, but should be provided with extraperitoneal drainage through a stab wound brought out the flank.

TRAUMA OF THE URETER

Trauma of the ureter is rare. At Parkland Memorial Hospital from 1965 to 1975, there were 1000 genitourinary trauma cases, 60 of which involved the ureter. When it occurs, it is usually secondary to a gunshot wound or stab wound, or is iatrogenic during the course of difficult pelvic or abdominal operation. Reasons for the low incidence of ureteral trauma are its small size, its excessive mobility, and the surrounding musculoskeletal protective structures—the psoas muscle posteriorly, the vertebral bodies medially, and the abdominal viscera anteriorly and laterally.

Diagnosis

In the patient who has sustained multiple simultaneous trauma, the diagnosis of ureteral damage should be suspected in patients with a stab wound, gunshot wound, or a penetrating injury along the course of the ureter. Physical signs usually occur late. Hematuria may be absent. A large mass may appear several days after the injury has occurred; this represents urinary extravasation. In the performance of the trauma series, described under the renal injury section, special care should be taken in every case of penetrating trauma to trace the course of both ureters from the kidneys to the bladder, looking for areas of extravasation, a cutoff of the column of contrast material, or ureteral dilatation. During the course of laparotomy for penetrating trauma, the ureters should always be explored, if in the path of the missile. Indigo carmine given 5 mL intravenously may sometimes show an area of extravasation. This does not totally rule out a ureteral injury, since the ipsilateral kidney may not be manufacturing urine to excrete the indigo carmine. When ureteral injury has occurred intraoperatively, the diagnosis should be made immediately and a prompt repair completed. If injury is not recognized at the operating table, the patient may develop chills, fever, mass, back pain, or pyuria several days postoperatively. An intravenous pyelogram confirms the diagnosis, demonstrating hydronephrosis of the affected side if the ureter has been tied, or urinary extravasation if the ureter has been severed.

Treatment

After the diagnosis of ureteral injury has been made, there are several ways to approach this problem. Hinman[10] and Weaver[31] have shown several principles which should be applied in the treatment of ureteral injury:

1 If one-third of the circumference of the ureteral mucosa is present, it will usually reepithelialize over a stent.

2 A ureteral stent is especially indicated if the affected ureter is infected or has been previously injured.

3 Nonabsorbable suture, in general, should not be used when attempting ureteral repair, unless a watertight closure is undertaken. The nonabsorbable suture may serve as a nidus for stone formation, and if urine extravasates, the suture can serve as a focus for chronic infection in this area.

4 It is preferable to use as few sutures as possible in ureteral repair.

5 Care should always be taken to straighten out any kinks which appear to be present in the ureter.

6 Healing is usually more efficient if the repaired ureter is wrapped in a sleeve of retroperitoneal or omental fat.

7 A ureteral stent adds little to the healing process.

8 The ureter should never be grasped with toothed forceps or any other large instruments. Vascular instruments are preferred for ureteral repair.

In the case of a gunshot wound which has partially severed the ureter, the blast effect is not easily detected at the operating table. The ureteral edges should be debrided back to bleeding, viable tissue, and a ureteroureterostomy performed. Methods of management of ureteral injuries are numerous. The procedure employed depends on the nature and location of the injury. In the multiple trauma victim, if a ureteral injury is recognized after several hours of surgery, then nephrostomy drainage with ligation of the damaged ureter will decompress the kidney and preserve the renal function. The ureteral reconstruction is performed at a later date. An alternative temporizing measure is to place a catheter in the lumen of the injured ureter and to bring the catheter out a cutaneous stab wound. These procedures allow prompt, effective urinary drainage without prolonging the operation of a critically injured patient.

When time permits, primary ureteral reconstruction should be attempted. If the injury has occurred in the upper one-third of the ureter, a ureteropyeloplasty or a ureteroureterostomy may be accomplished. If the injury has occurred in the middle one-third of the ureter, a ureteroureterostomy is preferred. To decrease the tension on the suture line, mobilization of the ureter with a psoas hitch may be necessary. If the injury has occurred in the lower one-third of the ureter, a ureteral reimplantation into the bladder by the technique described by Politano and Leadbetter is preferred. If there has been damage of a significant portion of the lower ureter and it will not reach the bladder, then a bladder flap with a tunneled ureteral reimplantation is usually employed. Alternate management of extensive destruction of the lower ureter is by transureteroureterostomy.[11]

Operative Techniques

For ureteroureterostomy, the ends of the ureter are debrided to viable, bleeding tissue. Each end is then spatulated approximately 7 mm longitudinally, and they are anastomosed using No. 5-0 chromic interrupted sutures through the muscular layers to exclude the suture from the ureteral lumen (Fig. 14-6). When performing a ureteroureterostomy, ureters should be adequately mobilized so that no tension is exerted on the suture line. This may usually be accomplished by simple proximal and distal dissection of the injured ureter. A psoas hitch may need to be performed; this consists of suturing the bladder adjacent to

the ipsilateral ureteral orifice to the psoas muscle to decrease the tension on the suture line. The technique of ureteral reimplantation has been adequately described by Politano and Leadbetter[22] and consists of a 2-cm submucosal tunneled placement of the ureter. The ureteral mucosa is sutured to the bladder with No. 4-0 interrupted chromic gut sutures (Fig. 14-6). If the lower ureter has been destroyed so that reimplantation is impossible, a bladder flap repair should be attempted by a modification of the technique of Boari[3] and Scott.[24]

In the construction of a bladder flap, the strip of bladder wall of appropriate length is incised and approximated to the viable ureter. Next, the ureter is placed in a 2-cm submucosal tunnel at the apex of the flap (Fig. 14-6). The flap is then tubularized with sutures of No. 3-0 chromic gut. A second adventitial layer of No. 3-0 or No. 4-0 chromic gut completes the repair. We feel that the method of a tunneled reimplantation of the ureter combined with a bladder flap will decrease the incidence of ureterovesical reflux with resultant infection and renal destruction.

Complications of Ureteral Injury

Immediate complications of a ureteral injury, particularly if it is overlooked, is gross urinary extravasation, flank mass, and infection which will require drainage and further surgery. Late complications usually related to ureteral stricture formation may result in hydronephrosis, necessitating further operative reconstruction. In the patient who has a bladder flap ureteroplasty or ureteral reimplantation, ureterovesical reflux should be sought,[27] and the patient should be carefully followed for any deterioration in renal function or chronic urinary infection.

BLADDER TRAUMA

Bladder injuries usually result from penetrating or blunt trauma. Although contusions may

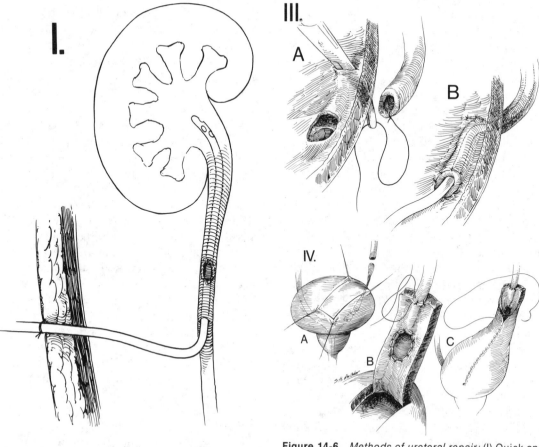

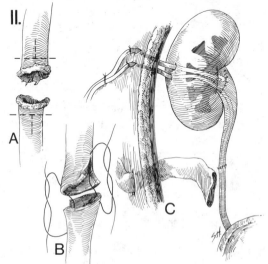

Figure 14-6 *Methods of ureteral repair:* (I) Quick and effective diversion with ureteral catheter when patient's critical condition does not permit definitive repair. (II) Repair of midureter. (*A*) Sharp debridement of ureter back to viable, bleeding tissue. (*B*) Suture of spatulated ureter with interrupted sutures. (*C*) Proximal diversion with nephrostomy and Silastic ureteral stent placed through repair. Penrose drainage out stab wound in flank. (III) Submucosal tunneled ureteral reimplantation for injury to lower third of ureter. (*A*) Creation of submucosal tunnel. (*B*) Completed repair with ureteral stent. (IV) Creation of bladder flap ureteroplasty for injury to lower ureter. (*A*) Incision of bladder flap. (*B*) Tunneled ureteral reimplantation placed at apex of reflected flap. (*C*) Closure of vesical defect.

occur as a result of blast effect of high-velocity missiles, the penetrating injuries are usually bladder lacerations with or without urinary extravasation. The blunt traumatic bladder injuries are usually divided into two types. The first type is extraperitoneal vesical rupture (Fig. 14-7), which constitutes about 80 percent of blunt bladder injuries. Bladder injuries of this type frequently result from a pelvic fracture with penetration of the bladder wall by a bony fragment. In most series of pelvic fractures, from 5 to 10 percent have associated extraperitoneal rupture of the bladder.[23] They are usually associated with a large amount of blood loss, especially in the patient with portal hypertension. The second type of blunt injury to the bladder is the intraperitoneal vesical rupture (Fig. 14-8). This usually occurs in the patient with a full bladder who has a sudden blow delivered to the lower abdomen. The bladder is acutely distended and tends to rupture at its weakest point, the dome. Subsequently, intraperitoneal leakage of urine occurs. These injuries account for approximately 20 percent of vesical ruptures.

Diagnosis

When seen in the emergency room, the patient should be questioned for suprapubic pain and time of last micturition. A clue to the diagnosis of ruptured bladder may be found in the patient's inability to void after the injury. A urine specimen is then examined for the presence of blood. After the plain film of the abdomen and pelvis has been viewed and urethral trauma has been excluded, a soft catheter is passed into the bladder; 300 to 400 mL of one-half strength iodine-containing contrast material, e.g., Renografin-60, is instilled into the bladder by gravity. A plain abdominal anterior-to-posterior film is then taken, and the size of the bladder can be determined. Any vesical irregularity or the presence of ureterovesical reflux should be

Figure 14-7   Pelvic fracture and an extraperitoneal rupture of the bladder.

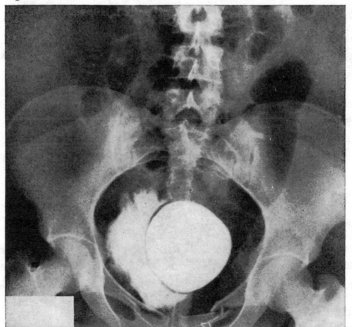

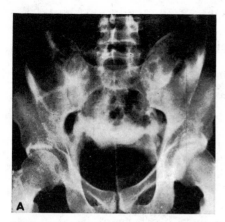

Figure 14-8 The usual picture of extraperitoneal rupture of the bladder and intraperitoneal rupture of the bladder is illustrated above. Fluid-covered loops of bowel are outlined by previously instilled contrast material after evacuation of the bladder by a urethral catheter.

noted. Next, a film is taken after drainage of the bladder since the bladder filled with contrast material may obscure small extravasations of urine. In the patient with extraperitoneal rupture of the bladder, there may be flamelike wisps of contrast material extravasated about the vesical neck. With intraperitoneal rupture, the urine is extravasated into the peritoneal cavity, and the bladder may contract and give the appearance of a normal but small-capacity bladder. Therefore, it is especially important that 300 to 400 mL of contrast material be instilled if intraperitoneal rupture of the bladder is suspected. If the bladder will hold only 25 to 50 mL, one should be suspect that a previous vesical rupture has occurred or that preexisting bladder disease is present.

Treatment

The patient with penetrating trauma will usually be surgically explored to rule out injuries to other abdominal viscera and vasculature. At this time, the bladder injury may be evaluated. After debridement, the vesical laceration is sutured with two layers of No. 2-0 or No. 3-0 chromic sutures placed in a continuous

interlocking fashion. A suprapubic cystostomy tube is usually left indwelling; a No. 30 French Pezzar or Malicot catheter is suitable. Penrose drains are left in the space of Retzius and should exist extraperitoneally. In most patients with extraperitoneal vesical rupture, the above technique is employed. However, in a female with clear urine and minimal injury in which no other surgery is contemplated, a urethral catheter may be inserted and left indwelling. Drainage of the space of Retzius should be performed under local anesthesia in these patients. In infants with bladder rupture, an alternative to suprapubic catheter drainage is cutaneous vesicostomy, which is easily performed since the bladder in infants is essentially intraperitoneal and easily approximated to the skin. In the intraperitoneal rupture of the bladder, the peritoneum should be thoroughly irrigated to remove all urine. The bladder defect is closed as mentioned previously and a suprapubic cystostomy tube is left in place.

URETHRAL TRAUMA

Injuries to the urogenital diaphragm usually result from blunt external force and pelvic fracture. They may be classified according to their location—superior or inferior to the urogenital diaphragm. Injuries superior to the urogenital diaphragm caused by blunt trauma constitute about 80 percent of the ruptures of the urethra. They result from external force when the patient has a distended bladder. The prostate is sheared from its attachments to the superior fascia of the urogenital diaphragm and the urethra severed either partially or totally (Fig. 14-9). Sphincteric activity of the vesical neck remains intact and may prevent bladder emptying. The bladder is subsequently found to be full of urine, and a large amount of urinary extravasation may not occur.

Injuries inferior to the urogenital diaphragm are usually the result of a straddle injury. The patient falls astride a bicycle or fence, or falls

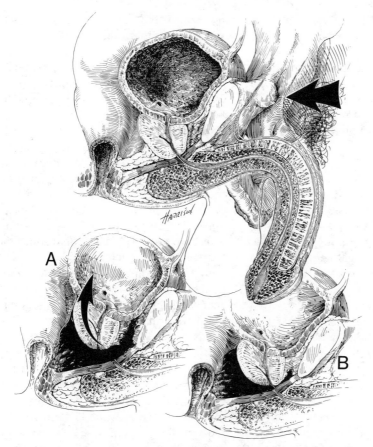

Figure 14-9 Rupture of urethra superior to urogenital diaphragm showing normal anatomy with arrow representing vector through which the force is applied. (*A*) Complete rupture of urethra with elevated prostate and large pelvic hematoma. (*B*) Incomplete rupture of urethra with less distortion of normal anatomy.

from a ladder or scaffolding, and a sharp blow is delivered to the perineum. It is important to recognize that many injuries to the urethra, both superior and inferior to the urogenital diaphragm, are not complete ruptures. In inexperienced hands, overzealous attempts to manipulate the urethra while inserting a catheter may convert the incomplete laceration to a complete tear.

Rupture of Urethra Superior to Urogenital Diaphragm

Diagnosis In patients subjected to blunt external force or sudden violent deceleration, rectal examination may disclose the prostate to be markedly elevated. If the prostate cannot be palpated, rupture of the urethra superior to the urogenital diaphragm should be suspected. In the female, rupture of the urethra superior to the urogenital diaphragm is frequently associated with a concomitant vaginal laceration. These lacerations are obvious on physical examination or seen when vaginal extravasation of contrast material is noted on the trauma series.

If one suspects a rupture of the urethra, full-strength water soluble contrast material, used for intravenous injection, is introduced through a catheter tip syringe placed in the urethral meatus, and an oblique roentgenogram is obtained (Fig. 14-10). If a soft catheter is already in place and urine is draining, water soluble contrast material may be injected alongside the indwelling catheter through a 16-gauge Angiocath and a urethrogram obtained. In this manner, urethral injury of serious magnitude may be noted, and proper alignment of the catheter may be assessed.

Treatment   After one ascertains that rupture of the urethra has occurred, there are several modes of treatment. Primary realignment of the urethra at the time of the injury may be accomplished by manipulation of the urethra with interlocking sounds and subsequent passage of urethral catheter. Traction on the catheter to hold the prostate against the superior surface of the urogenital diaphragm is then instituted.[18] Turner-Warwick[29] advocates primary realignment using a urethral catheter, but replaces catheter traction with perineal traction sutures through the bladder neck. Another surgical alternative is to perform primary anastomosis of the severed urethral ends at the time of the injury.[21]

At our institution, initial management of the rupture of the urethra superior to the urogenital diaphragm consists of suprapubic cystostomy *alone,* as suggested by Morehouse and MacKinnon.[14,15] One does not disturb the pelvic hematoma by extensive dissection or ma-

nipulation. No perivesical drainage is necessary, other than the suprapubic tube. This makes the initial management of a serious injury relatively simple. The patient with a pelvic fracture often has massive blood loss from the fracture sites, and this bleeding may be difficult to control during an operation. Exploration will only serve to increase bleeding, and an incomplete ureteral laceration may be converted to a complete disruption. After initial cystostomy, delayed reconstruction of the complete urethral rupture can be carried out 3 to 6 months later by either a perineal approach, as advocated by Morehouse,[14,15] Turner-Warwick,[28] and Johanson,[13] or by a transpubic approach as advocated by Pierce[20] and Allen.[2] This delay will allow the pelvic hematoma to resolve and the prostate to descend in proximity to the urogenital diaphragm so that only a short area of stricture exists.

If an indwelling catheter has been fortuitously positioned without surgery, the surgeon must decide whether to leave the catheter in place or, in addition, to do a suprapubic cystostomy. If the prostate is not resting in proximity to the urogenital diaphragm, a suprapubic cystostomy should be performed. The urethral catheter may then be removed, as it is anticipated from the work of Morehouse and MacKinnon[14,15] that the prostate will descend

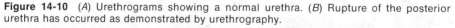

Figure 14-10   (*A*) Urethrograms showing a normal urethra. (*B*) Rupture of the posterior urethra has occurred as demonstrated by urethrography.

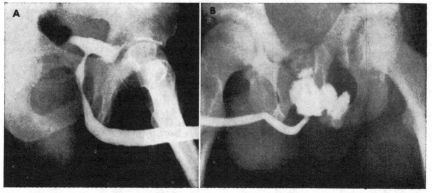

to the level of the urogenital diaphragm as the pelvic hematoma resolves. Urethral and genital complications of an indwelling urethral catheter, i.e., prostatitis, epididymitis, and stricture formation, are thus avoided. In those injuries which are not complete, the urethra often heals spontaneously, and voiding cystourethrography demonstrates the integrity of the urethra, obviating the need for surgical repair. This approach has greatly simplified the initial management of these otherwise difficult pelvic injuries. Historically, primary realignment with interlocking urethral sounds and subsequent catheter drainage and/or primary urethral reanastomosis have served usually to compound the degree of pelvic injury. The resulting incidence of impotence, stricture, and incontinence after additional urethroplasty has approached 37 percent,[8] 25 to 100 percent,[9,21,30,32] and 7 to 15 percent,[17] respectively. The more recent approach of cystostomy alone, followed by delayed definitive techniques of urethral repair, when necessary, has reduced the incidence of stricture, incontinence, and impotence to zero in some series.[14,15]

Rupture of Urethra Inferior to Urogenital Diaphragm

Diagnosis Injuries of the urethra inferior to the urogenital diaphragm usually result from straddle injuries. The perineum should be inspected for a butterfly hematoma (Fig. 14-11). Rupture of the urethra inferior to the urogenital diaphragm is often associated with a drop of blood at the meatus, which is carried there by a spasm of the bulbocavernosus muscle subsequent to the injury. Once again, the initial diagnostic approach should be the performance of an oblique urethrogram by injection of water soluble contrast material. If the catheter has already been inserted and one suspects urethral injury, then contrast material may be injected, as previously described, alongside the indwelling catheter and the magnitude of injury assessed.

Treatment If the injury is one of minor degree, the indwelling catheter is simply left in place. Major injuries require individualized surgical judgment. If urethral alignment is satisfactory, indwelling catheter drainage is adequate. If a severe rupture of the bulbous or membranous urethra is seen, suprapubic cystostomy is preferable to establishment of urethral catheter drainage. If massive extravasation is seen or there is any question as to whether the urethral catheter is in an extravesical position, suprapubic cystostomy is recommended. It is important to recognize the pathway of extravasation of urine and blood in ruptures of the urethra inferior to the urogenital diaphragm (Fig. 14-12). The blood and urine follow a path deep to Scarpa's fascia; they are limited by the attachment of the Scarpa's fascia to the fascia lata in the thigh and the coracoclavicular fascia in the axilla. Unrecognized urinary extravasation in the perineal area is serious, but if promptly recognized and drained, need not be fatal with modern antibiotic therapy.

INJURIES TO THE EXTERNAL GENITALIA

Injuries to the Penis

Injuries to the penile skin are usually secondary to a "power-takeoff" injury. In this type of injury, the clothing or the skin of the genitalia is caught in moving parts of a motor vehicle or of mechanical devices used in industry or farming. The principle in the management of injuries to the skin of the penile shaft is to discard any skin remaining distal to the point of injury, up to the coronal sulcus (Fig. 14-13). A thick split-thickness skin graft (0.015 in) is then applied from the proximal extent of the injury to the coronal sulcus. Efforts to save an inch of distal penile skin will result in tremendous lymphedema since the lymphatic drainage has been interrupted by the interposed graft.

Individuals who have placed various circumferential metallic objects about the penis

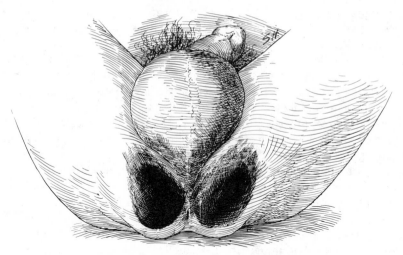

Figure 14-11   Butterfly hematoma in perineum of patient with rupture of urethra inferior to urogenital diaphragm.

Figure 14-12   Rupture of urethra inferior to urogenital diaphragm. (*A*) Rupture of urethra and tunica albuginea of the corporal bodies, but not Buck's fascia, showing limitation of urine and blood extravasation. (*B*) Rupture of urethra through Buck's fascia showing path of extravasation of blood and urine, limited posteriorly by Colles' fascial attachment at the perineal body and extending up the abdominal wall deep to Scarpa's fascia which is continuous with Colles' fascia anteriorly.

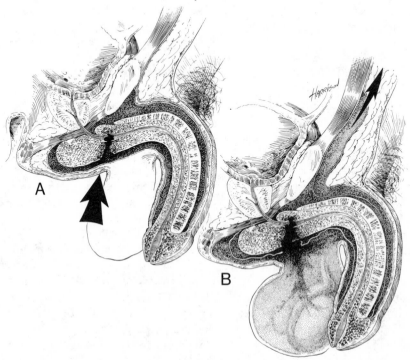

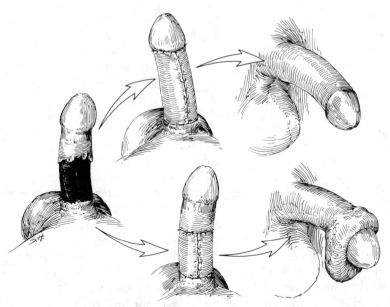

Figure 14-13 Correct (above) and incorrect (below) management of partial avulsion of penile skin. If distal remnant of penile skin is left in place, then lymphedema of distal segment will occur secondary to obstruction of lymphatic drainage.

for purposes of masturbation often present an acute problem. Appropriate treatment consists of removal of the object using a metal cutting instrument under light general anesthesia. Injuries to the prepuce, i.e., catching the prepuce in the zipper of the pants, may be treated by circumcision in conjunction with removal of the zipper. Metallic foreign bodies and other objects introduced into the urethra for the purpose of sexual stimulation may occasionally escape from the hands of their owner and present a problem in removal. Many objects can be removed simply by pushing them into the urinary bladder and removing them with an endoscopic grasping forceps. Many straight pins and needles in the distal urethra can be removed, simply by pushing them through the urethra and penile skin and removing them. Others may require grasping with endoscopic forceps through the cystoscope. If a pin or needle contains an enlargement on one end, the sharp or pointed end can

be pushed through the urethra and penile skin and levered so the enlarged end may be grasped through the meatus and removed.

Injuries to the Scrotum and Genitalia

Injuries to the scrotum and genitalia are classified as penetrating or nonpenetrating. The philosophy of management is to explore all penetrating injuries and perform proper debridement and cleansing. Blunt trauma to the scrotum requires individualized management. Exploration is often indicated because rupture of the testis may occur and salvage can be accomplished by immediate exploration and repair of that ruptured testis. Necrotic and extruded tubules are debrided sharply, and the tunica albuginea is closed with interrupted No. 3-0 chromic gut sutures. Drainage in a dependent area of the scrotum is provided. This approach has resulted in a higher salvage rate of testes than the conservative approach. Elevation and ice bag application has not only resulted in a high percentage of testicular loss, but prolonged the morbidity to the patient.

In scrotal injuries, when massive skin loss has occurred, coverage of the testis is needed. If not enough scrotal skin remains, one may implant the testis in a subcutaneous pouch in the thigh. Studies by Culp et al.,[6] at Iowa, have shown that the temperature is approximately 89°F in the superficial thigh pouch, as contrasted with 98°F in the abdominal or inguinal position. Regeneration of the scrotum is usually complete within 3 to 6 weeks after the injury, and the testis can then be returned to a resting scrotal position. In those cases in which the scrotum is completely avulsed, the testis can be left in the superficial thigh pouch. Chorionic gonadotropin may be administered in doses of 500 to 1000 IU 3 times a week to promote growth of the scrotal skin to cover the partially exposed testis.

Extensive scrotal lacerations are best handled by careful debridement and cleansing. If the tunica vaginalis is not opened, drains need not be used. Careful attention to closure of the dartos layer is of importance, since scrotal bleeding will be minimized by proper closure of this layer.

SPECIAL CONSIDERATIONS OF GENITOURINARY TRAUMA IN CHILDREN

Renal Trauma

Some considerations in the renal trauma patient are unique in children. The kidney is the most frequently injured visceral organ in children,[16] and there is an increased incidence of preexisting renal disease.[7] There is a higher incidence of hematuria when the patient is seen initially.[5,12] There is a lower incidence of rib fractures, probably due to the greater elasticity of children's bones.[16] The child who has sustained trauma is less apt to have exsanguination from major injuries. Emergency genitourinary evaluation should proceed in the manner previously described, with the injec-

tion of 1 mg/lb of iodine-containing contrast material. Arteriography should be approached more cautiously in children since there is greater risk of arterial thrombosis due to the smaller caliber of major arteries. Every effort should be made to preserve all viable renal parenchyma in children, since compensatory hypertrophy will occur, and to a greater extent than in the adult. On the intravenous pyelogram, compensatory hypertrophy is grossly observed in the opposite kidney when two-thirds to three-quarters of the damaged kidney is removed. However, it will occur functionally when any loss of renal parenchyma occurs.[1] Renal function studies have suggested that a glomerular filtration rate of more than 5 mL/min is necessary to avoid dialysis and allow medical management of renal failure. It appears that humans need approximately 25 percent of total renal mass to maintain life. This, however, is the lower limit and constitutes a reason for abstaining from total nephrectomy whenever possible. Growth is certain to be retarded if so little parenchyma remains that the child suffers from acidosis and azotemia.

Bladder Trauma

In management of bladder injuries in children, suprapubic diversion is preferable in boys with either extraperitoneal or intraperitoneal extravasation, because of the high incidence of complications secondary to the use of indwelling catheters in small urethras. Complications such as epididymitis, urethral stricture, and urethral fistula at the penoscrotal junction occur not uncommonly in boys following prolonged use of indwelling urethral catheters. In females with trauma to the bladder, urethral catheter drainage is sometimes satisfactory. In addition, cutaneous vesicostomy is particularly applicable to infants. A vesicostomy permits avoidance of foreign material in the urinary tract and lessens the incidence of infection and bladder spasm. A cutaneous vesicostomy will close spontaneously quite often and appears to be a more satisfactory method for lower urinary diversion in infants in whom the bladder is essentially an intraperitoneal organ.

External Genitalia

In considering trauma to the external genitalia, the preputial skin should be preserved as it represents skin with an unusual capacity for growth and may be used in reconstruction. When only a small bit of scrotum remains, it is especially important in children to place the testis in a subcutaneous pouch. Under hormonal stimulation, only a small remnant of scrotum may proliferate, and later a pouch may be constructed into which the testis may be reimplanted. Orchiectomy should be avoided if there is the slightest possibility that the testis is viable. Bleeding is a general but not infallible criterion of viability.

BIBLIOGRAPHY

1 Allen, T. D.: "Compensatory Renal Hypertrophy," in J. H. Johnson and W. E. Goodwin, *Reviews in Pediatric Urology,* Excerpta Medica, Amsterdam, 1974.

2 ———: The transpubic approach for strictures of membranous urethra, *J. Urol.,* **114**:63, 1975.

3 Boari: Contributo sperimentali alla plastica dell' uretere, *Atti. Accad. Sci. Med. Nat. Ferrara,* **68**:149, 1894.

4 Boeminghaus, H. and N. Goetz: Partial renal infarction and increased blood pressure resulting from ligature of aberrant renal vessels, (Abstract) *J. Am. Med. Assoc.,* **149**:1606, 1952.

5 Cass, A. S. and G. W. Ireland: Renal injuries in children, *J. Trauma,* **14**:719, 1974.

6 Culp, D. A. and W. C. Huffman: Temperature determination in the thigh with regard to burying the traumatically exposed testis, *J. Urol.,* **76**:436, 1956.

7 Esho, J. O., G. W. Ireland, and A. S. Cass: Renal trauma and preexisting lesions of the kidney, *Urology,* **1**:134, 1973.

8 Gibson, G. R.: Impotence following fractured pelvis and ruptured urethra, *Br. J. Urol.,* **42**:86, 1970.

9 ———: Urologic management and complications of fractured pelvis and ruptured urethra, *J. Urol.,* **111**:353, 1974.

10 Hinman, F., Jr.: Ureteral repair and the splint, *J. Urol.,* **78**:376, 1957.

11 Hodges, C. V., R. V. Moore, T. H. Lehman, and A. M. Behnam: Clinical experiences with transurectero-ureterostomy, *J. Urol.,* **90**:552, 1963.

12 Javadpour, N. et al.: Renal trauma in children, *Surg. Gynecol. Obstet.* **136**:237, 1973.

13 Johanson, B.: Reconstruction of the male urethra in stricture, *Acta. Chir. Scand. Suppl.,* 176, 1953.

14 Morehouse, D. D., P. Belitsky, and K. J. MacKinnon: Rupture of posterior urethra, *J. Urol.,* **107**:255, 1972.

15 ——— and K. J. MacKinnon: Urologic injuries associated with pelvic fractures, *J. Trauma,* **9**:479, 1969.

16 Morse, T. S.: Renal injuries in children, *Pediatr. Clin. North Am.,* **22**(2), May 1975.

17 Moulonguet, A.: Ruptures tramatiques de l'urethre posterieur, *J. Urol. Nephrol.,* **71**: Suppl. 38, October 1965.

18 Myers, R. P. and J. H. Deweerd: Incidence of stricture following primary realignment of disrupted proximal urethra, *J. Urol.,* **107**:265, 1972.

19 Page, I. H.: The production of persistent arterial hypertension by cellophane perinephritis, *J. Am. Med. Assoc.,* **113**:2046, 1939.

20 Pierce, J. M.: Exposure of membranous and posterior urethra by total pubectomy, *J. Urol.,* **88**:256, 1962.

21 ———: Management of dismemberment of the prostatic membranous urethra and ensuing stricture disease, *J. Urol.,* **107**:259, 1972.

22 Politano, V. A. and W. F. Leadbetter: An operative technique for correction of vesicoureteral reflux, *J. Urol.,* **79**:932, 1958.

23 Reynolds, B. M., N. A. Balsano, and F. X. Reynolds: Pelvic fractures, *J. Trauma,* **13**:1011, 1973.

24 Scott, F. B. and M. Greenberg: Submucosal bladder-flap ureteroplasty: Clinical experience, *South. Med. J.,* **65**:1308, 1972.

25 Straffon, R.: Personal communication, 1968.

26 Thompson, I. M., J. Baker, V. L. Robards, Jr., L. Kovacsi, and G. Ross, Jr.: Clinical experience with renal capsule flap pyeloplasty, *J. Urol.,* **101**:487, 1969.

27 ——— and G. Ross: Long-term results of bladder flap repair of ureteral injuries, *J. Urol.,* **111**:483, 1974.

28 Turner-Warwick, R.: Observations on the treatment of traumatic urethral injuries and the value of the fenestrated urethral catheter, *Br. J. Surg.,* **60**:775, 1973.

29 ———: The repair of urethral strictures in the region of the membranous urethra, *J. Urol.,* **100**:303, 1968.

30 Waterhouse, K. and M. Gross: Trauma of the genitourinary tract: A five-year experience with 251 cases, *J. Urol.,* **101**:241, 1969.

31 Weaver, R. G.: Ureteral regeneration: Experimental and clinical, *J. Urol.,* **79**:31, 1958.

32 Wilkinson, F. O. W.: Rupture of posterior urethra, *Lancet,* **1**:1125, 1961.

Chapter 15

Penetrating Wounds of the Neck

Robert F. Jones, M.D.

Although major wounds of the soft tissues of the neck are relatively uncommon in civilian surgical practice, the number of vital structures in the small volume of the neck makes it imperative that every penetrating neck wound be considered a serious surgical problem.

Prior to World War II the treatment of penetrating wounds of the neck was largely nonsurgical unless major bleeding or deep injuries were obvious. Reported mortality rates were 18 percent of 188 cases in the Spanish-American War and 11 percent of 594 cases in World War I. During World War II the mortality rate fell to 7 percent, probably because of a variety of factors, including earlier tracheostomy, earlier and more frequent surgical exploration, antibiotics, and

improvements in surgical and anesthetic techniques.[9]

In a study of neck wounds reported by Shirkey in 1963 it was noted that, of the 22 deaths which occurred, 6 were in the group in which exploration was either delayed beyond 6 h or omitted entirely.[20] Fogelman and Stewart had pointed out in 1956 that the mortality rate in their cases which were promptly explored was 6 percent, whereas in those in which surgical intervention was omitted or postponed the mortality rate was 35 percent.[7] After the initial phase of that series it became the policy of Parkland Memorial Hospital in Dallas to "treat the platysma like the peritoneum" and explore virtually all neck wounds that penetrated the platysma. In 1967 another series of 274 cases from Parkland Memorial Hospital was reviewed, and it was found that in 15 patients whose necks were explored in spite of wounds that appeared innocuous prior to surgery, i.e., with no visible bleeding, no visible hematoma, and no evidence of shock, there were several major vessel injuries and other significant trauma as noted in Table 15-1.[11]

In the same study there were 103 cases in which there were no significant injuries. In that group of negative explorations there were no deaths and no complications except one superficial wound infection which cleared promptly with drainage. Those patients were usually discharged within 72 h to a follow-up clinic if there were no associated injuries. The overall mortality rate in the Parkland series was 4 percent. Such cases which seem to be free of significant injury upon examination in the emergency room may later bleed massively on the ward when a blood clot is shaken loose, or other complications may develop from unrecognized injuries of the esophagus or pharynx. Also it is likely that injuries associated with damage only to subcutaneous tissues and muscles will heal faster with less chance of infection if hemostasis, debridement, and adequate drainage are performed. Several other series have been reported which support this policy.[1,4,5,6,10,12,15,17,22,23,26] Several other authors have recommended selecting certain cases with penetrating neck wounds for observation only.[3,8,15,18,20,24]

There is one reported case in which exploration was not done because of the "benign" appearance of the wound, and the patient died on the ward because of massive hemorrhage from the carotid artery into the trachea as a result of unsuspected injury to both structures.[24] Knightly reported complications in two patients with apparently innocuous wounds that might have been prevented had surgical exploration been done initially.[12] Sheely reported three deaths due to delayed exploration in which there were unrecognized perforations of the cervical esophagus.[19]

In view of the minimal morbidity from negative explorations and the risk of serious, sometimes lethal, complications in unexplored cases with occult injuries, the safest policy appears to be that virtually all penetrating wounds of the neck should be explored without delay, regardless of the preoperative opinion as to the extent and severity of the damage.

INITIAL TREATMENT

On admission to the emergency room, all patients with neck injuries are immediately evaluated regarding their systemic condition, i.e., airway and adequacy of ventilation, blood pressure, pulse, mental state, and peripheral signs of shock such as sweating, cold skin, and collapsed veins. If there is external bleeding, some type of pressure is applied for temporary hemostasis. If there is upper airway obstruction, an endotracheal tube is passed immediately or, if there is sufficient time, a tracheostomy is performed. Use of the fiberoptic bronchoscope has been described to facilitate endotracheal intubation in patients in whom airway obstruction has resulted from facial or neck trauma.[16] Meanwhile, one or two large-bore intravenous cannulas or needles are inserted in peripheral veins, and lac-

Table 15-1   Injuries in 15 Patients with Clinically "Negative" Neck Wounds
(No Visible Bleeding, Hematoma, or Shock)

Site of injury	Number of cases
Innominate vein	2
Subclavian vein	1
Internal jugular vein	6
Thyrocervical artery	3
Ascending pharyngeal artery	1
Thoracic duct	2
Esophagus (blast injury)	2

tated Ringer's solution is started while blood is drawn for typing and cross matching. If shock is present, the fluid is given rapidly and, if there is no evidence of significant blood loss, the intravenous infusions are kept going by slow drip. When indicated, whole blood is started as soon as it is available. Usually the salt solution will temporarily reverse the shock state until cross-matched blood is available. If shock is severe and is not improved promptly by the lactated Ringer's solution, type-specific or type O, Rh-negative low-titer unmatched blood is available. Plasma has also been used, but there is little advantage over salt solutions; i.e., both are helpful temporarily, and neither is a substitute for whole blood.

If it is apparent clinically that blood or air is free in a pleural cavity, closed-chest drainage is immediately instituted. If there is no clinical evidence of a pneumothorax or hemothorax, if the missile or blade could possibly have reached the pleura, and if the patient's systemic condition is stable, an upright chest film is obtained with a physician in constant attendance.

If the depth of the injury is not apparent, the wound is very gently probed with a small hemostat *only* to the depth of the platysma muscle. If the platysma has been penetrated, the probing is discontinued. Deep probing into nonbleeding neck wounds in an emergency room should not be done.

Arteriography may be useful in detecting vascular injuries and in planning operative management. This is especially true in the assessment of penetrating injuries near the base of the skull and the thoracic outlet. Preoperative detection of vascular wounds in these locations may allow the surgeon to more easily expose and control the involved vessels. When firm indications for operation are present, and the patient is hemodynamically unstable, it is usually best not to delay exploration for radiological studies, but to proceed with surgery.

The patient is then transferred to the operating room. No attempt is made to pass a nasogastric tube in the emergency room because of the danger of hemorrhage with coughing or gagging.

SURGICAL EXPLORATION

Anesthesia

Exploration should nearly always be done in the operating room under general anesthesia. Because the patients are often intoxicated, or have a stomach full of partially digested food, or have injury in or near the airway, it is essential that an orotracheal tube with an inflatable cuff be in place before exploration is begun.

The anesthetic agent used varies according to the specific problem: necessity for rapid induction, circulatory status, preexisting disease, etc. The anesthesiologist manages the fluids and blood, frequently consulting the operating surgeon. There are no specific contraindications in neck injuries per se to any of the commonly used anesthetic agents or relaxants.

The chest is again examined just prior to induction since pneumothorax or hemothorax may develop slowly following a neck wound, appearing an hour or longer after an initially negative chest x-ray. Wounds at the root of the neck following a downward path may barely penetrate the pleura, so that a pneumothorax is not apparent initially and may not become manifest until after the patient is intubated. This should be kept in mind as a cause for hypotension or hypoxia during anesthesia, especially if closed thoracotomy drainage has not been instituted.

Technique of Exploration

With adequate control of the ventilatory and cardiovascular systems, the surgeon can now safely and adequately explore the structures that are apparently or potentially injured.

The incision is planned to allow full exposure of the tract of injury. Proximal and distal control of the major vessels must also be considered in the length and position of the incision. The sternocleidomastoid muscle and/or any other neck muscles are transected whenever necessary to provide adequate exposure. An oblique incision along the anterior border of the sternomastoid muscle will usually provide access to the vessels and other important cervical structures. The tract of injury is followed to its depth, systematically examining each structure in or near the tract. It should also be pointed out that blast injury from gunshot wounds may not be immediately apparent in the tissues adjacent to the tract.

Specific Injuries

Blood Vessels   If injuries to the major vessels are suspected, umbilical tapes are passed around the vessels proximal and distal to the point of suspected injury *before* local clots are removed, if bleeding has previously occurred and stopped. This happens frequently with venous and occasionally with arterial injury. The vessels are then carefully inspected, all clots are removed, and repair is carried out by the techniques described in Chap. 9.

When the injury involves the low anterior neck, it may be necessary to resect a portion of the clavicle or to split the sternum to obtain proximal control and prevent uncontrollable hemorrhage. The medial segment of the clavicle is resected whenever necessary, disarticulating the sternoclavicular joint. There usually is no significant disability following this procedure, and if the periosteum is preserved, bony regeneration will often occur. When this does not adequately expose the great vessels for repair or for proximal control, the sternum is split with a sternal saw. The sternal incision may be extended laterally into the second or third intercostal space to avoid opening the full mediastinum unnecessarily. The sternum is closed later with stainless steel wire.

The internal carotid, common carotid, subclavian, and innominate arteries should be repaired if at all possible. An internal or external shunt may be utilized during carotid repair, as with carotid grafting or endarterectomy, or a large vessel such as the innominate artery is partially occluded with a curved vascular clamp to allow partial flow during repair. The vertebral artery is usually very difficult to repair in the bony canal, but may be controlled by prolonged pressure, suture ligatures, bone wax, or, occasionally, by proximal ligatures. The external carotid artery or its branches may be ligated, except in patients with carotid arteriosclerosis with an occluded common or internal carotid vessel. In these cases the external carotid may be a major source of collateral flow.

When the carotid arteries are to be handled or pressure applied to the bifurcation, the adventitia of the carotid bulb is infiltrated with a local anesthetic to prevent hypotension from reflexes originating in pressor receptors of the carotid sinus. Atropine may be given at intervals during the procedure when hypotension results from such stimuli.

The internal jugular vein is repaired if feasible, but may be ligated unilaterally if necessary without adverse sequelae. All other neck veins are routinely ligated if injured. Prompt pressure on an open vein and a slight head-down tilt to the table will minimize the risk of air embolism.

Larynx and Trachea   When laryngeal or tracheal injury is apparent in the emergency room, tracheostomy is performed promptly, prior to transfer of the patient to the main operating suite. If the injury is not apparent until the time of exploration, a tracheostomy is done during exploration. If the patient is hoarse or the wound is near the thyroid or larynx, indirect laryngoscopy is performed preoperatively when feasible to determine the integrity of the recurrent laryngeal nerve. Laryngeal blast injury without a visible opening may result from a bullet tract near the larynx; in such a case a tracheostomy is performed.

Subcutaneous air may be present with such injuries and may increase rapidly under observation. Air also may spread subcutaneously from outside via the entrance wound in the absence of tracheal, pharyngeal, or esophageal penetration. Cervical extension of mediastinal air from an injured bronchus or lung may also occur.

Clear lacerations of the trachea or larynx are closed using nonabsorbable suture. Beall recommends the use of Marlex or linear polyethylene and emphasizes careful mucosa-to-mucosa approximation to minimize tracheal stenosis.[2] If the defect cannot be closed primarily, a fascial flap may be used as a patch, or synthetic patch grafts such as Marlex may be used.

Larson and Cohn reported 30 cases of laryngeal injury, including 12 due to penetrating wounds. They emphasize the importance of anatomic repair of soft tissue injury, meticulous primary closure of mucosal laceration, open reduction of cartilaginous fractures, and the use of a soft stent, with a tissue graft when necessary.[13]

The tracheostomy is maintained until healing is complete and laryngeal or tracheal edema has subsided, usually 4 to 8 days. A competent laryngeal surgeon should see the patient during the operative procedure or as soon thereafter as possible to help ensure optimum management of laryngeal wounds.[25]

Pharynx and Esophagus These structures may be repaired primarily using chromic catgut suture, with debridement as necessary. It is vital to drain all such wounds, since infection and/or a salivary leak is not an infrequent complication. If a small esophageal injury is suspected but cannot be demonstrated during exploration, an anesthetic mask may be applied to the nose and mouth and positive pressure exerted while the wound is filled with saline solution. Bubbles may disclose the point of injury. This technique has been used successfully on several occasions when both esophagoscopy and surgical exploration have failed to demonstrate the esophageal penetration.

If there is massive loss of tissue, as with a close-range shotgun blast, it may be necessary to perform a cutaneous esophagostomy for feeding purposes and a cutaneous pharyngostomy for salivary drainage. A secondary plastic reconstruction will then be required after initial healing is complete.

A small plastic nasogastric tube is used for feeding purposes for 8 to 10 days following all cervical esophageal injuries, unless for some reason a gastrostomy is deemed preferable. Parenteral hyperalimentation is another alternative to a plastic feeding tube.

Nerves A preoperative neurologic examination is performed whenever possible to identify an injured nerve. The brachial plexus, deep cervical plexus, phrenic nerve, and cranial nerves are systematically tested. The vagus nerve can be checked by examination of the vocal cords. A hypoglossal or spinal accessory nerve injury is particularly easy to miss unless a preoperative neurologic examination is performed. An associated head injury or alcoholic intoxication will frequently complicate the neurologic evaluation. Whenever possible, all severed or lacerated nerves are debrided and repaired primarily, using interrupted fine silk sutures on the perineurium. If a motor nerve deficit is apparent, an expendable sensory nerve such as the great auricular nerve may be interposed as a nerve autograft to allow anastomosis without tension.

For more details of operative technique, see Chap. 11.

Thyroid After debridement of devitalized tissue, hemostasis may be secured by suture ligature. Adequate drainage is particularly important in the treatment of thyroid injuries, primarily to prevent the formation of a closed hematoma.

Thoracic Duct　Wounds near the inferior segment of the left internal jugular vein may sever the thoracic duct at or below the point of entry of the duct; the location is variable. Repair of the duct is not feasible because of its friability, but simple ligation is adequate treatment. Since the duct may divide just before entering the vein or there may be tributaries from the head and arm, multiple ligatures may be required for lymphostasis.

The area should be thoroughly dried and inspected before closing, since a large collection of lymph may occur postoperatively from even a small leak. If lymph does accumulate, incision and drainage with the application of a bulky pressure dressing will usually allow closure of the lymph fistula within a few days. The pressure dressing should be applied across the shoulder using elastic tape with adherent or tincture of benzoin compound applied to the skin to allow for steady, safe pressure across the injured area. Occasionally an injured right lymphatic duct is encountered on the opposite side in the same location and is treated in like manner.

Salivary Glands　If a major salivary duct is severed, it should be repaired if practicable. A sialogram may be used preoperatively to establish the diagnosis, or it may be determined during exploration. Injuries to the gland may be handled by debridement, hemostasis, and simple drainage. In the absence of ductal obstruction, a salivary fistula will rarely occur following injury to the gland substance. When the major duct is injured, it may be repaired with fine silk over a ureteral catheter stent. The catheter should be removed after repair is effected. When repair is not feasible because of the patient's critical condition or some

other compelling reason, the duct may be ligated and the gland allowed to atrophy or the duct may be reimplanted to the mucosa at a later time.

When the parotid gland is involved, the major facial nerve branches should be identified and repaired if injured. Primary repair has a better prognosis for nerve function than does delayed repair, unless there is gross bacterial contamination or massive loss of tissue.

Closure

Virtually all soft tissue neck wounds are drained for at least 24 to 48 h, using soft Penrose drains to prevent the accumulation of blood and serum. If the larynx, pharynx, trachea, or esophagus is injured, drainage is mandatory and is continued for 4 to 8 days. Failure to provide adequate drainage for such wounds can result in serious wound infections and, occasionally, mediastinitis, a potentially lethal complication.[12] All muscles are repaired, using nonabsorbable suture. In the case of massive gunshot wounds, such as a close-range shotgun injury, the wound is left wide open initially and delayed primary closure performed 3 to 4 days later if possible.

BIBLIOGRAPHY

1 Ashworth, C., L. F. Williams, and J. J. Byrne: Penetrating wounds of the neck, *Am. J. Surg.,* **121**:387, 1971.

2 Beall, A. C., Jr., G. P. Noon, and H. H. Harris: Surgical management of tracheal trauma, *J. Trauma,* **7**(2):248, 1967.

3 De La Cruz, A. and J. R. Chandler: Management of penetrating wounds of the neck, *Surg. Gynecol. Obstet.,* **137**:458, 1973.

4 Farley, H. H., R. Nixon, T. A. Peterson, and C. R. Hitchcock: Penetrating wounds of the neck, *Am. J. Surg.,* **108**:592, 1964.

5 Feraru, F.: Wounds of neck, *N.Y. State J. Med.,* p. 1789, July 1973.

6 Fitchett, V. H., M. Pomerantz, D. W. Butsch, R.

Simon, and B. Eiseman: Penetrating wounds of the neck, *Arch. Surg.,* **99**:307, 1969.

7 Fogelman, M. J. and R. D. Stewart: Penetrating wounds of the neck, *Am. J. Surg.,* **91**:581, 1956.

8 Getzen, L. C., S. B. Bellinger, and L. W. Kendall: Should all neck, axillary, groin, or popliteal wounds be explored for possible vascular or visceral injuries?, *J. Trauma,* **12**(10):906, 1972.

9 Hubay, C. A.: Soft tissue injuries of the cervical region, *Int. Abstr. Surg.,* **111**(6):511, 1960.

10 Hunt, T. K., F. W. Blaisdell, and J. Okimoto: Vascular injuries of the base of the neck, *Arch. Surg.,* **98**:586, 1969.

11 Jones, R. F., J. C. Terrell, and K. E. Salyer: Penetrating wounds of the neck: An analysis of 274 cases, *J. Trauma,* **7**(2):228, 1967.

12 Knightly, J. J., A. P. Swaminathan, and B. F. Rush: Management of penetrating wounds of the neck, *Am. J. Surg.,* **126**:575, 1973.

13 Larson, D. L. and A. M. Cohn: Management of acute laryngeal injury: A critical review, *J. Trauma,* **16**(9):858, 1976.

14 McQuaide, J. R. and D. de G. Villett: A four-year survey of penetrating wounds of the neck, *S. Afr. Med. J.,* **43**:1487, 1969.

15 Markey, J. C., J. L. Hines, and F. C. Nance: Penetrating neck wounds: A review of 218 cases, *Am. Surg.,* p. 77, February 1975.

16 Mulder, D. S., D. H. Wallace, and F. M. Woolhouse: The use of the fiberoptic bronchoscope to facilitate endotracheal intubation following head and neck trauma, *J. Trauma,* **15**(8):638, 1975.

17 Saletta, J. D., R. J. Lowe, L. T. Lim, J. Thornton, S. Delk, and G. S. Moss: Penetrating trauma of the neck, *J. Trauma,* **16**(7):579, 1976.

18 Sheely, C. H., K. L. Mattox, G. J. Reul, A. C. Beall, and M. E. DeBakey: Current concepts in the management of penetrating neck trauma, *J. Trauma,* **15**(10):895, 1975.

19 ———, K. L. Mattox, A. C. Beall, and M. E. DeBakey: Penetrating wounds of the cervical esophagus, *Am. J. Surg.,* **130**:707, 1975.

20 Shirkey, A. L., A. C. Beall, and M. E. DeBakey: Surgical management of penetrating wounds of the neck, *Arch. Surg.,* **86**:97, 1963.

21 Stein, A. and F. Kalk: Selective conservatism in the management of penetrating wounds of the neck, *S. Afr. J. Surg.,* **12**(1):31, 1974.

22 Weaver, A. W., S. Sankaran, S. H. Fromm, C. E. Lucas, and A. J. Walt: The management of penetrating wounds of the neck, *Surg. Gynecol. Obstet.,* **133**(1):49, 1971.

23 Weil, P. H. and F. M. Steichen: The treatment of penetrating injuries of the neck, *J. Trauma,* **11**(7):590, 1971.

24 Williams, J. W. and R. T. Sherman: Penetrating wounds of the neck: Surgical management, *J. Trauma,* **13**(5):435, 1973, Discussion by R. J. Freeark.

25 Yarington, C. T.: Immediate repair of blunt and penetrating trauma to the larynx and trachea, *Arch. Surg.,* **96**:403, 1968.

26 Yoder, R. L. and D. E. Merck: Innocuous appearing stab wounds to the neck: Is exploration always indicated, *South. Med. J.,* **62**:113, 1969.

Chapter 16

Principles of Fracture Management

William D. Arnold, M.D.

EXAMINATION OF THE MUSCULOSKELETAL SYSTEM IN THE INJURED PATIENT

At the time of the first examination of the multiply injured patient, identification of major skeletal and joint injuries allows for safe transportation to and within the hospital and for appropriate nursing management, sets the stage for later, planned, definitive treatment, and may prevent life- or limb-threatening complications. In addition to the obvious major injuries, equally serious but less obvious skeletal trauma must be recognized at this time if these objectives are to be accomplished.

A brief, systematic examination of the skeletal system should be performed at the earliest convenient moment. In the absence of neck

pain, lateral and anteroposterior (AP) manipulation of the cervical spine should be performed. A simple range-of-motion examination of the shoulders, elbows, wrists, and hands, with palpation of the intervening long bones, should be carried out. Localized swelling, pain, or restriction of the normal range of joint motion demands further evaluation. Palpation of the spinous processes of the thoracic and lumbar spine should be performed, and if the patient can lie on the side, gentle but somewhat forceful palpation with the closed fist over the spinous processes will elicit any discomfort due to localized injury in these areas. Asymmetry of the spinous processes may point to a fracture dislocation of the spine. An assessment of possible pelvic fractures may be carried out by direct palpation of the pubic rami and compression of the iliac crests toward the midline simultaneously. Fractures involving the sacral area or the wings of the ilium will be identified by this method.

It is important to examine both hips gently with passive motion, and in particular the hip should be stressed in internal rotation. Pain on internal rotation suggests a fracture of the femoral neck which may be impacted and not otherwise recognized, or a fracture of the pelvis not identified by other means. Ecchymosis about the trochanteric area suggests a fracture of the part, and ecchymosis in the scrotum and perineal region points to a fracture of the pelvis. Fractures of the femoral neck, since they are intracapsular, seldom have much, if any, blood loss and do not as a rule present any signs of ecchymosis in the surrounding soft tissues.

In the lower extremities, palpation of the long bones should be carried out to identify fractures of the femur or tibia. A gentle range-of-motion examination of both knees should be performed with manipulation of the patella and assessment of any significant knee effusion. Knee effusion requires an explanation and may indicate a fracture of the femoral condyle, proximal tibia or patella, or an internal derangement of the joint. Even in seriously injured patients, an assessment of ligamentous integrity of the knee is important since early definitive care is necessary to prevent later chronic instability of this joint. Ecchymosis over the medial aspect of the knee suggests a rupture of the medial collateral ligament. The knee should be stressed in varus and in valgus with the joint in slight flexion to determine whether there is opening of the joint either medially or laterally, indicating rupture of the corresponding collateral ligaments. More than 15° of opening either medially or laterally indicates serious damage to these ligaments. It is easy to compare the affected knee with the opposite joint to assess the degree of collateral ligament instability. More sophisticated orthopedic examination of the knee to determine injuries to the menisci and cruciate ligaments may be deferred at this time if the patient's condition does not warrant a careful examination of the joint. Completion of the examination of the skeletal system in the injured patient includes range-of-motion examination of the ankle and the subtalar joints, inspection for gross malalignment or swelling of the foot or ankle, and a test of ligamentous stability of the ankle, which is performed by inverting and everting the ankle and comparing it to its opposite member.

At the time of this examination, if it is suspected that there are injuries to the limbs, it is especially important to note and to record accurately the vascular and neurologic status of parts distal to the injury. In particular in the hand, a note of the radial pulse, the capillary filling of the fingertips, and a brief test of the integrity of all three nerves should be routine. In the foot the dorsalis pedis and posterior tibial pulses should be assessed, and the function of the peroneals, anterior tibial, and hallices longus tendons noted by simple eversion of the foot, dorsiflexion of the foot, and dorsiflexion of the great toe. It is particularly important to note normal results of such an examination. In a patient with a developing compartment syndrome following a fracture of the tibia, among the earliest signs are loss of sensation and weakness of dorsiflexion of the toes.

It should be remembered that shortly following major trauma, significant skeletal injuries may not be associated with much discomfort or may be overshadowed by other more painful injuries. Fractures of the lumbar spine or of the thoracic spine may produce symptoms mimicking visceral injury and be unrecognized unless palpation of the spinous processes is carried out as a routine in the early assessment of the injured patient. Severe ligamentous injuries of the knee, fractures of the carpus, and fractures about the shoulder are among those injuries often not identified at the time of the initial examination and in which relatively early definitive treatment is important in order to prevent later permanent deformity or disability.

In the unconscious patient it is equally important to identify major skeletal trauma. With a head injury, fracture of the cervical spine must be suspected, and the initial management of an unconscious patient with a head injury requires care in movement until at least a single lateral x-ray of the cervical spine, including specifically the C-7–T-1 level, confirms that there is no significant fracture or dislocation. A more detailed examination can be carried out at a later date, but this simple x-ray assessment is mandatory in the unconscious, injured patient to prevent possible spinal cord injury from an unstable cervical spine.

In the unconscious patient signs of skeletal injury are more difficult to identify because of the lack of patient response. Crepitus on range-of-motion examination of the joints is an important finding, indicating dislocation or fracture. The presence of subcutaneous hematoma, gross malalignment, and joint effusion should be noted carefully in such patients as a possible indication of skeletal injury. It is recommended that a similar examination to that described in the conscious patient be carried out in the unconscious patient, with particular stress on instability of joints and the presence of large joint effusions. Asymmetry of the spinous processes on palpation can also be helpful in the unconscious patient in identifying fractures or dislocations of the spine.

In addition to the recognition of the life-threatening complication of an unstable cervical spine injury, there are a number of fractures which may be associated with serious complications demanding early definitive

treatment. Among these may be mentioned a posterior dislocation of the knee—a lesion in which damage to the popliteal vessels occurs more than 50 percent of the time.[6] The recognition of this dislocation will alert the surgeon to the likelihood of damage to the popliteal vessels and the need for early assessment of this complication. Comminuted and displaced fractures of the pelvis by themselves seldom require definitive orthopedic care at an early date, but may be associated with major retroperitoneal blood loss. The identification of such a fracture will alert the trauma surgeon to the possiblity of retroperitoneal bleeding from the pelvis as a cause of shock. In addition, the recognition of segmental, bilateral fractures of the pubis or of significant widening of the pubic symphysis suggests the possibility of urethral damage and the need for the institution of appropriate diagnostic urologic procedures. The recognition of a displaced supracondylar fracture of the elbow in a child carries with it the possibility of major vascular impairment of the forearm musculature and hand unless reduction is carried out at an early moment. These are examples of injuries which if identified will alert the trauma surgeon to their potential complications and permit appropriate staging of treatment at an early date of those skeletal lesions which require management to prevent limb- or life-threatening complications.

PATTERNS OF SKELETAL INJURY

Certain patterns of trauma will suggest to the experienced surgeon likely areas of injury.

• A dashboard injury to the knee may not only result in a fracture of the patella and of the femoral shaft, but sometimes produce a posterior dislocation of the hip as well. Alertness to this possibility will lead the informed examiner to obtain an x-ray of the pelvis and thus identify this injury, which is sometimes overshadowed by the more distal fractures and which requires early reduction to prevent serious sequelae.

- In a patient who has jumped or fallen from a substantial height, fractures of one or both os calci are common. If such are present, an x-ray of the dorsal and lumbar spine should be performed since an associated fracture of the first lumbar vertebra is commonly found with this injury.

- The opposite knee should be examined in a patient with a bumper fracture of the tibia. If struck from the side, the more obvious fracture may overshadow a rupture of the lateral collateral ligament of the opposite knee, which occurs as a natural result of the same force producing the fracture of the tibia.

- A fall on the outstretched wrist may cause an obvious Colles' fracture, but also a not so obvious fracture of the radial head. In all such patients the elbow and shoulder should be carefully examined and x-rayed if there is any discomfort noted when a full range-of-motion examination is carried out.

It should be apparent that a study of the epidemiology of trauma enables the informed surgeon to recognize patterns of injury which regularly occur. This is of great potential value in the initial evaluation of the patient, and for the younger surgeon may be a substitute for experience.

Identification of major skeletal fractures will provide some guide to blood loss inherent in the multiply injured patient. For example, the average blood loss from a closed fracture of the femur or trochanteric area of the hip in an adult approximates 1000mL and may reach 2500mL. As noted, a greater blood loss is associated with comminuted fractures of the pelvis, and two units of blood loss or more may frequently be associated with fractures of the lumbar spine or even of fractures of the transverse processes of the spine. A simple fracture of the surgical neck of the humerus in an adult may lead to the loss of a unit or more of blood.[1]

In addition certain fractures are commonly associated with substantial ileus which may mask or complicate the assessment of visceral injury in the multiply injured patient. Among these are fractures of the lumbar spine and even nondisplaced fractures of the pelvis. This is particularly true in the more severe fractures in younger patients and in many fractures in the older population group. Failure to recognize a simple compression fracture of the lumbar spine may lead to the mistaken diagnosis of a visceral cause of the ileus and the institution of inappropriate treatment.

It is difficult to generalize concerning appropriate x-rays to be taken in the multiply injured patient. In addition to those necessary for evaluation of possible head and trunk injury, a lateral cervical spine x-ray is always required in the unconscious patient. In addition, if trauma to the spine is suspected, at least a lateral and AP x-ray examination of the dorsal and lumbar spine should be performed. A single AP x-ray of the pelvis to include the hip joints will be helpful in ruling out significant fractures to this area. In addition, an AP and lateral x-ray of any specific long bone or joint noted to be ecchymotic, swollen, or deformed or exhibit restriction of motion or crepitus on examination is required, and one must include the joints above and below the suspected injury.

IMMEDIATE MANAGEMENT OF CLOSED FRACTURES

In general, definitive management of skeletal injuries follows stabilization and management of other system injuries. Closed fractures of the long bones, if applicable, may be treated with the immediate application of plaster casts. If substantial swelling beneath the cast is to be expected, the cast should be bivalved down to the skin, including the padding beneath the plaster. This is especially true in patients with oozing wounds, since a blood-soaked stockinet or cotton padding will assume the consistency of plaster when stiffened with dried blood, and bivalving plaster without cutting through the underlying, hard, blood-soaked padding will not relieve circumferential pressure on an extremity. Unstable knee injuries may be immobilized in semiflexible splints, such as the modified Jordan splint. Fractures of the proximal femur may be temporarily managed by continuation of a traction splint, such as a Thomas splint, or by immediate skeletal traction with the insertion of a Steinman pin through the tibial tubercle. The application of a spica cast for fractures of the femur is not generally recommended in the multiply injured patient as a first procedure, since it makes it difficult to observe the patient for possible visceral injury. Skin traction applied to the calf for management of a femoral shaft fracture is unwise, and if applied temporarily, the weight should not exceed 6 lb, nor skin traction be continued more than 48 h because of the likelihood of damage to the skin and the inability to manage proximal femoral fractures with this method. Fractures of the femur should be stabilized early, even if further diagnostic procedures or surgical treatment of multiple injuries are required, inasmuch as continued displacement of these fractures will lead to further blood loss and extreme discomfort. Fractures of the upper extremities not immediately casted can be temporarily managed by a sling and swathe with bandaging of the arm to the chest. If there is any possibility of chest trauma, this method must not be used. Alternative means of stabilizing proximal humeral fractures include plaster splints fashioned to go over the shoulder as well as the elbow, and another splint to maintain the elbow in 90° flexion—the so-called "sugar-tongs" splint. This may permit some access to the chest in patients with chest or abdominal trauma. Alternatively, skeletal traction with a pin driven through

the olecranon process will maintain humeral shaft fragments in alignment and permit full access to the chest and abdomen.

When operative management of the traumatized patient is required for visceral injuries, simple closed reductions of fractures of the wrist, forearm, ankle, or tibia or about the elbow or shoulder may be performed at the same time without prolonging or unnecessarily complicating the original procedure. Simple reduction of most distal extremity fractures can be carried out under local or regional anesthetic, if required.

If major vascular surgery in the extremity is to be carried out in an area where a fracture of a long bone is in close approximation, stabilization of the extremity will be important for the management of the vascular repair. It is not necessary in most cases to fix internally such fractures, but reasonably effective immobilization can be obtained with skeletal traction, or in some instances with external fixation techniques. Specifically, the management of an open wound of the femur in which a fracture of the femoral shaft is complicated by a laceration of the femoral artery can be adequately managed in most instances by tibial tubercle pin traction with a Thomas splint and a Pierson extension, permitting knee flexion following surgical repair of the vascular lesion. When lacerations of the axillary or brachial arteries are complicated by fracture of the humerus, the fracture may be managed by skeletal olecranon traction, or sling and swathe immobilization in the absence of visceral injury. Occasionally in the uncooperative patient internal fixation of the fracture may be performed at the time of vascular repair.

In general, all dislocations should be reduced at the earliest feasible time. Even if accurate anatomic alignment of the fracture fragments cannot be carried out, as in the case of a displaced trimalleolar fracture of the ankle, reduction of the dislocation as soon as the patient is seen will prevent severe vascular, neurologic, and skin complications which result when dislocations persist unreduced. I would advocate reduction of grossly displaced joints even in the absence of x-ray, if obtaining x-rays of these areas will be delayed. A dislocated hip demands reduction as soon as possible to lessen the likelihood of later aseptic necrosis of the femoral head.

Closed fractures, especially those without major soft tissue injury, have a better prognosis than fractures associated with such injuries or than open fractures.[7] In general, the immediate management of closed fractures in patients with multiple injuries includes a systematic examination of the skeletal system, briefly but thoroughly, for the identification of significant skeletal injuries; immediate splinting or other simple immobilization of the injured part; reduction of any major dislocations prior to further assessment; the notation of the status of peripheral function distal to the injured part; and, finally, an appropriate plan of treatment in which early management of the skeletal injuries is included.

MANAGEMENT OF OPEN FRACTURES

By open fractures we mean compound fractures, preferring to discard the latter term as somewhat confusing to the uninitiated. Even to the initiated, however, the distinction between an open and a closed fracture is not always easy. A fracture with a laceration overlying it is not necessarily an open fracture if the laceration does not extend down to the fascia and periosteum overlying the bone. Furthermore, an open fracture may have contact to the skin at some distance from the fracture site. Fractures may be open in two ways, either from within out, as in the case of a spiral fracture of the tibia with the end of the sharp spiral fragment piercing the skin, or from without in, as for example a gunshot wound. Very substantial open fractures

caused by penetration of skin from within out by a sharp fragment of bone which then later withdraws into the soft tissues may present a very minor puncture wound at some distance from the fracture site. Blood loss may be minimal, and the appearance is that of a totally benign lesion. Do not be misled—this is every bit as much an open fracture as one with bone fragments exposed in a gaping wound. Occasionally even with close observation, it is impossible to tell whether a fracture is open or closed. Sometimes saline injected into the fracture site may escape through an open wound at some distance, thus confirming the fact that it is indeed an open fracture. A negative injection test does not rule out an open fracture, and if there is any doubt, it is better to treat the questionable fracture as open and to carefully debride the wound under general or regional anesthesia, exploring it to see if the wound communicates with the fracture site. Although there is always some risk inherent in creating an open fracture from a previously closed one, it is better than overlooking an open fracture and not rendering definitive treatment.

The early management of open fractures requires prophylaxis against gas gangrene, tetanus, and the more usual infections. Please refer to Chap. 6 for a detailed discussion regarding prophylaxis against gas gangrene and tetanus. Currently we recommend intravenous cephalothin for all open fractures or joint wounds. In a recent large study of severely contaminated fractures, the prophylactic use of cephalothin reduced the infection rate from 44 percent to approximately 9 percent.[2] It should be given pre- and postoperatively for at least 3 days in a wound closed primarily and in wounds left open until good granulation tissue without suppuration has developed.

Insofar as open fractures are concerned, the most important definitive treatment is wound debridement at the earliest possible time. We prefer that open fractures be debrided within 6 h from the time of the injury, if possible. Certainly closure of wounds involving open fractures beyond 12 h after injury is apt to be fraught with dangers of wound infection. In general, debridement of the skin is not of major importance, even in gunshot wounds where a margin of dirty skin fragments may prove to be viable and, even if not, are readily available to later debridement. Under good operative conditions adequate debridement of an open fracture will require little debridement of the skin, some debridement of obviously necrotic fascia, ruthless and complete debridement of any devitalized muscle, and careful, conservative debridement of bone fragments. Grossly contaminated fragments of bone, separated widely from the main bone structures, may be removed, but it is unwise to resect bone so widely as to leave a significant gap between fracture fragments. Loose bone fragments, not grossly dirty, should be replaced about the fracture site. Following debridement of open fractures and copious mechanical lavage of the wound, the remaining tissue should be seen to bleed actively. Except for the hand or where careful anatomic dissection is required, debridement should not be performed under a tourniquet, but if so, the tourniquet should be released before the wound is closed. It is important to plan for good skin closure over open fractures. If debridement is complete and thorough and adequate tissue is available for closure, a loose closure to approximate tissue over the open fracture can be carried out. Suction drainage is desirable if a substantial closed space is left. If it is not possible to obtain loose closure over the open debrided wound, then a releasing incision can be made at a distance from the wound to allow a loose closure with suction drainage if necessary. A skin graft of the released area may be performed at a later date, or even immediately if time permits. If the wound is still suspect after debridement,

closure is not advisable, and if possible, a muscle flap should be pulled into the wound to cover exposed bone, nerve, or vessels and then dressed loosely with a fine mesh gauze. About 5 days later the wound should be redressed completely, explored, and redebrided, if necessary. When good granulation tissue is apparent, skin grafting can be carried out or, if feasible, a secondary closure performed. In extensively contaminated wounds it is probably best not to attempt any primary closure.

When applying a plaster cast over an open wound, a window may be cut out over the wound for frequent inspection. It is important to replace the window after dressings are done to provide a firm compression of the limb and prevent "window edema," which may occur if the cast is left open over the site of the injury. This edema can cause pressure necrosis along the cut edges of the cast, slows wound healing, and is a hazard to grafts placed in this area. Should it be necessary for the wound to remain open for inspection, the cast should be bivalved or at least a much larger area opened to avoid the complication of edema.

When cast immobilization is not feasible, stabilization of an open fracture is best performed by external fixation or skeletal traction. Internal fixation directly in open fractures is to be discouraged except in unusual situations where the experienced surgeon may accept the risk of infection in order to gain stabilization of the fragments not possible by other means. Usually in open fractures of the femur, the wound may be debrided, appropriate prophylaxis against infection instituted, and the patient treated primarily in skeletal traction for a period of 10 days to 3 weeks. When the wound has healed without evidence of infection, then internal fixation with intramedullary rods or appropriate plates may be carried out. Better results have been achieved with delayed repair of femoral fractures than with immediate repair. It is possible that the internal fixation then coincides with a period of more active osteogenesis. This is a problem requiring expert surgical judgment based on experience. If grossly unstable, segmented, open, long bone fractures cannot be managed by other methods, internal fixation using intramedullary nails is preferable to plating.

OPEN JOINT WOUNDS

Open joint wounds, due to a penetrating object and/or secondary to an open fracture of a long bone extending into a joint, require specific early treatment for the joint itself. The complication most often experienced with these wounds is loss of joint motion as a result of adhesions with malunion of intraarticular fractures. In addition, fragments of bone and cartilage loose in a joint will lead to later derangement and the formation of loose bodies. For these reasons open wounds extending into joints will require, in addition to the routine debridement of the open wound, special attention to the joint itself. The joint should be clearly visualized at surgery, utilizing a standard arthrotomy incision and extensively irrigated to flush out loose fragments of bone and other debris. In practice this may mean up to 6 to 12 L of irrigating fluid, usually normal saline. It should be remembered that the synovial tissue poses no barrier to the transmissions of antibiotics from the bloodstream, so that intraarticular antibiotic therapy is not especially required. Following thorough lavage of the joint and careful removal of all loose bodies, consideration should be given to fixation of displaced intraarticular fragments to prevent joint incongruity and later degenerative changes. In many cases intraarticular fragments may be removed from the joint if this will not lead to significant later instability. Specifically, most of the capitellum, 70 percent of the olecranon, the radial head, the distal ulna, and a portion or all of the patella may be removed in open joint wounds,

often with a better prognosis than an attempt to repair and obtain osteosynthesis of these fragments, especially those in contaminated wounds. Following debridement of the joint, closure of the synovium and capsule is necessary. Leaving a joint open is an invitation for adhesions to form and leads to joint stiffness. In addition, leaving large drains in the joint may lead to compartmentalization of the joint. If the joint is unusually contaminated and dirty, a closed-tube irrigating system may be advisable. It is best to use a medium or large catheter with continuous irrigation from 6 to 12 L/day for about 48 h to insure meticulous mechanical lavage and irrigation of the joint.

The principles of management of open wounds of the joint are thorough debridement, removal of intraarticular fracture fragments which can be safely removed without causing joint instability, fixation of those intraarticular displaced fragments which are required for joint stability, and the restoration of an active range of motion as soon as possible. Occasionally this can be carried out as soon as 7 to 10 days following the injury, but in any event successful treatment of any injured joint will depend to a large degree on early institution of active joint motion, if not weight-bearing. Should the patient be placed in traction or be bedridden because of other injuries, the use of a Thomas splint with a Pierson attachment and a hand-pull device to allow the patient to carry out passive movement of the knee is of considerable use in restoring early joint motion to this joint. There are a number of techniques of fracture bracing available which also permit limited joint motion while supporting adjacent fractures of long bones.

TRAUMATIC AMPUTATION

The decision to salvage a traumatic amputation or a very extensive open wound with damage to bone, nerve, and vessel is one which should be made by a surgeon with considerable experience in the management of these wounds and a knowledge of the present status of limb reimplantation. This is especially true for the upper extremity, where salvage of even a partially functioning sensate hand is substantially better than any prosthetic device now available. In general, the rule of ascertaining whether the reimplanted or salvaged limb will function better than a prosthesis is a good one, and should be used to guide the surgeon to a wise decision. In the lower extremity, a badly damaged foot which is preserved will prove in most instances a far greater handicap than a well-functioning Syme amputation. Similarly a well-functioning below-knee amputation is preferable to an insensate, ununited, chronically infected and useless extremity, the result of a severe injury to the midtibial region. Present advances in prosthetic appliances for the lower extremity are such that it would be unwise to salvage a severely damaged lower extremity in which sensation is lost and circulation precarious, even if bony union could eventually be achieved. Since the primary demands upon the lower extremity are for pain-free, stable weight bearing, this can at times be accomplished more easily by a prosthesis. Surgeons considering attempts to reimplant a foot or ankle after traumatic amputation should bear this in mind.

In dirty, badly traumatized extremities in which reimplantation or salvage is deemed less satisfactory than prosthetic fitting, generally the original amputation should be in the nature of a guillotine debridement, leaving an open end with skin traction applied by a stockinet glued to the good skin above the amputation level. One or two dressings may be necessary with further debridement before a definitive amputation is carried out. An effort should be made to salvage sufficient limb length so that the amputation can be carried out at the normal elective site.

BASIC TECHNIQUES IN FRACTURE MANAGEMENT

Application of Casts in the Injured Patient

Immobilization of fractures should be a near first priority in the multiply injured patient, even though definitive treatment cannot be carried out. The application of a plaster cast in an unstable fractured extremity should not be undertaken by one person alone in the absence of a mechanical stabilizing device. In fact it is best to have two assistants (for example, when a cast is applied to a fracture of the tibia), one assistant to hold the thigh and one to stabilize the leg and foot, while the third operator applies a cast. In unconscious patients who cannot report on a possible tight cast or localized pressure, extreme care must be taken that such does not occur. It may even be necessary to completely bivalve the cast, inspecting the leg daily to be sure that pressure does not exist. In conscious patients with paraplegia or a neurologic deficit, extreme care must likewise be employed in the use of plaster to immobilize fractures, and again it will be necessary to inspect the area under the plaster regularly. It is easier in the multiply and acutely injured patient to use conventional plaster of Paris technique than to use any of the newer plastic or commercial types of plaster, which involve more elaborate equipment, present difficulty in manipulating the extremity to apply the plaster, or sometimes require the use of heat, which may not be tolerated by the injured, unconscious or neurologically impaired patient. When cutting casts with an oscillating saw in an unconscious patient, great care must be observed to avoid skin lacerations. Plaster casts applied over fractures which are in less than satisfactory alignment may be wedged at a later date under fluoroscopic control for more definitive management. An appropriate time for wedging casts to correct angulation is 10 to 14 days after fracture, when callus is just beginning to form.

Cast Bracing

Cast bracing is a technique of fracture immobilization permitting joint motion and weight-bearing before healing has occurred. This is accomplished by circumferential stabilization of the soft tissues about a long bone fracture, maintaining axial alignment of the fracture by the hydrostatic pressure of the soft tissue and the action of the surrounding musculature. Some motion and impaction of the fracture site occurs and may well be desirable with this technique. Transfer of weight through joints is permitted by brace mechanisms attached to the casts. Some weight is borne through the cast with ischial weight-bearing or patellar tendon weight-bearing techniques of application for femoral and tibial fractures, respectively. The cast braces are generally applied some weeks after initial treatment, when callus has begun to form, but occasionally can be used very early in treatment. Their great advantage is to permit more rapid mobilization of the patient and the joints in the injured extremity. Fractures most suitable for cast bracing are forearm fractures, low femoral fractures, and most tibial shaft fractures.[5]

External Fixation with Transfixation Pins

In massively traumatized extremities, in large open fractures in areas where inspection of soft tissues is required, when vascular repair has been carried out in an open wound, and in burns with underlying fractures, external fixation techniques may be useful with or without plaster immobilization.[3] In the upper extremity, the olecranon, the ulna, the distal third of the radius, and the second and third metacarpals are the usual sites for the insertion of pins. In the lower extremity, the supracondylar area of the femur, the region of the tibial tubercle, the supramalleolar area of the tibia,

and the os calcis are usually selected. In a comminuted tibia, for example, with a large soft tissue wound requiring debridement, fixation is secure with the insertion of two pins above the malleolus at distances approximately 1 to 2 in apart and two pins in the area of the tibial tubercle drilled through the tibia. These should be threaded Steinman pins of relatively large diameter inserted under x-ray or image-intensification fluoroscopic control, and then connected together with plaster or external fixation bars. Fixation will then be secure, the patient may be turned readily, and the wounds inspected and dressed with maintenance of alignment of comminuted fractures. A similar insertion of one or two pins in the supramalleolar area of the femur and one or two pins in the trochanteric area with fixation can help to stabilize a femur. The pins may be inserted with local anesthesia under simple sterile precautions in an emergency room.

Skeletal Traction

Skeletal traction is usually applied to a threaded Steinman pin of reasonably large diameter through the olecranon in dealing with fractures of the humerus or the os calcis and through the tibial tubercle or supramalleolar area of the femur when dealing with fractures of the tibia and femur, respectively. The supramalleolar area of the femur is not generally used, except in a situation where there may be extensive open wounds at the sites of elective pin insertion in the tibia. After introduction of these pins, traction is applied, and the limb is suspended in a Thomas splint with a Pierson attachment when dealing with fractures of the lower extremity. Occasionally, a fracture of the tibia may be suspended in a Bohler frame with traction applied to an os calcis pin. This may be a definitive method of treatment or, alternatively, a temporary method of treatment awaiting internal fixation at a later date. Skeletal traction is especially useful for fractures of the femur and severely displaced, unstable fractures of the humerus. In children, severely displaced supracondylar fractures of the humerus which can be difficult to reduce are often treated most effectively by skeletal traction utilizing an olecranon pin.

Internal Fixation of Fractures

Among the devices most commonly used for the internal fixation of fractures are intramedullary nails and compression plates. Intramedullary nails are more often used in fractures of the middle two-thirds of the femur, the humerus, and occasionally the tibia and forearm bones. They have the advantage of providing rather good fixation without stripping the periosteum, a major source of callus for the healing bone. Some techniques permit "blind nailing" without exposure of the fracture site, probably reducing the likelihood of postoperative infection.[8]

Plates applied to the cortex of bone provide rigid fixation, and with proper techniques, substantial compression can be applied to the fracture site, which may well speed healing. They are most suitable for fractures of both bones of the forearm and, less often, the humerus, tibia, and femur. Intraarticular fracture fragments, for example, malleolar fractures of the ankle, are best fixed by screws. A special case is certain hip fractures where prosthetic replacement for the femoral head or, occasionally, total joint replacement may be warranted.

The indications for open reduction and internal fixation of specific fractures depend far more on the experience of the treating surgeon than on any hard and fast recommendations that can be generalized. Usually, fractures that can be equally well treated with external fixation, skeletal traction, or plaster immobilization are best managed by these nonsurgical techniques. It is a matter of judgment based upon considerable clinical experience and a knowledge of fracture healing to determine

which specific fracture should be best approached by open reduction and which device should be used. At the risk of oversimplification, certain generalizations can be made regarding situations in which open reduction and internal fixation may be considered appropriate.

Very few children's fractures will require internal fixation. The exceptions to this rule are displaced fractures of the femoral neck, acute traumatic slipped capital femoral epiphysis, and some intertrochanteric fractures. These are best managed by multiple pin fixation, the latter fracture supplemented by a spica cast. In addition, certain fractures about joints where epiphyses are displaced and not amenable to closed reduction will require open reduction and internal fixation.

Multiple extremity fractures in severely injured patients are usually best managed by appropriately staged procedures to internally fix and stabilize the various long bone fractures. When several fractures must be stabilized surgically, it is usually best not to attempt too much, but to perform multiple operations fairly close together, limiting the surgical trauma and duration of anesthesia in each operation.

For example, a recent patient injured in a fall sustained a fracture of the right femoral neck, right midshaft femur, left femur, right open tibia, and left Monteggia fracture of the elbow, as well as severe chest and head trauma. Initial management included tracheostomy and respiratory assistance for 4 weeks, followed by a jejunostomy for feeding purposes, bilateral tibial tubercle traction, a left long arm cast, and a right short leg cast with external tibial pin fixation. Five days after admission, the Monteggia fracture was stabilized with resection of the radial head and intramedullary fixation of the left ulna. This permitted early active use of the left elbow. A few days after recovery from this procedure, the fracture of the right femoral neck was reduced and pinned percutaneously with Knowles pins. One week following this procedure, a double onlay plating of the right femur was carried out. One week following that procedure or approximately 3 weeks after the initial injury, a right angle plating of the supracondylar fracture of the right femur was performed. Initially the right tibia was treated with pins and plaster, and shortly after the completion of the last operative procedure, 6 weeks following the original trauma, the patient was mobilized with a patellar tendon weight-bearing cast for the right tibia. Although both femoral shaft fractures could have been treated in traction, open reduction and internal fixation was advisable in order to mobilize this extremely ill patient. In general, the more long bone fractures, the more important internal fixation of the specific fractures becomes.

Another indication for the use of internal fixation is in fractures occurring on both sides of a joint, so that the joint is left "floating." A typical example of this is a supracondylar fracture of the femur in association with a fracture of the midshaft of the tibia on the same side. Unless these fractures are treated with internal fixation and early knee motion, prolonged, if not permanent, restriction of knee motion would result from otherwise successful treatment by immobilization and/or skeletal traction.

In addition there are those fractures which by their very nature require internal fixation—for example, fractures of the femoral neck, intertrochanteric fractures of the hip, depressed fractures of the tibial plateau, and displaced fractures of the radial head. Intraarticular fractures generally will require open reduction and internal fixation unless accurate anatomic reconstruction of the joint surface is possible by closed means. Substantial deformity can be tolerated, for instance, in the midshaft of the femur, even in an adult, but little or no articular incongruity as a result of a

fracture can be tolerated without the later development of disabling arthritis, especially in a weight-bearing joint.

Finally, most pathologic fractures of long bones will require internal fixation, usually by intramedullary nail and sometimes with the supplemental use of methyl methacrylate cement. Joint replacement, especially femoral head or total hip replacement, is frequently employed for pathologic and certain other fractures of the femoral neck.

COMPLICATIONS OF FRACTURE MANAGEMENT

In the management of fractures there are certain complications which occur with sufficient frequency to warrant a brief discussion of them in a general review of this subject. Infection is perhaps the single, most serious complication in the management of fractures which will lead to a poor end result. In discussing open fractures, emphasis has been placed upon thorough debridement, and it is well to reemphasize the fact that definitive treatment of a fracture or late reconstruction of joints or long bones depends upon freedom from infection. It is therefore in the best interests of the patient at times to forgo early definitive management of a long bone fracture in order to assure oneself of a clean, well-healed wound. It is always possible to manage malunion and nonunion through normal tissue, but with an infected, draining sinus or chronic osteomyelitis there is little chance of reconstruction should union fail to occur.

Similar considerations hold for vascular damage in association with fractures. Mention has already been made of the supracondylar fracture of the humerus in children and posterior knee dislocations, which are frequently associated with severe vascular injuries. The recognition of major vascular injury is necessary so that immediate reconstruction of major vessels will preserve a viable extremity in which definitive fracture repair can take place. More subtle, more frequent, and often more difficult to manage are those compartment syndromes due to edema occurring within a tight fascial compartment usually in closed fractures about the elbow in children and of the tibia and fibula in adults. The early recognition of a compartment syndrome is of first importance in the management of this serious complication. Loss of sensation or motion in a digit previously noted to be intact or the development of severe pain, more than might be expected in an immobilized fracture, are important findings in this regard. It should be remembered that a fracture well immobilized in a cast should not be especially painful, and in such a situation the acute development of increasing pain strongly points to the possibility of early vascular impairment and may be the first sign of a compartment syndrome. In the upper extremity, pain in the forearm with passive dorsiflexion of the fingers is an ominous sign. Loss of the peripheral pulse may be a rather late sign of a compartment syndrome; but impairment of capillary fillings should be looked for, and if noted, definitive steps should be taken to improve the circulation. At this stage circular casts should be split down to the skin, and it is most important that a portion of the cast be removed. Limb compression cannot be relieved by a single univalving of a cast without splitting it widely. It is strongly recommended that in such a situation the cast not be singly split and then effort made to widen, which will simply cause increased pressure along the margins of the split, but instead the cast be bivalved and the anterior half removed using the posterior half as a splint. It is always possible to restore alignment of a fracture if it is lost as a result of opening a cast, but persistent vascular insufficiency, the result of a compartment syndrome, will lead to irreparable damage.

When a developing compartment syndrome is suspected, consideration should be given to measuring the fluid pressure within the closed compartment. This may be done by the wick technique, or by a more direct measurement manometer. If these tests indicate an increase in the fluid pressure in the closed compartment or, in the absence of such tests, if there is clinical evidence that such is developing, a fasciotomy should be performed. The possibility that a fasciotomy might be needed is usually the best indication for this procedure. Although this converts a closed fracture to an open one with all that this implies, a fasciotomy is necessary to prevent the compartment syndrome from progressing. There are a number of techniques for performing fasciotomy in the forearm and the leg, but it is important to open all four compartments of the leg, as well as both compartments of the forearm.[4]

A complication frequently noted in fracture management is phlebothrombosis and pulmonary embolus. This complication is particularly prevalent in patients with fractures of the pelvis, hip, and femur, particularly where prolonged immobilization is required. Depending upon the presence of other injuries, serious consideration must be given to anticoagulation therapy in patients with those fractures requiring prolonged recumbency. It is unusual for pulmonary embolization following fractures to occur until at least 2 or 3 days, and usually longer, after injury. However the classic signs of fat embolization are usually apparent within 1 to 2 days after injury. Tachypnea, tachycardia, fever, and mental confusion should alert the physician to this possibility, and the findings of a diminished arterial Pa_{O_2}, fat globules in the urine, and diffuse clouding of the lungs on x-ray tend to confirm the diagnosis. The current management of fat embolization includes steroid therapy and supportive measures.

A variety of neurologic complications may occur with specific long bone fractures. Among these may be noted radial nerve compression in fractures of the humerus, particularly those angulated in the distal third. Lesions of the sciatic nerve, especially of the perineal branch, may be associated with fracture dislocations of the hip in which a fracture fragment of the posterior acetabulum is driven into the sciatic nerve at this level. In addition, damage to the perineal nerve with fractures of the tibia and fibula, particularly proximal fractures of the fibula, is not uncommon and should be looked for in this type of injury. In general, satisfactory reduction of the fracture will relieve the stretch placed upon the nerve, since most of these injuries are due to traction upon a nerve rather than to a complete laceration. However a large fragment of bone adjacent to the posterior rim of the acetabulum in a sciatic nerve lesion deserves removal, and certainly consideration should be given to exploration of radial nerve in an angulated fracture of the distal humerus in which the nerve loss is complete and recovery has not occurred within a few weeks following fracture.

Late fracture complications, such as delayed union, malunion, nonunion, and chronic osteomyelitis are primarily matters of orthopedic reconstruction. Prevention of these complications, however, is best accomplished by avoiding errors in the early management of the injured patient. To accomplish this, and in summary of this subject, the following observations are worth emphasis.

1 Examine the injured patient systematically with the possibility of fracture always in mind. One may not discover what one does not suspect. Ignorance is no excuse.

2 Know the natural history of the fracture, the usual rate of healing, the frequently associated injuries, and the expected complications. Forewarned is forearmed.

3 Select that method of treatment which combines the lowest morbidity with the earliest possible return to function of the limb and the patient. When in doubt, be conservative.

BIBLIOGRAPHY

1 Clarke, R., F. G. Badger, and S. Sevitt: "Modern Trends in Accident Surgery and Medicine," in G. T. Shires (ed.), *Care of the Trauma Patient*, Butterworth & Co. (Publishers), Ltd., London, 1959.

2 Gustilo, R. B. and J. T. Anderson: Prevention of infection in the treatment of one-thousand and twenty-five open fractures of long bones: Retrospective and prospective analyses, *J. Bone J. Surg.*, **58A**:453–458, June 1976.

3 Karlstrom, G. and S. Olerud: Percutaneous pin fixation of open tibial fractures: Double-frame anchorage using the Vidal-Adrey method, *J. Bone J. Surg.*, **57A**:915–924, October 1975.

4 Mubarak, S. J. and C. A. Owen: Double-incision fasciotomy of the leg for decompression in compartment syndromes, *J. Bone J. Surg.*, **59A**:184–187, March 1977.

5 Sarmiento, A: Functional bracing of tibial and femoral shaft fractures, *Clin. Orthop.*, **81**:2–13, January-February 1972.

6 Shields, L., M. Mital, and E. F. Cave: Complete dislocation of the knee: Experience at the Massachusetts General Hospital, *J. Traum*, **9**:192–215, March 1969.

7 Van der Linden, W., H. Sungel, and K. Larsson: Fractures of the Tibial shaft after skiing and other accidents, *J. Bone J. Surg.*, **57A**:321–327, April 1975.

8 Wickstrom, J. and M. S. Corban: Intramedullary fixation for fractures of the femoral shaft: A study of complications in 298 operations, *J. Trauma*, **7**:551–583, July 1967.

Chapter 17

Specific Fractures and Dislocations

Louis H. Paradies, M.D.

Charles F. Gregory, M.D.

The contents of this chapter will be confined to the consideration of a relatively few fractures and dislocations. These injuries are chosen because of their tendency to include damage to vital soft tissue structures adjacent to the fracture or dislocation.

INJURY TO THE SPINE

The gravest problem which attends injury to the spine is concomitant damage to the spinal cord or spinal nerve roots. The definitive care of the combined injury is covered in Chap. 16. It remains then to consider the injured spine without involvement of the neural elements. One rule supersedes all others in dealing with either pattern of spinal injury: protect the cord and nerve roots against involvement or against further damage if they are already involved. The measures to protect the contents of the spinal canal begin at the scene of injury, and they must be vigilantly attended until the spine is stable enough that further threat to the cord or roots is not a problem.

The precepts of appropriate handling during first aid and transport of the patient with the spine injury are well known, but need frequent reiteration. Equipment is now available which can rigidly immobilize a victim, including the head relative to the body. This is the preferred method of transport for a suspect cervical spine injury. In the unusual case, if vomiting is a threat, a patient with a cervical injury may have to be transported in the prone position—head and chest supported so that the neck is not turned—rather than risk turning the head to prevent aspiration of vomitus.

It is significant that the upper cervical spinal canal has considerable space in excess of that needed by the cord, so that a fracture and/or dislocation, although markedly displaced, may not show neurologic involvement. (Indeed any involvement at all may well be fatal at this level.) Moreover, injury in this area of the cervical spine may be both unsuspected and undetected, especially in the patient with an associated head injury. A high index of suspicion will prompt the necessary x-rays, which usually reveal the presence of such an injury. The danger of serious or fatal late complications makes the identification and treatment of injuries in this area imperative. Initially, halter traction in a neutral position should be instituted, while the definitive treatment to be used is determined and begun.

If there is room to spare in the cervical spinal canal, there is none to spare in the thoracic canal. The appended rib cage plus a naturally limited range of motion between the thoracic vertebrae make dislocation in this segment of the spine uncommon. Yet any encroachment on the spinal canal in this region may result in cord or root involvement and demands the prompt attention outlined in Chap. 16. Splinting by recumbency on a firm bed (preferably a turning frame, which minimizes rotational stress also) should be instituted as early as practicable and used until definitive treatment of the spine is selected, should it be different from this regimen.

The first lumbar vertebra, when injured, may involve the conus and, below it, the elements of the cauda equina. These elements are most frequently involved when some degree of dislocation or fracture with dislocation is present. Even then, they usually produce an incomplete lesion, with spotty involvement. Holdsworth has referred to this as a "root-sparing" pattern. He urges selective open reduction and stabilization of an unstable dislocation to preserve the remaining intact neural elements. Most lumbar injuries are simple compression fractures without nerve involvement. Such injuries and also dislocations without nerve root involvement may be managed in most instances by simple recumbency in the supine position. The specific features of the individual fracture will determine the definitive treatment to be employed.

Compression fractures are prone to produce an ileus a few hours to a few days after injury. When severe, nasogastric suction may be required. It should be remembered for its potentiating effect upon symptoms arising incident to associated intraabdominal injury.

DISLOCATION OF THE SHOULDER

The most frequent structure injured in a shoulder dislocation, other than the musculoskeletal elements, is the axillary nerve. This injury is often occult because it is difficult to test the function of the deltoid muscle either before or after reduction of the dislocated shoulder. One must test for a sensory deficit in the area of distribution of the axillary nerve just below the point of the shoulder over the deltoid muscle, but absence of a positive finding, that is, a loss of sensation, does not guarantee integrity of the axillary nerve. As soon as the patient's shoulder is no longer immobilized, renewed attempts must be made to document, by careful muscle testing, whether or not the axillary nerve has been injured. Since this will be about 3 weeks after the injury, the time is about right for abnormalities to become manifest in the electromyogram. This test should be performed if there is any doubt as to the integrity of the axillary nerve. Any of the nerves that are formed by the brachial plexus and pass just medial to the coracoid process and from thence into the arm can be injured as the humeral head is forced under the coracoid process. Often there will be a temporary median, radial, or ulnar nerve palsy or a loss of function of all three nerves, which is quickly recovered after the reduction is accomplished. Occasionally, however, loss of neurologic function persists and must be dealt with later. Tears, partial and complete, of both axillary vein and axillary artery have been reported in association with dislocated shoulders. Evaluation of the vascular supply to the extremity involved is always a mandatory part of the examination before any manipulation is done. *Loss of the peripheral pulse that does not return immediately after reduction of the shoulder requires immediate exploration of the vessels.* In the case of the ruptured axillary vein, a palpable pulse may be present, but there is the rapid appearance of a large hematoma in the axilla. It should be remembered that although neurologic and vascular complications associated with shoulder dislocations are rather rare, they are often so disastrous that vigilance must not be relaxed in dealing with this injury.

HUMERAL SHAFT FRACTURES

It is not uncommon to see a humeral shaft fracture complicated by an associated radial nerve palsy. Since the radial nerve does not lie directly upon the bone in the musculospiral groove, it is usually not the midshaft fracture that involves the radial nerve, although this does occasionally happen. When a midshaft fracture is associated with a radial nerve palsy, many surgeons feel that treatment of the fracture and observation of the radial nerve palsy will result in a very high percentage of return of function. There is a particular fracture pattern, however, which is associated with more severe injury to the radial nerve. This fracture occurs at the junction of the distal third and middle third of the humerus and runs obliquely medially and inferiorly. The radial nerve is directly in contact with the bone at the lateral side of the humeral shaft at

about the junction of the middle third and distal third of the bone, so that it is occasionally insinuated into the fracture site in this particular fracture.[2] Either the patient has a radial nerve palsy immediately upon the initial examination, or he will develop it after manipulation of the fracture. The latter circumstance is an indication for open surgical exploration of the nerve and fracture site, careful identification and release of the nerve, and fixation of the fracture.

SUPRACONDYLAR FRACTURES OF THE HUMERUS

This fracture occurs in children of 5 to 10 years of age. The most common displacement is posterior, that is, the distal fragment is displaced posteriorly. This tends to stretch all the anterior neurovascular structures, the brachial artery, and the median nerve and radial nerve over the sharp distal end of the proximal fragment. Clinically one sees injuries to any one or all three of these structures. By the time these children are seen in the emergency room, there is almost always a great deal of swelling and the elbow appears as a large fusiform mass with absolutely no palpable landmarks. Obviously, the neurovascular status of the extremity distal to the fracture site must be promptly evaluated and recorded. A reduction is always mandatory, but is most urgent in the presence of physical findings which denote loss of function of either the nerves or the artery. Gentle reduction, *avoiding excessive traction and excessive hyperextension,* must be carried out as soon as possible. After the reduction of the fracture, the status of the neurovascular structures is again checked; if nerve deficits remain, the arm is immobilized, either in a plaster cast or in a traction device, and the extremity observed. If the radial pulse was not palpable initially and does not return in a reasonable length of time after the reduction (roughly $1/2$ h), the only safe course is to determine the nature of the arterial injury and take measures to restore the flow of blood to the forearm and hand muscles. This, of course, means surgical exploration of the vessels in the antecubital fossa. Once this has been done, it is probably indicated to fix the fracture itself with crossed Kirschner wires.

The major point in this particular injury is that *gangrene* of the extremity is seldom seen. The problem is much more subtle. The interruption of arterial flow to the muscles of the forearm and/or hand creates an ischemia of these muscles, which results ultimately in partial or complete replacement by fibrous tissue and marked contracture. This process gives rise to the ugly and disabling deformity known as Volkmann's ischemic contracture. Often, surgical exploration reveals that simple release of the lacertus fibrosus alleviates arterial spasm and allows return of flow to the forearm and hand.

DISLOCATION OF THE LUNATE BONE AT THE WRIST

A fall on the outstretched hand or some other injury which hyperextends the wrist sometimes results in a volar dislocation of the lunate bone. This injury is sometimes difficult to recognize on x-ray examination unless one is trained in observing the normal radiologic anatomy of the wrist. On a straight anteroposterior view, one sees a change in shape of the lunate bone from its normal trapezoid shape to a triangular shape. The lateral view, of course, reveals the volar displacement of the lunate bone. Since the proximal carpal row lies beneath the volar carpal tunnel, when this lunate bone is volarly displaced, it often compresses the median nerve up against the volar carpal ligament, producing pain and paresthesia in distribution of the medial nerve and sometimes loss of function of the nerve distal to this point. The treatment of this injury is

immediate, gentle manipulative reduction. This requires excellent anesthesia, traction, and hyperextension of the wrist with simultaneous pressure over the lunate bone. If this maneuver does not succeed, one should not procrastinate or make repeated attempts, but do an open reduction of the lunate, being careful to avoid additional damage to the median nerve in the process of reduction. Some of the soft tissue attachments to the lunate bone should be maintained since avascular necrosis is a complicating feature of this injury.

FRACTURES OF THE PELVIS

The pelvic ring, a rigid one, is composed of the two halves of the pelvis and the interposed sacrum. A single break results in no displacement, since it is a rigid ring, whereas a second or additional fractures may result in displacement, ranging to total disorganization. Fractures, though displaced, are stable when they heal. The dislocations which break the ring at the sacroiliac joint and the symphysis may lead to symptomatic instability if they are not reduced and maintained so. This is principally true when the displacement occurs in the weight-bearing arch of the pelvis, which passes from one acetabulum to the other across the sacrum and the two sacroiliac joints.

A number of soft tissue injuries may complicate the disorganized pelvis and pose an immediate and more serious threat to the patient.

1 Disruption of the genitourinary system, either as a bladder or urethral injury, is common in anterior arch injuries. Passage of a catheter into the bladder, cystogram, and urethrogram, if there is any question, ought to be carried out as soon as practicable (see Chap. 14, Trauma to the Genitourinary System).
2 Injury to the iliac vessels may occur where they lie in the pelvis or as they emerge from it and cross the superior rami. The signs

and symptoms of vessel injury should be sought in all pelvic disorganizations.

3 Fractures occurring in the iliac region may cause bleeding from the sinusoidal system of the marrow tissue and result in extensive blood loss into the retroperitoneal space. Such occult bleeding can be extensive and combined with other injuries, potentiate a refractory hypovolemia and continued shock (Table 17.1).

Initial treatment is to place the patient in a recumbent position on a firm surface. Traction may be applied as indicated. Since considerable traction force may be required, skeletal traction is often desirable from the outset. Care should be exercised in using pelvic slings, for they may aggravate displacement rather than relieve it. Some experience with their use or consultation of an extensive description of their application should precede the decision to employ one.

DISLOCATIONS OF THE HIP JOINT

Posterior dislocation of the hip is becoming a more and more common injury, since one of the mechanisms that produces this injury is a blow against the individual's knee as it strikes the dashboard in an automobile. This not only injures the knee, but often forces the femoral head posteriorly out of the acetabulum. As the femoral head is driven posteriorly, it can damage the sciatic nerve. This is said to occur in about 10 percent of the posterior dislocations of the hip, the injury involving sometimes the entire sciatic nerve or sometimes just the peroneal portion of the nerve. If sciatic palsy is present, an exploration of the posterior aspect of the hip joint is necessary. Careful dissection and isolation of the nerve and meticulous restoration and repair of the soft tissue structures in the area might enhance the chance for recovery of the nerve, since proliferation of fibrous tissue and scarring will be held to a minimum with this treatment. Sometimes, as the hip is driven posteriorly out of the acetabulum, a rim of the posterior acetabular bone is broken loose. This fragment of bone is sometimes wedged between the remaining acetabulum and the sciatic nerve. Removal of this fragment not only sets the stage for a more physiologic healing of this area, but its replacement in the posterior acetabulum and fixation there will probably add to the stability of the hip after its reduction. The larger the amount of articular cartilage that one finds on this broken piece, the greater is the need for it to be replaced in order to maintain a stable hip joint.

FRACTURES OF THE FEMUR

Femoral shaft fractures are sometimes associated with lacerations of the femoral artery.

Table 17-1

Injury	Range of blood loss, mL
Closed fracture of leg	500–1000
Closed fracture of femur	500–2000
Severe closed fracture of leg	500–2000
Severe closed fracture of femur	2000+
Closed fracture of forearm	500–750
Closed fracture of pelvis	1000–3000
Closed fracture of spine and/or ribs	1000–2000

Source: Modified from Clarke et al.[1]

Such lacerations are most often caused by sharply pointed ends of oblique and spiral fractures, but this is not necessarily the case. The author has seen a case in which the fracture was transverse and perfectly reduced when first seen; nevertheless, this fracture was associated with a lacerated femoral artery and an absent pulse distal to the site of injury. As in all fractures and dislocations, the status of the neurovascular structures distal to the point of injury should always be tested as the initial procedure in the physical examination of the traumatized patient.

The popliteal artery can be injured in supracondylar fractures, and in this type of injury, as in the femoral shaft fracture, the absent pulse distal to the fracture site requires open exploration of the artery. In fractures of this type, there is no point in reducing the fracture and awaiting return of the pulse, because of the likelihood that the artery actually has been lacerated by the sharp bone ends. Dislocations at the knee are so frequently associated with severe arterial damage that any question of blood supply distal to the knee should be resolved by an exploration of the popliteal artery and vein. The peroneal nerve is also frequently injured in knee dislocation, but the overwhelming problem is vascular. The role of arteriogram is debated; most surgeons feel that sufficient information is obtained to make preliminary arteriograms advisable. Five out of six recently reviewed knee dislocations had sufficient popliteal artery injury to require surgical exploration and repair. Two of the five cases with documented arterial lesions had palpable distal pulses according to the hospital record. Thus, in true knee dislocations, even the presence of palpable pulses distally does not alter the necessity for arteriogram and vessel exploration. In separation of the distal femoral epiphysis in children, since there are no sharp fragments and since the angular deformity is often great, the separa-

tion should be reduced and the distal pulses observed before surgical exploration.

TIBIAL FRACTURES

Separation of the proximal tibial epiphysis in children is a rather rare injury. Unfortunately, however, it is associated with a high percentage of damage to the popliteal artery, and the mere presence of this injury should alert the surgeon to a careful evaluation of the vascular status of the extremity distal to the injury. Again, any question of the vascular supply distal to the point of injury should be resolved by open surgical exploration.

Tibial fractures are so common as to be treated in a rather routine fashion. When the fracture is in the proximal tibia, it does not ordinarily arouse much concern, because it is often easily reduced and the reduction maintained by a plaster cast. Also, nonunion and malunion are not outstanding problems in proximal tibial fractures. This particular fracture will on occasion, however, be associated with a severe vascular problem. When the fracture in the proximal tibia is severely comminuted, it indicates that a large amount of kinetic energy was dispersed at this point in the extremity. As the popliteal artery descends behind the knee and reaches the highest point of the interosseous membrane, the anterior tibial artery branches off at a right angle and enters the anterolateral compartment of the leg. It is at this point—when excessive amount of energy is imparted to the leg resulting in a badly comminuted fracture—that the arterial lesions can occur. Thus, these seemingly rather simple injuries should alert one to a careful evaluation of the vascular status of the extremity distal to the injury. Even when there is no direct arterial damage, a severely comminuted proximal tibial fracture often causes severe bleeding into tight fascial compartments, resulting in extremely high pressures within the fascial envelopes which contain the muscles of the leg. These patients will complain of severe pain, out of proportion to what one would expect from the proximal tibial fracture. They may have rather severe swelling and/or a bluish discoloration of the toes. When one sees this sequence of events, the cast should be immediately split, the entire extremity examined, and the possibility kept in mind of doing a fasciotomy of the anterolateral compartment and/or of the posterior compartments of the leg. The aim is to relieve excess pressure and to prevent the ischemia which could cause later contracture and severe functional loss.

FOOT AND ANKLE FRACTURES

These fractures are seldom associated with direct damage to neurovascular structures. In this area, however, there is very little overlying muscle, and the blood supply to the overlying skin is poor. Severely displaced and badly comminuted fractures of the foot and ankle should always be regarded as a dangerous threat to the integrity of the overlying skin. Immediate reduction should be obtained, and after reduction is obtained under adequate anesthesia, the skin should be given a regular surgical cleansing and covered with some type of sterile dressing before the plaster cast is applied. In this way, if there is break in continuity of skin or loss of skin, the risk of infection is minimized. It is in association with severe injuries around the foot and ankle that one commonly sees the infamous blebs which are sometimes white and sometimes red. These blebs are a manifestation of the severe underlying trauma and interference with the circulation to the skin. When one or more of these blebs overlying a fracture site are red (that is, filled with blood), the fracture is best assumed to be open, since most often the blood which fills the bleb comes directly from a small opening in the skin which communicates with the fracture. Because of the organisms resident in the sweat glands and hair follicles, this type of fracture could be contaminated.

Because of the paucity of tissues with adequate blood supply in the ankle area, and because this distal part of the lower extremity may be involved with peripheral vascular disease, *open* fractures and fracture dislocations of the distal tibia and ankle joint are to be considered with the utmost respect. Every one of these injuries represents a potential loss of limb because of possible infectious complications. They should be carefully debrided; the joint, in the case of an open ankle fracture, must be carefully inspected and irrigated. Care must be taken with extending or accessory incisions not to damage blood supply to already precariously supplied skin, as even minor skin loss here can be disastrous.

FRACTURES AND THE PATIENT WITH MULTIPLE SYSTEM INJURIES

The treatment which may be selected for a fracture as a solitary injury is usually based solely upon the nature of the injury without reference to extraneous factors. Yet treatment of the same fracture occurring as a part of a complex of injuries involving several systems may require modification because of the overriding concern for other, perhaps more threatening injuries. Priorities have been considered elsewhere, and the principle of life before limb has been clearly stated. Neither fractures nor dislocations can be disregarded for long, and indeed to treat and thereby dispose of them often has a distinct advantage in the continued care of other more serious injuries. The principles of fracture care in these circumstances remain the same, but the technique and the timing may be altered.

As an example, consider a patient with a

suspected abdominal injury and a known dislocated hip. The latter is characteristically painful, and by the nature of the deformity (flexion, adduction, and internal rotation of the involved extremity) the patient cannot gain a comfortable position, and grows restless and apprehensive, all of which make examination of the abdomen difficult, and often inconclusive. Should abdominal exploration become abruptly necessary, a reduction of the dislocation would be required at once to facilitate the laparotomy. Moreover, the subsequent manipulation of the patient might well hazard redislocation, a departure from the more ideal management of the hip, had it been the only injury. The point is that in selecting the form of treatment, the surgeon must consider the *probable* course of subsequent events and select that method least likely to be disturbed by necessary activity of the patient. Such activity may be volitional or may result from manipulation by the surgeon for diagnosis or treatment.

When a closed method of dealing with a long bone fracture is selected, and either a cast or splint is used to maintain the manipulative reduction, the surgeon assumes that no violent effort will be made which might dislodge the reduced fragments and that the reduction is intrinsically stable enough to withstand the usual forces which are brought to bear upon it in ordinary nursing care. This is not much of a problem in most unconscious patients. However, certain patients with head injuries develop a maniacal state and become physically quite active. Seemingly insensitive to the pain produced by moving the fracture fragments (or perhaps stimulated to some extent by it), these patients quite regularly displace the fracture fragments, disrupt the reduction, and favor the development of malunion or nonunion. On occasion, they may convert a closed fracture to an open one by bone end extrusion through the skin. Anticipa-

tion of this state may permit internal fixation of fractures when it is practical and thereby either prevent or lessen those complications.

The infrequent burn patient who also has a major fracture may benefit from internal fixation when it is possible to do so. Such internal stability may render the whole patient more mobile and comfortable and thereby facilitate the patient's general care or the specific care of the burned areas. Recently, extensive use of skeletal pin fixation devices such as the Roger Anderson equipment has greatly facilitated the care of fractures associated with gross soft tissue injuries or burns. Basically, pins are inserted above and below the fracture and then fixed together externally by rods in multiple planes.

The almost limitless combination of injuries, including fractures and dislocations, makes it difficult to be specific about any given case. Yet the underlying guide consists of arranging treatment of the involved bone or joint so that the general needs of the patient are met first. Thereafter, expediency in the care of a limb can be considered. The various methods of dealing with the injured bone must be at the surgeon's disposal to cope with all the possibilities which may present themselves.

ASSOCIATED NEUROVASCULAR INJURY

Among the multiple system injuries which may be encountered in limbs are those which occur in the same anatomical location and chiefly concern nerve and blood vessel injury in conjunction with open or closed fractures and dislocations. The principles of diagnosis and treatment of nerves and vessels are considered in Chap. 11. Significant vascular injury clearly takes precedence over bone or joint injury and as often as not may determine how the bone shall be dealt with. An artery which has been recently repaired requires considerable stability while healing. When there is an associated adjacent fracture, stability must be imposed, usually through internal fixation. On the contrary, a repaired artery lying adjacent to an unstable joint may require no more than a splint or a cast to stabilize the joint and protect the artery. Should more stability be indicated, especially if the patient has other injuries, so that manipulation of the involved extremity will be required, pins may be inserted into involved bones and in turn incorporated in a plaster cast. In either case (that is, a fracture or a dislocated joint), the limb can be arranged to permit free manipulation of the patient, if that is required, with assurance that the arterial repair site will be free of undue stress and strain.

Apart from special considerations similar to those which have been outlined, fractures and dislocations occurring in the patient with multiple system injuries are not different from the fracture which is an isolated injury. Any difference in the course of events in such injuries usually relates to the impact of additional trauma on the patient as a whole or because of special treatment made necessary by requirements extraneous to the fracture.

Fractures are usually accompanied by soft tissue injury and blood loss. Wray[3] has shown that the volume flow per minute into the limb of an experimental animal rises when a fracture is produced in it. A number of studies[1] have shown that the amount of blood shed into the soft tissues around the bone ends of a displaced fracture is variable, but usually far greater than had been suspected (Table 17-1). The phenomenon of increased volume flow into the injured limb may well enhance such loss. Although the losses outlined in Table 17-1 might be adequately compensated for in single injuries, in others, notably the disorganized pelvis or flank injury associated with transverse process fracture, the rate of loss may continue and the volume lost may be-

come very high. Such patients become hypovolemic, and shock may very well occur.

Where trauma has involved a number of systems, or more than one limb, blood loss may be very rapid and a hypovolemic state established quickly. Perhaps even before significant hematoma occurs about the fractures themselves, such a limb may show rather weak or absent pulses, not at all in keeping with the phenomenon of increased volume flow in the injured limb. The unwary may conclude that an artery has been damaged. Generally it is better to interpret the decreased or absent pulse as due to major arterial injury only when the patient is in a normotensive state and preferably out of shock. Often pulseless limbs show normal pulses once the shock has been corrected. Yet with the reestablished arterial inflow, the opportunity now occurs for sequestration of blood at the site of injury, and hypovolemia may become reestablished. In such cases, the use of splinting and compressive dressings on open wounds becomes clearly evident. Splinting suppresses pain and further bleeding, both of which may aggravate a preexisting state of shock.

Closed fractures in the patient with multiple system injuries require no special consideration except that the treatment chosen should not prejudice the patient at the time it is administered, nor the patient's further care. At the outset it is best to stabilize the unreduced fracture while the patient is made physiologically stable, then restabilize the *reduced* fracture in preparation for its healing. Dislocated joints will not become comfortable until they are reduced. Most dislocations do not bleed very much, unless a major adjacent vessel has been damaged, and so do not contribute significantly to hypovolemia. The disjointed pelvis may be an exception. The dislocation's chief effect is continued pain and a deformity which may alter the patient's position and interfere with moving the patient about, either for diagnosis or for treatment of other injuries. A reduced dislocation becomes fairly comfortable at once, and since reduction must be done, it may as well be carried out as soon as possible. When a dislocation compromises circulation at the knee or ankle, it must be reduced at once in the interest of survival of the distal parts. Reduction can often be accomplished with a minimum of anesthetic, or none at all, in the severely traumatized patient.

BIBLIOGRAPHY

1 Clarke, R., F. G. Badger, and S. Sevitt: *Modern Trends in Accident Surgery and Medicine,* Butterworth & Co. (Publishers), Ltd., London, 1959.
2 Holstein, A. and G. B. Lewis: Fractures of the humerus with radial-nerve paralysis, *J. Bone J. Surg.,* **45A**:1382, 1963.
3 Wray, J.: Personal communication.

Chapter 18

Injuries to the Hand

Louis H. Paradies, M.D.

Severe hand injuries can be baffling problems because of the complexity of the hand as an organ and its great importance in the function of the human individual. The picture can never be oversimplified, but falls into proper perspective when one considers that there is one *primary* objective which overshadows every other aspect of the problem. This objective, simply stated, is the *earliest* possible *complete* healing of the wound. No matter what are the associated bone, joint, tendon, or vascular injuries, no matter what complex reconstructive problems are visualized for the future, the initial wound must heal rapidly and completely if there is to be any prospect for *functional* recovery. The acknowledgment of

this first principle and its application will allow even surgeons not trained in reconstruction surgery of the hand to give adequate initial care to the injured part.

The sine qua non of initial treatment of the traumatized hand is thorough, meticulous debridement. This is the only way to achieve the objective of early, complete primary healing. The more severe the injury, the *more* time it will take to accomplish a meticulous debridement and the *less* consideration there will be for associated injuries, such as fractures and severed tendons. In severely traumatized hands, fractures and tendon injuries become secondary considerations and often cannot be definitively treated at the initial operation.

Needless to say, vascular lesions must be treated initially, and many authorities believe that the peripheral nerves, including digital nerves, should be sutured at the time of the initial debridement. A simple guide for the surgeon inexperienced in reconstruction procedures is to save all viable parts and digits, *provided* that there is nothing remaining to interfere with the early primary complete healing of the wound. One point remains to be qualified: primary healing does not necessarily mean that all wounds of the hand must be linearly closed. There will be times when in order to save a digit that is otherwise well vascularized, one will be forced to use either split-thickness skin dressings or free full-thickness grafts with the subcutaneous fat removed and cut to the exact size of the defect to be covered. Skin dressings are acceptable, either in the initial treatment or where their application must be delayed 4 or 5 days. Split-thickness skin dressings and free full-thickness grafts must not be placed over joints or tendons. When these structures must be covered, the surgeon must use local flaps, or sometimes even resort to abdominal or cross-forearm flaps in unusual cases when damage to the hand is severe and the goal is to salvage a few remaining structures.

The problem of the initial care of hand injuries cannot be considered without due emphasis on the importance of the conservation of skin. Every digit is important; the thumb, of course, holds a position of prime importance. One should not be overawed, however, by the hand as a mechanical unit. The marvelous complexity of tasks that can be performed by the human hand is not the product of the efficiency of the hand as a mechanical unit, but of the human intelligence and cortical control of the hand.[4] The cortical control of the hand is completely dependent upon normal sensation. Only *normal hand skin* mediates all components of sensation,

and herein lies the importance of saving *all normal* skin that is salvageable.[5]

When the surgeon enters upon the initial care of the traumatized hand prepared to make certain decisions as to what parts shall be saved and what parts shall be discarded, the occupation of the patient must be known. The importance of saving digits or parts of digits is obviously greater in a violinist than it is in a laborer.

EVALUATION OF THE INJURED HAND AND INITIAL CARE

Cursory inspection of the injured hand in the emergency room can give one some idea of the amount of tissue lost and the parts salvageable, but this estimation and evaluation are best done in the operating room. A decision must sometimes be made as to whether the hand can be cared for in the emergency on an outpatient basis or whether the patient must be taken to the operating room. If the patient is alert enough to cooperate, the *wound is covered* with a sterile dressing and *functional tests* are used to determine the extent of the damage to neurovascular structures and tendons. The sight of a physician intently probing a hand wound in semicasual emergency room surroundings should never occur in institutions where the surgeons are even remotely aware of the problems associated with hand injuries. If the functional evaluation reveals no neurovascular damage and no loss of tendon function, the wound can be cared for in the emergency room if the skin loss or damage is minor. If, on the other hand, there is major skin damage or examination does not *conclusively rule out* tendon or neurovascular damage, the patient must be brought to the operating room, where instruments, drapes, light, and personnel are optimum to evaluate and treat the injured hand adequately. If functional examination reveals definite neurovascular or tendon injury, the patient must, of course, be taken to the operating room, where, under completely formal surgical conditions, the injured hand must be prepared and draped carefully, the wound explored, and the decision made as to the proper initial definitive treatment.

OPERATIVE MANAGEMENT

Once the patient is brought to the operating room, the injured hand is carefully prepared with soap or detergent solution. These solutions are used to clean the intact skin. They are to be kept out of the open wound. The wound itself can be lavaged with saline solution, both before and after draping. Tourniquet control is an absolute requisite for inspection, evaluation, and debridement of the wound. The tourniquet should be applied loosely enough so that it can be released and reapplied with simple elevation during the surgical procedure if necessary. A tight tourniquet requires a compressive bandage to empty the limb of venous blood, and this tight wrapping may be undesirable in the severely injured hand. In deciding whether a particular piece of skin is viable, it is helpful to release the tourniquet and see if blood returns to the particular part of skin in question. If the area flushes satisfactorily, then the hand can be elevated, the tourniquet reinflated, and the procedure continued, saving the area in question.

Meticulous debridement must be carried out. The hand is compact, and being compact, it has almost no tissue that does not have specific function. Tendons, nerves, vessels, and important muscles lie in close juxtaposition to one another. Some type of magnification of the surgical field can materially aid this process of evaluation and debridement. The importance of the skin already has been emphasized. The debridement must be done under tourniquet control. It must be slow,

careful, and complete. Intermittent irrigation is helpful in revealing small tags of devitalized tissue. After thorough debridement, primary linear closures are attempted whenever possible, but split- and full-thickness grafts, and occasionally flaps, can be used as discussed above. Depending on the magnitude of soft tissue injury, the wound may be closed and pressure dressings applied before the tourniquet is released. It is often advisable, however, when there is much soft tissue injury and consequently major debridement, to release the tourniquet before the wound is closed, tie significant bleeders, and then close the skin. As an alternative, one can elevate the hand after ligation of bleeding vessels, reinflate the tourniquet, do the necessary closure, apply a pressure dressing, and then release the tourniquet again.

TENDON INJURIES

Extensor Tendons

A laceration of an extensor tendon can be a relatively minor injury, but certain considerations are worthy of note. The extensor tendon lacerated in an area that does not overlie a joint can usually be repaired successfully in an emergency room, the only precaution being the use of atraumatic technique and as small a suture as will satisfactorily hold the tendon together. The wound must heal with a minimum of inflammatory response and a minimum of adhesions between the tendon repair site and surrounding structures. Extensor tendons lacerated over any of the finger joints must be considered *open joint injuries* and treated if at all possible in the operating room. Here again, the tendons are sutured together, using as little suture material as possible. There is no need for any complex suturing technique. The tendon ends must be turned up and the joint inspected for foreign material and irrigated before the tendon repair is accomplished. Most extensor tendon lacerations are held in semicomplete extension for approximately 3 weeks before motion is gradually begun.

Flexor Tendon Injuries

The fundamental principles pertaining to injuries of the flexor tendons of the hand and wrist were laid down many years ago by surgeons with a great deal of experience in this field. Such authors as Boyes,[2,3] Pulvertaft,[8,9] and Potenza[6] should be studied before dealing with even the initial care of flexor tendon injuries.

Briefly the problem is this: Tendons heal by proliferating, invading fibroblasts from surrounding tissues and structures. In the hand and wrist, and especially in the fingers, there is a minimum of loose or areolar tissue surrounding the flexor tendons. In the fingers, in the area known as "no man's land," for instance, the only available tissue is the synovial sheath which lines the fibroosseous tunnel. This "tunnel" is rigid, immovable, and tends to prevent the normal gliding of the tendon if attached to it by firm, fibrous adhesions. The prime objective of the surgeon who first treats the injury is to obtain a primarily healed wound with *minimal* inflammatory reaction and *minimal* proliferative response. Only this result in the healing of the original wound is acceptable, both from the standpoint of success of immediate repair and of future reconstructive work. Since every fresh wound is an unknown quantity, the surgeon is forced to judge the likelihood of primary healing in each individual injury. A marked proliferative response is called forth with even slight trauma to a tendon or synovial sheath.[10] The added trauma incident to a tendon repair—the drying effect of the open wound, the handling of the tendons with tissue forceps, and the placement of foreign bodies (sutures)—is such a great surgical risk that more often than not, especially in constrained areas like the fibroosseous tunnels of the fingers, the surgeon should elect to defer definitive repair of the flexor tendon laceration and simply cleanse, debride, and close the wound.

Some basic guidelines are used in dealing with tendon lacerations of the hand and wrist. Lacerations of the fingers lie almost entirely in "no man's land." This is an area from the distal palmar crease to about the middle of the middle phalanx. In this area the sublimis and profundus glide within a closely fitting fibroosseous tunnel. Here no primary tendon repair work is done, unless all conditions are optimal, including the presence of an experienced hand surgeon. Just distal to this area, if the profundus tendon is lacerated within about 1 to 1.5 cm from its insertion, the distal stub may be excised and the proximal end advanced to be inserted in the base of the distal phalanx.

In the palm, when multiple tendon lacerations occur, primary repair of all tendons can be accomplished if conditions permit. Minimal trauma, minimal contamination, and maximum surgical skill are the prerequisites for primary repair.

The initial treatment of severe volar wrist lacerations depends on the same variables. Today's surgeon must see to it that radial and ulnar arteries and nerves are repaired (in most instances primarily) by experienced hands using *microscopic techniques.* Nothing less than this is optimal treatment. The accompanying tendon lacerations are usually repaired at the same time, but may be delayed if conditions of the wound and/or operating time so dictate. Sometimes only the profundus tendons are repaired primarily.

OTHER INJURIES

Fingertip Injuries

Most fingertip injuries can be resolved into two main problems. The first involves a laceration of the fingertip which is almost, but not completely, through the distal portion of the fingertip, being held by a small intact pedicle of soft tissue. This injury is best handled by two or three loosely placed sutures, which are usually enough to secure the partially severed fragments back in place. If necessary for stability of this distal portion of the fingertip, a small Kirschner wire can be passed through the tip of the finger and into the proximal portion of the distal phalanx. It should be emphasized that it is better to stabilize this fragment with a small Kirschner wire than to suture the wound tightly closed, no matter how tempting this may be. A tight wound closure will obstruct venous drainage and thereby increase tissue tension to the point that the small trickle of arterial blood that was sufficient to nourish the fingertip will be stopped and the fingertip will become gangrenous. If a portion of the nail remains, it can be held together with one suture and will form an excellent splint for the remainder of the soft tissue.

The other problem is the complete severance of part of the distal phalanx from the remaining digit. It should be stated at the outset that it is probably never wise to resuture a completely severed part of a digit except possibly in children. Reimplantation surgery is in its infancy and is to be attempted only by experienced surgical teams. The simplest and most economical solution in terms of time is simply to shorten the remaining bone of the distal phalanx and perform a primary linear closure of the wound in such a manner that the incision falls transversely across the fingertip on its most dorsal aspect. This procedure shortens the finger rather markedly, but it has the great advantage that the remaining skin is completely normal palmar skin. If part of the nail remains here, the palmar flap can be sewed up under the remaining nail. If it is desired to maintain as much length as possible in the fingertip, the wound will have to be covered with a skin graft. In children, it is probably best to use a small split-thickness graft as a skin dressing without any shortening of the distal phalanx. With growth of the child, and normal contraction of the wound, the area that is covered by split-thickness skin will practically disappear. In adults, it is probably necessary to use a free full-thickness graft to cover wounds of this nature. This is easily obtained from the forearm using local anesthesia and cutting an exact pattern of full-thickness skin according to the defect that is to be covered. The biggest advantage of this approach to the problem is probably cosmetic, in that there is much less shortening of the distal phalanx. If bone is exposed, of course, it cannot be covered with a free graft of any kind. Either the digit must be shortened to the extent that the bone is covered with soft tissue, or else some other type of flap procedure will have to be considered. If the patient is a laborer who is not concerned about cosmesis, the simplest procedure is to shorten the bone and do a primary linear closure as described above. A patient treated in this way should be back to work in 2 or 3 weeks at the most. If the patient does extremely delicate work with his or her fingers, the problem becomes more critical. The surgeon will have to analyze the patient's occupation very carefully in each individual situation. The patient who does delicate work or handles very tiny instruments or parts will probably function better with a shortened fingertip but one that has normal palmar skin covering the end. A fingertip of more normal length but covered by a full-thickness graft will regenerate protective sensation but never approach normal two-point discrimination or stereognosis. There are occupations, however, in which it is mandatory to save length.

Partial Amputations of Digits

The care of partial amputations is similar to that described for the partially lacerated distal fingertip. Obviously, however, the situation becomes more critical as the laceration becomes more proximal. As a general rule, if one attempts to save a partially amputated digit, one should follow the rules laid down in the previous section concerning loose suture of the laceration. In addition to this, however, added stability will almost always be required in the form of intramedullary wire fixation of the fractured phalanx. This not only aligns the fracture for ultimate optimum function, but it immobilizes the soft tissue and is conductve to earlier primary healing.

If the laceration is in the middle phalanx, it is probably worthwhile to attempt to save the finger, even if both tendons and the bone are severed, as long as the arterial supply to the fingertip remains. The bone can be fixed with intramedullary wire, the extensor tendon repaired, and the skin very loosely repaired with two or three sutures. If nothing more is done, the patient will have adequate use of the finger and will lack only the flexion of the distal phalanx. If necessary this problem can be handled most simply by tenodesis of the distal flexor tendon stump or a distal interphalangeal joint fusion.

If the laceration is in the proximal phalanx, the matter becomes more complex. One may attempt to save a finger that has both extensor and flexor tendons and bones severed, but the prognosis for function becomes greatly reduced. The probable approach would be, again, intramedullary fixation of the fracture site with a small Kirschner wire, repair of the extensor tendon, and loose repair of the skin. Of course, adequate arterial supply to the distal part of the finger is mandatory; usually one intact neurovascular bundle is sufficient. It is probably wise to do primary suture of one digital nerve. Repair of digital nerves requires microsurgical techniques for optimum results. If both digital nerves are severed along with all the structures named above, the prognosis is extremely poor for adequate function of this finger. If the surgeon has undertaken to save a digit that has been injured in this manner, has

fixed the bone, extensor tendon, and digital nerve, and has loosely sutured the skin and if all goes well, a flexor tendon graft will have to be performed after the wound is solidly healed. In such cases, the surgeon should discuss the problem preoperatively with the patient. In most instances, although cosmetically not as satisfactory, completing the amputation is by far the simplest and most economical procedure. A complete or partial ray resection can also be done, either primarily, if the wound is fairly clean, or later.

WRINGER INJURIES

Although wringer injuries are becoming less frequent, their potential severity and occult nature make them worthy of special mention. There are two general types of wringer injuries. One results from the standard washing machine wringers that are used to squeeze clothes dry, and the other from the so-called mangle or ironing device. The latter injuries tend to be extremely severe, being frequently associated with second- and third-degree burns. Most of the following comments will be related to the type of wringer injury not associated with heat.

Five types of injury may occur when a person's hand and arm are caught in washing machine wringers, or as a matter of fact, in any device with a similar action.

1 There is a possibility that if the limb comes to a stop and the wringers continue to roll, they will cause direct injury to underlying major nerves and vessels.

2 When the extremity comes to a stop and the wringers continue to turn, there is always some degree of abrasion or burnlike injury from the friction and pressure being localized to one spot.

3 Perhaps the most important injury, because of its occult nature, is the mechanism of *compression,* wherein soft tissues, especially muscles in the forearm and arm, are crushed.

4 There is a marked tendency for the rollers to slide the various layers of tissue so as to produce cleavage planes between subcutaneous tissue and fascia, between various layers of muscle, and between muscle and bone.

5 Occasionally, fractures are produced.

The treatment of the direct neurovascular injuries, fractures, and abrasions and burns caused by the spinning rollers is not particularly unique as far as the wringer injury is concerned, and the same principles described elsewhere would hold true. The problems that are unique to the wringer injury are the crushing and compressing effect of the rollers and the tendency for them to cause abnormal cleavage planes between tissues. The results of this type of mechanical trauma are ischemia and sloughing of areas of skin and severe muscle ischemia which can result in contracture. The patient, usually a child, who is admitted shortly after having his or her hand caught in a wringer more than likely will have no evidence of injury whatsoever. *This* patient is the patient for whom a rather rigid routine must be adopted since there is no way of predicting the extent of the damage that has occurred within the planes of the forearm or arm or to the muscle tissue itself. If we are to prevent large areas of skin loss and the adverse effects of muscle ischemia which are secondary to the swelling produced by the crushing trauma, we must treat each patient as if the maximum amount of damage to the soft tissues has occurred.

The classic treatment for this injury is the application of a massive pressure dressing. The rationale behind the use of pressure dressings is that the cleavage planes produced by the stripping and sliding action of the rollers on the soft tissue fill with hematoma, which will further dissect abnormal planes and render certain tissues, especially skin, ischemic and therefore augment the damage done, with resultant greater necrosis and slough. It is hoped, then, that compression dressings will maintain viable tissue in contact with viable tissue, prevent further dissection by bleeding and hematoma, and minimize at least some of the loss of skin that would ordinarily result without this treatment. There is some evidence, furthermore, that early compression may restore the circulatory imbalance in the tight fascial compartments.[1] Poulos[7] has suggested that compression dressings, rather than being a necessary feature of the treatment of the wringer injury, are not only unnecessary but may interfere with the accurate observation of the extremity and lead one to neglect a more vital part of the injury, namely, that of the increasing pressure within the tight fascial compartments of the forearm. Poulos' writings are invaluable in that they have served to emphasize what is, after all, the most important part of the pathologic change and that part which is responsible for the most severe disabilities in this type of injury. Nonetheless, it is felt that there is some rationale behind the use of compression dressings and that they do indeed tend to minimize the swelling, edema, and dissection of fascial planes which result in large areas of skin loss. The following routine then is advised for the treatment of wringer injury.

The patient should be admitted to the hospital as an inpatient, the bone and joint damage evaluated, and the skin cleansed utilizing a standard surgical preparation. Sterile dressings are then applied. A large bulky compression dressing (preferably with rolls of cotton) is applied, and the arm is elevated, with the patient at complete bed rest. The patient's tetanus immunization status is evaluated and a booster tetanus toxoid shot given if necessary. The entire dressing will then have to be taken down approximately every 3 h for about the first 9 h to check the forearm and arm compartments for undue swelling and tension. If firm, hard swelling of the forearm is noted, then surgical fasciotomies should be performed. These may be done in any way that the surgeon chooses, the simplest being through a short skin incision, splitting the forearm fascia in both proximal and distal directions. There are extensor and flexor compartments in the forearm, it should be recalled, and both these compartments must be decompressed. A word of caution should be sounded in that it is extremely dangerous—especially in the swollen forearm—to make a short skin incision over the *flexor* surface and then simply run the scissors up and down the forearm fascia. The radial artery is very superficial, especially with a swollen forearm, and could easily be damaged with this maneuver. The periods of observation can be reduced to approximately every 6 h after the first 9 h period, and if after 48 h no untoward results are noted, the patient is discharged. If complications have ensued, however, the patient must, of course, be kept in the hospital for additional treatment.

BIBLIOGRAPHY

1 Athol, Parks: Treatment of traumatic tension ischemia of muscle and nerve, *J. Bone J. Surg.,* **41B**:628, 1959.

2 Boyes, J. H.: Flexor tendon grafts in the fingers and thumb, *J. Bone J. Surg.,* **32A**:489, 1950.

3 ———: "Operative Techniques in Surgery of the Hand," in Charles H. Pease (ed.), *Instructional Course Lectures, American Academy of Orthopaedic Surgeons,* J. W. Edwards, Publisher, Incorporated, Ann Arbor, Mich., 1952, vol. 9, p. 181.

4 Jones, Frederic Wood: *The Principles of Anatomy as Seen in the Hand,* 2d ed., Baillière, Tindall Cox, Ltd., London, 1946.

5 London, P. S.: Simplicity of approach to treatment of the injured hand, *J. Bone J. Surg.,* **43B**:454, 1961.

6 Potenza, Capt. Austin D.: Tendon healing with the flexor digital sheath, *J. Bone J. Surg.,* **44A**:49, 1962.

7 Poulos, Ernest: The treatment of wringer injuries, *Am. Surg.,* **24**:458, 1958.

8 Pulvertaft, R. G.: Flexor tendon grafts, *J. Bone J. Surg.,* **418**:629, 1959.

9 ———: Tendon grafts (editorial), *J. Bone J. Surg.,* **43B**:421, 1961.

10 Skoog, T. and B. T. Persson: Experimental study of early tendon healing, *Plast. Reconstr. Surg.,* **13**:384, 1954.

Chapter 19

Facial and Extracranial Head Injuries

James E. Bertz, D.D.S., M.D.

Robert V. Walker, D.D.S.

Severe injuries to the maxillofacial region are common in today's accidents which involve high-velocity vehicular acceleration and deceleration. Of the many causes of wounds, the most spectacular and drastically mutilating maxillofacial injuries result from automobile accidents. Serious injury to the face and jaws is commonplace following autobile accidents. As the maxillofacial region is the prime focus of appearance and encompasses the key portals for respiration and feeding and the highly specialized functional areas for sight and smell, care of these wounded parts is of major significance and can be lifesaving.

The facial bony skeleton is a highly functional apparatus. It provides channels for the passage of air, receptacles to house the units of vision, chambers for producing resonance to the voice, anchorage for the dental structures and chewing, and symmetrical support of the overlying soft tissue. If any of these key functions is altered by injury to the maxillofacial skeleton or adjacent soft tissue, the earliest possible repair is indicated and desirable.

Following injury, the old axiom admonishing one to preserve and restore normal function and appearance has a unique coetaneous application in regard to facial injuries. Appearance and function are so intimately related in this area that the two objectives are hard to separate, and many times they need not be. A badly fractured and displaced mandibular or maxillary fracture seriously interferes with respiration and mastication and concurrently produces disharmony of facial appearance. Correct alignment of displaced fragments and adjustment of the occlusion to a functional position relieves the airway and chewing problem and, in most instances, restores symmetry and order to the face. A simple-appearing depressed and inferiorly displaced zygoma produces a flat side to the face and an ungainly downward position of the eye. Concomitantly, vision is altered and the mandible is deflected from its usual excursive pattern by the overlying bony impingement. Raising the zygoma to a reduced position restores facial symmetry, normal binocular vision, and mandibular function. These uncomplicated examples point out the closeness with which function and appearance are related to each other in the total utility of the maxillofacial unit.

The extravagant vascularity to all parts of the maxillofacial complex, the remarkable interconnections and cross communications of the terminal arborization of the facial nerve, the lack of long tendinous insertions, an extensive lymphatic drainage network, generous subcutaneous tissue, highly mobile and relaxed skin, and a static bony framework (excepting the mandible) are exceptional regional advantages that favor good results in the treatment of maxillofacial injuries.

Soft tissue wounds in the region are no different than other soft tissue injuries except that vascularity is abundant and predisposes to favorable healing. Even with the generous blood supply, there are few large vessels which can lead to troublesome and dangerous hemorrhage. Most of the vessels are small in caliber and usually well supplied with elastic fibers. If transected or cut, they usually retract within bony canals and are occluded by thrombosis.[8] Bleeding from the most gaping laceration usually stops spontaneously without special treatment or is controllable by pressure. An occasional partially transected facial artery may require forceps control. When completely severed, the facial vessels generally retract and are not a source of difficulty. The general principles of thorough cleansing and removal of impregnated dirt and debris is paramount. This may be accomplished with irrigation, scrubbing with surgical scrub brush and/or with a pulsating, irrigating device. Meticulous debridement of soft tissue injuries is important and may be done with a scalpel, scissors, or other instruments. Only obviously devital tissue is generally removed from facial injuries. However, the wound edges in general should be squared so as to allow the best healing opportunity. Surgical principles of hemostasis and elimination of dead space are fundamental in these closures. Appropriate suture material of No. 4-0 chromic, No. 5-0 plain gut, or other surgical sutures may be used in the deeper tissue. Smaller suture material such as No. 6-0 black silk which has been siliconized and No. 6-0 monofilament nylon in an interrupted or continuous fashion are the indicated skin sutures. A firmly anchored pressure dressing helps control capillary ooze, lessens edema and hematoma formation, and supports the wound for better patient comfort. Drains are not generally necessary unless segments of underlying bone or soft tissue have been avulsed at the time of injury.

Severe maxillofacial trauma produces a shocking appearance to the patient. Such a garish countenance suggests that other vital areas may, also, be disturbed and require immediate attention. Unconsciousness, hemorrhage, respiratory embarrassment, shock, and pain are well-recognized concomitant problems and are covered in earlier chapters. Only acknowledgment of their significance is given here. The importance of a thorough physical examination and an evaluation of the neurologic status of each traumatized patient cannot be overemphasized.

Loss of airway, head injury, thoracic injury,

and marked alteration of the hemodynamic status are the common severe complications which carry an immediate threat to the life of the facially injured patient. Early and continued assessment of physical findings related to these injuries are, therefore, mandatory. Shock in the severely injured patient is common, but even in the presence of head injury should not be presumed to be due to cerebral injury until proved otherwise.[5] Shock demands immediate attention and should be treated as such under any circumstance of its occurrence.

The greatest single immediate threat to the life of the patient with a facial or jaw injury is lack of an airway. Provision of an airway is, obviously, given the number one priority in treatment.

The tongue receives anterior support from the mandible. Any fracture of the mandible which causes the jaw to fall posteriorly at the same time allows the tongue to occupy a more posterior position in the pharynx (Fig. 19-1A and B). It takes very little posterior displacement of the tongue to seriously obstruct the pharyngeal airway. With the addition of edema or bleeding in the tongue, obstruction can become acute rapidly and asphyxiate the patient.

The mouth and pharynx should be suctioned quickly. With adequate illumination, a tooth, bone, prosthesis, or other foreign body loose within the oral cavity or pharynx that might be aspirated can be seen. If illumination is not available, the jaw may be held forward with one hand and the oral cavity and pharynx quickly explored with the forefinger of the opposite hand. Any foreign body encountered may be carefully removed.

If other injuries permit, the patient should be rolled to the prone position so that gravity will aid in holding the jaw and tongue forward. Additionally, this position aids in removal of secretions from the mouth by the same princi-

Figure 19-1 Bilateral condyle fractures and comminuted fractures of the mandibular symphysis due to automobile accident. *(A)* Gaping open-mouthed attitude of the patient with marked posterior displacement of the multiple mandibular fragments allowing the tongue to fall back into the pharynx. Immediate tracheostomy is necessary to relieve the airway. *(B)* Lateral x-ray view demonstrating the multiple fractures.

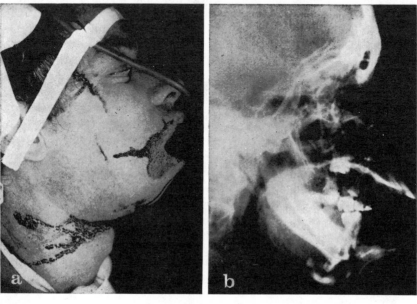

ple and prevents aspiration of these pooled secretions.

If the patient has to remain in the supine position, an oral airway may be tried. If this is not tolerated, gentle pull on the jaw to a forward position may be used, thereby holding the teeth lightly in contact. If the patient can breathe comfortably with the jaw in this attitude, the upper and lower teeth may be ligated securely together with whatever is available. Suitable for this purpose is 22- to 26-gauge wire. Of importance is the fact that moving the jaw forward and stabilizing it improves the airway, and in many instances the patient is made a great deal more comfortable by thus controlling the flailing jaw. If both maneuvers fail to improve the airway, a tracheostomy must be performed at once. These deliberations and efforts should take very little time.

Fractures of the upper jaw almost always involve the nasal fossa or pharynx. However, the patient does not often have immediate airway difficulty following this injury. The upper jaw generally is displaced posteriorly, and the molar teeth are jammed against the lower molar teeth. This produces a tilting open of the anterior teeth so that the patient is seen with a marked open-mouthed attitude (Fig. 19-9 A and C). With this wide open oral airway the patient is not dependent on the clogged nasal passages or a closed nasopharynx for respiration. However, the need for a tracheostomy following reduction and treatment of these fractures is far greater than the need following reduction and fixing of mandibular fractures.

The presence of a full complement of teeth markedly influences the need of a tracheostomy if fractures extend across the nasal airway.[24] Patients show evidence of severely distorted nasal anatomy and obstruction to these passages. However, on admission to the hospital they may have no airway difficulty when the mouth is held or propped wide open. Only when the fractures are reduced and the full complement of teeth are wired in occlusion does the critical compromise of the airway become apparent. The teeth completely fill or occlude the intermaxillary space, and buccal edema plugs the clefts behind the last teeth. The nasal mucosa is already engorged and blocks the nasal aperture. Air movement becomes exceedingly difficult or impossible. These patients require prophylactic tracheostomies.

If the patient has only a few remaining teeth or many have been avulsed by the traumatic episode, tracheostomy will rarely be required regardless of the extent of the midface insult. A large-bore airway is available via the intermaxillary spaces formerly occupied by teeth even if the few remaining ones are wired in occlusion.

Tracheostomies are required in about one of every two patients when midface fractures not associated with mandibular fractures extend across the nasal airway at some point and treatment requires wiring of the teeth in occlusion.[24] Very few have been required when the patient is initially seen in the emergency room. This is especially true if the patient is conscious; however, the converse is true in the unconscious patient. The conscious patient will find a head position to allow adequate respiratory exchange, but not the unconscious patient. Gunshot wounds to the floor of the mouth and base of tongue area will require tracheostomies. There may be no initial respiratory distress; however, edema secondary to the blast effect and the few limiting anatomical boundaries will lead to edema in a few hours that will result in the need for a tracheostomy. It should be done early to eliminate the emergency tracheostomy that will be needed. Most tracheostomies are done electively at the time of the facial surgical procedure to facilitate management of anesthesia during the procedure and control the airway afterward. Occasionally, it is necessary to perform a tracheostomy following the surgical intervention to relieve an embarrassed airway that was not anticipated.

Appraisal of head injury in regard to the timing for repair of facial fractures is not too well defined. This evaluation, however, many times determines the optimum remedy which may be used for the facial injuries. There is little disagreement that early repair of most injuries is advisable for precise management.

Little agreement on timing for treatment has been established for the unconscious patient. Thompson[21] states, "Unconsciousness is not a single clinical state but rather a series of stages like the rungs of a ladder. At the top of the ladder there is full consciousness and at the bottom is the stage of permanent unconsciousness, death." The top and bottom rungs of such a ladder offer little problem in choosing the correct time for treatment. The top rung, or the conscious patient, would receive immediate or early treatment in most institutions. No thought has to be given the patient representing the bottom rung. The rungs in between are the gray areas. As soon as the maxillofacially traumatized patient who is unconscious is seen in the receiving area, immediate determinations of blood pressure, pulse, respiration, and response to verbal and physical stimuli should be made and recorded for convenient reference. At regular 15-min intervals these determinations should be repeated and recorded. With the advent of cerebroangiography and the CAT (computerized axial tomography) scanner, the evaluation of the neurologically impaired patient has been greatly sophisticated. The CAT scanner has shortened the period of angiography evaluation and lessened the morbidity secondary to the angiography studies. It has also made the evaluation of the neurologically injured patient more accurate. By utilizing the physical evaluation of the patient along with the radiographic studies and CAT scanner we can carry out the definitive correction of the facial injuries with general anesthesia in many instances during the acute phase. Of course, if there is

marked fluctuation in the patient's general physical condition or neurological status and the CAT scan or other evaluating devices show deterioration, the maxillofacial surgical intervention should be delayed until proper treatment has intervened or the condition has stabilized.

This simply means that head injury alone without evidence of a progressive intracranial mass lesion is not a contraindication to an early general anesthetic and a reparative surgical procedure. It is difficult to predict when the unconscious patient will awake, and to wait may mean that the advantage of an early repair is irretrievably lost.

Beck and Neil[2] reported a series of 39 consecutive patients with multiple trauma and a varying degree of head injury who were taken to the operating room immediately (within a 2- to 6-h period following injury) and given a general anesthetic. These patients included 12 with facial fractures and other serious injuries. The neurologic status of these patients varied from being awake to being unconscious. None of the patients worsened as the result of the general anesthetic, and most demonstrated slight improvement of their general physical and neurologic status. The postoperative morbid complications were minimal in these patients.

A more complete discussion of shock, head injury, and chest injury is given in Chaps. 1, 11, and 12.

THE MANDIBLE

Mandibular Dislocation

Anterior dislocation of the mandible is the usual jaw dislocation without fractures, but this injury is not common. It results from blows to the face, an abnormally wide yawn, holding the jaw wide open for long periods of dental treatment, attempting to open the jaw sufficiently to bite a large sandwich or apple, or any excessive jaw-opening excursion. In these movements, the condylar head advances foward beyond the articular eminence. In this forward position, spasm of the jaw-closing muscles occurs and jams the condyle superiorly above the lowest point of the articular eminence. In this position, the patient cannot retract the condyle back into the articular fossa. The mouth is literally locked in this wide-open position, and the patient cannot close it. The patient experiences severe pain because of acute myospasm of the muscles which close the jaw. The continuing spasm keeps the jaw dislocated. Hysteria, anxiety, pain, and discomfort perpetuate the spasm.

Treatment is not difficult. From a mechanical standpoint, the physical maneuvers which created the dislocation in the first place are simply reversed. The jaw has to be drawn downward to get the condyle at least to the level of the articular eminence. The jaw should then be moved posteriorly to allow the condyle to return to the articular fossa. It may snap into the fossa with resounding authority. As these movements are carried out by placing the thumbs on the lower molar teeth with the fingers grasping the lower border of the jaw, the thumbs should be protected by wrapping with a towel or gauze to prevent them from being mashed between the teeth if the jaw does suddenly snap into place.

The patient should be adequately sedated with an analgesic to make the reduction easier. This calms the patient and lessens the discomfort. Infiltrating the internal pterygoid, masseter, temporalis, and external pterygoid muscles with a local anesthetic directly relieves the spasm of these muscles and greatly facilitates reducing the dislocation. Rarely is a general anesthetic required to reduce a dislocated mandible. However, reducing a long-standing chronic dislocation may require general anesthesia supplemented with a short-acting skeletal muscle paralyzing agent. It is advisable to "rest" the jaw for a 2- or 3-week period following reduction of an acute dislocation. This is most effectively done by wiring the teeth in occlusion. More aggressive ma-

neuvers may be necessary to control the chronic dislocating mandible.

Avulsed Teeth and Alveolar Ridge Fractures

Teeth and alveolar processes may be injured alone or in combination with fractures of the jaws or facial bones.

In most instances, anterior teeth are involved. These injuries appear to occur with greatest incidence between 7 and 11 years of age. At this age the permanent anterior teeth have erupted into positions of isolated prominence and are exposed to injury. Teeth may be avulsed partially or completely. In the cases of recent partially avulsed teeth, the offended teeth are simply reseated in their sockets. After reseating, the teeth should be immobilized if unstable when reseated in the socket. The immobilization can be accomplished with orthodontic appliances, splints, and/or arch bar. When several teeth or a large segment of the alveolus is involved, intermaxillary fixation may be indicated to prevent further injury by the occlusion of teeth.[11]

In all cases of partially or completely avulsed teeth, roentgenographic examination prior to treatment is indicated. When anterior teeth are involved, periapical or occlusal film examinations are helpful. Posterior teeth and the posterior alveolus can be examined best by lateral oblique films of the jaws.

In cases of complete avulsion of teeth, when the injury is very recent and the teeth are intact, root canal fillings may be done prior to reseating the teeth in their sockets. The teeth should be placed in saline solution while preparations are made to complete the procedure. The teeth should be handled gently while removing the pulp tissue and cleaning the pulp canal. These pulp chambers should be completely occluded with some filling material such as gutta-percha. The teeth are then immobilized as previously described.

In some cases a large segment of alveolar bone may be fractured from basal bone of the jaw. In this situation, if the segment contains stable teeth, these teeth may be used to immobilize this part to the other stable parts of the dental arch. In cases where it is doubtful that the teeth will ever become stable but large segments of alveolar bone are involved, immobilization is still indicated. This at least allows the bone to heal and conserves an important segment of the dental arch (Fig. 19-2A–C). The teeth can be removed in 6 to 8 weeks if they do not become stable. The conserved alveolar bone is useful for later support of prosthetic appliances. Coverage of the involved bone in these cases with adequate soft tissue flaps is of prime importance.

At the time of initial examination, one may decide not to save grossly avulsed or damaged teeth. In this instance, conservation of bone and soft tissue is even more important. Adequate debridement of devital tissue, cleansing with copious saline solution irrigations, and meticulous suturing are essential and neces-

sary. In removal of the teeth, care must be taken not to displace bone fragments attached to periosteum or to tear vital skin flaps. In suturing soft tissue, coverage of the bone is very important.[20]

In cases where the edges of teeth are fractured and the pulp is exposed, these teeth should be removed unless root canal treatment or pulpal dressings can be made available in the near future.

Follow-up roentgenographic and clinical examinations are indicated during treatment and at 6-month to 1-year intervals. These are essential, as pulpal necrosis and periapical involvement at a later date are distinct possibilities. As a general rule, the teeth of young children and those in their early teens have a better chance for survival because the apical foramens of their teeth are larger, which allows quicker revascularization.

Antibiotic coverage is indicated in many

Figure 19-2 Severe comminuting of large segments of alveolar bone displacing teeth in all directions. *(A)* Displacement of tooth-bearing segments of bone on admission to the hospital. *(B)* Reduction of the various segments by placing the teeth in proper occlusion and immobilizing the jaw with intermaxillary wiring. *(C)* Slight shift in occlusion over long-term follow-up, but the occlusion remains stable and functional with no additional loss of teeth.

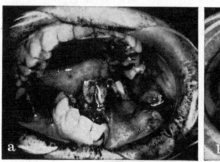
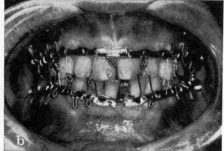
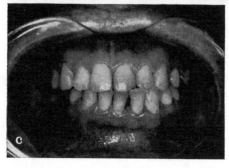

cases, but judgment should be used to determine which cases require such coverage.

Local or general anesthesia may be used depending on the individual case.

Mandibular Fractures

The mandible is a somewhat horseshoe-shaped rim of bone that furnishes key support for the lower chewing platform. A fracture at any point along the mandible will disrupt the fitting of this lower table against its upper counterpart and seriously interfere with normal chewing.

The lower teeth normally occlude with the upper in a balanced and precise manner. In reducing and immobilizing mandibular fractures, great care is needed to reestablish this precise meshing of upper and lower teeth. Fracture reductions, therefore, have to be exact, as malalignment of only a millimeter or so can prevent the teeth from occluding properly. However, the very presence of teeth makes the accurate reducing and fixing of mandibular fractures a great deal easier. If the upper jaw is intact and a normal dentition is present, these teeth furnish an accurate pattern or key into which the lower teeth can be fitted. If the occlusion is reestablished snugly, the fractures will be in good alignment; otherwise, the teeth would not be allowed to fit together properly. Additionally, the teeth furnish convenient places of attachment for fixation devices such as wiring, arch bars, or splints. Fortunately, the largest percentage of mandibular fractures can be treated by this highly accurate and simple technique of wiring the teeth in occlusion.

Fractures of the edentulous mandible are a two-sided consideration. Many require no reduction or fixation. On occasion, however, they present difficult problems in reducing and immobilizing or fixing the fragments. There are no teeth protruding from the bone to serve as anchors for the attachment of fixation devices. Elaborate splints, plates, pins, or wiring are often required to control the frag-

ments adequately. However, since occlusion of teeth is not involved, great accuracy of fracture reduction is not always required.

Therefore, the presence or absence of teeth in mandibular fractures creates a paradoxical situation. When teeth are present, responsibility is great for reestablishment of correct occlusion. Even though an extremely correct reduction is required, the job is made infinitely easier by the very presence of the teeth. When teeth are absent and responsibility for a precise reduction of the fracture is greatly lessened, the job is infinitely more difficult as teeth which could serve as a purchase on the underlying bone are missing. Elaborate fixation devices may then be necessary to control and fix the fragments.

Mandibular fractures result from the trauma of fights, automobile accidents, falls, athletic accidents, kicks, occasional train and airplane accidents, and multiple random causes.

Fractures of the Mandible with Teeth   The mandible containing a fairly full complement of teeth is most commonly fractured at the cuspid area, the third molar area, and the condyle neck area. There are reasons for this.

The cuspid tooth is extremely long and reaches far into the mandibular bone. Therefore, there is less total bone here than in immediately adjacent areas, and the alveolus of the tooth serves as a line of cleavage for radiating stresses distributed in the area. Additionally, the cuspid's location in the jaw is where a great deal of the mandible's horseshoe-shaped curve is developed. Following blows to the jaw, intense stresses and strains usually accumulate at this curve regardless of their external origin on the jaw.

Fractures at the third molar occur for somewhat similar reasons. This tooth is frequently impacted and as such is situated deeper in the mandible than erupted teeth. Here again tooth is replacing bone, and jaw strength is somewhat weakened by the tooth's presence. Of equal or greater importance in this area is the form of the jaw. Even though the mandible appears horseshoe- or U-shaped from above or below, it is not perfect in this regard. At the posterior limit of the tooth-bearing part of the jaw (the alveolus), the bone flares laterally to join the vertical ramus. A mechanical weakness exists at this abrupt change in the mandible's form. An addition to the problem here is the heavily padded vertical ramus. The lower half of the vertical ramus is well insulated by soft tissue padding of the masseter and internal pterygoid muscle attachments whose anterior borders greet this slightly flared conjoining area of bone to the ramus. The three factors, third molar tooth, change in direction of bone, and exposure at the anterior of a thickly padded portion of the ramus, lead to frequent fractures in this area.

The condylar neck is the thinnest force-supporting part of the mandible. All stresses of mastication or blows to the jaw are eventually radiated to this connecting link with the jaw's fulcrum, the condyle. When the jaw is closed, the condyle lies in the articular fossa. The floor of the articular fossa and the middle cranial fossa share a lamina of relatively thin bone which separates them. However, the articular fossa is rarely fractured regardless of the immensity of jaw trauma as the condylar neck yields to fracture before allowing the condyle to be driven into the middle cranial fossa. The shock-absorbing qualities of the meniscus and other soft tissue lining structures within the temporomandibular joint, of course, contribute to lack of fractures within the joint, but the relatively frail condylar neck is the greatest single safety-valve mechanism preventing fracture of the cranial base at the joint. Thus, in driving blows to the jaw, the last link that prevents frequent cranial injury from the mandible is the condylar neck. It plays its role well as it is probably the most common jaw fracture. Mandibular fractures lead in percentage of occurrence in many reported series, as in those of Dingman (36

percent),[7] Walker (44 percent),[24] and Rowe and Killey (45 percent).[16]

Fractures occur, of course, at any place along the mandible, depending on the variables of direction of force, type of trauma, intensity of trauma, and jaw position at the moment when struck. These fractures are not common about the ramus or coronoid process because of heavy muscle attachments at these areas. Even if the ramus or coronoid process is fractured, it is rarely displaced because of widespread muscle attachments.

Multiple fractures of the mandible occur more than 50 percent of the time. If a fracture is noted at any point along the jaw, the patient and available x-rays should be closely inspected because of the 1 in 2 chance that additional fractures are present. The cause of the multiple fracturing is the contrecoup effect of radiating forces and stresses about the curved bone to a point opposite the area where trauma was received. Common combinations include body (cuspid area) and opposite angle (third molar area), body (cuspid area) and opposite condyle, symphysis and angle (third molar area), and symphysis and condyle.

Most jaw fractures along the tooth-bearing portions are open fractures. Antibiotic coverage is indicated for these contaminated fracture wounds. Antibiotics have greatly lessened the incidence of morbid complications of jaw fractures. Following jaw fracture, bleeding around the neck of a tooth, a detached mucoperiosteal flap behind a second molar, and/or the obvious protrusion of bone into the oral cavity are all fairly reliable signs that the fracture wound opens into the oral cavity's contaminated environment. A fractured end of bone exposed through an overlying cutaneous laceration is an additional obvious indication of a compound wound. Such lacerations should be explored carefully prior to closure as the existing portal to the fracture may be used in the placement of fixation devices.

Ecchymosis in the floor of the mouth is pathognomonic of a mandibular body fracture. Because of the mylohyoid muscle's wide attachment around the entire medial surface of the mandibular body, there is no way that external bruising or ecchymosis can migrate superiorly past the mylohyoid's sealinglike attachment. It prevents this ecchymosis from appearing in the floor of the mouth. Fractures through the mandibular body, even hairline ones, tear periosteum above and below the mylohyoid's attachment. Bleeding or oozing is then allowed to seep into the loose areolar tissue of the floor of the mouth.

Condylar neck fractures present several problems. Beginning with a child or young patient, thought has to be given to the growth potential of the condyle. Of all the growth areas about the jaw, the condyle's cartilaginous cap is the foremost. It compares with an epiphyseal plate in long bones but differs enough to make it a unique growth area. It lacks a bony plate on either side, it never closes or "seals" completely, and it is separated from the articular fossa only by a heavy fibrous covering. Its growth is elaborated in an epiphyseal-like endochondral fashion. Thus, if the condyle is fractured, dislocated, and displaced, the mandible's chief growth mechanism might be considered severely crippled by its malposition.

Clinical and laboratory experience shows, however, that fracture dislocations of the condylar process in the young patient should be managed conservatively.[24] Such treatment may consist of wiring the teeth in occlusion for 10 to 14 days or allowing the patient immediate use of the jaw with no period of immobilization. There is no evidence to indicate that either method is superior to the other. The jaw will shift forward slightly on the fracture side so that the raw ramus stump is opposite the articular eminence and a new arthrosis will form at this point. The slight forward shift of the ramus stump to the articular eminence probably prevents a great immediate loss of ramus height as the ramus is not drawn up into the articular fossa. The medially

displaced condyle resorbs, and a new condylar head forms at the fracture site on the ramus (Fig. 19-3 A–E). Remarkably, a new cartilaginous cap covers this re-formed condyle head. The cartilage is well oriented and apparently contributes to continued growth of the jaw. The total growth scheme is only temporarily disrupted during the condylar re-formation period. This takes 6 to 24 months. Only the slightest shortening of the jaw on the fracture side is produced. Jaw function may be anticipated to be excellent.

Open reduction of these condylar fractures in young patients will also produce excellent results when done well. However, there is no evidence that the patient fares any better than with conservative treatment or that uninterrupted growth of the jaw is enhanced by the procedure.

Fractures which occur quite low on the condylar neck below the sigmoid notch level deserve more aggressive attention than those occurring at a higher level. These low condylar neck fractures with dislocation in the young patient have a great deal less tendency to re-form a condylar head and cartilaginous growth center. For these fractures, open reduction and fixing of the condyle in an upright position are required. There seems to be a gradient in that the lower the fracture of the condylar neck down the ramus with marked dislocation and displacement of the condyle, the less favorable is the prognosis for continued growth or the re-forming of a condyle. Therefore, these low condylar neck fractures require open reduction.

In the adult, fracture dislocation of the condyle can result in foreshortening of the ramus and slight shift of the jaw to the involved side. The great pull of the jaw's closing muscles (masseter, internal pterygoid, temporalis) tends to pull the ramus upward into the space vacated by the displaced condyle. Deviation to the fractured side occurs because the external pterygoid muscle's anterior contractural pull is lost (having ac-

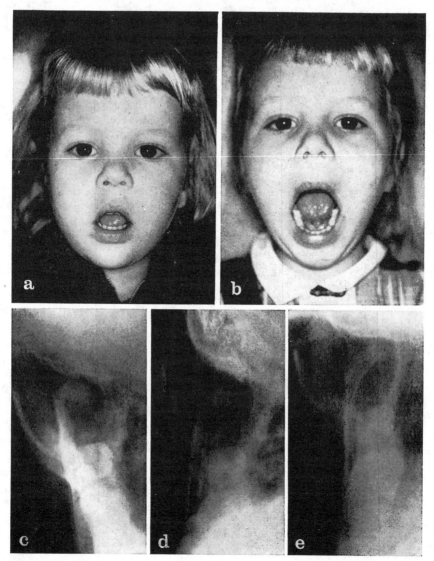

Figure 19-3 Mandibular condyle fracture dislocation caused when a child fell from a tricycle and struck her chin on the curb. *(A)* A 2½-year-old-girl with the jaw held in the most comfortable position following fracture dislocation of the mandibular right condyle. No treatment or immobilization of the jaw was used. *(B)* One year later following the no-treatment regimen. No deviation is seen on widest opening. Occlusion is stable and correctly aligned. *(C)* Transorbital view of fractured and dislocated condyle immediately following injury. *(D)* Transorbital view of condyle 4 weeks later showing rounding and beginning resorption of the fragment. *(E)* Transorbital view 1 year later showing complete resorption of the old condyle fragment and re-formation of a new condylar segment in an upright position. Function is excellent. Growth disturbance is minimal or absent.

companied the condyle to its point of displacement), and the opposite external pterygoid tends to pull the jaw to the side where its antagonist to such pull has been lost. Rather obvious jaw assymmetry is produced which seriously interferes with occlusal relationships. If an adequate number of posterior teeth are in occlusion, simple immobilization of the jaw is indicated for a 4- or 5-week period. The formation of a new arthrosis is anticipated and desired. If there are no opposing posterior teeth on the side of the fracture dislocation, an open reduction and fixing of the condyle in anatomic position are indicated to prevent displacement of the ramus superiorly and the concomitant loss of interocclusal space. Immobilization of the jaw by wiring any remaining teeth in occlusion is indicated. Immobilization has to be maintained for a minimum of 6 weeks since the aim of this treatment is good bony union at the fracture site to prevent relapse of the condyle to a dislocated position. This of course would lead to shortening of the ramus and closure of the intermaxillary freeway space again.

Fractures of the Edentulous Mandible   The edentulous mandible is probably more prone to fracture than the jaw with teeth in it. Edentulous jaw fractures usually occur in older patients, and all bones are more susceptible to fracture as individuals age. After teeth are lost, the alveolar bone resorbs markedly and reduces the overall size of the jaw. Particularly, the vertical depth of the mandibular body is lost, and most fractures of the edentulous mandible occur within this body area. If the intraoral mucoperiosteum is not torn, there often is very little displacement of the fragments. Gentle splinting of the jaw to prevent excessive jaw movement may be all that is necessary to provide satisfactory healing. If pain or discomfort is intolerable, more aggressive immobilization may be necessary.

Some of the most markedly displaced mandibular fractures occur in the edentulous jaw.

Bilateral fractures within the mandibular body which result in tearing of the oral mucoperiosteum are apt to be badly displaced. As these fractures are anterior to the masseter and internal pterygoid muscle attachments, the proximal fragments are drawn far upward and inward. There are no opposing teeth to prevent it. The single distal fragment is subjected to the full contractural pull of the suprahyoid group of muscles. The digastric, geniohyoids, genioglossi, and mylohyoid all tend to tip the symphysis inferiorly. A gaping separation at the fracture sites is thus produced. This patient is apt to be in immediate serious respiratory trouble. Not only is anterior support for the tongue lost, but the excessive traumatic edema and ecchymosis that accompany this fracture are accentuated in the elderly patient because of poor capillary integrity which allows increased permeability and transudation of plasma. Ecchymosis or edema may extend long distances through the loose areolar tissue of the floor of the mouth. The floor of the mouth may be raised by the edema, the tongue may become distended, and the pharyngeal areas may become ecchymotic and engorged (Fig. 19-4A–C).

Immobilization and Fixation for Jaw Fractures   The reasons for stabilizing or immobilizing jaw and facial fractures are no different than those for other skeletal fractures. If the bone is kept relatively still and in correct alignment, it simply heals better and quicker.

When teeth are present and can be wired in occlusion via arch bars or one of the various interdental wiring techniques, immobilizing the mandible is not difficult. The procedure is simple and effective. As a rough rule of thumb, if a fracture occurs within this tooth-bearing area, a closed reduction of the fracture and immobilization of the jaw via interdental wiring is the treatment of choice. If the fracture is proximal to the tooth-bearing area, there is no control of the proximal fragment by interdental wiring. The fragment may be

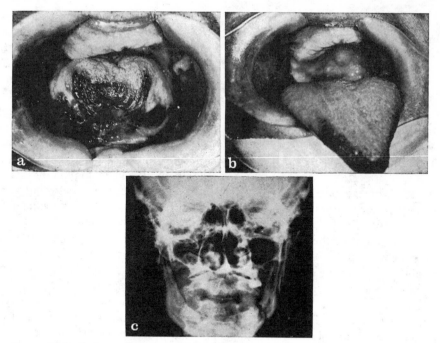

Figure 19-4 Ecchymosis and swelling of the tongue and pharynx in an elderly patient with minimal displacement of mandibular fracture fragments. *(A)* Severe ecchymosis and swelling of the tongue and floor of the mouth secondary to fracture of the left body of the mandible. *(B)* Tongue pulled forward, demonstrating extension of the ecchymosis and swelling of the right pharynx and maxilla secondary to a mandibular right condyle fracture. *(C)* Posteroanterior x-ray view demonstrating the minimally displaced fragments producing the extensive ecchymosis.

significantly displaced by the powerful closing muscles of mastication. Again as a rough rule of thumb, those fractures posterior to the tooth-bearing area generally require an open reduction to control the proximal fragment. There are exceptions, of course.

Open procedures allow direct visualization of the fracture, and precise adjustment of the fragments is therefore possible. Stainless steel wiring placed across the fracture line and secured in holes drilled in both fragments is the easiest method to aid in maintaining the realigned bone. Bone plates are rarely indicated in fixing fragments of the dentulous jaw. Plates, however, are of real value in maintaining fragments of the fractured edentulous mandible.

Fixing or immobilizing fractures of the edentulous jaw can be a problem. Wiring the patient's artificial dentures together in correct occlusion, after securing the lower plate to the mandible by circumferential wiring and the upper plate to the maxilla via peralveolar wiring or circumzygomatic suspension wiring, can provide positive immobilization of the lower jaw. This has been a common and successful method of immobilizing the edentulous lower jaw. If the patient has no dentures, Gunning type splints can be made from impressions of the patient's upper and lower jaws and used in lieu of the dental plates. If these two alternatives are not possible, open reduction of the fracture with secure wiring or plating of the bone ends in good apposition is advisable. An additional method is the placement of pins through the skin into the bone on both sides of the fracture, attaching them firmly together via a series of locking devices of an external skeletal appliance. These devices hold the fragments in alignment and prevent their movement even though the jaw is allowed limited motion. A last alternative is the driving of a Kirschner wire or pin through bone across the fracture site to skewer the fragments in reasonably close apposition. In some hands this method has been widely used with success. The patient enjoys the advantage of being able to open and close the jaw during treatment.

Fracture of the pencil-thin mandible is a particularly tough edentulous jaw fracture to control. Extreme atrophy has diminished the mandibular body size to an inordinately frail wisp of bone that seems to do nothing more than serve as a connector between the two vertical rami. The jaw is too dainty to accommodate the screws of a stainless steel plate without splintering. Stainless steel wiring is inadequate, because there is not enough interface of bone at the fracture site to prevent the fragments telescoping or tilting as the wire is tightened down. Circumferentially wiring a denture or Gunning type splint across the fracture line in the mouth is not always successful, because there usually is an abundance of hyperplastic and hypertrophied tissue overlying these ridges. The thickness of this tissue prevents good adaptation of the denture or splint to the ridge and allows movement of the bone ends regardless of how well and secure the wires seem to be placed. The tiny fragments are hard to skewer with Kirschner wires or pins.

Extraoral skeletal control of mandibular fractures using stainless steel pins, usually two on each side of the fracture, and a connecting acrylic bar has been useful in maintaining fragments in proper position. This biphasic system has been useful in comminuted fractures and long-term fixation. Accurate placement and securing of the pins, however,

is difficult. Placing a rib graft or iliac crest bone with both cortices intact across the fracture site should receive consideration. The graft can be bound to the bone by circumferential wires at a distance from the fracture. The graft itself offers support and splinting for the fracture.[19]

As evidenced by the multiple treatment modalities suggested, there is no 100 percent positively effective method for stabilizing the edentulous fragments. The need of each situation must be kept objectively in mind. Adapt the technique that will best control the variables of fracture displacement, the size of the fracture fragments, the patient's psyche, and the patient's morphologic makeup.

THE ZYGOMA

The zygoma articulates with the frontal, maxillary, and temporal bones rather superficially and with the greater wing of the sphenoid in a deeper plane. It is the prominent "cheekbone" and helps form the lateral and inferior orbital rims. The eye's lateral canthal ligament, continuing medially as the orbital suspensory ligament, attaches to the zygoma's frontal process. Additionally, the zygoma contributes to the floor of the orbit laterally and anteriorly and forms a large part of the antral roof. The temporalis muscle passes beneath it for attachment to the mandible. On opening and closing and in lateral excursive movements of the jaw, the coronoid process moves freely beneath the zygoma. This firmly attached bone, when markedly fractured and displaced, can thus alter facial symmetry and ocular, mandibular, or antral function. Its prominent facial position leads to frequent fracture and the several altered conditions listed.

The usual direction of displacement is inward, downward, and posteriorly with a separation occurring at the zygomaticofrontal suture and a step defect occurring along the infraorbital rim. A separation and slight inward displacement may occur along the zygomatic arch. A portion of the body may be impacted into the underlying antrum. Comminution of its orbital floor extension and along its long interface with the maxilla is not uncommon.

Common clinical signs of fracture of the zygoma may include:[16]

1 Flatness of the usually rounded cheek area

2 Limited mandibular movements (secondary to direct mechanical impingement of the coronoid process or myospasm of the temporalis)

3 Anesthesia of the cheek, ala of the nose, upper lip, and gingiva (secondary to fracturing at the infraorbital foramen)

4 Unilateral nosebleed (bleeding into the antrum by the fracture drains into the nose via the maxillary ostium)

5 Altered vision (eye position changed by enlarged orbit as the zygoma is depressed—diplopia is very common)

6 Circumorbital and subconjunctival ecchymosis

7 Intraoral tenderness and unevenness at the zygomatic process of the maxilla (upper first molar area)

8 Palpable step defects along the infraorbital rim and at the zygomaticofrontal attachment area

Reduction and Fixation   Acute fractures of the zygoma usually may be reduced without great difficulty. Many fractured zygomas snap into position with a positive click when raised to a reduced position. This indicates that very little tissue was interposed in the fracture lines and the bone was allowed to key sharply into its normal position. The bone tends to stay securely in the reduced position following such a reduction. If the zygoma tends to migrate from a reduced position immediately following its adjustment, soft tissue probably is interposed at some area along the fracture lines and needs to be manually moved or

reduced to its usual position. This requires visualization via an open approach. The areas which commonly require this maneuver are the separations occurring at the zygomaticofrontal suture and the zygomaticomaxillary suture along the infraorbital rim.

A convenient technique for controlling the bone during manipulation is by grasping the zygoma via a firmly seated Carroll-Girard screw driven into the heaviest portion of the body. It allows positive bone control for moving the zygoma in any direction during adjustment of the bone. A stab incision made directly over the heaviest palpable part of the zygoma permits a small hole to be started in the bone with a No. 6 dental burr. The Carroll-Girard screw may also be inserted through the infraorbital incision when one is made, thus eliminating the need for the stab incision over the zygomatic bone. The larger diameter screw is then inserted into this starter hole and turned 3 or 4 times until a firm purchase between screw and bone is established. The extended part of the screw has a T bar attached at the outer end for grasping the instrument. The firmly anchored screw furnishes a handle to the bone which permits the zygoma to be manipulated in any required direction (Fig. 19-5A–D). Directions of movement are not limited, as occurs when various devices are inserted beneath the zygoma for levering. With levering, outward and upward movements are the principal directions possible. Placement of the screw takes only 1 or 2 min. The technique is useful for closed or open procedures. Frequently, the simple lifting of the zygoma is all that is required, and the total operative procedure can be completed in a very few minutes. If open operation is required, the screw lends itself well to continuous control and support of the bone during the various hole-drilling maneuvers at the parts needing supplemental wire fixation.

Exposure of the zygomaticofrontal suture line may be gained via an incision approxi-

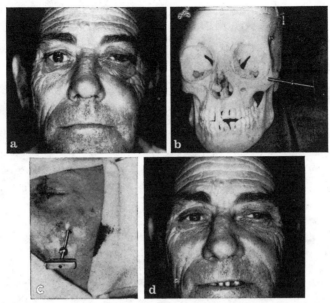

Figure 19-5 Simple depressed fracture of the left zygoma caused by a blow with a fist: *(A)* Immediate postinjury view of the patient, showing flatness at the malar eminence area. *(B)* Skull showing a Carroll-Girard screw anchored in the heaviest part of the body of the zygoma for easy manipulation of the bone. *(C)* Patient with the screw inserted percutaneously into the left zygoma. *(D)* Postoperative view of the patient with symmetry restored to the flat side of the face by reducing the zygoma.

mately 2 cm long made directly over the articulation. The incision parallels the fibers of the orbicularis oculi and usually extends into the lateral part of the eyebrow. However, the eyebrow is *not* shaved. Good control of the markedly displaced or rotated zygoma can be achieved by wiring the frontal process of the zygoma snugly to the zygomatic process of the frontal bone. This bone is secure and is not generally fractured other than at the point where the zygoma has become disarticulated from it. Holes are drilled through each of these bony processes about 0.5 cm from the fracture line. The holes are directed into the orbit, but the orbital contents are protected by an elevator placed subperiosteally on the orbital side. A 24- or 26-gauge stainless steel wire may be used to fix the two parts together. The wire is passed laterally through the lower hole. This may be attached to a doubled 32-gauge wire passed through the upper hole. The medial ends of the heavier and lighter wires should next be attached to one another. The heavier wire then can be drawn up through the medial opening of the upper hole by the lighter wire to complete the wiring directly across the fracture line.

The sequence of wire passage is practical, because the greatest pull is needed in drawing the 26-gauge wire belayed to the 32-gauge wire from the inaccessible medial side to the outer side. Since the 32-gauge wire is threaded through the hole in the zygomatic process of the frontal bone, great traction can be made against this fixed point. By reversing the order in wire placement, the traction would be placed against the zygoma which is already quite movable because of the fracture. It is not desirable to create extra motion or displacement in an already well-traumatized area.

The zygoma may then be manipulated into position with the Carroll-Girard screw. Twisting the 24- or 26-gauge wire tightly down to bone furnishes secure fixation as there is a broad interface of bone in this area that prevents rotation of the bone even with the one-wire fixation.

Exposure of the infraorbital rim and floor of the orbit is generally made via an infraciliary incision or one in the most superior natural crease of the lower lid. Less scarring and possible binding down of the incision to the underlying bone may be anticipated by one of these approaches. Exposure of the bony rim is made under the skin muscle flap dissection. Incising of the periosteum overlying the inferior orbital rim is done below the attachment of the septum orbital to prevent herniation of the orbital fat into the surgical field. Bone of the orbital rim itself is fairly heavy, but bone of the orbital floor and anterior maxillary wall is quite thin and friable. Wiring in this area, therefore, is slightly different from areas where broad surfaces of bone can be brought together. Advantage has to be taken of the rim because this is the only bone of integrity in the area. A figure-of-eight wiring across the fracture line and the inferior orbital margin offers the best support. Holes should be drilled on both sides of the fracture from the anterior wall of the maxilla directed in a slightly superior and posterior direction. These holes may be controlled to come out on the same side of the fracture in the orbital floor as the side on which they were started. The holes pass through the superior part of the underlying antrum, which is of no consequence, and beneath the inferior orbital margins. A 24- or 26-gauge wire may be passed through these holes in a figure-of-eight fashion and twisted tight. This lashes these parts together far more securely than lighter-gauge wire passed directly across the fracture but anchored in thin bone.

Antral Packing Supporting the fractured zygoma by antral packing is a long-established and acceptable method of controlling the bone's reduced position. It is a particularly useful technique when there is extensive comminuting of the body of the zygoma or orbital floor.

The antrum may be approached via an incision along the buccal sulcus in the mouth. A generous mucoperiosteal flap should be raised to expose the entire anterior antral wall. Removal of bone comprising the anterior antral wall should not be difficult as fractures of the zygoma frequently radiate across the anterior maxilla. Even if the wall is intact, a chisel or burr can be used to start a hole into the antrum safely above the roots of the teeth. Enlargement of the opening may be done with chisels, but Kirschner back-biting rongeur forceps give greater control and are more convenient for this maneuver. After widening the window sufficiently to allow insertion of a forefinger or blunt instrument, the multiple small fracture fragments can be molded into place along the orbital floor and infraorbital rim, and the larger part of the body of the zygoma can be lifted into correct position. A space-occupying pack within the antrum is necessary to maintain the reduced fragments in place. A continuous strip of ribbon gauze (preferably a plastic gauze such as Adaptic) should be systematically wound and built up within the antrum with a free end left outward to allow its eventual easy removal (Fig. 19-6 A–E). The appearance and hygiene of the antrum determine whether this free end is trailed out through the nasal cavity or the oral cavity. If the antral membrane is grayish and friable and has several polyps attached to it, a chronic sinusitis probably exists and some provision should be made to adequately drain and irrigate the antrum after removal of the pack. A window or antrostomy should, therefore, be established in the medial wall of the

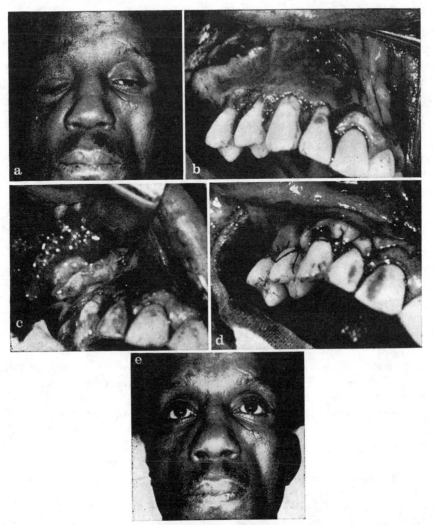

Figure 19-6 Badly displaced and comminuted fracture of the right zygoma caused by a blow from a bottle across the right face. *(A)* Preoperative view of the patient showing flatness and loss of symmetry to the right face. *(B)* Intraorally, a generous mucoperiosteal flap raised from the height of the buccal sulcus or from around the necks of the teeth allows exposure of the anterior maxillary wall and fracture of the zygoma. *(C)* Enlarging a hole in the antral wall permits the comminuted fragments of the zygoma to be reduced and maintained in a corrected position with a space-occupying pack within the antrum. *(D)* The trailing end of the antral pack may be led from the antrum through a stab incision in the overlying mucoperiosteal flap as in this case. The mucoperiosteal flap should be sutured back in position. Hygiene of the antrum determines whether the antral pack is led from antrum via the oral cavity or through an opening beneath the inferior turbinate in the nasal cavity. *(E)* Postoperative view of the patient with the zygoma in a corrected position.

antrum that opens anteriorly in the nasal fossa beneath the inferior turbinate. The end of the antral pack should be led out through this nasal opening. If the antral membrane is pink, shiny, and healthy, good antral hygiene probably prevails, and there is little need to establish an additional bony opening for postoperative antral drainage. The end of the antral pack may be led into the oral cavity through a stab incision made in the mucoperiosteal flap that overlies the anterior maxillary wall. The pack should be left in the antrum for 10 to 14 days. It is removed by whatever route the end was trailed from the antrum. Whichever exit was used, the pack is easily drawn from the antrum through either the intraoral stab incision overlying the antral wall or the nasal antrostomy without great discomfort to the patient. Daily sterile saline solution irrigations through the intraoral stab incision are desirable for 3 or 4 days after the pack has been removed. The opening will close over and heal quite rapidly, and the orifice usually will not be patent for much longer than these 3 or 4 days. The diseased antrum should be irrigated for 7 to 10 days through the nasal window following removal of the pack.

Although open reductions and the direct wiring of bone are much in favor at the moment, antral packing still has much to offer in the management of fractured zygomas and other midface fractures.

Orbital Floor Fractures

Loss of the orbital floor through extensive comminuting of zygomaticomaxillary complex fractures and the unique "blowout" fracture have received recent wide attention. The floor offers support to much of the orbital soft tissue, and if its continuity is destroyed or markedly displaced, the position of the eye is changed. If the orbital soft tissue is not returned to a normal position and the floor is not repaired, ocular function can be seriously altered and a cosmetic blemish produced. The globe of the eye is lowered. Soft tissue including the inferior extraocular muscles may be trapped in the defect. If left unattended, some degree of diplopia is virtually ensured and ocular motility will be seriously impaired. As healing progresses, fat atrophy and maturing of the fibrous healing have a tendency to draw the eye inward and downward, thus increasing the original deficiency.

The true blowout fracture of the orbit occurs with a sudden increase in intraorbital pressure. The fractures occur at weak areas of the bony structure of the orbit. The resulting blowout is a result of the hydraulic pressure of soft tissues on the weak areas of the bony orbit. In the true blowout fracture, the orbital margin and zygomatic complex remain intact. The trauma which produces this type of injury is blunt and is directed at the globe and lids. The injury is usually caused by a fist, large ball, or some other nonpenetrating object which is slightly larger than the orbital inlet.[6]

The other type of orbital floor fracture which occurs is not a blowout in the true sense of the word. In this type there is severe comminution of the orbital floor as a result of telescoping of the strong bony structure of the inferior orbital rim. This fracture is usually a part of the zygomaticomaxillary complex type which involves the infraorbital rim.

The orbit is a pyramidal-shaped space with contributions from seven bones entering into the formation of its walls. These bones are the frontal, zygomatic, sphenoid, palatine, ethmoid, lacrimal, and maxillary. The floor of the orbit is directly in a line of weakness of the Le Fort type II fracture. The anterior half of the orbital floor is extremely thin and is further weakened by the infraorbital groove or canal. The floor is partially formed anteriorly by the orbital surface of the maxilla, laterally and anteriorly by the zygoma, and medially and posteriorly by the palatine bone. The floor gently slopes upward toward the medial wall. The lamina papyracea of the ethmoid bone which makes up a large portion of the orbit's medial wall is another area of great fragility.[9,15]

Radiographic Findings A true blowout fracture of the orbit may be missed without a careful radiographic and clinical examination. The Waters' view, stereoscopic Waters' view, and laminograms, when coupled with clinical examination, are useful in diagnosing orbital floor fractures.

The roentgen findings in blowout fractures may indicate: (1) protrusion of orbital soft tissue into the maxillary sinus, (2) fragmentation of the orbital floor with depression of bony fragments, (3) fracture of the medial orbital wall with protrusion of orbital soft tissue into the ethmoid air cell area, and (4) emphysema of the orbit.[14]

The bony fragments of the fractured floor may be seen as a depressed, irregular, semilunar mass superimposed over the upper one-half of the maxillary sinus. This mass may represent bony fragments and soft tissue or just soft tissue alone. The protrusion of soft tissue alone may represent a trapdoor-type fracture of the orbital floor. In this case the sudden increase in intraorbital pressure causes the bone fragment to become displaced enough to allow protrusion of the orbital fat. However, after the soft tissue has been expelled, the bony fragment snaps back into an approximately normal position. The extruded soft tissue is trapped in the maxillary sinus by a three-sided crack in the bony floor. This hinged bony lid is kept wedged slightly open in a downward position because of the soft tissue between its edges. This herniated soft tissue will appear as an opaque gray to white soft tissue density on the radiograph (Fig. 19-7).

There may be masking of a blowout fracture in chronically diseased maxillary sinuses or in cases of massive hemorrhage into the maxillary sinus.[6]

Clinical Signs and Symptoms Enophthalmos, diplopia, impaired ocular motility, infraorbital nerve anesthesia or hypothesia, periorbital edema and ecchymosis, subconjunctival hemorrhage, and periorbital emphysema are helpful signs in the clinical diagnosis of blowout fractures. The signs and symptoms vary, of course, with the length of time between injury and when the patient is first seen.

Enophthalmos usually occurs after the edema or ecchymosis has resolved. It occurs because (1) the orbital fat is now contained in a much larger cavity and cannot support the eye in its normal position, (2) scar formation may pull the remaining orbital soft tissue posteriorly and inferiorly, and (3) periorbital fat atrophy occasionally occurs.

Diplopia is another significant finding in the blowout fracture. It may occur immediately following injury or may appear after the edema has subsided.

Impaired motility of the eyeball may result from: (1) herniation of orbital soft tissues into the antrum, (2) direct trauma to the inferior oblique and inferior rectus muscles, (3) scar tissue partially or completely immobilizing the eye in certain movements (usually a late occurrence), or (4) direct trauma resulting in motor nerve injury to the extraocular muscles.[17]

Treatment The objectives in treating comminuted orbital floor fractures are: (1) correction of enophthalmos, (2) relief of restricted extraocular muscle function because of incarceration by bony or soft tissue, (3) elevation of the lowered eye, and (4) correction of diplopia.

The two principal methods of treating orbital floor fractures are: (1) maxillary sinus packing and (2) orbital floor reconstruction.[3,4] In some cases both approaches may be found useful and necessary to obtain the best possible result.

Historically, control of the multiple small

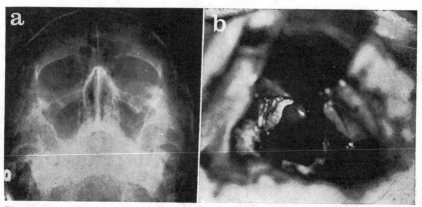

Figure 19-7 Classic example of a blowout fracture of the orbit caused by a ball striking the patient directly over the orbit. *(A)* Waters' view x-ray showing intact bony rims of both orbits. An opaque rounded gray mass hanging beneath the left infraorbital ridge in the antrum furnishes a hint as to the true extent of the orbital damage. *(B)* Direct visualization of the herniated orbital soft tissue hanging in the superior part of the maxillary sinus seen through a large intraoral antral opening.

fragments comprising the orbital floor has been achieved via an antral approach. Through an opening made in the anterior maxillary sinus wall, the fragments can be molded back to a reasonably normal position and then maintained with an antral pack or some other space-occupying material. This approach gives limited visual access to the orbital floor, but the technique is still an excellent method for treating the injury.

A great deal of attention currently is directed to approaching the orbital floor wound from the inferior orbital margin route. The approach is precisely the same as that used for wiring infraorbital ridge fractures. By this approach a defect in the floor can be easily visualized for lifting the orbital contents back within the orbital confines. After evaluating the size of the orbital floor defect, a disk-shaped material may be fashioned to the desired form and fitted over the opening in much the same manner as a manhole cover plugs a hole in the street (Fig. 19-8*A–B*). Homogenous and autogenous grafts of bone, cartilage, and fascia lata have been used to cover these orbital floor defects. Alloplasts of tantalum mesh, acrylic, Teflon, polyethylene, and

Silastic are all currently popular and are used for the same purpose. Silastic seems to be the most desirable alloplast from many standpoints. It can be sterilized by autoclave, is inert, does not warp, can be cut and shaped at the time of the surgical procedure, and can be used to cover defects of unlimited size. Importantly, it saves the patient extra surgical treatment and anesthesia time by eliminating the need for taking the patient's own bone.

The alloplastic implant should be placed subperiosteally on edges of bone on both sides of the floor defect. Judgment is needed in deciding on the particular thickness and size of each implant. The periosteum should be resutured with care at the infraorbital rim as this closes the fracture wound and furnishes immobilization for the alloplast. Muscle, subcutaneous, and skin layers may then be closed in their usual order.

FRACTURES OF THE MIDDLE THIRD OF THE FACIAL SKELETON

Fracture detachments of the maxillas and/or associated bones are designated as fractures of the middle third of the facial skeleton and

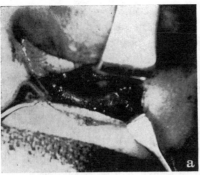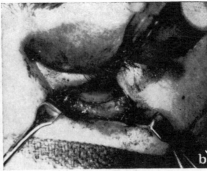

Figure 19-8 Orbital floor blowout fracture treated by placing a Silastic implant over the floor defect. *(A)* Orbital floor visualized via an inferior orbital rim approach. Broad flat Army-Navy retractor is placed subperiosteally and lifts the eye during adjustments of the orbital floor. *(B)* Silastic implant carved and fitted over the floor defect.

are commonly referred to as midface fractures. The region extends on a horizontal plane from the two zygomaticofrontal suture lines across the frontomaxillary and frontonasal sutures downward to the incisal and occlusal plane of the teeth.[16]

Detachment of any midface bone or combinations of midface bones may produce a painful and annoying flail at the point of detachment, or the bones may become rigidly impacted and difficult to reduce.

The separated midface fracture may vary from a horizontal detachment of the maxilla at the level of the floor of the nasal fossa (called a Le Fort type I fracture) to all combinations of facial segments above this arbitrary line. A common, severe, in-between segmental fracture of the midface is termed a pyramidal fracture and is frequently designated as the Le Fort type II fracture. The whole central region of the face including the maxilla, half of the antrum, medial half of the infraorbital ridge, medial portion of the orbit and orbital floor, nasal fossa, and nasal bones is violently torn from the cranial base.

The classic end of this scale in detachment of the facial bony skeleton is the total craniofacial disjunction, the Le Fort type III fracture. This massive injury includes detachment of both zygomas, the maxillas, nasal bones, ethmoids, vomer, and all lesser facial bones from the cranial base. The face sags and presents an elongated aspect. Many of the bones are extensively comminuted and displaced. Airway, bone, drainage ducts, occlusion, spinal fluid leaks, and ocular support all become involved in the shifting, tearing, and mangling of tissue. Such a complex injury requires considerable ingenuity and judgment in the final realigning, fixing, and repair. There can be unilateral or bilateral involvement with all combinations of these segmental fracture patterns.

The facial bony skeleton has to be reestablished in a nearly symmetric and normal attitude. The logical course to follow in repair of these wounds begins with the mandible. Mandibular fractures, if they exist concomitant to the facial fractures, have to be properly aligned and stabilized first. Open reductions and direct bony wiring may be required to establish a rather firm mandible and occlusal table against which to build. If the mandible escapes being fractured by the blow which smashes the midface, the job is easier. Once a relatively rigid mandible is established, the level of the midface fracture is determined and everything is rebuilt from the mandible up to this level and fixed to the first stable bone superiorly. The maxilla or multiple maxillary segments are brought forward, and the maxillary and mandibular teeth are fitted together in occlusion. A functional chewing table is thus established, but in so doing much of the maxilla and many of the bone fragments attached to it are drawn into a corrected and anterior position. A fair appraisal of the correct anterior position for midface can be estimated from these initial adjustments.

Most cases of a horizontally detached maxilla at the level of the nasal fossa floor are handled satisfactorily by the simple expedient of wiring the teeth in occlusion. There is nothing fancy about this procedure, but it is highly effective. If there is great comminution along the fracture lines and the maxilla is difficult to stabilize, all bony structures cephalad to this level are solid and can be used to attach fixation wires or appliances. After the teeth are wired in occlusion, the attached unit of maxilla and mandible can be moved vertically to the desired facial position. Suspension wiring can be utilized to secure the mandible in this position during the period of fracture healing (Fig. 19-9*A–D)*. The suspension wires may be attached bilaterally to the lateral walls of the nasal fossa or to the infraorbital rim. They may also be looped around the zygoma (circumzygomatic wiring) (Fig. 19-9*D)* or secured directly to the maxillary process of the zygoma. The cortical bone at the lateral wall of the nasal fossa or along the infraorbital rim is adequate to support a suspension wire. After attachment to a secure bone above the fracture, the wires on both sides are drawn into the oral cavity and attached to the mandibular arch bar. The mandible should then be anchored in the position deemed appropriate for the occlusal plane of the teeth. This fracture does not commonly produce great disturbance to the nasal airway or air movement as it is at the lowest part of the nasal fossa. However, there will be varying degrees of nasal mucosal edema and ecchymosis. Therefore, thought has to be given to the airway as it is

liable to become compromised by this edema or by possible hematoma formation.

Problems of pyramidal and complete craniofacial disjunction type fractures will be discussed jointly because they both share common severe complicating features. The immense and savage trauma required to rip these whole facial segments from the cranial base leaves complex and intricate damage. A thoroughly plugged airway, distorted and torn nasolacrimal drainage apparatus, collapsed maxillary antrums, cracks in the cranial base leaking cerebrospinal fluid, minced orbital floors, mangled canthal attachments, and splintered and separated segments of dental occlusion all suddenly loom as taxing facets of the repair picture.

The compromised airway and the crack at the cranial base allowing the cerebrospinal fluid leak are the injuries most likely to produce early complications. As stated earlier, about one out of every two patients with middle face fractures involving the nasal passages requires a tracheostomy. The incidence is higher as the extensiveness and comminution about the nasal fossa increase. These massive disarticulations fall into this category. Even though the patient may not require immediate airway help because of a propped-open mouth, a tracheostomy is indicated as soon as these facets of the injury have been assessed. This will make respiration easier during the acute early phases of the injury, and it provides a convenient route for the administration of anesthesia when facial repairs are made.

Cerebrospinal Fluid Rhinorrhea Cerebrospinal fluid rhinorrhea is a common complicating feature of severe midface trauma. Blunt trauma received directly in the midface causes shearing, telescoping, or impacting of the bones in the interorbital area along the cranial base. Fractures of the sphenoid sinus or more frequently through the ethmoid's cribriform

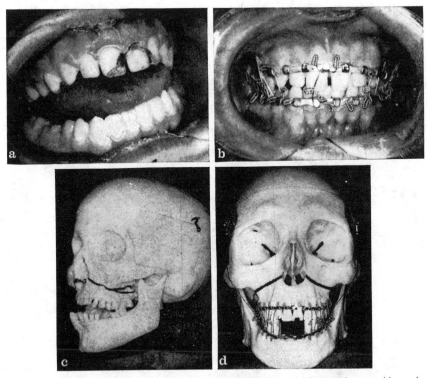

Figure 19-9 A transverse fracture of the maxilla (Le Fort type I fracture) caused by a sharp blow with the heavy end of a pool cue stick across the lower midface. *(A)* Preoperative view of the maxilla tilted superiorly at the front and displaced posteriorly, resulting in premature occluding of the molar teeth. The mouth is thus propped open. *(B)* Postoperative view of the realigned maxilla into proper occlusion. The mandible is immobilized via circumzygomatic wires seen entering the oral cavity at the highest point of the mucobuccal fold on both sides. *(C)* The Le Fort type I fracture reproduced on a skull, demonstrating the posterior displacement of the maxilla, the premature occluding of the molar teeth, and the anterior open bite. *(D)* Demonstration of the reduced fracture and fixation appliances on a skull. The scheme of the circumzygomatic suspension wires may be noted.

plate lead to dural tear and a spinal fluid leak.[13] Less frequently the leak comes from a fracture of the posterior wall of the frontal sinus. The dura overlying the sphenoid sinus and particularly the cribriform plate is tightly adherent and tears easily. In childhood the dura is more loosely attached in these areas and is not so readily torn as in skull fractures of adults.[1] Cerebrospinal fluid rhinorrhea occurs in about 25 to 30 percent of patients with fractures involving the interorbital area (Figs. 19-10A, 19-11A, 19-12).[10,24]

Diagnosis In cases of nasal, facial, or skull trauma, almost any persistent thin nasal drainage should be looked at suspiciously and considered to be cerebrospinal fluid rhinorrhea until proved otherwise.

Roentgenographic studies are usually inconclusive and not always helpful. However, in some cases air may be seen intracranially, and air in the cranium indicates an anterior fracture and dural tear or a fracture of one of the paranasal sinuses.[10] Bending the head forward, compressing the jugular veins, or having

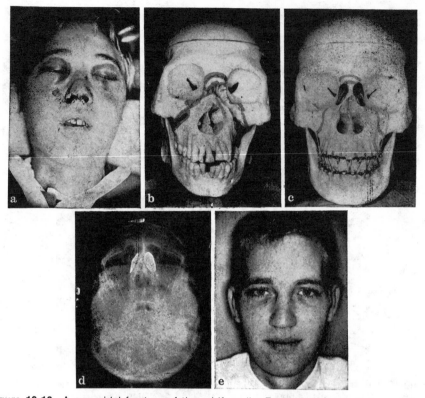

Figure 19-10 A pyramidal fracture of the midface (Le Fort type II fracture) caused by an automobile accident. *(A)* Preoperative view of the patient, showing open-mouth attitude caused by posterior tilting of the whole midfacial bony segment, widening of the interorbital area caused by fracturing and outward splaying of the interorbital bones, thin, watery nasal discharge suggesting cerebrospinal fluid rhinorrhea, and extensive circumorbital ecchymosis—all characteristic of extensive midface fractures. *(B)* Skull with fractures demonstrating the pyramidal type fractures incurred by the patient. *(C)* Demonstration of the reduced fractures and fixation appliances on a skull. The scheme or suspension wires attached to an intact inferior orbital margin and the lower arch bar may be noted. Crimping and fixing the interorbital bones medially and upwardly in correct position is demonstrated, using malleable lead plates. *(D)* Postoperative Waters' view x-ray depicting the appearance of the appliances in place and the alignment that may be maintained. *(E)* Postoperative appearance of the patient.

the patient strain all increase intracranial pressure and speed up the rate of flow—but these maneuvers are not recommended to confirm a cerebrospinal fluid leak. If there is a persistent nasal discharge, consider it as spinal fluid and proceed with treatment.

Large doses of antibiotics should be started immediately on becoming suspicious of or confirming a cerebrospinal fluid leak. Patients with cerebrospinal fluid rhinorrhea should not have the upper nasal passages packed as an aid in maintaining fragments following reduction unless there is a life-endangering hemorrhage that cannot be controlled otherwise. Even though such packs aid in the control of small fragments, the tamponading effect hinders the flow of all fluids and secretions from this area. Open drainage is one of the best methods of preventing infection in the midface. If damming up occurs high in the nasal

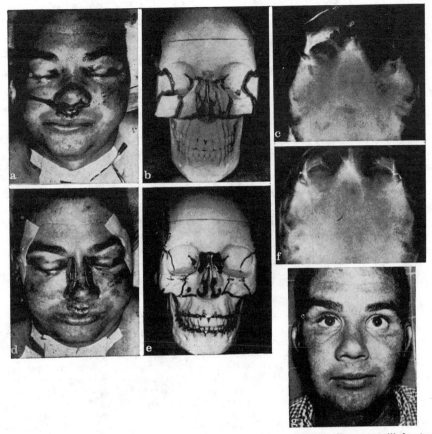

Figure 19-11 Patient with complete craniofacial disjunction (Le Fort type III fracture) caused by an automobile accident. *(A)* Preoperative view of tracheotomized patient showing typical widespread facial edema, widened and flattened interorbital area, and thin, watery nasal discharge. *(B)* Patient's extensiveLe Fort type III fractures reproduced on skull. *(C)* Preoperative Waters' view x-ray demonstrating disarticulation and separation on the various facial bones involved. *(D)* Immediate postoperative appearance of the patient. *(E)* Scheme of the fixation and wiring appliances utilized to secure the multiple fractures. Suspension wires extend from both zygomatic processes of the frontal bone to the lower arch bar, thus supporting the comminuted facial skeleton between the mandible and cranial base. Thin Silastic orbital floor implants have been inserted to occlude the orbital floor defects. Direct wiring of the separated segments along the infraorbital rim and at the zygomaticofrontal suture lines has been done. Maintenance of the interorbital skeletal framework has been secured by the lead plates and transnasal wiring after the bones were lifted and molded to a corrected position. *(F)* Postoperative Waters' view x-ray showing the realigned and wired facial skeleton. *(G)* Follow-up appearance of the patient with suspension wires still in place.

vault, the propagation of virulent organisms even higher via this convenient pabulum becomes a hazard that need not be provided.

A key aid to stopping cerebrospinal fluid rhinorrhea is to reduce and fix the multiple facial fractures as early as possible. Since the whole central unit of the midface is detached, it moves with each swallowing effort, during attempted phonation, and when the mandible is closed against the maxillary teeth. The

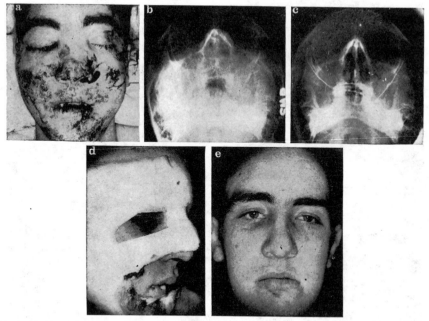

Figure 19-12 Greatly widened and flattened interorbital area secondary to large laterally splayed fracture segments. *(A)* Preoperative view of patient with craniofacial disjunction, Interorbital area is flattened and widened. *(B)* Preoperative Waters' view x-rays showing splayed interorbital bones in addition to the other Le Fort type III fractures. *(C)* Postoperative Waters' view x-ray showing the realigned interorbital bones which were held in place by the plaster strips demonstrated in Fig. 19-12*D.* *(D)* Following the lifting and reduction of larger and less comminuted nasoorbital segments, passage of a transnasal wire may be difficult. Fixation and control of the segments may then be achieved by using narrow, dampened plaster strips which are molded over the frontal, nasal, and cheek areas and allowed to harden as demonstrated. *(E)* Follow-up appearance of the patient with narrowed interorbital area and built-up nasal bridge.

movement is transferred to the fracture line and many times acts in a ball-valve manner at this point to perpetuate the flow. Securing the facial skeleton prevents this movement.

Elevating the patient's head approximately 40 to 60° above the horizontal also contributes to an early cessation of cerebrospinal fluid flow by allowing tissue on the cephalad side of the fracture to rest on or herniate into the dehiscence. This mechanical plugging probably hastens fibrous healing across the defect on both the caudad and cephalad sides. The patient should be instructed to avoid nose blowing, sneezing, and coughing.[23] Cessation of the cerebrospinal fluid flow may be antici-

pated in 5 to 12 days following fixation and securing of the facial skeleton.

The patient with cerebrospinal fluid rhinorrhea should be watched carefully for a minimum of 48 h. The patient can have insidiously slow bleeding from an intracranial vessel and not manifest the usual increasing blood pressure, slowing pulse, and slowing respiration to indicate a building cranial mass lesion. These clinical signs are absent because the cerebrospinal fluid leak maintains decompression of the brain while the hemorrhage continues. No indication of an increase in intracranial pressure is given. Such a situation may result in sudden and unexpected death. For this reason the patient requires close attention for at least the first 48 h and at cessation of the cerebrospinal fluid flow.[12]

Fracturing across the "bridge" of the nose which is damaging enough to produce cerebrospinal fluid flow usually causes extensive comminution in the interorbital area (Figs. 19-10A, B, 19-11A, B, 19-12). These fractures are frequently called nasoorbital fractures. The small bones deep behind the nasal bones and the frontal processes of the maxillas are not of great substance and easily splay outward and laterally or telescope inwardly under immediate influence of the trauma. Secondarily, the small comminuted fragments may tend to migrate laterally. With its bony anchorage destroyed, the medial canthal ligament lacks resistance to the slight lateral pull of the orbicularis oculi, and the globe of the eye is allowed to shift laterally. The intercanthal distance is thus widened (Figs. 19-10A, 19-11A, 19-12A, 19-13A). The triad of a widened nasal bridge, an increased intercanthal distance, and ocular hypertelorism with the eyes far apart are the clinical signs associated with nasoorbital fractures. If these injuries are not recognized and repaired early, they become an exceedingly difficult and sometimes impossible secondary repair.

The crippled interorbital area may be corrected by judicious intranasal manipulation of the multiple small bones in an upward and forward direction and molding them across the interorbital area between the thumb and forefinger. A blunt instrument should be used intranasally. The reduced fragments should be fixed by crimping them between a nonyielding material that will prevent the fragments from collapsing in a lateral direction. Lead plates contoured to the medial canthal areas and secured by a through-and-through transnasal 24- or 26-gauge stainless steel wire mattress suture is a suggested method (Figs. 19-10C and D, 19-11C and D). The wire mattress suture should pass beneath or through the frontal

processes of both maxillas to help hold these important structures up and forward. It may occasionally be impossible to pass the wire suture as described. Small holes should then be drilled through the frontal processes of the maxillas to accommodate passage of the wire. In many instances direct wiring of the medical canthal ligaments to the anterior lacrimal crest of the lacrimal bone will be needed to prevent rounding of the medial portion of the palpebral fissure. In addition to direct wiring of nasal bones to each other, the frontal process of the maxilla or frontal bone may be indicated to reconstruct the interorbital area. This is done with 24- or 26-gauge wire with proper placement of small intraosseous holes. The approach may be through a vertical midline incision or an H-shape incision over the nasal bridge. In most instances nasal plates are used in addition to the direct wiring procedure to secure the realigned nasoorbital skeleton. A suggested compromise technique is the use of dampened narrow orthopedic plaster strips which are contoured to the repaired interorbital form and are allowed to set. When properly placed, the hardened plaster effectively retains the reduction.[24]

Reestablishment of a patent nasal airway can usually be accomplished during the various molding maneuvers necessary to raise, align, mold, and fix the injuries across the interorbital area. A blunt forceps or instrument carried along the floor of the nasal fossa until it passes the posterior choanae is a help in gently repositioning comminuted fragments bulging into the nasal cavity. The bones that make up this posterior oval opening—the horizontal plate of the palatine bone, the posterior free border of the vomer, the medial plate of the sphenoid's pterygoid process, and the inferior surface of the body of the sphenoid bone—are not situated for convenient visual inspection. Molding them into the desired position is, therefore, a blind procedure and largely dependent on the operator's tactile

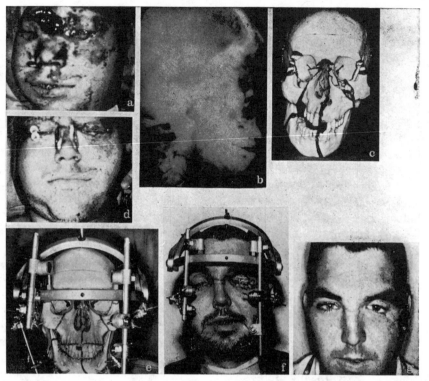

Figure 19-13 Massive comminution, disarticulation, and shearing to one side of the facial skeleton. *(A)* Preoperative view of torn and mangled face. *(B)* Preoperative lateral x-ray view of facial skeleton showing the bony parts dangling from the cranial base. *(C)* Fractures reproduced on demonstration skull. Comminution of the facial bone at all articulations with the cranial base are important complicating features that make immobilization of the parts difficult. *(D)* Immediate surgical repairs consisted of reestablishing the normal occlusion, doing an open reduction at the right angle of the mandible, rebuilding the nasal and interorbital area with fragments of bone in the area, closing the extensive high midface laceration, and enucleating the partially avulsed left eye. *(E)* Skull depicting the cranial and pin fixation devices utilized to stabilize and secure the multiple floating parts. *(F)* The cranial and pin devices affixed to the patient for firm immobilization of the floating parts. *(G)* Follow-up facial view of the patient with ocular prosthesis in place. Minor lid and scar revisions on the left were subsequently done to improve the cosmetic result about the left eye.

sense. Since the nasal cavity is rarely packed in the face of a cerebrospinal fluid leak, maintenance of these fragments in a reduced attitude can be helped by placing a nasal airway or large suction catheter in each side of the nasal fossa. These tubes should be of equal caliber and reach slightly beyond the posterior choanae. Their presence aids in holding the cartilaginous septum and vomer in a good vertical position while restraining the bones

comprising the nasal fossa's lateral wall from migrating into the reestablished patent air corridor.

The nasolacrimal apparatus is frequently involved when there is massive interorbital trauma. If damage to the system goes unrecognized and is not repaired, scar tissue closes or constricts the patency of the duct, sac, or canaliculi and the patient is subjected to a most annoying posttraumatic epiphora or tearing. Correcting the underlying cause at a later date is very difficult to do satisfactorily. The nasolacrimal sac and duct are fairly well protected in the recess formed by the lacrimal bone and frontal process of the maxilla and by the overlying medial palpebral ligament. Moderate blunt trauma and superficial lacerations rarely affect the system. When a canaliculus is transected or torn following a powerful blow to the region or as the result of a laceration extending across the medial canthal area, conventional repairs can be made. Most often the canaliculus leading from the upper or lower lid is transected between the punctum and the lacrimal sac. Under these circumstances, the torn medial and lateral ends of the canaliculus are located and cannulized with a suture to guide a polyethylene or Silastic stent into the canaliculus. A small stainless steel rod with swedged-on No. 3-0 or No. 4-0 black silk may also be used as a stent. The silk is less likely to cause scarring at the punctum opening and can be easily removed following healing of the canaliculus. Placement of this stent in proper position for the repair is usually easier with the following method:

This maneuver may be done by passing a small round needle backward through the upper punctum and canaliculus and thence downward through the lower canaliculus until it is exposed in the laceration of the lower lid. A silk suture should be attached to the eye of the needle. As the needle is backed out along its original route and removed, the suture accompanies it back through the upper punctum. The suture now lies within the lumen of the upper canaliculus with one end trailing out of the medial portion of the lower canaliculus and the opposite end leading out of the upper punctum. The eye end of the small round needle should next be placed into the lower punctum for traversing the lateral portion of the lower canaliculus. The eye of the needle now projects into the laceration.[18] The previously placed suture dangling from the medial

part of the canaliculus may be attached to the eye of the needle. On withdrawing the needle, the suture is drawn from the lower punctum, which completes continuity of the suture across the transected lower canaliculus. This small first placed suture may be used as a traction apparatus to guide a small polyethylene or Silastic stent through the lumen of the canalicular system. The stent serves to keep the torn ends of the canaliculus properly aligned. The free ends of the stent should be tied into a loop and attached to the patient's forehead or cheek with adhesive tape. Closure of the muscle layers, lid, and skin may proceed in the usual manner. Patency of the duct may be maintained through daily traction on the stent by moving it approximately 8 to 10 mm back and forth within the canaliculus. It is advisable to leave the stent in place for 2 to 6 weeks.[22] This maneuver is not easy even when the transection is produced by an incisional type wound.

The extremes of trauma often leave the area in a pulverized, macerated mess with few identifiable landmarks. When severe blunt trauma is received directly over the interorbital area, massive comminuting of the relatively thin and fragile bones of the area occurs. At the moment of impact, the instantaneous inward and sometimes upward telescoping of the parts avulses much of the soft tissue apparatus in the area (Fig. 19-14A). The more important entities here include the medial palpebral ligament attachment and the entire medial portion of the lacrimal drainage apparatus. The ends of both upper and lower canaliculi are frequently torn from the lacrimal sac and upper end of the nasolacrimal duct, which are completely mulched and not identifiable. Judgment and ingenuity are requisites to salvaging workable parts from this calamitous injury.

As reestablishment of an intact canalicular anastomosis with the lacrimal sac or duct is highly improbable and unlikely, an attempt

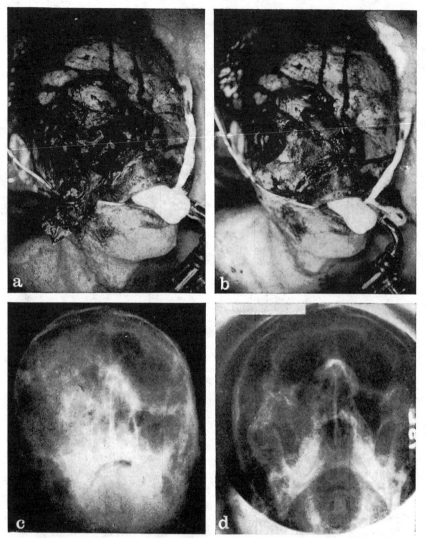

Figure 19-14 Tearing and ripping of the midface away from usual soft and bony attachments. (A) Preoperative view of patient with right face torn laterally, beginning just to the left of the midline. Nasal septum and right half of the nose is included in traumatic flap. Nasolacrimal sac and duct are avulsed by trauma. (B) Soft tissue flap is turned medially to a near-normal position. Cartilaginous septum is turned upward. (C) Preoperative Waters' view x-ray showing destruction of bony integrity of right orbit, zygoma, and maxilla. Most of the comminuted bony parts remained attached in various parts of the soft tissue flap. (D) Postoperative Waters' view x-ray demonstrating the scheme of multiple wiring required in fitting the comminuted fragments back in place. The anterior part of the perpendicular plate of the ethmoid and the cartilaginous septum were attached by wire to the undersurface of the nasal and frontal bones. The lower linear length of the cartilaginous septum was secured to the vomer's still intact anterior border with No. 1–0 chromic gut suture. (E) Postoperative view of patient showing No. 4–0 silk suture guided through the lower punctum and torn canaliculus and thence downward through the nasal fossa to emerge beneath the inferior turbinate and out the anterior naris. The two ends of the suture are tied together. This is a compromise technique to provide a tract for the drainage of tears when the nasolacrimal sac and duct are avulsed at the time of the accident.

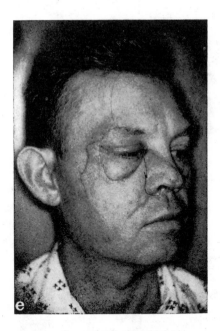

should be made to establish a tract for nasal drainage of the tears. The puncta can usually be located. Once again, the back end of a small round needle threaded with a fine suture should be passed through the lower punctum to the torn or cut end of the canaliculus. From this point medially, there probably are few distinguishable landmarks or identifiable tissue. The suture emerging from the cut end of the canaliculus may now be changed to the eye of a quite large round needle. This needle should then be threaded backward by its blunt end into the nasal fossa and thence downward to emerge beneath the inferior turbinate and out the anterior naris. Little resistance to passage of the needle should be encountered because of the extensive bony comminution along the path. The trailing suture serves as a traction device to guide a polyethylene (Fig. 19-15) or Silastic stent over the route just traversed by the suture. The ends emerging from the punctum and the anterior naris are looped together and taped to the patient's forehead or cheek (Fig. 19-14E). Movement of the stent back and forth daily is desirable as an aid in keeping the tract patent. The stent should be left in place for 2 or 3 months in anticipation of the tract's becoming epithelialized and able to maintain its own patency.

The medial palpebral ligament is superficial to the lacrimal apparatus and should next be sought out. A 30- or 32-gauge wire may be used as a mattress-type suture for attaching to the ligament. After as much of the bony architecture of the nasoorbital region has been raised and positioned as possible, the two fine wires fastened to the medial canthal ligament may be threaded through the ligament's former attachment at the comminuted medial orbital wall and carried across the nasal fossa and out through the skin of the opposite side. Here the wire should be fixed to a small lead plate contoured to the form of the canthal area. Two holes in the lead plate allow the separate ends of the wire to be drawn through the holes for tightening by twisting. By direct visualization, the correct medial position for the medial palpebral ligament can be determined and the ligament secured by the wire mattress suture.

Expert ophthalmologic consultation and assistance are imperative for proper appraisal and management of these complicated wounds.[25]

Fractured Maxillary Antrums

Collapsed or mashed-in maxillary antrums are frequently recontoured best by sinus packing. This procedure has already been described. However, caution has to be exercised when packing an antrum with several or all walls fractured and comminuted. It is not difficult to inadvertently displace an antral floor too far downward, a nasal wall too far medially, or an orbital floor too far superiorly with injudicious jamming in of gauze. Just enough gauze packing should be used to act as a filler and prevent fragments from closing or diminishing the size of this air chamber.

Internal Skeletal Fixation (Suspension Wiring) Support of these disarticulated facial segments consists of sandwiching the loos-

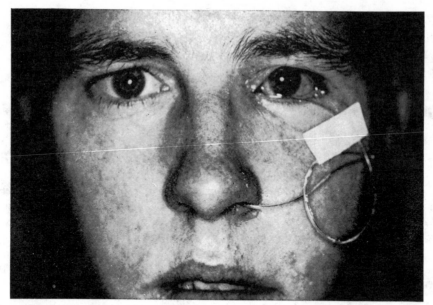

Figure 19-15 Polyethylene catheter used as a stent for maintenance of a tract for the drainage of tears after healing, scarring, and binding down of an old laceration through the nasolacrimal apparatus.

ened fragments in their correct position between the mandible and the unfractured parts of the face or cranial base and immobilizing them in this position. As the mandible is the only part that normally moves, immobilizing it with the middle facial parts reassembled in correct relation to and fixed to the lower jaw effectively stabilizes the whole facial unit. Internal skeletal fixation wires suspended from unfractured facial and cranial bones that are fastened at the lower end to arch bars or splints on the mandibular teeth are positive means of controlling mandibular movement. These wires are relatively simple to place and are more comfortable for the patient than headcaps.

The usual types of internal suspension wiring include:

1 Pyriform fossa wiring[16]
2 Maxillary peralveolar wiring
3 Zygomaticomaxillary buttress wiring
4 Inferior orbital rim wiring
5 Circumzygomatic wiring
6 Frontal bone wiring (zygomatic process)

Pyriform fossa wiring is used chiefly for suspending low, unstable horizontal fractures of the maxilla or as an aid in stabilizing fractures of the edentulous mandible when the patient's dentures are used in fixation. The wires may be quickly placed via an incision high in the mucobuccal fold under the upper lip. The incision should extend through the mucoperiosteum down to bone for sharp reflection of the mucoperiosteal flap up to the level of the pyriform fossa's lateral wall. Cortical bone comprises this lateral wall and is far more substantial than bone at the floor of the fossa. Wires should thus be attached to the lateral wall for security. The nasal mucosa may be reflected gently and protected with a periosteal elevator as a hole is drilled through the lateral wall beneath the inferior turbinate.

A 24-gauge wire threaded through the hole completes the wiring. Both ends of the wire should be led into the oral cavity through the incision and secured to the lower arch bar or splint.

Peralveolar wiring is used principally for attaching a maxillary denture to the maxilla. These wires are usually placed through holes directed from high in the mucobuccal fold at the cuspid-bicuspid area diagonally downward and toward the midline through the maxillary alveolar bone to emerge in the hard palate. A small hand awl or motor-driven burr can be used to burrow out the small hole. A 24-gauge wire may be guided through the hole, which can then be threaded through holes of the patient's upper denture or splint. Twisting the wire tight lashes the denture securely to the maxilla. Wiring from other areas may then be fastened to the fixed denture. Suspension wiring from the zygomaticomaxillary buttress area is advantageous because the wire span is shortest of all methods, there is thick cortical bone for placement of the intraosseous hole, and it is easily accomplished from an intraoral approach.

Inferior orbital rim suspension wires are useful in helping stabilize pyramidal-type midface fractures (Fig. 19-10). The zygomas are usually unfractured, and their inferior orbital rim extensions are quite secure. Attachment of a suspension wire to these stable rims should be made via the usual incision for work along the inferior orbital margin. Holes drilled from the maxillary side beneath the rim to emerge in the orbital floor provide secure anchorage around the whole cortical infraorbital ridge. A 24-gauge wire is suggested as a reliable size to thread through the hole. The two free ends should be attached to the eye of a large straight needle to direct the wires into the oral cavity. The point of the needle should be kept in contact with the anterior maxillary wall as it descends into the oral cavity to emerge through the mucobuccal fold at the cuspid-bicuspid area. After pulling the two wire ends taut, they may be fastened to the mandibular arch bar or splint.

Circumzygomatic suspension wires are useful for supporting horizontal fractures of the maxilla, pyramidal-type fractures of the midface, or combinations of the two. In these instances, the zygoma is unfractured and offers stable support for wiring. No incision is necessary to loop a wire around the zygoma. After locating the L-shaped junction of the frontal and temporal processes of the zygoma by palpation, a 3- or 5-in half-curved postmortem needle may be used for percutaneous insertion down to bone. The point of the needle should be "walked" off the back edge of the bone precisely at the junction of these two processes and directed beneath the zygoma. By keeping the point of the needle in contact with the undersurface of the zygoma, it may be safely passed beneath the zygomatic process of the maxilla into the oral cavity at the height of the mucobuccal fold opposite the bicuspid teeth. The deep wire is thus led into the oral cavity attached to the end of the postmortem needle. The opposite free end may be attached to a straight needle and brought into the oral cavity along the outer surface of the zygoma. The long straight needle should be inserted into the same puncture hole made by the postmortem needle. The straight needle should also contact bone at the junction of the frontal and temporal processes and then be directed across the outer surface of the zygoma. It is important to keep the point of the needle in contact with bone during this traverse to prevent facial nerve damage. Stretching of the skin at the point of needle entry allows sufficient maneuverability to maintain this contact and to keep the needle directed to enter the oral cavity near the deep wire. The two wires in the oral cavity should now be grasped and secured snugly against the zygoma with a sawing motion. The wire should be sufficiently long to permit the work-hardened wire immediately next to the bone to be drawn away and eliminated. Attachment of the two free ends to a lower arch bar or splint completes the procedure.

Suspension wires attached to the zygomatic process of the frontal bone are useful in supporting many total facial fracture disarticulations from the cranial base (Fig. 19-11*D* and *F)*. The zygomas are loose and nonstable as are all facial bones beneath. The frontal bone is the last remaining stable bone in a cephalad direction. Attachment to the zygomatic process of the frontal bone should be made via the usual approach to the zygomaticofrontal suture line. A hole for anchorage in this angular process of the frontal bone may be made in the manner explained earlier for securing detached zygomas. A lengthy piece of stainless steel wire may be threaded through this hole and both ends affixed to a 5-in half-curved postmortem needle. The postmortem needle should be passed beneath the zygoma into the oral cavity in the same manner as was the deep circumzygomatic wire. Both frontal suspension wires, however, pass beneath the zygoma. The two free ends in the oral cavity may be fastened to the lower arch bar or splint (Fig. 19-11*D)*.

External Skeletal Fixation Headcap fixation is still an important tool in treating fractures of the middle third of the facial skeleton. Many comminuted disarticulations of the facial skeleton require anterior traction and support or stabilization of segments in which broad interfaces of connecting bone have been destroyed. These fractures are better controlled via headcaps or pin devices. Among those injuries requiring headcap type fixation are:

1 Craniofacial disjunctions where there is wide comminution of bone along the edges of key connecting bones between the facial skeleton and cranial base (Fig. 19-13*C)*. Direct wiring or suspension wiring may be impossible at these areas. These segments should be moved to a correctly aligned position and then stabilized with rods or pins connected to a headcap. Fibrous healing between the bony fragments may be all that can be anticipated, but it will be adequate if the parts are in an acceptable position.

2 Badly comminuted facial fractures with concomitant fracturing of the mandible at the symphysis and both condyles. It would be desirable to reestablish an intact mandible by open reduction of the various mandibular fractures against which to build the facial skeleton. However, these procedures would be too prolonged to precede the pending lengthy midface repairs. Rods or pins connecting the mandible to a solidly seated headcap can securely maintain the mandible, prevent foreshortening of the rami at the condyle fracture areas, and control splaying of the rami laterally because of the condyle and symphysis fractures. This mandibular fracture is difficult to treat alone, but when combined with extensive midface fractures, it becomes an enormous problem. A Kirschner wire passed from one inferior portion of the body of the mandible through the floor of the mouth to the opposite body of the mandible in second bicuspid area may be a helpful method of stabilizing bilateral condyle fractures and a mandibular symphysis fracture. This is done through a small stab incision and is rapidly accomplished. The pin is placed with the jaws in occlusion and the angles compressed medially to prevent flaring of the mandibular angles.

3 Severely impacted maxillary fractures which require anterior traction plus support at the tuberosity areas.

4 Split maxillary fractures that require lateral traction for maintenance of two or more segments in acceptable positions.

Headcaps securely anchored to the cranium with pins (Fig. 19-13*E* and *F)* are most useful because they do not shift with scalp movements or during moderate activity by the patient. Positive, firm control of fixation devices connected to them is possible. However, accurately constructed and placed plaster of Paris headcaps still have something to offer and should therefore be a part of the available armamentarium.

BIBLIOGRAPHY

1 Adson, A. W.: Cerebrospinal rhinorrhea: Surgical repair of cranio-sinus fistula, *Trans. Am. Surg. Assoc.*, **59**:457, 1941.

2 Beck, G. and L. Neil: Anesthesia for associated trauma in patients with head injury, *Anesthesia Analgesia*, **42**:6, 1963.

3 Browning, C. W. and R. V. Walker: Polyethylene in post-traumatic orbital floor reconstruction, *Am. J. Ophthalmol.*, **52**:5, 1961.

4 —— and ——: The use of alloplastics in 45 cases of orbital floor reconstruction, *Am. J. Ophthalmol.*, **60**:684, 1965.

5 Clark, K.: The incidence and mechanisms of shock in head injury, *J. Southern Med. Assoc.*, **55**:5, 1962.

6 Converse, J. M.: *Reconstructive Plastic Surgery*, W. B. Saunders Company, Philadelphia, 1964, vol. II, p. 549.

7 Dingman, R. O. and P. Natvig: *Surgery of Facial Fractures*, W. B. Saunders Company, Philadelphia, 1964.

8 Douglas, B. L. and G. J. Casey: *A Guide to Hospital Dental Procedures*, American Dental Association, Chicago, 1964.

9 Duke-Elder, W. S.: *Textbook of Ophthalmology*, The C. V. Mosby Company, St. Louis, 1954, vol. 6.

10 Kahn, E. A.: Neurosurgical complications of facial fractures, *Trans. Am. Acad. Ophthalmol.*, September-October 1958.

11 Kruger, G.: *Textbook of Oral Surgery*, The C. V. Mosby Company, St. Louis, 1964, Chap. 17.

12 Lewin, W.: Cerebrospinal fluid rhinorrhea in closed head injuries, *Brit. J. Surg.*, vol. 42, July 1954.

13 —— and H. Carius: Fractures of sphenoidal sinus with cerebrospinal fluid rhinorrhea, *Brit. Med. J.*, **1**:16, 1951.

14 Lewin, J. R., D. H. Rhodes, and E. J. Pavsek: Roentgenographic manifestations of fractures of the orbital floor, *Am. J. Roentgenol.*, **83**:628, 1960.

15 Morris, H.: *Human Anatomy*, McGraw-Hill Book Company, New York, 1953, p. 135.

16 Rowe, N. L. and H. C. Killey: *Fractures of the Facial Skeleton*, The Williams & Wilkins Company, Baltimore, 1955.

17 Smith, B. and J. M. Converse: Early treatment of orbital floor fractures, *Trans. Am. Acad. Ophthalmol.*, **61**:5, 1957.

18 Stallard, H. B.: Early surgery of injuries of the eyelids, *Trans. Ophthalmol. Soc. U.K.*, vol. 79, 1959.

19 Stewart, F.: Personal communication.

20 Thoma, K. H.: *Oral Surgery*, 4th ed., The C. V. Mosby Company, St. Louis, 1963.

21 Thompson, R. K.: Traumatic unconsciousness, *Maryland Med. J.*, **2**:3, 1953.

22 Viers, E. R.: Obstruction of lacrimal system, *Am. J. Ophthalmol.*, **56**:6, 1963.

23 Vrabec, D. P. and D. E. Halberg: Cerebrospinal fluid rhinorrhea, *Arch. Otolaryngol.*, vol. 80, August 1964.

24 Walker, R. V.: Unpublished data.

25 Zaydon, T. J. and J. B. Brown: *Early Treatment of Facial Injuries*, Lea & Febiger, Philadelphia, 1964.

Chapter 20

Eye Injuries

John R. Lynn, M.D.

The purposes of this chapter are to relegate eye injuries to a proper perspective in patients with multiple injuries, to detail those points of an eye examination which can be carried out without specialized equipment, and to outline some accepted principles of ophthalmologic management as goals to be sought, not thwarted, in the original care given the patient.

The circumstances leading to emergency examination usually prompt the physician to suspect a certain type of injury. When the injury involves the eye, its evaluation should be carried as far as the limits of safety to the eye and the patient's cooperation permit. Whenever possible, some estimate of the patient's visual acuity should be obtained.

For the sake of convenience in using this chapter as a quick reference, the general types of eye injury will be discussed in the following order: abrasions, superficial foreign bodies, blunt injuries, lacerations, penetrating foreign bodies, and burns. The factors which most influence the long-term visual prognosis will be covered initially under each type of injury.

ABRASIONS

Cornea

The symptoms of corneal abrasion are pain, lacrimation, photophobia, and spasm of the lids.

When inspecting the globe for abrasions, the examiner should open the lids by pushing the soft tissue against the upper and lower orbital rims, carefully avoiding any pressure against the eye itself. The force which abraded could have ruptured the globe, and until adequate examination establishes the contrary, every suspected eye injury should be treated with as much respect as if it were known to be a penetrating wound. When a penetration is suspected, general anesthesia may be necessary for the examination of uncooperative patients, such as frightened children.

To find the abrasion, a bright, well-focused light should be directed constantly onto the eye while the light is being moved slowly into various positions of obliquity (Fig. 20-1). A light directed straight into the eye along the visual axis is not as helpful diagnostically, and it is certainly less comfortable for the patient. One should look with a magnifying loupe (spectacles) for irregularities in the corneal reflections of the light as indications of epithelial defects. Shadows are also cast on the iris by almost invisible corneal lesions.

Analgesics Following an abrasion of the cornea, the epithelium returns by migration and mitosis over a period ranging from a few hours to 3 or 4 days, depending on the severity of the injury. One should not hesitate to use topical analgesics such as proparacaine to obtain cooperation for adequate diagnosis. These agents, however, do slow down the regenerative processes; so topical analgesics should not be prescribed for the patient to use at home. Though cocaine is an extremely potent topical analgesic, it softens the cornea and permits loss of even more epithelium than was originally denuded. Butacaine causes a high incidence of allergic reaction.

Staining After it has been established that there is no obvious penetration, fluorescein strips and irrigation may be safely used to stain the cornea's epithelial defects. Bottled fluorescein drops are easily contaminated and act as good culture media for *Pseudomonas*,

Figure 20-1 Examination of the cornea with a well-focused flashlight. Corneal abrasions, ulcers, or foreign bodies may be invisible on simple inspection. These lesions may often be detected by an irregularity in the corneal reflection of the rays from a slowly moving pen light which also produces a slightly magnified shadow of the corneal defect on the iris. The shadow moves in a direction opposite to the motion of the light, as shown by the inset.

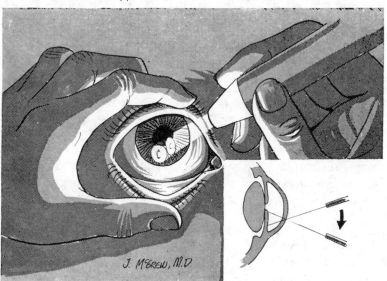

one of the most virulent organisms attacking the eye. Individually packaged fluorescein-impregnated paper strips are commercially available as sterile Fluori-strips.

Complications Fingernail abrasions of the cornea often lead to recurrent erosions, manifest as pain on awakening as long as several weeks after the original injury. These apparently result from a better adhesion between the lid and the corneal epithelium during sleep than that between the newly migrated epithelium and Bowman's membrane, the most anterior layer of corneal stroma. Prophylaxis for this condition includes the use of a bland, inexpensive ophthalmic ointment such as 4 or 5% boric acid for lubrication in the injured eye at bedtime. This lubricant and a word of caution to the patient about opening the eyes slowly on awakening are continued for a few months. When these measures fail, the ophthalmologist may denude the epithelium and patch the eye for several days.

Herpes Simplex Keratitis Herpes is said to be the most common cause of corneal ulcers. Twigs, leaves, fingernails, and other such contaminated fomites lead to about 10 percent incidence of this virus infection of the cornea in the characteristic branching or dendritic ulcer pattern. When a branching pattern is seen, corneal sensitivity should be compared with that of the other eye. The technique of this examination consists of having the patient look upward while the examiner alternately stimulates both corneas with separate wisps of cotton (Fig. 20-2). A single piece of cotton is especially dangerous for performance of this test because it may inoculate the healthy cornea with the organisms, causing an ulcer in the other eye.

If the corneal sensitivity is definitely decreased in the eye with foreign body sensation and branching or "dendritic" pattern, the presumptive diagnosis of herpes simplex keratitis

can be made. Though many cases heal spontaneously, others may be difficult to treat successfully. These virus infections can be treated by the ophthalmologist with IDU (2-iodo-5-deoxyuridine) during the early phase, resulting in a slight improvement in the percentage of remission.

Superficial herpes infections of the eye (which still take a stain) should never be treated with topical corticosteroids, for this therapy somehow lowers resistance to stromal involvement, with resultant deep scarring and possible perforation of the cornea.

Mycotic Keratitis If the history of injury implicates cornstalk, cotton stubble, twigs, or other agricultural material as the abrading agent, the possibility of a secondary fungus infection of the cornea is increased, especially when topical corticosteroids have been used following the injury. At the first sign of infiltration or prolonged failure to heal, these lesions should be promptly scraped for culture on blood agar and Sabouraud's medium. Treatment with an appropriate antifungal or antibacterial agent should be started immediately and altered, if necessary, by sensitivity results. Some fungal ulcers do not respond to any medications, so visual function is frequently lost or the eye may even have to be removed. Any damage to subepithelial corneal tissues, whether due to the original injury or to secondary infection, will result in scarring and a corresponding decrease in vision, most marked if the scar is located centrally.

Treatment of Abrasions Corneal abrasions should be irrigated with normal saline solution, oral analgesics should be administered, and the eye should be firmly patched with two eye pads for 24 to 48 h, although some patients are more comfortable without the patch after an hour or so. If the lesion is deep, 1% cyclopentolate (Cyclogyl) 4 times daily or 2% homatropine 3 times daily may be prescribed

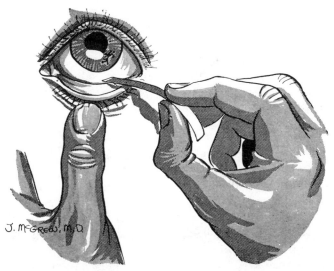

J. McGrew, M.D.

Figure 20-2 Staining with fluorescein to demonstrate the typical dendritic pattern of herpes keratitus. The branching superficial pattern and a decreased corneal sensitivity are characteristic of herpes. Sterile paper strips impregnated with fluorescein provide a source of stain which is safer than bottled fluorescein, for these are not so easily contaminated. Patients with known corneal ulcers have a relatively high rate of complications and sequelae; so they usually deserve referral.

for a few days. Atropine should be avoided as its action of 2 weeks duration is unnecessarily prolonged. A topical antibiotic solution such as bacitracin, neomycin, or polymyxin B or a sulfonamide may be added. Ointments are not used because they mechanically delay healing.

Corneal abrasions usually heal within 2 or 3 days. When, instead, the eye remains red and uncomfortable and the abraded area continues to stain and develops a gray-white ring of infiltration under and around the original site, a deep corneal ulcer must be suspected. Therapy should then be directed toward scraping the ulcer itself with a sterile spatula for smears and culture, followed by appropriate antibiotic therapy.

When the wound is deep and overlies the pupil, binoculuar patches and bed rest are helpful. Therapy should include use of the antibiotic solution until the lack of both stain and scratching pain indicates that the wound is healed. The cycloplegic should be continued until any residual iritis, as manifest by redness, photophobia, and deep pain, has cleared.

Lids and Conjunctiva

When severe (third-degree) "brush-burn" abrasions occur on the lids, some authors advocate immediate debridement and thin full-thickness skin grafting to obtain the best functional and cosmetic results.

Conjunctival abrasions should be suspected of hiding the scleral wound of a penetrating foreign body. Therapy of uncomplicated conjunctival wounds is a single application of sulfonamide solution.

SUPERFICIAL FOREIGN BODIES

The patient who complains of "something in the eye" may have a loose eyelash or foreign body in the cul-de-sac, a bit of foreign material embedded in the cornea or stuck to the inner surface of the upper lid, an abrasion, a flash burn, a recurrent erosion, or a corneal ulcer such as herpes simplex.

Examination Bright, well-focused light and loupes are used first to inspect the eye's injection pattern. A sector of limbus with a deep flush is often an indicator of corneal pathologic change in the same region. The cornea's reflection of the light should be observed as the light remains directed onto the eye and is moved slowly into various oblique positions with respect to the eye. Abrasions and ulcers cause irregularities in the usually smooth mirror surface of the cornea and consequent distortions of the minified image of the light which is being observed. Even though the cornea is essentially clear, the epithelial interruption will cast a shadow on the iris. This iris shadow also demonstrates small foreign bodies or lacerations as it magnifies their images. The shadow moves in a direction opposite to the one in which the light is slowly moving.

Lacerations which enter the globe do not usually cause a great deal of pain. Before assuming that "something in the eye" is innocuous and that the eye can be manipulated freely, one should be relatively certain that a penetrating wound has been ruled out by the history; otherwise the eye must be examined with this possibility in mind.

If the history is reassuring and the flashlight has been fully utilized without touching the eyelids, the patient may be asked to look up while the lower lid is retracted by pressing a finger against the lower orbital rim and sliding the skin downward. This will expose the lower conjunctival cul-de-sac, which should be searched for the foreign body.

Upper Lid Eversion The upper cornea can be inspected in a similar manner, but examination of the upper conjunctival cul-de-sac requires a maneuver which everts the lid (Fig. 20-3). This should always be done when no foreign body is found originally but discomfort has persisted and there is a corneal abrasion, especially one with a vertical orientation, for the upper tarsus may harbor one or more foreign bodies. To prove or disprove this possibility, the upper lid may be everted. The procedure of upper lid eversion is: (1) have the patient look downward so that the sensitive cornea will not be stimulated by manipulation of the upper lid, (2) grasp the lashes of the upper lid with one hand while (3) pushing the top of the tarsus inward and downward from the outside of the lid with a finger or cotton-tipped applicator. The stiff tarsus in the upper lid measures about 10 or 11 mm vertically and can often hold the lid in its "flipped" position once the lash traction is released.

If no foreign body is then seen by using loupe magnification and a bright light, a drop of fluorescein may be instilled. This is provided by moistening a sterile dye-impregnated paper strip with saline solution and using the strip to touch the inner surface of the lower lid. The excess may be removed by irrigation with saline solution or by waiting 2 or 3 min for tears to dilute it.

Double Lid Eversion Vertical green lines on the cornea after fluorescein staining strongly suggest a foreign body partially embedded in the upper tarsus, and the technique of double lid eversion should be performed to allow visualization of the entire upper cul-de-sac. This consists of (1) using a vein retractor with its handle directed downward, its blade touching the lid at the upper edge of the tarsus, (2) a gentle pull on the upper lashes while the patient looks down, (3) depression and backward pressure on the retractor to evert the tarsus, and (4) swinging of the retractor handle in an arc upward to the brow doubly to evert the lid.

Other epithelial defects also stain green, and

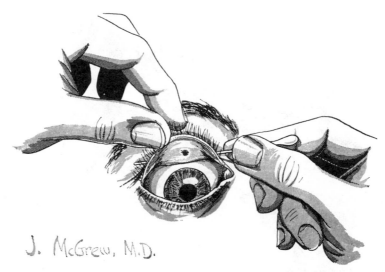

J. McGrew, M.D.

Figure 20-3 Eversion of the upper lid. The maneuver consists of five steps: (1) Ask the patient to look downward, (2) grasp the upper lashes, (3) position an object such as a cotton-tipped applicator against the upper lid about 1 cm above the lid margin, (4) simultaneously pull the lashes outward while pressing backward and downward with the applicator, and (5) allow the lid margin to move backward while removing the applicator.

their patterns may be helpful. The branching pattern of herpes keratitis has been discussed under the heading of Abrasions.

Technique of Removal Foreign bodies which cannot be dislodged with analgesic and focal irrigation with saline solution should be removed with bright light, loupes, or by biomicroscopic magnification (Fig. 20-4). Before attempting removal of a foreign body, adequate topical analgesia is obtained with proparacaine, instilled 2 or 3 times, and a hand is braced on the patient's face so that, if the patient moves, the hand cannot move toward the patient and cause an additional injury. While the patient looks steadily at some object for fixation, a sterile 20-gauge hypodermic needle or an eye spud is introduced barely deep to the foreign body to lift it straight out. When used for foreign body removal, cotton-tipped applicators cause widespread denudation of the cornea.

Treatment after Removal of Foreign Body The use of a topical antibiotic or sulfonamide solution is helpful in preventing ulcers, which are especially likely to occur if the lesion was caused by contaminated material. Ointments are avoided because they may retard wound healing. Patching for 4 to 24 h and cycloplegia with homatropine 2% will help the patient's comfort, but if antibiotics are indicated, the patch period must be brief so that the drops may be used at hourly intervals during the day, less frequently at night, and be continued until no stainable lesion or pain persists.

Rust-ring Removal When the foreign body contains iron and is present for some time, a red-brown rust ring may develop around the foreign body. This should be removed as it may interfere with adequate healing over the area. A small, round dental burr may be used directly on the cornea. This may be found

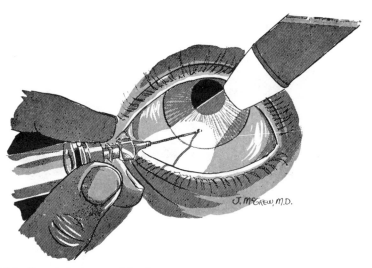

Figure 20-4 Removal of corneal foreign body. After topical proparacaine drops, administered 3 times, the patient fixes his or her gaze on an immobile object to help keep both eyes open and stationary. Some foreign bodies may be freed by focal irrigation, but when this is not successful, they should be lifted straight out, not wiped, depressed, or broken and scattered by other techniques. A bright light source and magnification help in adequate visualization of the foreign object and in the placement of a sterile No. 20 hypodermic needle just deep to it. The hand holding the needle should be braced against the patient's face before inserting the needle tip.

helpful at times when the spud does not dislodge the rust ring along with the foreign body. An alternative method is to touch the ring with a cotton-tipped applicator which has been dipped in 1% silver nitrate solution and well wrung out. The eye is then irrigated and patched for 24 h. The day following this treatment, the ring can be lifted out like a simple foreign body.

Multiple Foreign Bodies Numerous foreign bodies which are not metallic or chemical may be allowed a day or two to extrude themselves so that the cornea is not endangered by the repeated use of a spud. Antibiotic solutions, cycloplegics, and patching should be utilized during the early waiting period to allow relative comfort and safety while most of the foreign bodies are extruded spontaneously. The remaining ones can be removed the following day in a routine manner.

Corticosteroids The use of topical corticosteroids following the removal of foreign bodies is not of real value, for such wounds do not become vascularized and the extent of scarring depends almost exclusively on the amount of damage to the subepithelial cornea. The increased propensity to infection with viruses, bacteria, and fungi plus the possibility of secondary glaucoma from cortisone therapy are unnecessary hazards.

BLUNT INJURIES

The term "contusion" embraces only those effects of blunt injury which are due to rupture of small vessels, whereas "laceration" denotes a gross rent or separation of tissues.

The classical "black eye," though often considered only for its antisocial significance, can hide a ruptured sclera or choroid; edema of the posterior pole, which can lead to macular degeneration; dislocated lens; or hemorrhage into the vitreous or anterior chamber, which can, in turn, mask a retinal detachment, lead to secondary glaucoma, or result in blood staining of the cornea. These and a variety of other lesions may influence the patient's visual function profoundly with the passage of time.

When a patient is seen with lid ecchymosis, the first consideration is the visual acuity, which should be obtained accurately on admission. A subsequent change in vision may be of considerable clinical significance.

Skull Fractures An ocular sign of skull fracture can become evident if free blood is not originally present in the lids. Ecchymosis appearing in the upper lid 1 to 3 days after the injury usually signifies a fracture of the orbital roof. In the lower lid, the same late appearance of blood suggests a fracture of the base of the skull. Abrupt loss of vision in an eye at the time of injury without signs of damage to the globe can be explained at times by trauma to the optic nerve related to a fracture into the optic canal. Exploration of the orbital apex by the neurosurgeon is debatably effective, for the damage may be on a vascular basis or be due to transection as well as the therapeutically amenable entity of nerve compression.

Scleral Rupture The care during examination to prevent extrusion of the ocular contents through a ruptured sclera must be doubly exercised in examining the eye with a blunt injury. The likelihood of rupture is increased because the blunt injuries are directed more specifically toward the globe than is the case in abrasions.

Complete or partial scleral rupture is suggested by a poor or absent red reflex, decreased vision, and a soft globe. The uniform red fundus reflex may be seen normally through an ophthalmoscope set on 0 from a distance of a foot or more. Scleral rupture is most commonly located at the limbus (junction of cornea and sclera) in the upper nasal quadrant as a result of an inferior temporal quadrant blow (the one least guarded by the bony orbit), but it may occur deep to any of the rectus muscles. These sites of predilection are caused by: (1) a weakness resulting from the presence of the outflow apparatus, (2) changes in curve of the coats as the cornea joins the sclera, and (3) a tendency for expansion of the globe at a right angle to the direction of force, with maximum stress localized in a circle around the globe, about 17 mm from the point of impact.

One should always be suspicious that the source of blood in subconjunctival hemorrhages may be intraocular structures and that the blood itself is hiding the rupture site. If the globe is obviously quite soft, such an eye should be considered for subconjunctival exploration, especially if other signs of rupture such as free blood inside the globe or decreased vision are concomitantly present.

Management of Ruptured Globe If rupture or penetration of the globe is suspected, the eye should be protected with a large dressing which does not compress it. The patient should be referred to an ophthalmologist as an emergency. Tension examination should never be performed on patients with known penetrations.

When partially prolapsed uveal tissue is noted beneath the conjunctiva at the time of surgical exploration, it must be excised and a primary wound repair performed if such an eye is to have optimal chances for recovery. If not discovered and repaired, the prolapsed tissue or poorly reapposed sclera can cause a weak area which may herniate and result in sympathetic ophthalmia (discussed under Lacerations below).

Ocular Hypotony A low intraocular pressure may indicate a partial rupture of the globe's wall, not necessarily including the conjunctiva. These ruptures usually begin inside the limbus at the chamber angle where the outflow channels represent a weakness of the fibrous coat. The tears then extend obliquely and posteriorly to emerge through the sclera 3 or 4 mm behind the limbus, where a dark bulge may sometimes be seen. When the intraocular pressure is very low, small perforating wounds of the sclera and lacerated globes from blunt injuries should be suspected. Though traumatic ocular hypotony and retinal detachment are both associated with reduced intraocular pressure, the magnitude of this reduction is relatively small, for the pressure is likely to be measurable with the Schiotz tonometer, whereas in most cases of perforating scleral injuries, it is too low to be recorded with this instrument.

Retinal Detachment The ophthalmoscopic appearance of a retinal detachment is generally a gray mound protruding into the eye, disturbing at least a part of the red fundus reflex (Fig. 20-5). The surface of the elevated retina may show ripplelike fine striae and larger folds as well. The whole structure often undulates with the slightest motion of the eye. The vascular pattern of the choroid is obscured in the area involved by the detachment. The retinal vessels in the detached area are out of focus with the lens which shows the disk best. They can be well seen by the addition of a few more diopters of plus power and appear smaller and darker than the vessels in normal retina of the other eye.

Detachments begin in the retinal periphery when a hole in the retina allows fluid from the vitreous to pass into the potential space between retina and pigment epithelium. Finding the hole which led to the detachment is often difficult, if not impossible, with the direct ophthalmoscope because the location of the hole is so far anterior, especially when the cause of the detachment is trauma. The binocular indirect ophthalmoscope discussed under

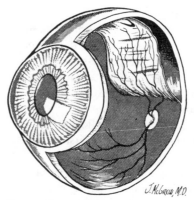

J. McGrew, M.D.

Figure 20-5 Retinal detachment not involving the macula. The ophthalmoscopic appearance of a detached retina can be partially understood by this cutaway drawing. The retina above the disk is abruptly separated from the underlying vascular choroid, causing it to change from the usual pink color to faint gray-pink and go out of focus. In this collapsed position, the retina is not taut; so it undulates and is wrinkled, even folded. The horeshoe-shaped tear in the periphery above looks red and allows fluid from the vitreous to go between the retina and choroid, causing the detachment. When the patient with a detachment can still read newsprint with the involved eye, the macula is intact and the patient deserves an emergency referral.

Penetrating Foreign Bodies is very helpful in evaluating patients with retinal detachment. The peripheral vision in the corresponding quadrant (opposite the detachment) is diminished; for example, a superior nasal detachment shows an inferior temporal defect in the visual field.

Macular Involvement in Retinal Detachment It is most important to diagnose retinal detachment before it reaches the macula, for high-grade visual acuity depends upon macular function, which is usually permanently impaired after the macula has been detached. Although a detached retina involving the macula can be reattached surgically, the state of nutrition at this critical area is diminished during the period of detachment, presumably because of impaired osmosis from the choroid. The inertia of appreciable free fluid behind the retina can dissect the macula off when combined with a normal rapid glance. For this reason, a partially detached retina not involving the macula should be reattached as soon as possible. If there is uncertainty about the presence of macular detachment, a good test is visual acuity; i.e., if the patient can read the newspaper, the macula is intact. The already limited prognosis for visual acuity is not appreciably diminished if reattachment of the macula is achieved within 1 week after its detachment, although the prognosis becomes gradually poorer if surgical treatment is delayed longer.

The patient with a retinal detachment which does not involve the macula is a candidate for emergency referral who should have the eyes immobilized by patching and bed rest until repair can be performed.

Traumatic Edema of the Retina Edema of the posterior pole of the retina becomes manifest early by a white appearance ophthalmoscopically. It may clear completely without sequelae or lead to macular cysts and holes with marked diminution in visual acuity. Treatment, though inconsistently effective, is 30 to 40 mg of prednisone per day, bed rest, tranquilizers, and analgesics.

Hyphema Moderately severe blunt injuries to the globe often cause hemorrhage into the anterior chamber of the eye, or hyphema. This is associated with a recession of the chamber angle in about 71 percent of cases, indicating a tear in the iris root or ciliary body without external communication or penetration. The different inertias of the several intraocular tissues must allow for individual rates of movement in response to the shock wave of an injury. In the vast majority of cases hyphema is due to minor blunt trauma, perhaps forgotten by the patient, not to bleeding or clotting disorders. Spontaneous hyphema oc-

curs with certain granulomatous diseases and with some neoplasms, but the lack of a good history of trauma does not preclude injury as the cause. Bleeding and clotting studies should be instituted on admission if the history is unreliable or suggests a blood dyscrasia. If an abnormality in the clotting mechanism is discovered, appropriate therapy should be started promptly.

The presence of even a small amount of free blood inside the eye should be noted early, for such a hyphema can disappear in a matter of minutes. Although most eyes that have suffered blunt injuries with hyphema recover without appreciable permanent effects, recurrent hemorrhage may occur. Of those eyes which do hemorrhage secondarily, about 50 percent develop glaucoma, experience degeneration to very poor vision, or undergo removal. When the initial hyphema goes unrecognized, the additional activity accorded a patient without this problem can lead to a secondary hemorrhage with the poor prognosis noted above.

Bleeding into the eye usually stops spontaneously because of vessel retraction and tamponade from the increasing intraocular pressure. If the anterior chamber is then filled with blood, a prolonged elevation of intraocular pressure or a little damage to the corneal endothelium will lead to the passage of blood decomposition products forward into the stroma of the cornea, producing a green opacity there. This "blood staining" later turns white and may absorb over a period of weeks to months, effectively eliminating good vision for that period. If the patient is a preschool child, this period of virtually total elimination of form vision will often lead to "occlusion amblyopia," which is a drop in vision without demonstrable organic damage to the refractive media, retina, or optic nerve. The eye may have organic damage caused by associated traumatic sequelae, namely, dislocation or opacification of the lens, hemorrhage into the vitreous, iris rupture or dialysis, or retinal detachment. Cataracts and edema of the posterior pole changing to cysts and/or holes in the macula account for most of the cases of hyphema which suffer ultimate visual decrease (about 15 to 25 percent). Those cases of hyphema which bleed only 1 time with the initial trauma fare significantly better than the group in which rebleeding occurs. The recurrent hemorrhage takes place 2 to 5 days after the original injury, and much therapy is directed toward its prevention.

The blood in the anterior chamber is apparently absorbed from the surface of the iris and from the aqueous outflow channels. This process requires a few minutes to a few weeks. Other debris resulting from the trauma also has egress by these routes. When an obstruction to normal aqueous flow occurs, the intraocular pressure becomes elevated and a state of secondary glaucoma exists. The blood staining which follows this is the primary indication for lowering pressure, although the optic nerve can be damaged by marked increases in intraocular pressure. These are not the only early complications of hyphema, for fibrin in the clotted blood may become organized to form posterior or anterior synechiae, and sympathetic ophthalmia may rarely occur after blunt trauma without external communication. The late complications are an atrophic iris or optic nerve, hemophthalmitis, and heterochromic iritis.

Cautery or ligatures have been utilized occasionally to close off the bleeding vessel. These procedures could possibly damage a previously intact lens and should be avoided.

Uncontrolled studies suggest that Premarin 10 mg intravenously and 5 mg/day in children under 12 years old or twice this dosage in adolescents and adults may diminish the incidence of secondary hemorrhage.

Hyphema Therapy   The conservative therapy of hyphema is bed rest, preferably in a hospital, and bilateral patching, with sedation,

analgesia, and tranquilizers if necessary. No drops are used early, but after 6 or 7 days when iritis and a tendency toward formation of synechiae are present, a cycloplegic such as homatropine or hyoscine is employed. Topical steroids may be used before and after this period for iritis. If secondary glaucoma occurs early, the initial medical therapy is acetazolamide. This is followed, if necessary, by the addition of an osmotic agent such as oral glycerol (1.5 g/kg every 6 h) or intravenous urea or mannitol. When none of these is successful and the pressure is still elevated, topical miotics and sympathomimetics are employed. If the pressure still remains elevated, the eye surgeon must do a paracentesis and possibly irrigate the anterior chamber with saline solution or fibrinolysin, an enzyme which can, after about 30 min of repeated washing, dissolve much of the clot.

If rebleeding occurs, the only change in therapy would be the discontinuation of any cycloplegic being used, for these tend to have a vasodilator effect.

Orbital Fractures   When subjected to blunt trauma, the semisolid contents of the orbit obey the laws of hydraulics, exerting equal forces in all directions and resulting in the well-named "blowout" fracture into the ethmoid sinus, or, more commonly, into the maxillary antrum (Fig. 20-6). The orbital contents are edematous and diffusely hemorrhagic early so that no drop in the level of the globe or enophthalmos is noted in the first few days or weeks, but these signs appear as late sequelae of such fractures. One helpful sign in cooperative patients is diplopia on up and down gaze with fusion on looking directly to the right and left. This is caused by trapping of the inferior rectus muscle in an antral hole. The inferior rectus cannot contract effectively to achieve down gaze because of its new "short" origin, and it can no longer stretch easily to allow other muscles to effect upward

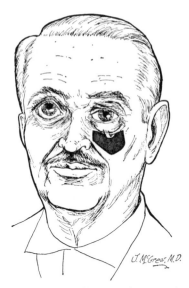

J. McGrew, M.D.

Figure 20-6 Blowout fracture due to blunt trauma. The thin bony floor of the orbit gives way to expansile forces, and orbital fat plus the inferior rectus muscle herniate into the maxillary antrum, where they remain trapped until surgically freed. The patient cannot move the involved eye fully in either up or down gaze and so sees double at these times. The patient can often fuse in horizontal excursions and straight ahead. This patient deserves surgical treatment if x-ray signs are positive or improvement does not progress with clearance of the edema.

gaze. When air enters the orbit from a sinus following a blowout fracture, palpation of the orbit may demonstrate crepitus. The patient should be started promptly on antibiotics to prevent orbital cellulitis or cavernous sinus thrombophlebitis and should be warned not to blow his or her nose. The diagnosis of blowout fracture is sometimes easily substantiated by sinus x-rays, but occasionally the most elaborate tomograms are ineffective in confirming a definite clinical impression. In this instance, the clinical findings are given more weight than the x-rays. Treatment consists of an orbital implant after freeing the incarcerated tissue in adults or of packing the antrum after freeing these tissues in children.

Another orbital injury which may result in

diplopia is the dislocated trochlea. This pulley for the superior oblique muscle is located at the upper nasal corner of the anterior orbit, just under the rim. On x-ray pictures the dislocated structure may or may not be visualized as a bit of calcified material free in the anterior upper orbit medially. The patient with malfunction of one superior oblique muscle often is seen with the head tilted toward the contralateral side, for this permits binocularity in spite of the injury. The trochlea can be restored by suturing the periorbita to it original position.

When a fracture at the inferior medial angle of the orbital rim occurs, the possibility of obstruction to the nasolacrimal duct is present. Early canalization from punctum via the sac into the nose with a small polyethylene or Silastic tube may, by acting as a stent for 4 to 6 weeks, prevent a stricture with its associated chronic tearing.

Avulsion of the optic nerve results when blunt objects such as fingers gouge beneath the globe, forcing it outward.

When pulsating exophthalmos and orbital bruit are noted as a late sequel to orbital trauma, they usually indicate the presence of an arteriovenous shunt. The care of this lesion should be referred to a neurosurgeon.

Displaced fractures of the orbital rim are treated by restoration of position and fixation by wiring, as described in Chap. 19, "Facial and Extracranial Head Injuries."

Lens Contusions If the iris trembles when the eye moves, the lens must be partially dislocated or totally absent from its normal position behind the pupil. If a dislocated lens leads to secondary glaucoma, treatment is medical until such measures are unsuccessful, then surgical.

The lens may be recognized as a clear ovoid mass about two-thirds the size of the cornea. It may be located in front of the iris, subconjunctivally after a scleral rupture or far posteriorly, free in the vitreous. The lens may become cloudy as a result of contusions, but this opacity often does not reach its peak for several weeks. Traumatic dilation of the pupil is not uncommon after blunt trauma, and its significance is poorly understood.

Corneal Trauma   Corneal opacity can result from blunt trauma. The differential diagnosis includes striate keratopathy due to hypotony, overall edema due to ocular hypertension (or glaucoma), ruptures in Descemet's membrane, deep keratitis (which appears 5 to 7 days after trauma and may require drainage of necrotic cells), dendritic keratitis, and rupture of the cornea, either complete or partial. Therapy for all but the last two conditions is expectant and symptomatic. Ruptured corneas require surgical repair because they are penetrating injuries; herpes keratitis is discussed under Abrasions.

Choroidal Rupture   Blunt trauma can lead to rupture of the choroid, sometimes leaving both retina and sclera intact. The ophthalmoscopic picture of a crescent-shaped white area generally concentric to the disk is characteristic. The resultant visual field defects correspond to the white crescents.

Lid Contusions   Contused lids can be treated locally with cold for 24 h and then with heat. Enzymatic therapy has not been dramatically impressive, and gluteal sloughs have been reported.

LACERATIONS

When the lids are lacerated, the most important question is whether or not the eye itself has also been injured. If the globe has been cut, this wound clearly should be repaired before considering therapy for the lids.

Fibrous Coat of the Eye   The signs of perforation of the cornea include a faint gray ring of corneal edema around the wound opening and blood in the anterior chamber of a soft eye (Fig. 20-7). When blood is absent or scanty, the iris may be visualized as it bows forward to make a shallow or flat anterior chamber as a result of leakage of aqueous. There may also be pupillary distortion in the direction of the shallowest part of the chamber. In the early period following a penetrating wound, uveal tissue appears brown or black, but after a few hours the ischemic tissue becomes decolorized so that it resembles mucus. When a transparent jelly protrudes, this is likely to be lens or vitreous. All the prolapsed contents are usually mixed with blood so that the first natural reaction of wanting to wipe away a clot is dangerous because it may cause further prolapse. For this reason, when a global laceration is strongly suspected, the eye should be carefully patched until the patient is asleep on the operating table, at which time the lids can be separated without the patient squeezing and rotating the eyes with resultant extrusion of intraocular contents.

Pus may be present as a sign of fibrous coat perforation if the penetrating wound is several hours old and, though the prognosis is guarded, an attempt should be made to culture the purulent material at the time of the surgical procedure; large doses of antibiotics such as subconjunctival methicillin and polymyxin B should be started immediately and modified later as sensitivities indicate.

Unlike the neat categories of rupture sites seen with contusions, the locations of global lacerations are completely unpredictable except for those associated directly with wounds of the overlying lids.

Preparation   Prior to intraocular operative procedures, the lashes should be trimmed to remove the reservoir of bacteria which would be contained there both pre- and postoperatively. The patient's face from above the brow to the upper lip and from midnose to ear should be scrubbed with pHisoHex for about

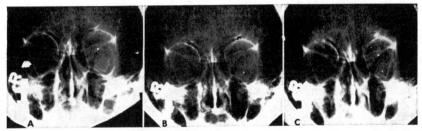

Figure 20-9 Orbital x-rays with the eyes turned up, then down, to show an intraocular foreign body. In x-rays *b* and *a*, the eyes are turned up and down as indicated by the arrows. A foreign body is seen in both *b* and *a* but in different positions. Superimposition of both x-rays in *c* confirms the disparity of position and establishes the strong suspicion that since the foreign body is higher with the eyes rotated downward, and lower with the eyes up, the foreign body must be located behind the center of rotation of the globe. These scout films should be taken before dilating the pupil, when an intraocular foreign body is suspected, for the formal localization which follows is usually more accurate with a small pupil.

widely dilated with 10% Neo-Synephrine and the fundus explored with first a direct, then an indirect ophthalmoscope. Observation of the posterior pole of the eye by means of the usual hand ophthalmoscope has the advantage of a 15 times magnification of the structures at or near the disk. This magnification also applies to foreign bodies, so that their identification as such is usually easy once they are spotted. Axiomatically, to see what extends above one's field of view with the direct ophthalmoscope, one asks the patient to look up; when looking at retina to the patient's right, one asks the patient to look right. This rule, of course, applies for all fields of gaze.

The actual breadth of the magnified field seen with the direct ophthalmoscope is rather small; so fairly gross lesions can be overlooked by this method. Also, the anterior extent of the retina routinely visualized by the use of this instrument is the equator of the globe. This is located about 4 or 5 mm behind the ora serrata, which is the junction of the retina and the ciliary body. Most retinal tears that lead to detachment occur between the equator and the ora. The limitations of the direct ophthalmoscope can be overcome by the skilled use of the binocular indirect ophthalmoscope and scleral depression. Some

practice is necessary in the use of this instrument, which is worn on the head and used with a hand-held lens. Magnification is only about 5 times, depending on the power of lens used, but the field of view is much larger. The indirect ophthalmoscope requires a large pupil, and patients frequently object to its bright light source.

When scout x-ray films with eyes up and eyes down show a foreign body inside the eye, the pupil should not be dilated until x-ray localization is complete. When the radiologist uses a contact lens or other technique which does not depend upon visual centration with reference to the pupil, this point may be ignored, but the usual Sweets localization can easily be thrown off by the thickness of the sclera when the pupil is too large to center the markers accurately, resulting in a false localization inside or outside the eye. If possible while the radiologist is doing the formal localization, a friend or relative should be sent to find a piece of whatever material is reasoned to be in the eye, including both the object which was struck and the instrument used to hit it.

If the material inside the eye is ferrous, a giant eye magnet can be used to retrieve the foreign body, either anteriorly via the cornea, through the pars plana of the ciliary body, or posteriorly through the retina. The anterior approach is certainly favored for anterior chamber particles. The intermediate route is advantageous for posterior foreign bodies since it does not involve pulling a sharp object across a delicate lens capsule to extract it anteriorly, and it does not cause a detachment by creating a hole in the retina. Both the posterior and intermediate routes routinely receive electrodiathermy to prevent this complication. The formation of inflammatory exudates around the foreign body can prevent the necessary mobility of the foreign body which aids in its operative localization and removal by "tenting" when the electromagnet receives current. This problem, plus the inability to attract nonmagnetic metallic particles, can be overcome by the use of the Berman or, more recently, the Wildgren metal localizer. These instruments set up weak magnetic fields, and when a foreign body lies within the field and influences the lines of force, these change the current's resistance and lead to an audible change in pitch of the tone being produced as a baseline. A small or weakly magnetic foreign body bound down by exudates so that it does not tent the sclera can be localized by this means and, after scleral incision, be finally drawn out with the magnet.

Removal of nonmagnetic foreign bodies is being done under direct visualization through the pupil, by direct, self-illuminated instruments posteriorly, and more recently by forceps which are guided to their target electronically with the help of sonar.

Copper and iron must be removed, as must contaminated vegetable matter, but certain inert sterile materials can be left in the eye with more safety than they can be removed. The reason for removing copper and iron is the destructive effect their ions have on ocular tissues.

Corneal foreign bodies which penetrate the anterior chamber yet remain partially embed-ded in the cornea present an interesting technical problem, but more important, they can easily be mismanaged (Fig. 20-10). Attempts at removal of such material in a room used for minor surgical procedures should be discouraged, for the foreign body may be broken, lost in the anterior chamber, or most significantly, it may be partially dislodged, allowing the escape of aqueous with a resultant anterior shift of lens and iris. This anterior shift is equivalent to pushing the foreign body slightly inward, for in either case, the intact lens may be injured, resulting in a cataract. These problems can be approached more effectively in an operating room with facilities for intraocular surgical procedures. Emergency referral of such patients, with no medication except perhaps topical antibiotic solution, with a large loose bandage, a stiff shield, and much tape will save their eyes from iatrogenic or inadvertent patient-inflicted cataract. The patient may be transported sitting but should not be permitted any exertion.

Systemic antibiotic therapy should be instituted promptly in all perforating wounds of the eye. Penicillin, chloramphenicol, erythromycin, and Declomycin are known to penetrate the eye well.

Prevention of foreign body injury to the eye involves the use of safety-hardened glass or, better, plastic lenses in home workshops, in small industry, or in the yard, especially while using power mowers. The effectiveness of such measures has been well proved by required safety measures in large industries. The only reason such lenses are not prescribed routinely is their higher cost and the ease with which plastic can be scratched.

BURNS

Chemical Burns When a patient with a chemical burn is seen initially, the only history obtained before treatment is begun should be the fact that a chemical entered the conjuncti-

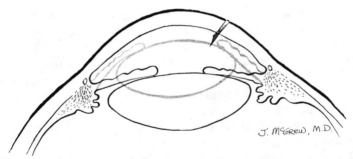

Figure 20-10 Penetrating foreign body of cornea, still embedded in the cornea. A partially penetrating object, once dislodged by attempts at emergency removal, may result in leakage of aqueous and resultant forward shift of the iris-lens diaphragm. This may lead to perforation of the lens capsule and a needless cataract. This can best be avoided by completion of the examination and any necessary manipulation in the operating room.

val cul-de-sac. The first treatment to be instituted is copious irrigation with whatever innocuous fluid is available, without much regard for its sterility or composition. This irrigation should utilize at least 2 L of fluid and continue for at least 30 min or until all the dissolved and particulate chemical is gone. Analgesia may be necessary to obtain cooperation for the irrigation. If particulate matter cannot be removed by irrigation, it should be removed with forceps, using proparacaine (Ophthaine) or other topical analgesics if necessary. When the chemical agent causing the burn is a solid, the upper lid must be double everted (as described above under Superficial Foreign Bodies) so that irrigation and inspection for particles can include all the upper cul-de-sac.

Irrigation should not be delayed to wait for any special solution, for time is extremely important in these injuries. This is especially so when alkaline agents cause the burn, for these agents continue to coagulate tissue as long as they are present. Acids tend to coagulate tissue, and they are then incapable of penetrating it to do further damage. While the irrigation is under way with a liter of normal saline solution, a bottle of 2.5% hypertonic saline solution can be obtained. When the original liter of normal saline solution is about one-third gone, keep it going but add 100 mL of 2.5% NaCl to the original bottle. This approximates a 1.12% solution which can be used comfortably without causing edema of the cornea such as results when solutions of lower osmotic tension are used for a long period.

Paracentesis has been recommended by a few authors who advocate it as a means of removing alkali from the anterior chamber. The pH is increased in the fluid so obtained, but experiments with NaOH have shown that the pH returns to normal within a few minutes after the alkali is removed from the cul-de-sac. The rapid equilibration presumably means that the base is rapidly fixed to the tissues; so violation of the anterior chamber in these cases is probably of little value.

Neutralization of the chemical causing eye burns has not proved of much value over ordinary rapid irrigation, and waiting for an appropriate neutralizing agent has done considerable harm. After prolonged washing, the instillation of fluorescein from a sterile paper strip will allow some estimate of the damage. If one-third or more of the cornea stains or if it appears gray before staining, a topical cycloplegic such as hyoscine 0.2% or homatropine 2% used 3 times a day will be necessary along with antibiotic solutions every 1 to 2 h. When healing is not likely to be complete in a few days, topical steroids may be helpful in the prevention of scarring and vascularization.

Where the conjunctiva has become gray or white and no vascular bed is evident, the sclera is likely to rupture and may require support by grafting with eye bank sclera or some other material. The same prognosis in the cornea is signified by an apparent rapid clearing of the corneal cloudiness. In reality, the cornea is only becoming thinner. This, too, may require grafting with eye bank material. If none is available, a conjunctival flap may be pulled over the cornea (as described above under Lacerations) to give it better nutrition. Further support in the form of a tarsorrhaphy (anastomosis of the upper and lower lids) is also helpful in preventing imminent rupture.

The late complications of chemical burns include dacryostenosis, ectropion, and symblepharon. The closure of the lacrimal drainage apparatus by scarring may be prevented by inserting a stent of fine Silastic tubing which contains a fine steel wire. This stent is softer than polyethylene; so it is less likely to necrose the sphincter of the punctum. Lid scarring and resultant ectropion are minimized by an early tarsorrhaphy, although the lid may still require early or late skin grafting. The adhesion of lids to globe, termed symblepharon, may be helped early after the burn by the frequent instillation of bland ointments; by the use of a conjunctival stent or conformer made of wax, soft rubber, or plastic; by instructing the patient to move the eyes frequently and through as wide a range as possible; and by mechanically separating adhesions as they form.

Thermal Burns   Burns from flames, hot grease, or boiling water involve the lids more commonly than the globe, but their treatment is similar to the burn caused by acids. Cyclo-plegic, antibiotic, and corticosteroid drops are used if the cornea is involved. An antibiotic ointment may be used on the skin with no other dressing. Crusts should be removed three or four times daily by the use of warm, moist compresses and gentle swabbing. If corneal exposure becomes a problem and a tarsorrhaphy is not feasible or desirable, a bland agent such as 5% boric acid ointment will provide the needed protection from drying.

Radiation Burns   Sunburn of the skin is familiar enough so that it is not usually a cause for consultation, but ultraviolet burns of the cornea often bring the patient to a physician. A history of exposure some 4 to 6 h before onset of pain may implicate such sources as sunlamps, welding arcs, germicidal lamps, or the sun. The association with these agents may not occur to the patient because of the long period without pain.

The patient may describe pain severe enough to have wakened him or her. Topical analgesics may be required before the patient will permit an examination. The cornea is usually slightly dull when examined by a bright well-focused light, and it takes a diffuse punctate stain with fluorescein. Photophobia, tearing, spasm of the lids, and red conjunctiva are present without appreciable discharge or crusting.

The patient should be told the cause, that he or she may be unable to work for a day or two, and that no scarring or ultimate visual loss should be expected. The treatment should not include topical analgesics as these retard healing, but oral analgesics such as aspirin or codeine are helpful. Sedatives, ice packs, and short-acting cycloplegics are also valuable. Antibiotic solutions may or may not be used in these cases, depending on the amount of contamination, the patient follow-up anticipated, and the severity of the burn.

BIBLIOGRAPHY

1 Blanton, F. M.: Anterior chamber angle recession and secondary glaucoma, *Arch. Ophthalmol.,* **72**:39, 1964.
2 Duke-Elder, W. S.: "Injuries," in *Textbook of Ophthalmology,* The C. V. Mosby Company, St. Louis, 1954, vol. VI, p. 5717.
3 Gordon, D. M.: "Ocular Injuries," in *Medical Management of Ocular Disease,* Paul B. Hoeber, Inc., New York, 1964, p. 363.
4 Havener, W. H.: "Diagnosis and Management of Eye Injuries," in *Synopsis of Ophthalmology,* 2d ed., The C. V. Mosby Company, St. Louis, 1963, p. 44.
5 Hogan, M. J. and L. E. Zimmerman: *Ophthalmic Pathology—An Atlas and Textbook,* 2d ed., W. B. Saunders Company, Philadelphia, 1962.
6 Keeney, A. H., et al.: *Industrial and Traumatic Ophthalmology, Symposium of the New Orleans Academy of Ophthalmology,* The C. V. Mosby Company, St. Louis, 1964, p. 44.

Part Four

Management in the Posttraumatic and Postoperative Period: Complications

Chapter 21

Postoperative Fluid Management

G. Tom Shires, M.D.

Fluid and electrolyte management in the post-operative and convalescent periods after major traumatic injury is an important aspect of surgical care. Severe trauma imposes a greater impact on body physiology than most elective surgical procedures, and may involve directly (i.e., head injury) or indirectly (shock, renal failure) the function of organs vital to the normal regulation of fluid balance. As in other surgical complications, understanding of the metabolism of salt, water, and other electrolytes will result in prevention of fluid disorders and in early diagnosis and successful therapy when such disorders develop.

The selection of appropriate fluid therapy depends upon the knowledge of the anatomy of body fluids, the physiologic principles governing both gains and losses, and the movement of salt as well as of water and other electrolytes between body compartments. An attempt will be made to present a usable classification which has both physiologic and therapeutic meaning.

The Anatomy of Body Fluids Water constitutes 50 to 70 percent of total body weight. The actual figure, which is remarkably constant in a given individual, is a function of lean body mass. That is leanness is associated with a high and obesity with a low total body water (TBW). Young adults average 63 percent for men and 52 percent for women, which correlates with the sex trend toward subcutaneous adipose tissue. Total body water increases with age at either extreme. The highest proportion is found in infants (near 80 percent) and in the elderly (near 70 percent).

The water of the body is divided into three functional compartments, diagrammed in Fig. 21-1. The fluid within the body's diverse cells (intracellular water) is between 30 to 40 percent by weight. The extracellular water is 20 percent by weight and is divided between the intravascular fluid (plasma 4.5 percent) and the interstitial or extravascular extracellular fluid (16 percent).

The chemical constituents of each of the various compartments is shown in Fig. 21-2. The difference in ionic composition between the intracellular and extracellular fluid (ECF) is maintained by the cell wall, which functions as a semipermeable membrane. The total number of osmotically active particles is 297 to 310 miliosmols (mOsm) in each compartment. A change in the effective osmolarity in one compartment is compensated for by the passive movement of water across the cell wall until the total osmolarity of each compartment is equal. Any solution containing the same number of osmotically active particles as that of the body fluids is said to be *isotonic*.

The principal cation of the extracellular space is sodium, and that of the intracellular space is potassium. The concentration of each ion is maintained by an active pump mechanism present within the cell membrane, which is known to be influenced by changes of the extracellular fluid.

Electrical neutrality is maintained in the extracellular fluid principally by bicarbonate and chloride; the proteins and phosphates plus a small concentration of sulfate constitute the anionic neutrality intracellularly.

All losses and gains of body fluid are directly from the extracellular fluid volume phase. Thus, the intracellular fluid shares in losses which involve a change in concentration of cations (Na^+) or composition (anion) of the extracellular fluid, but usually not in changes involving volume alone.

Classification of Body Fluid Changes The foregoing concepts can be expressed as an anatomic and physiologic classification that allows the diagnosis of fluid disorders as in other diseased states and thus dictates the indicated therapy for these disorders.

If an isotonic salt solution is added or lost to the body fluids, only the *volume* of extracellular fluid will change. If water alone is added or lost to the extracellular fluid, the *concentration* of osmotically active particles will change. Sodium ion accounts for 90 percent of the osmotically active particles in the extracellular fluid, and these principally determine the tonicity of all body fluid compartments.

Figure 21-1 Functional compartments of body fluids.

% BODY WT.

Plasma	5%
Interstitial Fluid	15%
Extracellular Vol.	20%
Intracellular Vol.	40%
Total	**60%**

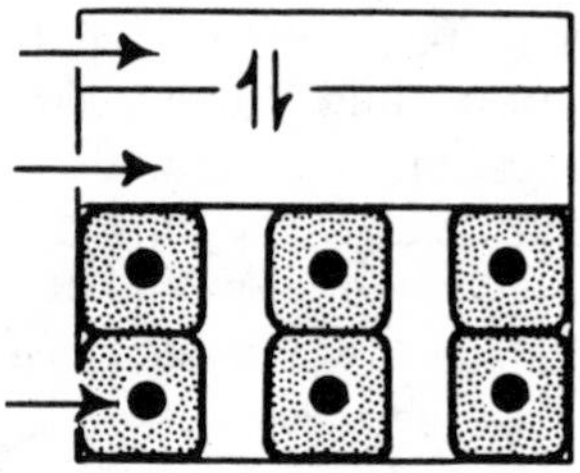

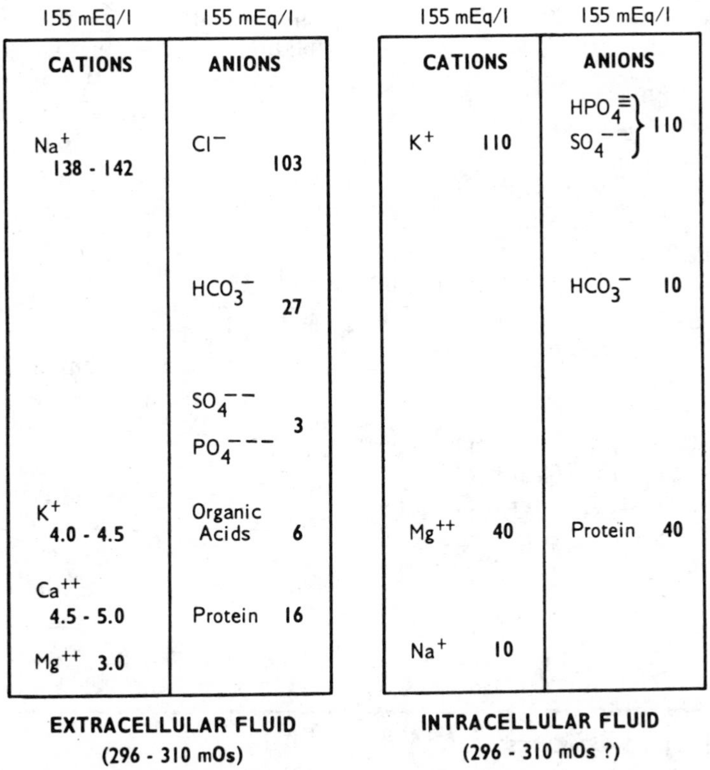

155 mEq/l	155 mEq/l	155 mEq/l	155 mEq/l
CATIONS	**ANIONS**	**CATIONS**	**ANIONS**
Na^+ 138 - 142	Cl^- 103	K^+ 110	$\left.\begin{array}{l}HPO_4^{=}\\ SO_4^{--}\end{array}\right\}$ 110
	HCO_3^- 27		HCO_3^- 10
	SO_4^{--} 3 PO_4^{---}		
K^+ 4.0 - 4.5	Organic Acids 6	Mg^{++} 40	Protein 40
Ca^{++} 4.5 - 5.0	Protein 16		
Mg^{++} 3.0		Na^+ 10	
EXTRACELLULAR FLUID (296 - 310 mOs)		**INTRACELLULAR FLUID** (296 - 310 mOs ?)	

Figure 21-2 Chemical composition of body fluid compartment.

The concentration of all other ions within the extracellular fluid can be altered without significant change in the total osmotically active particles, thus producing only a *composition* change.

An internal loss of extracellular fluid into a nonfunctional space, such as the sequestration of isotonic fluid in a burn, peritonitis, or ascites or following muscle trauma or hemorrhagic shock, is termed a *distributional* change. The transfer or functional loss of extracellular fluid internally may be extracellular (e.g., peritonitis) or intracellular (e.g., as probably occurs in hemorrhagic shock). In any event all distributional shifts or losses result in a contracted functional extracellular fluid space.

In order to determine the status of body fluids, it is necessary to know the intake of fluid and electrolytes by all routes (oral, parenteral, rectal, etc.) and to measure all available losses. Since sodium concentration (270 to 280 mOsm) determines primarily the osmolarity of the extracellular space (290 to 310 mOsm), the serum concentration will indicate the isotonicity of body fluids. Since compositional changes may occur in bicarbonate, chloride, calcium, magnesium, acids, or products of metabolism (urea, nonprotein nitrogen), determination of these ions will indicate the compositional changes which have occurred. Unfortunately, volume deficits or excesses cannot be diagnosed by any chemical laboratory procedure, only by clinical signs.

NORMAL EXCHANGE OF FLUID AND ELECTROLYTES

The basic principles governing both the internal and external exchanges of water and salt are directly applicable to the traumatized patient in the postoperative period. The wide range of physiologic compensation in maintaining a constant internal fluid environment which is accomplished by the kidney, brain, lung, skin, and gastrointestinal tract may be compromised by shock or direct damage to any one of these organs.

Normal Water Exchange   The normal man consumes roughly 2100 to 2600 mL of water per day; 1000 to 1500 mL of water is taken by mouth, 650 mL is extracted from solid food (Fig. 21-3). The daily water losses equal the amount gained—250 mL in stools, 1000 to 1500 mL as urine, and approximately 750 mL as insensible loss. A patient deprived of all external access to water must still excrete a minimum of 500 to 800 mL of urine/day in order to excrete the products of catabolism and will in addition lose 700 to 1000 mL/day insensibly through the skin and lungs.

The posttraumatic patient will gain between 350 to 800 mL of water from excessive catabolism, depending on the degree of trauma, the operation, and the complications occurring in the postoperative period. Thus the net water loss per day will be 1200 to 2000 mL, or roughly that volume of urine required to excrete the catabolic end products (800 to 1000 mL/day) plus insensible losses.

Insensible loss of water occurs through the skin (75 percent) and the lungs (25 percent)

Figure 21-3   Daily water exchange (60- to 80-kg man). *Sodium content may vary from 10 to 90 meq/L. †Greater losses represent sweat which may evaporate and not be appreciated.

H₂O GAIN - ROUTES	AVERAGE DAILY VOLUME	MINIMAL	MAXIMAL
Sensible			
Oral Fluids	800 - 1500	0	1.5 l/hr
Solid Foods	475 - 725	0	1500
Insensible			
Water of oxidation	250	125	375
Water of solution	0	125	250
H₂O LOSS - ROUTES			
Sensible			
Urine	800 - 1500	300	14 l/hr (diabetes insipidus)
Intestinal	0 - 250	0	500
Sweat	0	0	4.5 l/hr *
Insensible			
Lungs	100 - 350	50	1000
Skin	150 - 450	50	750 †

and is increased by hypermetabolism, hyperventilation, and heat (fever). The water loss through the skin cannot exceed approximately a liter per day since sweating will supervene. An unhumidified tracheostomy may with hyperventilation result in insensible losses up to 1 to 1.5 L/day. When excessive heat production (or excessive environment heat) results in fever, the capacity for insensible loss is exceeded and sweating occurs. These losses may, but seldom do, exceed 250 mL/day per degree of fever.

Salt Gain and Losses In the normal ambulatory man, the salt intake per day varies between 3 to 5 g (56 to 90 meq/day) as NaCl (Fig. 21-4). Balance is maintained mainly by the normal kidneys, which excrete a similar quantity. Under conditions of reduced intake or extrarenal losses, the normal kidney can reduce sodium excretion to less than 1 meq/day within 24 h after restriction.

Although a small quantity of salt may be lost in sweat and in urine, in a previously healthy individual normal losses are virtually free of salt for practical consideration. All gastrointestinal losses are isotonic,* and their replacement must be by an isotonic salt solution. It is important also to reiterate that distributional or sequestration losses at any point in the posttraumatic course also represent isotonic sodium losses.

FLUID VOLUME CHANGES AFTER TRAUMA

Changes in the volume of extracellular fluid are the most frequent and important abnormalities encountered in the surgical patient. They occur as a result of gains or losses of isotonic fluids and are not reflected in changes in the concentration of electrolytes per liter. The diagnosis of volume changes is made almost entirely from the clinical signs and symptoms. The signs and symptoms of volume deficiency in the various organ systems are shown in Fig. 21-5. The signs which will be present in an individual patient depend not only upon the relative or absolute quantity of extracellular fluid which has been lost, but on

*Slightly hypotonic.

Figure 21-4 Daily NaCl (salt) exchange (60- to 80-kg man). *Calculated loss of 4 L/h in an unaclimatized man (75 meq/L). **Urine sodium reduced to less than 1 meg within 24 h when salt intake was zero. †Salt-wasting renal disease may have obligatory sodium excretion of 100 to 140 meq/L. Salt-loaded normal kidneys may excrete 200 to 250 meq/L. ††Diarrhea, ileostomy, high intestinal fistulas.

SODIUM EXCHANGE	AVERAGE	MINIMAL	MAXIMAL
Sodium Gain			
Diet	90 mEq/day	0	75 - 100 mEq/hr (oral)
Sodium Loss			
Skin (sweat)	0	0	300 mEq/hr*
Urine	10 - 80 mEq/day	0**	110 - 240 mEq/l†
Intestines	0 - 20 mEq/day	0	300 mEq/hr††

	CNS	GASTROINTESTINAL	CARDIOVASCULAR	TISSUE SIGNS	METABOLISM
Moderate	Sleepiness Apathy Slow (appropriate) Responses Anorexia Lose thirst Cessation of activity	Progressive decrease in food consumption	Orthostatic hypotension - Tachycardia Weakness Collapsed veins Collapsing pulse	Soft, small tongue Longitudinal wrinkly tongue Sticky skin (decreased elasticity)	Mild decrease 99 - 97° Ⓡ
Severe	Decrease tendon reflexes Anesthesia distal extremities Stupor Coma	Nausea, vomiting Refusal to eat Silent ileus and distention	Cutaneous lividity Hypotension Distant heart sounds Cold extremities Absence peripheral pulse	Atonic muscles Sunken eyes	Marked decrease 98 - 95° Ⓡ
Arbitrary division - Signs depended on rate of loss also. Moderate, acute losses may be suddenly lethal.	Signs are similar to barbiturate intoxication. CNS signs and cardiovascular signs occur early with acute rapid losses.		Appears early with acute losses. In recumbent positions hypotension - tachycardia are signs of severe loss.	These signs occur more slowly and may be absent with acute, rapid losses.	Often obscures febrile response to infection.

Figure 21-5 Signs and symptoms of extracellular fluid volume deficiency.

the rapidity with which it is lost and the presence or absence of an associated disease.[9]

In many instances of internal fluid volume shifts, it is not known whether the sequestration is intracellular or extracellular. In either case, the net result is a deficiency in the normal functional amount available to tissues.

After major traumatic injury, volume abnormalities are commonly observed both in the immediate postoperative period and later in the clinical course. The causative factors and the presenting signs are quite different in each. Immediately after a surgical procedure, extracellular fluid volume depletion occurs as a result of continued losses of fluid into sites of injury or into sites of operative trauma, such as into the wall of the small bowel. Several liters of extracellular fluid may be deposited into such areas within a period of a few hours or more slowly in the first day or so from the time of injury.

The sequestered fluid is as nonfunctional as if it were to be lost externally. In a few injuries, this type of loss may be quantitated.

For example, an increase of 1 in in diameter of a midthigh represents a fluid volume loss of 1 to $1\frac{1}{2}$ L. Unfortunately, most injuries do not manifest such an obvious loss.

Unrecognized deficits of extracellular fluid volume during the early postoperative period are manifest primarily as *circulatory* instability. The signs of volume deficiency in other organ systems are delayed for several hours in this type of fluid loss. Diagnosis of the cause of hypotension and tachycardia postoperatively and appropriate therapy are generally required. The generally accepted adequacy of blood pressure of 90/60 and a pulse rate of less than 120 in postoperative patients may not be sufficient to prevent renal ischemia unless, in addition to lack of signs of shock, urine flow is adequate.

In the immediate postoperative period, reliance on a single clinical sign to determine the absence or presence of circulatory insufficiency is fraught with considerable error. Evaluation of the level of consciousness, pupillary size, airway patency, breathing patterns, pulse rate and volume, skin warmth and color, and body temperature, and a 30- to 50-mL hourly urine output combined with a critical review of the injury and the operative fluid management are usually rewarding. For example, reliance upon only a good hourly urinary volume, although usually a good index of volume replacement, may be totally misleading. The excessive administration of glucose (more than 50 g in a 2- to 3-h period) may result in an osmotic diuresis because of the inability of the body to metabolize glucose under anesthesia. Other osmotic agents tend to increase the urine output at the expense of the vascular volume (see Chap. 23, Acute Renal Insufficiency). Chronic renal disease or incipient acute renal damage occurring as the result of shock and injury may be associated with inappropriately high urine volumes.

Since most major trauma involves a loss or transfer of significant quantities of whole blood, plasma, and/or extracellular fluid which can be only grossly estimated, circulatory instability is most commonly caused by an underestimation of the initial losses or insidious concealed continued losses. Operative blood loss is usually estimated by the operating room surgeon as 15 to 42 percent less than the isotopically measured blood loss from that patient. In addition, literally liters of extravascular extracellular fluid can be sequestered in areas of injury and be manifest only by oliguria and mild depression of the blood pressure with a rapid pulse. For example, laparotomy involving considerable handling of the small bowel in the presence of acute chemical peritonitis may result in the functional loss or distributional shift of 6 to 7 L of isotonic fluid into the peritoneum and small bowel.

Completion of the surgical procedure implies control of hemorrhage and often infers the cessation of isotonic fluid losses. The most common cause of postoperative circulatory embarrassment is continued loss either exter-nally or internally of whole blood, plasma, or extravascular extracellular fluid. Common examples are continued swelling in an extremity following a fracture with the loss of both whole blood and extracellular fluid volume; reconstituted arterial injury producing ischemic edema of mostly extravascular fluid; or contusion to a muscle mass which produces a moderate amount of continuing hemorrhage and a large sequestration of extravascular extracellular fluid. Gunshot wounds of the stomach and small bowel result in extensive peritonitis and a remarkable amount of isotonic fluid sequestration. Unless the volume loss is whole blood and very rapid, hypotension due to these causes tends to be latent (6 to 12 h) following operative correction of the injury.

The problem of circulatory instability when such volume losses have been recognized and approximately replaced is often difficult. Further volume replacement of an additional 1000 mL of fluid, while determining whether continuing losses or concomitant contributing causes are present, will often resolve the circulatory instability. Vigorous pursuit of contributing causes with all diagnostic aids discussed elsewhere (Chap. 5, Anesthesia Considerations) must be carried out before excessive harmful volumes of fluid have been administered.

The problem of volume management during the postoperative convalescent phase is one of measurement and replacement of all losses. In the otherwise healthy individual, this usually involves the replacement of measured and collected losses of gastrointestinal origin. The concentration and composition of various types of gastrointestinal drainage fluid are shown in Fig. 21-6. Most fluids are essentially isotonic with few exceptions. When the estimated loss is either slightly above or below isotonicity, appropriate corrections can be made in the daily water administered while

	VOLUME (ML./24 HR.)	NA (MEQ./L.)	K (MEQ./L.)	CL (MEQ./L.)	HCO₃ (MEQ./L.)
Salivary	1,500 (500–2,000)	10 (2–10)	26 (20–30)	{ 10 (8–18)	30
Stomach	1,500 (100–4,000)	60 (9–116)	10 (0–32)	130 (8–154)	
Duodenum	(100–2,000)	140	5	80	
Ileum	3,000 (100–9,000)	140 (80–150)	5 (2–8)	104 (43–137)	30
Colon		60	30	40	
Pancreas	(100–800)	140 (113–185)	5 (3–7)	75 (54–95)	115
Bile	(50–800)	145 (131–164)	5 (3–12)	100 (89–180)	35

Figure 21-6 Daily volume and composition of gastrointestinal sections.

isotonic solutions are used to replace these losses volume per volume.

Appreciation of volume deficits which occur as a most frequent fluid derangement is extremely important. As Moyer[1] has pointed out, oxygen consumption decreases in a linear fashion with increasing extracellular fluid volume deficits (or decreases in exchangeable sodium mass). The clinical signs of volume loss may appear only after deficits of 3 to 5 meq/kg (roughly, 350 meq or 2½ L) have been incurred. Since recognition of volume depletion is purely on the basis of clinical signs, it is important to recognize their potential development prior to the development of severe deficits.

Most important is the fact that changes in composition and concentration are less likely to occur and can be corrected much more readily when the functional volume of body fluid compartments is kept near normal. These observations are at least in part explained by clinical experiments showing that "postoperative salt intolerance" does not occur if extracellular fluid volume deficits are prevented[14]

and others showing normal excretion of a water load after operation if extracellular fluid volume is restored prior to water loading.[19]

VOLUME EXCESSES

The administration of isotonic solutions in excess of volume losses (external or internal) will result in overexpansion of the extracellular fluid spaces. The otherwise normal patient in the postoperative state tolerates an acute overexpansion extremely well. Excesses administered over a few days will soon exceed the kidney's ability to excrete sodium, and since water losses continue, hypernatremia (concentration excess) will ensue. Therefore it is important to determine as accurately as possible from intake and output records, and serum sodium concentrations, the actual need of the patient managed over a period of several days postoperatively.

Attention to the signs and symptoms of overload usually will render this fluid abnormality uncommon. It most frequently arises in an attempt to meet excessive volume losses which are not measurable, such as those occurring through a fistula where drainage is not totally controlled. Several liters of excess extracellular fluid must be present before edema is manifest.

The earliest sign of overload is a weight gain (when obtainable) during the catabolic period when the patient should be losing $1/4$ to $1/2$ lb/day. Heavy eyelids, hoarseness, and dyspnea on exertion may rapidly appear. Circulatory and pulmonary signs of overload are late in appearance and represent a massive overload. The use of central venous pressure is of limited usefulness in following volume replacement. A rise in central venous pressure above normal is indicative of too fast a rate of fluid administration, but does not establish the volume status of the patient.

CONCENTRATION ABNORMALITIES AFTER TRAUMA

Significant changes in serum sodium concentration following trauma are not frequently observed if adequate volumes of isotonic salt solutions have been given following hemorrhage and surgical intervention (see Chap. 1, Principles in the Management of Shock). The kidneys retain the ability to excrete moderate excesses of salt water administered in the early postoperative period. Shires et al.[14] have shown by sodium balance studies that patients do excrete sodium when the functional deficit incurred by the shift to extracellular fluid has been replaced. The normal capacity to excrete water postoperatively has been demonstrated by Wright and Gann,[19] when isotonic salt solutions were administered prior to a challenge with a water load. Thus the commonly described "hyponatremia" associated with surgical intervention and traumatic injury is obviated by replacement of extracellular fluid shifts.[8] The daily maintenance of normal osmolarity is then simplified to the replacement of observable losses of known sodium con-

tent.[3] A few abnormal situations are encountered with specific types of trauma.

Hyponatremia Hyponatremia may easily occur when water is given to replace losses of sodium containing fluids, or when water administration consistently exceeds the water losses. The latter may occur with oliguria or in association with decreases in water loss through the skin and lungs, intracellular shifts of sodium, or the cellular release of excessive amounts of endogenous water. Severe or refractory hyponatremia is difficult to produce if renal function remains normal.

Replacement of Sodium-Containing Fluid Losses with Water A most common error is replacement of gastrointestinal fluid losses with only water or a hypotonic solution. Patients after head injury[17] or patients with preexisting renal disease (loss of concentrating ability) may elaborate urine with a high salt concentration. Both types of patients may have a normal daily urinary volume containing 50 to 200 meq (normal less than 30 meq) of sodium/L. Replacement of these urinary losses with water for a short time will result in hyponatremia usually accompanied by symptoms of water intoxication.

Decreases in Urinary Volume Oliguria from whatever cause (prerenal or renal) reduces the daily water requirements if not corrected. The metabolic acidosis produced by the retention of nitrogenous waste products increases the cellular release of water. Therefore the gain of endogenous water decreases the total water requirements beyond that expected when urinary volume is low.

Decreased Insensible Loss Cutaneous vasoconstriction from any cause decreases both insensible and evaporative water loss by this route. This situation is most commonly encountered with the use of generalized hypothermia.

Endogenous Water Release The patient maintained on intravenous fluids will, between the fifth and tenth day, release the intracellular water solutions as cells disrupt, thus decreasing the quantity of exogenous water required per day.

Intracellular Shifts   Systemic bacterial sepsis is often accompanied by a precipitous drop in serum sodium concentration. This sudden change in extracellular fluid sodium concentration is poorly understood, but is thought to represent loss of extracellular fluid volume either as interstitial or intracellular sequestration. This condition is best treated by withholding water and initiating treatment for the sepsis.

Many hyponatremic states are asymptomatic until the serum sodium falls below 120 meq/L.[5] The moderate, asymptomatic hyponatremia however signifies inappropriate therapy or points to the diagnosis of the basic underlying condition. Symptomatic hyponatremia or water intoxication is difficult to produce if renal function is normal. Convulsions and apnea from uncorrected water excesses occur most often in children and elderly persons. Within the limits imposed by the circulatory apparatus, these deficits should be corrected by the administration of hypertonic salt solutions until the serum sodium is at least above 130 meq/L.

Hypernatremia   Hypernatremia (serum sodium above 150 meq/L), although uncommon, is a dangerous concentrational abnormality. In contradistinction to decreased serum sodium concentration, hypernatremia is easily produced when renal function is normal. In other words, renal compensation for water shortage is poor.

The extracellular fluid hyperosmolarity results in an intracellular water shift to the extracellular fluid. Then presence of a high serum sodium denotes a significant deficit of total body water.

In traumatized patients, hypernatremia arises most often from excessive or unexpected water losses, although it may occur as a result of the use of salt-containing solutions to replace water losses. The following classification of these water losses may be helpful in preventing and treating this abnormality.

Excessive Extrarenal Water Losses   With increased metabolism from any cause, but particularly that associated with fever, the water lost through the evaporation of sweat may reach 200 to 300 mL/h (i.e., 3 to 3½ L/day). Patients with tracheostomies in a dry environment can (with excessive minute volume air exchange) lose as much as 2 L/day by evaporation. The increased evaporation of water from a granulating surface is of significant magnitude in the thermally injured patient in whom water losses may be as great as 3 to 5 L/day.[7]

Increased Renal Water Losses   Extremely large volumes of solute-poor urine may result from hypoxic damage to the distal tubules and collecting ducts or loss of antidiuretic hormone (ADH) stimulation from damage to the central nervous system.[18] In both instances, facultative water reabsorption is impaired. The former occurs in high output renal failure (see Chap. 23, Acute Renal Insufficiency) and in our experience is the most common type of renal failure following injury. The latter occurs with extensive head injuries (usually cerebral and closed) where a temporary state of diabetes insipidus occurs (see Chap. 11).

Solute Loading   High-protein diets may produce an increased osmotic load of urea which necessitates the excretion of large volumes of water. Hypernatremia, azotemia, and decreased volume deficits follow. In general, this can be prevented by furnishing 7 mL of water/g of dietary protein.

Excessive glucose administration results in a large volume of water being required for excretion.[16] In this case, hypernatremia occurs more rapidly.

In addition, all osmotic diuretics, such as mannitol and urea, result in the obligatory excretion of a large volume of water as well as increasing the urinary sodium output. Isotonic salt solutions if used to replace water losses rapidly produce hypernatremia.

COMPOSITIONAL ABNORMALITIES AFTER TRAUMA

Although the metabolism of all the remaining electrolyte and nonelectrolyte substances in the body fluids may change to some extent after injury,[6] only the metabolism of potassium and the acid base balance[4] are important in producing clinical entities requiring therapy during the postoperative period.

The important compositional changes in body fluids occurring during resuscitation and surgical intervention such as the administration of calcium during massive blood replacement (to prevent citrate bleeding), prompt complete resuscitation of shock to prevent the accompanying metabolic acidosis, and the management of airway and ventilation mechanics are discussed elsewhere (see Chaps. 5, 12, dealing with anesthesia, chest trauma, etc.).

Acid-Base Derangements Acid-base derangements are frequently observed in surgical patients.[4,10] Significant problems of acid-base control in traumatized patients occur with chest injuries, with injuries in which pulmonary complications develop, with hypoxic renal damage, and with abdominal injuries requiring prolonged parenteral fluid management. The respiratory control of acid-base derangements is described in Chap. 12, Trauma to the Chest. The metabolic control of acid-base balance is concerned with renal function and the therapy of gastrointestinal losses.

Renal damage may interfere with the important role of the kidneys in the regulation of acid-base control (see Acute Renal Insufficiency, Chap. 23). The kidneys serve a vital function in the normal maintenance of acid-base equilibrium through the excretion of nitrogenous waste products and acid metabolites by the reabsorption of bicarbonate and excretion of chlorides.[13] Exchange of H^+ for Na^+, ammonia formation, and potassium excretion occur in response to acid loading. If renal damage occurs and these functions are lost, a rapidly developing metabolic acidosis ensues. With normal kidneys, acidosis or alkalosis develops when the capacity of the kidneys in handling chlorides and bicarbonate is exceeded.

Most metabolic derangements of acid-base balance occur in patients who are maintained on parenteral fluids for several days. Such derangements also occur when there is excessive loss of gastrointestinal fluids from nasogastric suction, fistulas, ileostomies, or diarrhea. The administration of isotonic fluids with an inappropriate chloride-bicarbonate ratio will not correct the pH changes. The pH of gastrointestinal secretions is usually related to the concentration of chloride or bicarbonate in the fluid. The concentration of ions in various gastrointestinal fluids is shown in Fig. 21-6.

The composition of various parenteral fluids available for administration is shown in Fig. 21-7. Isotonic sodium chloride solution contains 155 meq of sodium and 155 meq of chloride/L. The high concentration of chlorides above the normal serum concentration of 100 meq/L imposes upon the kidney an appreciable load of excess chloride, which cannot be rapidly excreted. Thus a dilutional acidosis develops.[15]

The best available isotonic salt solution is Ringer's lactate solution, which contains 130 meq of sodium balanced by 104 meq of chloride and 26 meq of bicarbonate (44 meq of lactate convertible to 26 meq of sodium bicarbonate). The chief disadvantage of lactated Ringer's solution is the slight hypoosmolarity with respect to sodium. Each liter of Ringer's

SOLUTIONS	ELECTROLYTE CONTENT mEq/l							
	CATIONS					ANIONS		
	Na	K	Ca	Mg	NH$_4$	Cl	HCO$_3^-$	HPO$_4^-$
Extracellular Fluid	142	4	5	3	.3	103	27	3
Lactated Ringer's	130	4	3			109	28	
Ringer's Solution	147	4	4.5			155.5		
.9% Sodium Chloride (Saline)	154					154		
M/6 Sodium Lactate	167						167	
M (molar) Sodium Lactate	1000						1000	
3% Sodium Chloride	590					590		
5% Sodium Chloride	980					980		
.9% Ammonium Chloride					169	169		
2.14% Ammonium Chloride					400	400		

Figure 21-7 Composition of extracellular fluid and of commonly employed (commercially available) electrolyte solutions.

lactate solution furnishes approximately 100 to 150 mL of free water. This presents little or no clinical problem if this fact is considered in the calculation of water loss replacement. For mild metabolic acidosis which occurs with excessive bicarbonate loss, $^1/_6$ molar lactate (130 meq/L each of sodium and bicarbonate) may be employed.

One molar sodium lactate or $2^1/_2$ or 5% sodium chloride is used for the correction of symptomatic hyponatremic states. The choice of which anion (lactate or chloride) to use is determined by the accompanying acid-base derangements. In any case, the total sodium deficit should be calculated (deficit in meq/L × L of total body water) and one-half of this amount administered slowly. Reevaluation of the patient clinically and chemically should be carried out before further administration of sodium.

Potassium Abnormalities Although 98 percent of the potassium is located within the intracellular compartment, the small amount in the extracellular fluid is critical for cardiac and neuromuscular function. Although the total extracellular potassium is only 56 meq in a 70-kg man (4 meq/L × 14 L), the turnover rate through this compartment may be extremely rapid.

The intracellular and extracellular distribution of potassium is influenced by many factors. While significant amounts of intracellular potassium move extracellularly in response to injury, surgical intervention, acidosis, and the catabolic state, dangerous hyperkalemia (greater than 6 meq/L) is rarely encountered if renal function is normal. Following severe trauma, however, normal or excessive urinary volumes may not reflect the ability of the kidney either to clear solutes or excrete potassium (see Chap. 23, Acute Renal Insufficiency).

The common problem is hypokalemia which may occur as a result of (1) increased renal excretion or the movement of potassium into cells; (2) renal excretion of potassium (although reduced 10 to 20 meq/day) continuing after the intake of potassium is reduced to zero, and (3) administration of large quantities of "potassium-free" fluid.

Potassium plays an important role in the regulation of acid-base balance.[2,10,11] Increased excretion occurs with both respiratory and metabolic alkalosis. Potassium is in competition with hydrogen ion for excretion in exchange for sodium ion. Thus in alkalosis the increased potassium ion excretion in exchange for sodium ion permits hydrogen ion conservation and increases K^+ excretion. Low serum K^+ produces a metabolic alkalosis since an increase in excretion of H^+ ion occurs when K^+ is not available in the tubular cell. In a metabolic acidosis, the excess hydrogen ion exchanges for sodium, and potassium is reabsorbed in greater amounts. However, hyperkalemia seldom occurs if parenteral K^+ is withheld.

Excretion of potassium ion increases when increased quantities of sodium are available for excretion. The more sodium available for reabsorption, the more potassium is exchanged for it in the lumen. Potassium requirements for prolonged or massive isotonic fluid volume replacement are increased, probably on this basis. The same mechanism may also explain the increased potassium ion excretion with steroid administration.

In summary, most of the factors which tend to influence potassium metabolism result in excess excretion. A tendency toward hypokalemia is usually found in the traumatized patient whether or not the patient has undergone surgical intervention, except when shock and/or acidosis interferes with the normal renal handling of potassium.

The renal excretion of potassium may be small when compared with the potassium contained in gastrointestinal secretions. The amount per liter of various types of gastrointestinal fluids is shown in Fig. 21-6. In the replacement of these fluids, it is safer to assume the upper limits of loss since an excess is readily handled by the normal kidneys.

BIBLIOGRAPHY

1 Allen, K. G., H. N. Harkins, C. A. Moyer, and J. E. Rhoads: *Surgery Principles and Practice,* J. B. Lippincott Company, Philadelphia, 1961.
2 Berliner, R. W., T. J. Kennedy, Jr., and J. Orloff: Relationship between acidification of the urine and potassium metabolism, *Am. J. Med.,* **11**:274, 1951.
3 Berry, R. E. L.: The pathophysiology and management of complex problems of body fluid homeostasis attending surgical disease states, *Surg. Clin. North Am.,* **41**:1143, 1961.
4 Crandell, W. B.: Acid-base balance in surgical patients: I. A survey of 62 selected cases, *Ann. Surg.,* **149**:342, 1952.
5 DeCosse, J. J., H. T. Randall, D. V. Halif, and K. E. Roberts: The mechanism of hyponatremia and hypotonicity after surgical trauma, *Surgery,* **40**:27, 1956.
6 Mark, J. B. D. and M. A. Hayes: Studies of calcium and magnesium metabolism during surgical convalescence, *Surg. Gynecol. Obstet.,* **113**:213, 1961.
7 Moncrief, V. A. and A. D. Mason: Water vapor loss in the burned patient, *Surg. Forum,* **13**:38, 1962.
8 Moore, F. D. and M. R. Ball: *The Metabolic Response to Surgery,* Charles C Thomas, Publisher, Springfield, Ill., 1952.
9 Moyer, C. A.: *Fluid Balance,* Year Book Medical Publishers, Inc., Chicago, 1954.
10 Randall, H. T. and K. E. Roberts: The significance and treatment of acidosis and alkalosis in surgical patients, *Surg. Clin. North Am.,* **36**:315, 1956.
11 Roberts, K. E., G. Magida, and R. F. Pitts: Relationship between potassium and bicarbonate in blood and urine, *Am. J. Physiol.,* **172**:47, 1953.
12 ———, H. T. Randall, H. L. Sanders, and

M. Hood: Effects of potassium on renal tubular reabsorption of bicarbonate, *J. Clin. Invest.*, **34:**666, 1955.

13 Rush, B. F., Jr. and H. T. Randall: Postsurgical anuria: An experimental study of fluid and electrolyte changes, *Surgery,* **44:**655, 1958.

14 Shires, G. T. and D. E. Jackson: Postoperative salt tolerance, *Arch. Surg.,* **84:**703, 1962.

15 —— and V. Holman: Dilutional acidosis, *Ann. Intern. Med.,* **28:**551, 1948.

16 Soroff, H. S., E. Peorson, G. K. Arney, and C. P. Artz: Metabolism of burned patients: An estimation of the nitrogen and potassium requirements, *Research in Burns,* No. 9, AIBS Publishers, Washington, D.C., 1962.

17 Stern, W. E.: Problems in fluid replacement and cerebral edema in the management of surgical lesions of the central nervous system, *Am. J. Surg.,* **100:**303, 1960.

18 Wise, B. L. and V. J. Pileggi: Fluid and electrolyte balance following injuries to the head, *Am. J. Surg.,* **97:**205, 1959.

19 Wright, Hastings K. and Donald S. Gann: Correction of defect in free water excretion in postoperative patients by extracellular fluid volume expansion, *Ann. Surg.,* **158:**70, 1963.

Chapter 22

Ventilatory Management

Leonard D. Hudson, M.D.

This chapter deals with ventilatory management of the trauma patient with acute respiratory failure. Ventilatory management is based on an understanding of the pathophysiology in this patient, discussed in Chap. 32, "Postinjury Acute Pulmonary Failure." Ventilatory therapy is supportive: it improves oxygenation and prevents further alveolar collapse and filling with fluid. It does not replace careful management of the underlying condition and complications (such as sepsis) which led to the respiratory failure and, if left untreated, may propagate further lung injury.

Ventilatory management has become quite technical in certain aspects. However, the goals and principles of ventilatory management remain simple in concept and must be understood and controlled by the attending physician. The attending physician should not abdicate the responsibility of supervising the respiratory aspects of the patient's care. Important supporting personnel have been developed who can help immensely in the care of the patient requiring ventilatory support. Respiratory therapists can be particularly helpful with the technical aspects of such care. The purpose of this chapter is to review the principles and practice of ventilatory management of the trauma patient in order to help the primary care physicians carry out their supervisory role.

INDICATIONS FOR VENTILATORY SUPPORT

The point in a patient's course at which ventilatory support should be instituted remains a clinical decision. Guidelines can help in making this decision but should not be considered as being absolute. Helpful guidelines have been reviewed in the previous chapter (see Chap. 32).

In general, ventilatory support should be initiated early in the trauma patient, when developing respiratory failure is first recognized. For reasons already reviewed (describing the pulmonary responses to trauma), the primary manifestation of the lung injury is a failure in oxygenation rather than failure in CO_2 removal. Therefore, the presence of hypoxemia is an important factor in determining the need for ventilatory support. In general, if an adequate Pa_{O_2} (for example, a Pa_{O_2} of 65 mmHg) cannot be maintained by nasal oxygen or a face mask from a source delivering 40% oxygen, ventilatory support should be considered. If oxygenation is marginal, the fraction of inspired oxygen (FI_{O_2}) should be increased until airway control is established by endotracheal intubation. Intubation allows more precise control of the FI_{O_2} and provides the route for assisted or controlled ventilation, if necessary. If adequate oxygenation cannot be achieved with the patient breathing 40% O_2 from a T piece attached to the endotracheal tube, or if respiratory acidosis (or failure to compensate for a metabolic acidosis) is present, mechanical support of ventilation must be considered. If hypoxemia is clearly progressing, ventilatory support should be considered even if an arbitrary level of hypoxemia has not yet occurred. In this clinical situation, early institution of ventilatory support may prevent the need for a long period of support later in the patient's course.

CONTROL OF OXYGENATION

The causes of hypoxemia have been reviewed in detail in Chap. 32. Briefly, there are four physiological processes involving the lung which cause hypoxemia: hypoventilation, ventilation-perfusion mismatch, shunting, and diffusion limitation. Hypoventilation is un-common in trauma patients and can be easily recognized by an increased Pa_{CO_2}. Diffusion limitation is not an important cause of hypoxemia and for practical purposes can be ignored. Ventilation-perfusion mismatch and shunting are the major causes of hypoxemia associated with trauma. Shunting can be thought of as one extreme of a ventilation-perfusion imbalance; i.e., *no* ventilation is present but perfusion continues, effectively causing shunting of blood from the right side of the heart to the left without ever being exposed to an opportunity to take up oxygen. The practical aspect of the difference between ventilation-perfusion mismatch and pure shunt involves the FI_{O_2} required to achieve adequate oxygenation of the arterial blood. A relatively small amount of supplemental inspired oxygen will allow an adequate Pa_{O_2} if a ventilation-perfusion mismatch is the problem, but a high inspired FI_{O_2} will be required if the hypoxemia is caused by shunting. The pathological pulmonary processes which most commonly occur in association with trauma are diffuse alveolar edema and diffuse focal areas of atelectasis. Both result in no ventilation but continued perfusion. Thus, pulmonary shunting is the most common cause of hypoxemia in the trauma patient. The remainder of this section will deal with the methods which should be considered in the control of hypoxemia.

Effect of Tidal Volume

The use of relatively large tidal volumes (V_T) is important. Small tidal volumes (5 mL/kg of body weight) during anesthesia have been shown to result in progressive hypoxemia, presumably due to progressive areas of focal alveolar atelectasis.[2,21] If the V_T is 10 mL/kg of body weight or greater, hypoxemia does not develop.[63,65] Since diffuse alveolar atelectasis is one of the pathological features in acute respiratory failure associated with trauma, the use of high tidal volumes both for treatment and prevention is logical. In fact, evidence exists that high tidal volumes in combination with other ventilatory modalities are helpful in improving oxygenation in an animal model of ARDS.[25] Therefore, tidal volumes in the range of 10 to 15 mL/kg of body weight are recommended. There are potential adverse effects of applying excessively high tidal volumes. First, there is experimental evidence that extremely high tidal volumes may result in the reduction of surfactant activity.[27] However, the volumes associated with this effect are far in excess of those recommended for use in patients, so this complication is probably not of clinical significance. Second, and much more real, is the possibility of lung rupture leading to pneumothorax or pneumomediastinum. In a study of patients receiving mechanical ventilation, pneumothorax was found to be associated with excessive tidal volumes.[7] An extension of this study showed that the tidal volumes associated with increased risk of the lung rupture could easily be determined by a simple measure of total compliance.[6]

Compliance (change in volume/change in pressure) is a measure of lung stiffness; the stiffer the lungs the lower the compliance. Alveolar atelectasis results in decreased compliance. Compliance will increase if an increase in tidal volume recruits atelectatic alveoli. If the tidal volume is increased further, at some point the open alveoli will become relatively overdistended. At this point, the lung behaves as if it were stiffer, and compliance decreases. A measurement, usually called total static compliance or effective total static compliance (C_{eff}), which reflects lung compliance is easily measured in patients receiving mechanical ventilation.[5]

Determining compliance requires measuring the change in volume and the change in pressure. The change in volume is equal to the tidal volume used. The change in airway pressure is shown by the pressure dial on the ventilator. However, the peak airway pressure achieved during tidal volume delivery consists both of the pressure required to overcome airway resistance and the pressure required to hold the lung at that volume. In order to eliminate that pressure required to overcome airway resistance, the airway pressure must be measured during a period of no air flow. This can be easily accomplished by occluding the exhalation line at peak inflation. The pressure on the ventilator manometer dial will then fall from the peak pressure to the pressure required to maintain the lung and the chest wall at the tidal volume employed. Compliance is easily calculated by dividing the corrected exhaled tidal volume by the inhalation hold pressure. If positive end-expiratory pressure is being used, the end-expiratory pressure must be subtracted from the inhalation hold pressure to obtain the *change* in pressure during the ventilatory cycle. The resulting compliance (C_{eff}) is an indication of compliance of the lung and chest wall (thus the term "total compliance"). Changes in total compliance in the acutely ill patient primarily reflect changes in the compliance of the lungs. Therefore, C_{eff} can be used to pick the optimal tidal volume for the individual patient.

By measuring C_{eff} at increasing tidal volume, a curve can be constructed plotting compliance against tidal volume. Usually the compliance will initially increase but eventually begin to decrease. It has been suggested that the appropriate tidal volume to use would be that which coincides with the peak compliance (i.e., the highest tidal volume that can be achieved before alveolar "overdistention," decreased compliance, and increased risk of lung rupture occurs).[5]

Some ventilators can provide a sigh breath, that is, a periodically delivered breath larger than the usual tidal volume. A sigh capability was designed for two reasons. First, progressive atelectasis may occur when small tidal volumes are used, as discussed above. Second, sighs occur in a normal spontaneous breathing pattern. However, a normal breathing pattern also consists of smaller tidal volumes than are usually used with mechanical ventilation. When tidal volumes in the range of 10 to 15 mL/kg of body weight are used, there is no evidence that sighs are necessary. Therefore, routine use of sighs is not recommended.

Respiratory rate and flow rates affect oxygenation only through an effect on CO_2 regulation and will be discussed in the section on control of Pa_{CO_2} and pH. Variations in flow rates in the ranges available on most ventilators have not been found to result in measurable changes in distribution of ventilation or oxygenation.[23]

$F_{I_{O_2}}$

The fraction of inspired oxygen ($F_{I_{O_2}}$) is extremely important in control of arterial oxygenation. An increase in $F_{I_{O_2}}$ is often the most rapid way of improving oxygenation. The toxic effects of oxygen (except for reduced respiratory drive in the chronic obstructive pulmonary patient) are time-dose related and do not appear acutely. Therefore, one should err on the high side of $F_{I_{O_2}}$ in *initial* respiratory adjustments. Hypoxemia is the most life-threatening aspect of acute respiratory failure, and control of hypoxemia is of paramount importance. If an extremely high $F_{I_{O_2}}$ is required to avoid dangerous hypoxemia, then it must be used initially. On the other hand, since parenchymal oxygen toxicity can occur, efforts must be made to adjust the $F_{I_{O_2}}$ to the lowest level which provides adequate arterial oxygenation (oxygen saturation of hemoglobin greater than 90%). Lung injury from high $F_{I_{O_2}}$ is related to the alveolar P_{O_2} (PA_{O_2}) and not the arterial P_{O_2} (Pa_{O_2}) achieved.[67] This lung injury is nonspecific and similar to that which has already been described as occurring in trauma patients (see Chap. 32). This type of toxicity is related both to time and dose but is variable from patient to patient. Clinically significant parenchymal oxygen toxicity at an

$F_{I_{O_2}}$ of 1.0 requires at least 24 h of exposure. Lower levels require a longer period of time for toxicity to be manifest. The level of $F_{I_{O_2}}$ which is considered "safe" is debatable. Significant oxygen toxicity has been demonstrated at an $F_{I_{O_2}}$ of 0.7.[10] A $F_{I_{O_2}}$ of 0.4 in dogs for several days has produced demonstrable pathological changes, but the clinical importance of these are unknown.[48] Even relatively short periods of 100% oxygen can impair mucociliary clearance mechanisms[14,54] and have been shown to inhibit alveolar macrophage activity in animal models.[34] The clinical significance of these effects is not clear. In terms of parenchymal oxygen toxicity, a $F_{I_{O_2}}$ of 0.4 to 0.5 is generally considered relatively safe.

In order to determine the lowest $F_{I_{O_2}}$ which still allows adequate arterial oxygenation, arterial blood gases must be monitored. Any adjustment of the $F_{I_{O_2}}$ must be related to changes in Pa_{O_2}. Arterial blood gas analysis should be repeated after the adjustment has been made. As noted above, hypoxemia in the trauma patient is primarily due to shunting of blood through the lung. When a large shunt is present, a high $F_{I_{O_2}}$ is required to improve the arterial Pa_{O_2}. Over the long term, other methods must be considered to lower the $F_{I_{O_2}}$. Also, when a large shunt is present, a large change in $F_{I_{O_2}}$ may have relatively little effect on the Pa_{O_2}. Therefore, if a $F_{I_{O_2}}$ of 1.0 results in a Pa_{O_2} of 80 mmHg, it may be possible to lower the $F_{I_{O_2}}$ with a relatively small change in Pa_{O_2}. For example, in this situation a $F_{I_{O_2}}$ of 0.7 may result in a Pa_{O_2} of 70 mmHg.

One further factor that may occasionally play a role in the adjustment of $F_{I_{O_2}}$ is the mixed venous oxygen saturation. In some situations the mixed venous oxygen saturation is a relatively good reflection of overall tissue oxygenation. Therefore, it may be possible to lower $F_{I_{O_2}}$ even with borderline values of Pa_{O_2}, if there is no decrease in the mixed venous oxygen saturation value. This fine adjustment of $F_{I_{O_2}}$ would only be wise if the mixed venous oxygen saturation could be readily monitored (i.e., a pulmonary artery catheter is in place) and high $F_{I_{O_2}}$ has been required for more than one day.

Positive End-Expiratory Pressure

If high $F_{I_{O_2}}$ alone is used to support oxygenation in the trauma patient with diffuse lung injury, a therapeutic dilemma is created. First, if shunting is severe, even a $F_{I_{O_2}}$ of 1.0 may not result in adequate correction of hypoxemia. Second, even if initial improvement in the Pa_{O_2} is achieved, the $F_{I_{O_2}}$ required may result in further lung injury with eventual progression of hypoxemia. Therefore, other steps to support oxygenation and also to allow reduction in potentially toxic levels of $F_{I_{O_2}}$ are obviously important. Positive end-expiratory pressure (PEEP) is currently the major ventilatory technique which results in improved oxygenation. PEEP improves ventilation of poorly ventilated or nonventilated segments and prevents further alveolar filling or collapse.

PEEP consists of maintaining a positive airway pressure throughout the entire respiratory cycle rather than just on inspiration as with usual positive pressure ventilation. In its original use, PEEP was primarily employed to allow a reduction in the $F_{I_{O_2}}$ from potentially toxic levels.[1,39,45,47] Currently there is great interest in whether PEEP also results in a change in the natural history of the acute respiratory failure and its pathophysiology. Recent reports have suggested using extremely high levels of PEEP, which result in maximum improvement in oxygenation even if the $F_{I_{O_2}}$ could be lowered to that of room air.[8,36] It has been suggested that this method results in improved survival.[36] At the time of this writing, firm evidence that this method results in a significant improvement in the course of the pathophysiology is not available. Therefore, this section will deal with PEEP as used in the standard or "traditional" application. The goal of the standard method of applying PEEP will be defined as supporting oxygenation so that

the $F_{I_{O_2}}$ can be lowered to a safe level, generally considered to be 0.4 or less.

The use of positive end-expiratory pressure is indicated if a high $F_{I_{O_2}}$ (greater than 0.4) is required for adequate oxygenation in the trauma patient with acute respiratory failure due to diffuse lung injury (adult respiratory distress syndrome). PEEP should always be initiated under a protocol by which the beneficial and potential adverse effects can be evaluated. This will be discussed below. PEEP is usually not effective when there is a localized pulmonary abnormality, such as lobar pneumonia, as the cause of hypoxemia.

There may be a potential prophylactic effect of PEEP in patients with high risk of developing acute respiratory failure. A lower prevalence of the development of the adult respiratory distress syndrome in surgical patients with severe disease randomized to prophylactic PEEP has been reported.[59] One method of applying this information until it is confirmed would be to employ PEEP with more liberal criteria in the multiple trauma patient. If the patient with trauma requires an airway for other purposes and has even mild hypoxemia, a low level of PEEP (for example, 5 cmH_2O) is reasonable and may prevent further progression to acute respiratory failure. Other patients at high risk for ARDS for whom prophylactic PEEP may be indicated are listed in Chap. 32. Firm recommendations regarding prophylactic PEEP must await further investigation in this area.

The major beneficial effect of PEEP is improvement in Pa_{O_2}. This is related to an increase in lung volume.[24,47] Both diffuse alveolar edema and focal atelectasis, the underlying pathological abnormalities in these patients, result in decreased lung volume. If either of these processes can be reversed, lung volume should improve. The association of improvement in Pa_{O_2} with increasing lung volume suggests that PEEP reverses one or both of these processes. No acute change in the total amount of lung water has been shown with PEEP application, although Pa_{O_2} acutely improves.[14,31] This indicates that the major improvement in both lung volume and Pa_{O_2} is due to recruitment of atelectatic alveoli. A change in distribution of lung water or pulmonary edema fluid also remains a possible mechanism.

The level of PEEP is limited primarily by reduction of cardiac output. PEEP potentially can lower cardiac output in two ways. PEEP necessarily results in an increased intrathoracic pressure. This pressure may be transmitted to the pleural space resulting in an increased intrapleural pressure. As the great veins return to the heart through the thorax, they are exposed to pleural pressure. Thus, an elevated pleural pressure may result in impaired venous return and reduced cardiac output.[12,29] With increased lung stiffness, less of the pressure applied to the airways is transmitted to the pleural space. Therefore, this effect is less apparent in patients with adult respiratory distress syndrome (with reduced compliance) than it would be in normal subjects. However, it still can clearly occur, especially in the patient with hypovolemia, and is a significant concern in trauma patients. The second potential cause of cardiac output decrease is related to the effect of PEEP increasing lung volume. If alveolar distention of a significant proportion of alveoli becomes excessive, i.e., some alveoli are relatively "overdistended," a narrowing and stretching of the capillaries supplying those alveoli results. This will cause an increase in pulmonary vascular resistance, resulting in a decreased cardiac output.[29,47] A third possible cause of a PEEP-related reduction in cardiac output is a direct depressive effect on left ventricular function.[9,49,53] Any effect on left ventricular performance may be due to a decrease in filling volume.[17]

Another potential adverse effect of PEEP is possible lung rupture. Pneumothorax and pneumomediastinum have not been shown to be definitely related to PEEP.[40] However, if PEEP is increased until alveolar overdisten-

tion occurs, the potential of lung rupture remains a concern.

In applying PEEP to any patient, the major responsibility of the clinician is to ensure the beneficial effect of improved oxygenation while minimizing the potential of adverse effects, especially reduction in cardiac output. When PEEP is initially applied, two questions must be answered:

1 Is PEEP beneficial in this patient?
2 What is the best level of PEEP for this patient?

In order to answer these questions, it is imperative that PEEP be applied in a systematic fashion and appropriate observations be made. This systematic application and evaluation of PEEP will be referred to as the "PEEP trial." A PEEP trial should include the following elements:

1 PEEP should be the only variable changed.
2 PEEP should be increased by steps.
3 The period of time at each step before evaluation should be relatively short.
4 At each step, evaluation for beneficial effect (increased Pa_{O_2}) and adverse effects (decreased cardiac output and its clinical results) should be carried out.

PEEP should be the only variable changed in order to assure that any improvement (or deterioration) may be reasonably related to PEEP. Therefore, the patient should be on a $F_{I_{O_2}}$ which will assure reasonable (not dangerous) levels of arterial oxygenation. This $F_{I_{O_2}}$ need not be 1.0, which has been commonly used in the past during PEEP trials. If a $F_{I_{O_2}}$ of 1.0 is used, the amount of shunt can be measured in percent.[66] However, for clinical purposes significant improvement in oxygenation can be recognized on any $F_{I_{O_2}}$, and percent shunt need not be measured. In addition, a $F_{I_{O_2}}$ of 1.0 may result in absorption atelectasis with worsening of the shunt.[4,28,30] This occurs because nitrogen is no longer present in areas of lung with partially compromised ventilation. The oxygen may be taken up by the blood more rapidly than it can be replaced through ventilation, and alveolar atelectasis can result. Therefore, it is recommended that the PEEP trial be done on any $F_{I_{O_2}}$ which will provide a safe level of Pa_{O_2} (preferably greater than 60 mmHg). It is important that the $F_{I_{O_2}}$ and tidal volume remain constant throughout the remainder of the PEEP trial.

PEEP should be increased by steps; 5 cmH_2O is a convenient increment to use. If larger steps are used, the PEEP level which is best for an individual patient may be inadvertently passed. In fact, oxygenation which may have been improved at a lower level of PEEP may actually worsen at high PEEP levels.[33] The shorter the period of time at a given PEEP level, the more likely any major changes would be related to the PEEP instead of a change in the underlying condition of the patient (unrelated to PEEP therapy). On the other hand, the time should be long enough to allow a reasonable chance of improved oxygenation. Early in ARDS, PEEP has a significant beneficial effect on oxygenation within 10 to 15 min;[39] 15 to 30 min at any given PEEP level is a reasonable period of time to allow a beneficial effect and reduce the chance of significant changes in the underlying pathophysiology that are not PEEP related. This period of time may not allow the maximal oxygenation effect at a given PEEP level to be manifest. It may also miss beneficial Pa_{O_2} increases in "slow responders." However, it seems to be a reasonable compromise. Therefore, 15 to 30 min at each PEEP level is recommended in a standard PEEP trial. Clinicians should be aware that considerably longer periods of time may be required for a beneficial response to be demonstrated late in the course of the adult respiratory distress syndrome.[43]

Arterial blood gases are analyzed at each PEEP level to show the beneficial effects of PEEP. Which parameters should be monitored to determine whether PEEP has had an adverse effect on hemodynamics is a more difficult question. This must be individualized to the specific patient and to the available facilities. However, certain generalizations can be made. Parameters which are practical to measure include clinical parameters reflecting cardiac output such as blood pressure, pulse amplitude, and urine output; laboratory measurements which reflect cardiac output such as mixed venous oxygen saturation; and direct measurements of cardiac output (for example, by the thermodilution method). Obviously the easily measurable clinical parameters should always be followed. These may be sufficient measures of hemodynamics in relatively stable patients without evidence of potential blood volume or cardiac abnormalities and in whom a relatively low level of PEEP is anticipated. However, in the unstable patient, the patient with a questionable volume or cardiac status, or the patient in whom it is likely that relatively high levels of PEEP (15 cmH_2O or greater) will be required, more direct measurements of cardiac output should be obtained. Since the blood volume status is often unclear in the patient with severe trauma, these other measurements of cardiac output are definitely recommended if the patient has severe hypoxemia.

Mixed venous oxygen saturation may reflect cardiac output and tissue oxygenation. As cardiac output falls, more oxygen is taken up from the hemoglobin at the tissue level and mixed venous oxygen saturation will decrease. This value is related to cardiac output through the Fick principle, in which

Cardiac output = oxygen consumption/arterial O_2 content − mixed venous O_2 content.

In this relationship, changes in arterial oxygen content are likely to be minimal since a $F_{I_{O_2}}$ is usually employed at which almost complete saturation of the hemoglobin is already present; therefore, even large increases in Pa_{O_2} will have relatively little effect on the arterial oxygen content, as this is mainly dependent on oxygen saturation of hemoglobin. If oxygen consumption remains unchanged, cardiac output will be reflected by mixed venous oxygen saturation, which is the major factor in determining mixed venous oxygen content. However, in the acutely ill, unstable patient, to assume that oxygen consumption remains unchanged may not be valid. Also, changes in distribution of cardiac output will affect both oxygen consumption and mixed venous oxygen saturation. Therefore, if a more direct measurement of cardiac output is available, this is preferable. Since mixed venous oxygen saturation measurement requires a pulmonary artery catheter (in order to avoid the streaming effect which occurs when blood is drawn from the superior vena cava),[32] it seems reasonable to measure cardiac output by the thermodilution method if thermodilution pulmonary artery catheters and a thermodilution cardiac output computer is available.[26] This method allows safe, rapid serial measurements of cardiac output.

One study has suggested that the measurement of effective total static compliance (C_{eff}) during a PEEP trial reflected cardiac output and oxygen transport (cardiac output times arterial oxygen content).[62] Mean data from this study indicated that the highest C_{eff} occurred at the best cardiac output and maximum oxygen transport values. However, C_{eff} was not found to be helpful in picking the PEEP level at which cardiac output and oxygen transport were best when this concept was applied to individual patients.[35] The majority of patients have a significant (20 percent) decrease in cardiac output at a PEEP level before there is a significant (10 percent) decrease in compliance.[35] Therefore, compliance cannot be relied on to determine changes in cardiac output, and some more direct measure of cardiac output must be followed.

Compliance may be useful in another regard. The same reasoning discussed above in using compliance to predict the most benefi-

cial tidal volume can also be applied to a PEEP trial. If a fall in C_{eff} indicates the PEEP level at which a significant proportion of alveoli are being "overdistended," this may also be the level at which lung rupture is more likely to occur. Although this concept has not been tested (and, indeed, would be most difficult to test in these critically ill patients), it is certainly logical to consider a large fall in C_{eff} as a criterion for terminating the PEEP trial and returning to the previous level of PEEP tested.

PEEP Withdrawal

Less attention has been paid to the appropriate method of PEEP withdrawal as compared to PEEP institution. However, it has been demonstrated that if PEEP withdrawal is premature, adverse pulmonary effects can occur, resulting in falls in Pa_{O_2}.[42] When PEEP is reinstituted, some patients require a higher level of PEEP than was previously required or may require more than 24 h to return to the previous level of oxygenation. Although specific criteria for PEEP withdrawal are not yet available, some general guidelines are clear. PEEP withdrawal should not be attempted when the patient is unstable. Even if the respiratory status is relatively stable, PEEP withdrawal should not be attempted if the underlying cause of respiratory abnormality is ongoing, for example, uncontrolled sepsis. Oxygenation should be stable or improving before PEEP withdrawal is considered. In a retrospective review of PEEP withdrawal, failure was associated with worsening oxygenation as indicated by a decreased Pa_{O_2}/FI_{O_2} ratio over the 12 h prior to PEEP withdrawal. Failure was also more likely if a patient had been at a particular PEEP level for a short period of time (less than 6 h). The greatest number of PEEP withdrawal failures occurred at the step from 5 to 0 cmH_2O PEEP.[42] Sudden reduction of PEEP from high values to zero may result in a sudden increase in pulmonary blood volume (autotransfusion phenomenon) resulting in a transient increase in pulmonary edema and worsening pulmonary function.[50]

The following guidelines for PEEP withdrawal are recommended:

1 The patient should be clinically stable before PEEP withdrawal is attempted.

2 Oxygenation should be improving as indicated by a rising $Pa_{O_2}/F_{I_{O_2}}$ ratio.

3 The $F_{I_{O_2}}$ should be 0.4 or less before PEEP withdrawal is attempted.

4 PEEP should be lowered by steps (again, 5 cmH_2O is convenient).

5 After each decrease in PEEP arterial blood gases should be checked initially (within 30 min).

6 Arterial blood gases should be measured again just before the next PEEP decrease is attempted.

7 The patient should have stable or improving arterial blood gases for at least 6 h at each PEEP level before another lowering step is attempted.

8 Special caution should be used when reducing the PEEP from 5 to 0 cmH_2O.

CONTROL OF Pa_{CO_2} AND pH

Control of Pa_{CO_2} is important primarily in relation to its effect on pH, both of arterial blood and cerebrospinal fluid. The Pa_{CO_2} is determined by the balance between CO_2 production and ventilation. Although CO_2 production may be increased in the trauma victim with ARDS, usually there is a low Pa_{O_2} as the severe hypoxemia stimulates increased ventilation. The Pa_{CO_2} can be lowered by hyperventilation because of the difference in the dissociation curves of O_2 and CO_2. The areas of relatively well preserved alveoli are hyperventilated to such a degree that considerable CO_2 can be removed. This is usually in excess of the CO_2 which is retained in the areas of poor ventilation-perfusion or shunting; the end result is a Pa_{CO_2} which is lower than normal. However, little O_2 can be added, as the O_2 saturation in blood perfusing the well-ventilated areas approaches 100 percent even before hyperventilation begins.

Occasionally hypercapnia does occur with extremely severe adult respiratory distress syndrome. Also, hypercapnia may be a problem if the trauma victim has previously existing chronic obstructive pulmonary disease or requires heavy sedation. Manipulation of the Pa_{CO_2} may be important if a severe metabolic acidosis is present which is not adequately compensated by the patient's spontaneous ventilation. The goal of ventilatory management in controlling Pa_{CO_2} and pH is to result in a relatively normal pH. One exception would be the patient with severe head trauma. Early in management of this patient a respiratory alkalosis may be of benefit by decreasing cerebral blood flow and reducing cerebral edema. However, the cerebrovascular response to respiratory alkalosis is relatively short-lived and does not justify maintenance of an alkalosis for several days, as alkalosis has other harmful effects.

The level of Pa_{CO_2} is directly related to alveolar ventilation. Appropriate management of the complications such as sepsis may reduce CO_2 production, but the most direct way to affect Pa_{CO_2} is to change the minute ventilation. Minute ventilation is a product of tidal volume times respiratory rate. Since Pa_{CO_2} is related to alveolar ventilation rather than total minute ventilation (alveolar ventilation plus dead space ventilation), the same minute ventilation produced by differing combinations of tidal volume and rate may result in differing levels of alveolar ventilation and, thus, differing Pa_{CO_2} values. For example, in a given patient with a dead space of 200 cc, a ventilatory pattern of 1000 mL tidal volume at a respiratory rate of 10 would result in the same minute ventilation as a tidal volume of 500 mL at a respiratory rate of 20. However, the alveolar ventilation would be quite different. In the first case alveolar ventilation would be 8 L/min (1000 − 200 mL = 800 mL × 10), whereas in the second case an alveolar ventilation of 6 L/min would result (500 − 200 mL = 300 mL × 20). In general, a larger tidal volume at a lower rate is more efficient and preferable.

Most ventilators allow variation in inspiratory flow rate. In this setting, flow rate is important only as it affects the patient's comfort. Tachypneic patients may require a fast inspiratory flow rate, and this should be adjusted for patient comfort. However, in the presence of chronic obstructive pulmonary disease, inspiratory flow rate may be a factor. A long expiratory phase may be required in order to allow enough time for exhalation of the tidal volume. When adequate time for exhalation is not allowed, progressive air trapping will result. A longer exhalation phase at the same respiratory rate will result from shortening inhalation. Also, respiratory rate may be slowed when a rapid inspiratory flow rate is provided. Therefore, if severe obstruction is present, a rapid inspiratory flow rate should be used and tidal volume and respiratory rate adjusted until complete exhalation of each inspired tidal volume is achieved.

Ventilatory rate and tidal volume should be adjusted primarily according to the Pa_{CO_2} and pH. In addition, effective compliance (C_{eff}) (discussed above under Control of Oxygenation) should be taken into account. If respiratory alkalosis is present while ventilation is being controlled (i.e., the patient is not initiating the ventilator breaths), the respiratory rate should be decreased first without changing the tidal volume (for the reasons discussed above under Control of Oxygenation). If an alkalosis is still present when the lower limit of rate for the ventilator being used is reached, tidal volume may be decreased. If it is felt desirable to maintain a certain lower limit of tidal volume, then dead space tubing can be added to the ventilator to control respiratory alkalosis. This method of controlling alkalosis does not apply to the patient who is initiating ventilator breaths, resulting in a respiratory alkalosis; this situation will be discussed below.

ASSISTED VERSUS CONTROLLED VENTILATION

In the patient with intact ventilatory drives, ventilation may be either assisted or controlled. Ventilation is assisted when the patient initiates all or most ventilator breaths. A spontaneous breath attempt results in a decrease in airway pressure, which triggers the ventilator. Controlled ventilation refers to delivering all ventilator breaths at a set rate and not allowing any spontaneous breaths or patient-initiated ventilator breaths. In general, assisted ventilation is the preferred pattern. Controlled ventilation may allow a reduction in CO_2 production, particularly if it is accompanied by drug-induced muscular paralysis. However, the resulting disadvantages of complete patient immobility, difficulty in following neurological course, and possible psychological effects outweigh any potential advantages. Therefore, muscle paralysis and controlled ventilation should be only used as a last resort in the patient who is "fighting the ventilator" with resultant ineffective ventilation or in the patient with severe, potentially dangerous respiratory alkalosis which cannot be corrected by other means.

The patient may be breathing out of phase with the ventilator or may be triggering the ventilator with what appears to be an inappropriately high rate. This may result in either ineffective ventilation or in excessive ventilation, causing respiratory alkalosis, which in turn may lead to arrhythmias, decreased cardiac output, or seizures. The cause of the patient's agitation must be sought. An arterial blood gas should be checked to exclude hypoxemia. Also, respiratory acidosis may be present, and a high minute ventilation may be required for CO_2 removal. In this case, a higher tidal volume should be tried. If adequate oxygenation and a respiratory alkalosis are confirmed by the arterial blood gas, other conditions in the patient which could cause hyperventilation should be checked. Pain, sepsis, and alcoholic withdrawal can all cause hyperventilation. Once these factors have been excluded, an attempt should be made to adjust the ventilator to more comfortable settings for that patient. The inspiratory flow rate should be adjusted and the patient questioned whether breathing is more comfortable. If the patient is out of phase with the ventilator, an attempt at "capturing" the patient's respirations by increasing the respiratory rate for a short period of time and then gradually slowing the rate until the patient occasionally triggers the ventilator should be tried. Intermittent mandatory ventilation should also be tried (see below). If these maneuvers are unsuccessful, sedation or tranquilization should be attempted. A pharmacological agent with which the physician is most familiar should be used, starting with small doses and gradually increasing the dose to see if a more appropriate ventilatory pattern can be established. Muscular paralysis with pharmacological agents should only be attempted once all of these steps have failed. Most patients can be managed without muscle paralysis for control of ventilation.

INTERMITTENT MANDATORY VENTILATION

Intermittent mandatory ventilation (IMV) is a ventilation method in which intubated patients spontaneously breathe a controlled oxygen mixture and also receive mechanically delivered breaths at preset intervals.[19] IMV is now provided as an integral ventilation mode on many ventilators and can be achieved through adaptation of any existing volume- or pressure-limited respirators.[15] Proponents for IMV claim several advantages over controlled mechanical ventilation. Proposed advantages include: (1) facilitation of weaning,[18,19,20,38,52] (2) prevention of acute respiratory alkalosis seen with controlled mechanical ventilation by allowing Pa_{CO_2} to be determined by the patient's own spontaneous breathing,[18,20,38] (3) prevention or restoration of loss of neuromus-

cular coordination and respiratory muscle tone,[13,20,38] and (4) prevention of loss of ventilatory drives during mechanical ventilation.[18,20] Nearly all studies have compared IMV with controlled ventilation rather than assisted mechanical ventilation. Allowing the patient to determine the ventilator rate by initiating ventilator breaths (assisted ventilation) may already provide some of the advantages claimed for IMV without extra equipment and monitoring. Use of positive end-expiratory pressure with the IMV mode will be discussed separately below.

Potential disadvantages of IMV include the additional time, equipment, and monitoring by the respiratory therapist which is required (although this is not extensive), increased resistance to breathing if the required one-way valves become moist and malfunction, and an unnecessary increase in the work of breathing. Primarily because of the potential for an increase in the work of breathing, we recommend that IMV be reserved for specific indications. These include during the weaning process in the patient in whom weaning difficulty is anticipated, especially in the patient recovering from long-term paralysis. Also, IMV may be helpful for the control of pH if continuing respiratory alkalosis is present.

The combination of IMV with maintenance of positive pressure during expiration of the spontaneous breaths (termed continuous positive airway pressure or CPAP) has been recommended in the application of PEEP.[37] IMV with CPAP results in lower mean intrathoracic pressure and thus less reduction in cardiac output. In a controlled study comparing IMV with CPAP to assisted mechanical ventilation with PEEP, we found this advantage in approximately one-half the patients. In the other half, cardiac output fell equally on IMV with CPAP as compared to AMV with PEEP. Also, it could not be predicted which method would promote the best oxygenation in the individual patient. Therefore, it is recommended that the initial PEEP trial be conducted with assisted mechanical ventilation. If a fall in cardiac output is demonstrated before the desired improvement in oxygenation is obtained, IMV with CPAP should be tried at the same PEEP level and blood gases and cardiac output remeasured. IMV, particularly with very low mandatory rates, should be avoided in the severe, long-term ARDS patient, unless this has been shown to be associated with better cardiac output at a given PEEP level, until the patient is ready for weaning. In the unstable patient, an inappropriately low rate of mandatory breaths results in an unnecessary increase in the work of breathing at a time when the patient's CO_2 reduction is already excessive.

MONITORING DURING VENTILATORY MANAGEMENT

Appropriate monitoring is the key to successful ventilatory management. Pulmonary monitoring is reviewed in Chap. 31. "Postinjury Acute Pulmonary Failure," and specific aspects of monitoring are discussed in the appropriate sections of this chapter. However, a word of emphasis on the importance of monitoring is in order. Each change in ventilatory management should be considered a therapeutic trial. Although each management change has a desired outcome, it is not known whether this outcome will be achieved in the individual patient. Considering each change as a therapeutic trial implies that a therapeutic goal or desired effect as well as possible adverse effects must be identified prior to each change in therapy. Only then can beneficial and adverse effects be appropriately monitored. Using this method, each step in the ventilatory management can be justified by objective data. This allows application of general therapeutic principles such as discussed in this chapter to individual patients while taking into account the effect of the many variables possible from patient to patient on the outcome of the therapeutic modality applied. The extent

of monitoring necessary can vary widely. Simple means of monitoring, such as systematic recording of easily obtained clinical observations, should not be overlooked when they can provide pertinent answers in favor of "more sophisticated" techniques which may not be appropriate for the clinical situation.

OTHER VENTILATORY SUPPORT MEASURES

Airway Management

A closed system is necessary when providing continuous ventilation by intermittent positive pressure breathing. An endotracheal tube with a cuff or balloon to occlude the airway is initially placed. The decision to change from an endotracheal to a tracheostomy tube is based on the estimated length of time of ventilatory support. Since complications at the site of the tube cuff are similar for both tubes, the decision is based on the risk of laryngeal complications from the endotracheal tube versus the morbidity and mortality associated with tracheostomy. Therefore, a tracheostomy should be considered when the risk of laryngeal, pharyngeal, or nasal injury from the endotracheal tube substantially increases. With the use of newer materials and careful respiratory care, it appears that this period of time has increased to 1 to 2 weeks. Therefore, if it is estimated that ventilatory support will be required for less than 1 week, tracheostomy is not necessary. However, if the period of ventilatory support will be significantly longer than 2 weeks, tracheostomy should be performed early in the course of ventilatory support.

The choice between oral versus nasal route of intubation is largely one of personal preference. Secure external fixation is important with either type of endotracheal tube. Both laryngeal and cuff complications are increased by movement of the tube.

Complications at the cuff site are related to the pressure exerted by the cuff on the tracheal mucosa and the resulting effect on blood flow. This, in turn, is related to the pressure within the cuff. If the pressure transmitted by the cuff to the tracheal wall exceeds capillary pressure, blood flow to the mucosa is compromised and tracheal erosions and/or subsequent fibrosis with tracheal stenosis can result. The likelihood of these complications has been lessened by the development of low pressure, high residual volume cuffs. The cuff–tracheal wall pressure can be monitored by measuring the pressure within the high residual volume cuff. The pressure in the cuff should be measured and recorded at least once each shift. Emergency medical personnel sometimes prefer use of tubes with small volume, high pressure cuffs for emergency intubation. When this type of airway is required for more than 1 day, the tube should be changed to one with a high volume, low pressure cuff.

Secretion Control

The management of airway secretions should be individualized in each patient. Most trauma patients with ARDS either have few secretions or have thin watery secretions representing pulmonary edema. The patient with little or no secretions does not require frequent suctioning. Following the commonly ordered "hourly suctioning" protocol may only traumatize the airways, causing secretions to be produced as well as creating the potential of hypoxemia and vagal stimulation during suctioning. On the other hand, if the patient has secretions from pulmonary infection or preexisting chronic obstructive pulmonary disease, suctioning must be performed as frequently as necessary (sometimes much more often than hourly) in order to control the secretions.

Patients with airway secretions often have endotracheal tubes left in place for the purpose of "control of secretions" after ventilatory support is no longer necessary. Suctioning through the endotracheal tube only removes secretions from the central airways, usually the trachea and one main-stem bronchus. The patient must still cough to raise secretions to the central airways. Cough is not maximal with an endotracheal tube in place, as the glottis cannot be closed. This patient can usually clear secretions better if the endotracheal tube is removed once ventilatory support is no longer necessary. Patients with airway secretions must be stimulated to cough and deep-breathe periodically.

Mobilization

The patient receiving ventilatory support is often kept in one position, usually supine. This is particularly true when hemodynamic monitoring with its prerequisite catheters is required. However, frequent position changes are mandatory for optimal pulmonary function and should be done routinely.[11] Once the patient is hemodynamically stable and if traction is not required, the patient can sit up in a chair while ventilatory support is still necessary. In the patient requiring prolonged ventilatory support, muscular exercise including both passive range of motion and active exercise is important in order to maintain muscular strength. This can include walking with ventilatory support via an anesthetic or self-inflating bag with an oxygen source.

WITHDRAWAL FROM VENTILATORY SUPPORT

Withdrawal from ventilatory support represents another important step in the ventilatory management. Several criteria have been proposed as physiological guidelines predictive of successful withdrawal from mechanical ventilation.[3,51,55,56,57,61] However, few studies have vigorously tested these guidelines, and the decision to withdraw ventilatory support largely remains an arbitrary clinical decision. The patient's clinical situation is extremely important. Withdrawal of ventilatory support should not be attempted while the patient remains unstable. Adequate nutrition and maintenance of muscular strength are critical to successful withdrawal of support. These factors should be addressed early in the patient's course, while ventilatory support is still necessary. These subjects are covered in other chapters. Once the patient's condition has improved and stabilized, evaluation for withdrawal of ventilatory support can be performed. The following easily measured criteria are suggested:

1 $F_{I_{O_2}}$ of 0.4 or less with adequate arterial oxygenation
2 Tidal volume greater than 5 mL/kg
3 Vital capacity greater than 10 mL/kg
4 Maximal inspiratory force $-30\ cmH_2O$ or less (more negative)
5 Resting minute ventilation less than 10 L/min
6 Maximum voluntary ventilation (MVV) more than twice minute ventilation

A stable patient meeting these criteria can almost certainly breathe spontaneously without further support. Other criteria which require more complicated technical measurements have been proposed. These include arbitrary alveolar-arterial oxygen gradient $[D(A\text{-}a)O_2]$ values while breathing a $F_{I_{O_2}}$ of 1.0 and measurement of the dead space–tidal volume ratio (V_D/V_T).[46] $D(A\text{-}a)O_2$ at $F_{I_{O_2}} = 1.0$ adds little to the finding of an adequate Pa_{O_2} on $F_{I_{O_2}}$ of 0.4. The latter is a useful and practical test of oxygenation since a $F_{I_{O_2}}$ of 0.4 can be achieved by nasal prongs or face-mask oxygen. V_D/V_T of less than 0.6 may be a useful additional parameter.[46] However, a resting minute ventilation of less than 10 L/min will usually correlate with an adequate V_D/V_T ratio. In a patient with borderline resting minute ventilation, measurement of V_D/V_T may be of interest. Whether it offers further practical information not given by the resting minute ventilation and maximum voluntary ventilation is unclear.

The criteria of a resting minute ventilation of less than 10 L/min and a MVV which doubles resting minute ventilation has been tested in a prospective study.[56] Patients with adequate oxygenation who met these criteria could all be removed from ventilatory support. Patients who failed to meet these criteria were also tested for ability to breathe spontaneously. Some of these patients had adequate spontaneous ventilation despite failing to meet the criteria. When these patients were compared with those who failed the criteria and could not maintain adequate spontaneous ventilation, two differences were apparent. In the patients able to successfully withdraw from ventilatory support, values of the test criteria were borderline—either minute ventilation was slightly over 10 L/min or the patient could not quite double this with a MVV maneuver. Also, these patients had a greater inspiratory force than the patients who could not breathe spontaneously. A combination of the easily measured criteria listed above are usually adequate to determine physiological ability to successfully be removed from ventilatory support.

Most patients who meet these physiological guidelines can be placed on a short trial of spontaneous breathing via a T piece while breathing a $F_{I_{O_2}}$ of 0.4. Long T-piece trials (greater than 2 h) are not recommended. A long trial of spontaneous breathing through an endotracheal tube, particularly if it is of relatively small diameter with increased airway resistance, may place the patients at a disadvantage when they could be successfully extubated.[57] Therefore, arterial blood gas analysis should be performed and a decision on extubation made within 2 h. Most patients can be withdrawn from support in this simple fashion. Application of the term "weaning" to these patients may not be appropriate, as weaning implies gradual removal. However, patients who have required long periods of ventilatory support or patients with significant underlying lung or neuromuscular disease may require weaning from supported ventilation. IMV has been suggested as being helpful in these patients.[18,19,20,38,52] Current reports of weaning using IMV are anecdotal, and controlled studies are not available. However, IMV does appear to be useful in selected patients if properly applied. It is recommended that IMV be tried in the patient found to be difficult to withdraw from supported ventilation. Its routine use in all patients for this purpose is unnecessary.

Most studies have not separated the step of withdrawal from ventilatory support from that of removal of the endotracheal tube. Adequate arterial blood gases during spontaneous breathing is important in evaluation of both. If the patient is able to be successfully withdrawn from ventilatory support, there are additional factors to be considered in evaluation of extubation. These include the patient's state of consciousness, ability to protect the airway, and ability to clear secretions. If the patient is awake, has an active gag reflex, and can cough adequately to clear secretions, the endotracheal tube can be removed.

FLAIL CHEST

Flail chest is defined clinically by the observation of paradoxical chest wall motion in the trauma patient. Ventilatory management of flail chest in the trauma patient deserves special attention. Earlier methods of mechanical stabilization of the unstable chest wall segment by external means or by internal fixation with rods are outmoded and unnecessary. The standard management of flail chest at most centers consists of internal fixation by mechanical ventilatory support via an endotracheal or tracheostomy tube.[16,22,44,57,58] This method has been in vogue since 1956 and is widely accepted at the present time. This conventional ventilatory management consists of controlled mechanical ventilation without patient-initiated breaths and continuation of ventilatory support until rib fractures heal sufficiently and no paradoxical motion occurs.

Recently, new methods of flail chest management have been advocated.[13,60,64] These new approaches are based upon the premise that the fundamental disorder is contusion of the underlying lung or adult respiratory distress syndrome and not chest wall instability. Conventional physiological criteria for withdrawal of ventilatory support are followed regardless of the state of the flail segment. Three studies have evaluated various aspects of this general approach. Two of these studies use historical controls differing from the study group in several aspects of general management.[13,64] All three lack follow-up studies on lung mechanics and functional status of the patients.

This approach to ventilatory management of flail chest based upon physiological derangement rather than observable flail segment is worthy of further study. Until controlled studies are available, conventional ventilatory support is recommended until healing of the flail segment occurs. This may require 7 to 21 days of supported ventilation. In practice, patients with small flail segments, particularly flail sternal segments, may not require ventilatory support.

SUMMARY

Ventilatory management of the trauma patient is based on an understanding of the pulmonary pathophysiology. Management can be divided into those aspects affecting control of oxygenation and control of Pa_{CO_2} and pH. Control of oxygenation is of primary concern. Important management techniques include use of high tidal volumes and appropriate application of positive end-expiratory pressure (PEEP). PEEP must be systematically applied and evaluated, with monitoring of oxygenation and hemodynamic status. A standard approach to PEEP withdrawal should also be followed.

Control of Pa_{CO_2} and pH is dependent on alveolar ventilation. Alveolar ventilation is controlled by tidal volume and respiratory rate. Assisted ventilation is preferable to controlled ventilation in most circumstances. Ancillary pulmonary and general care aspects are important in successful ventilatory support and in allowing withdrawal of ventilatory support once the patient is stable. Several easily measured physiological guidelines are predictive of successful withdrawal from ventilatory support.

Appropriate monitoring is instrumental in ventilatory management. Each change in ventilatory management should be considered a therapeutic trial with monitoring for the desired effect and possible adverse effects. In this way, the therapeutic principles described in this chapter can be appropriately applied to the individual patient.

BIBLIOGRAPHY

1 Ashbaugh, D. G., T. L. Petty, D. B. Bigelow, and T. M. Harris: Continuous positive pressure breathing (CPPB) in the adult respiratory distress syndrome, *J. Thorac. Cardiovasc. Surg.*, **57**:31, 1969.

2 Bendixen, H. H., B. Bullwinkel, J. Hedley-Whyte, and M. B. Laver: Atelectasis and shunting during spontaneous ventilation in anesthetized patients, *Anesthesiology*, **25**:297, 1964.

3 ———, L. D. Egbert, J. Hedley-Whyte, et al.: "Management of Patients Undergoing Prolonged Artificial Ventilation," in *Respiratory Care*, The C. V. Mosby Company, St. Louis, 1965, pp. 149–150.

4 ———, J. Hedley-Whyte, and M. B. Laver: Impaired oxygenation in surgical patients during general anesthesia with controlled ventilation, *N. Engl. J. Med.*, **269**:991, 1963.

5 Bone, R. C.: Compliance and dynamics characteristics curves in acute respiratory failure, *Crit. Care Med.*, **4**:173, 1976.

6 ———: Pulmonary barotrauma complicating mechanical ventilation (abstract), *Am. Rev. Respir. Dis.*, **113**:118, 1976.

7 ———, P. B. Francis, and A. K. Pierce: Pulmonary barotrauma complicating positive end-expiratory pressure (abstract), *Am. Rev. Respir. Dis.*, **111**:921, 1975.

8 Carter, G. L., J. B. Downs, and F. J. Dannemul-

ler: "Hyper"-end-expiratory pressure in the treatment of adult respiratory insufficiency: A case report, *Anesthesiology*, **54**:31, 1975.

9 Cassidy, S. S., W. L. Eschenbacher, C. H. Robertson, Jr., et al.: Effects of IPPB and PEEP on cardiovascular function and pulmonary circulation in normal human subjects (abstract), *Am. Rev. Respir. Dis.*, **115**:313, 1977.

10 Clark, J. M., and C. J. Lambertsen: Pulmonary oxygen toxicity: A review, *Pharmacol. Rev.*, **23**:37–133, 1971.

11 Clauss, R. H., et al.: Effects of changing body position upon improved ventilation-perfusion relationships, *Circulation* (Suppl. II), **37** and **38**:214, 1968.

12 Cournand, A., H. L. Motley, L. Werko, et al.: Physiological studies of the effects of intermittent positive pressure breathing on cardiac output in man, *Am. J. Physiol.*, **152**:162, 1948.

13 Cullen, P., J. H. Modell, R. R. Kirby, et al.: Treatment of flail chest: Use of intermittent mandatory ventilation and positive end-expiratory pressure, *Arch. Surg.*, **110**:1099, 1975.

14 Demling, R. H., N. C. Staub, and L. H. Edmunds, Jr.: Effect of end-expiratory airway pressure on accumulation of extravascular lung water, *J. Appl. Physiol.*, **38**:907, 1975.

15 Desautels, D. A. and J. L. Bartlett: Methods of administering intermittent mandatory ventilation (IMV), *Respir. Care*, **19**:187, 1974.

16 Diethelm, A. J. and W. Battle: Management of flail chest injury: A review of 75 cases, *Am. Surg.*, **37**:667, 1971.

17 Dorethy, J. F. and V. Lam: The effect of positive end-expiratory pressure on left ventricular function in patients with respiratory failure (abstract), *Chest*, **72**:398, 1977.

18 Downs, J. B., A. J. Block, and K. B. Vennum: Intermittent mandatory ventilation in the treatment of patients with chronic obstructive pulmonary disease, *Anesth. Analg.*, **53**:437, 1974.

19 ———, E. F. Klein, Jr., D. Desautels, et al.: Intermittent mandatory ventilation: A new approch to weaning patients from mechanical ventilators, *Chest*, **64**:331, 1973.

20 ———, H. M. Perkins, and H. A. Modell: Intermittent mandatory ventilation: An evaluation, *Arch. Surg.*, **109**:519, 1974.

21 Egbert, L. D., M. B. Laver, and H. H. Bendixen:

Intermittent deep breaths and compliance during anesthesia in man, *Anesthesiology,* **24**:57, 1963.

22 Elberty, R. E. and J. M. Egan: Blunt trauma to the chest, *Am. Surg.,* **42**:511, 1976.

23 Fairley, H. B. and G. D. Blenkarn: Effect on pulmonary gas exchange of variations in inspiratory flow rate during intermittent positive-pressure ventilation, *Br. J. Anaesth.,* **38**:320, 1966.

24 Falke, K. J., H. Pontoppidan, A. Kumar, et al.: Ventilation with end-expiratory pressure in acute lung disease, *J. Clin. Invest.,* **51**:3215, 1972.

25 Flint, L., G. Gosdin, and C. J. Carrico: Evaluation of ventilatory therapy for acid aspiration, *Surgery,* **78**:492, 1975.

26 Forrester, J. S., W. Ganz, G. Diamond, T. McHugh, D. W. Chonette, and H. J. C. Swan: Thermodilution cardiac output determination with a single flow directed catheter, *Am. Heart J.,* **83**:306, 1972.

27 Greenfield, L. J., P. A. Ebert, and D. W. Benson: Effect of positive pressure ventilation on surface tension properties of lung extracts, *Anesthesiology,* **25**:312, 1964.

28 Haab, R., J. Piiper, and H. Rahn: Attempt to demonstrate the distribution component of the alveolar-arterial oxygen pressure difference, *J. Appl. Physiol.,* **15**:235, 1960.

29 Harken, A. H., M. F. Brennan, B. Smith, et al.: The hemodynamic response to positive end-expiratory ventilation in hypovolemic patients, *Surgery,* **76**:786, 1974.

30 Hlastala, M. P., P. S. Colley, and F. W. Cheney: Pulmonary shunt: A comparison between oxygen and inert gas infusion methods, *J. Appl. Physiol.,* **39**:1048, 1975.

31 Hopewell, P. C. and J. F. Murray: Effects of continuous positive pressure ventilation in experimental pulmonary edema caused by increased left atrial pressure and/or saline infusion, *J. Appl. Physiol.,* **40**:568, 1976.

32 Horovitz, J. H., C. J. Carrico, and T. G. Shires: Venous sampling sites for pulmonary shunt determinations in the injured patient, *J. Trauma,* **11**:911, 1971.

33 Horton, W. G. and F. W. Cheney: Variability of effect of positive end expiratory pressure, *Arch. Surg.,* **110**:395, 1975.

34 Huber, G., M. LaForce, and R. Mason: Impairment and recovery of pulmonary antibacterial defense mechanisms after oxygen administration (abstract), *J. Clin. Invest.,* **49**:37a, 1970.

35 Hudson, L. D., J. Tooker, C. E. Haisch, and C. J. Carrico: Does compliance reflect optimal oxygen transport with positive end-expiratory pressure? (abstract), *Chest,* **72**:401, 1977.

36 Kirby, R. R., J. B. Downs, J. M. Civetta, et al.: High level positive end-expiratory pressure in acute respiratory insufficiency, *Chest,* **67**:156, 1975.

37 ———, P. C. Perry, H. W. Calderwood, et al.: Cardiorespiratory effects of high positive end-expiratory pressure, *Anesthesiology,* **43**:533, 1975.

38 Klein, E. F., Jr.: Weaning from mechanical breathing with intermittent mandatory ventilation, *Arch. Surg.,* **110**:345, 1975.

39 Kumar, A., K. T. Falke, G. Geffin, et al.: Continuous positive pressure ventilation in acute respiratory failure, *N. Engl. J. Med.,* **283**:1430, 1970.

40 ———, H. Pontoppidan, K. Falke, et al.: Pulmonary barotrauma during mechanical ventilation, *Crit. Care Med.,* **1**:181, 1973.

41 Laurenzi, G. A., S. Yin, J. J. Guaneri: Adverse effect of oxygen on tracheal mucus flow, *N. Engl. J. Med.,* **279**:333, 1968.

42 Luterman, A., J. H. Horovitz, C. J. Carrico, P. C. Canizaro, D. Heimbach, C. Phillips, and J. Colocousis: Withdrawal from positive end expiratory pressure, *Surgery,* in press, 1977.

43 Lamy, M., R. J. Fallat, E. Loeniger, et al.: Pathologic features and mechanisms of hypoxemia in adult respiratory distress syndrome, *Am. Rev. Respir. Dis.,* **114**:267, 1976.

44 Lewis, F., A. N. Thomas, R. M. Schlobohm: Control of respiratory therapy in flail chest, *Ann. Thorac. Surg.,* **20**:170, 1975.

45 Nicotra, M. B., P. M. Stevens, J. Viroslav, et al.: Physiologic evaluation of positive end expiratory pressure ventilation, *Chest,* **64**:10, 1973.

46 Pontoppidan, H., M. B. Laver, and B. Geffin: "Acute Respiratory Failure in the Surgical Patient," in C. E. Welch (ed), *Advances in Surgery,* Year Book Medical Publishers, Inc., Chicago, 1970, vol. 4, pp. 163–254.

47 Powers, S. R., R. Mannal, M. Neclerio, et al.: Physiologic consequences of positive end-

expiratory pressure (PEEP) ventilation, *Ann. Surg.* **178**:365, 1973.

48 Pratt, P.C., A. P. Sanders, and W. D. Currie: Oxygen toxicity and gas mixtures: Morphology, *Chest,* **66**, July, Supplement: 8S, 1974.

49 Prewitt, R. M. and L. D. H. Wood: Positive end-expiratory pressure (PEEP) decreases myocardial function (abstract), *Am. Rev. Respir. Dis.,* **115**:153, 1977.

50 Quist, J., H. Pontoppidan, R. Wilson, et al.: Hemodynamic response to mechanical ventilation with PEEP: The effect of hypervolemia, *Anesthesiology,* **42**:45, 1975.

51 Radford, E.P., Jr., B. G. Ferris, Jr., and B. C. Kriete: Clinical use of a nomogram to estimate proper ventilation during artificial respiration, *N. Engl. J. Med.,* **251**:877–884, 1954.

52 Rappa, D. J. and R. N. Lavery: Psychological dependence on mechanical ventilation resolved by sigh-breath intermittent mandatory ventilation, *Respir. Care,* **21**:708, 1976.

53 Robotham, J. L., W. Lixfeld, L. Holland, et al.: Effect of PEEP on left ventricular performance (abstract), *Am. Rev. Respir. Dis.,* **115**:371, 1977.

54 Sackner, M. A., J. Landa, J. Hirsch, and A. Zapata: Pulmonary effects of oxygen breathing: A six-hour study in normal men, *Ann. Intern. Med.,* **82**:40, 1975.

55 Safar, P. and H. G. Kunkel: "Prolonged Artificial Ventilation," in P. Safer (ed.), *Respiratory Therapy,* F. A. Davis Company, Philadelphia, 1969, pp. 126–128.

56 Sahn, S. A. and S. Lakshminarayan: Bedside criteria for discontinuation of mechanical ventilation, *Chest,* **63**:1002–1005, 1973.

57 ——, S. Lakshminarayan, and T. L. Petty: Weaning from mechanical ventilation, *J. Am. Med. Assoc.,* **235**:2208, 1976.

58 Sankaran, S. and R. F. Wilson: Factors affecting prognosis in patients with flail chest, *J. Thorac. Cardiovasc. Surg.,* **60**:402, 1970.

59 Schmidt, G. B., W. W. O'Neill, K. Kotb, et al.: Continuous positive airway pressure in the prophylaxis of the adult respiratory distress syndrome, *Surg. Gynecol. Obstetr.,* **143**:613, 1976.

60 Shackford, S. R., D. E. Smith, C. K. Zarins, et al.: The management of flail chest, A comparison of ventilatory and non-ventilatory treatment. *Am. J. Surg.,* **132**:759, 1976.

61 Stetson, J. B. (ed.): *Prolonged Tracheal Intubation,* Little, Brown and Company, Boston, 1970, vol. 8, pp. 767–779.

62 Suter, P. M., H. B. Fairley, and M. D. Isenberg: Optimum end-expiratory airway pressure in patients with acute pulmonary failure, *N. Engl. J. Med.,* **292**:284, 1975.

63 Sykes, M. K., W. E. Young, and B. E. Robinson: Oxygenation during anaesthesia with controlled ventilation, *Br. J. Anaesth.,* **37**:314, 1965.

64 Trinkle, J. K., J. D. Richardson, J. L. Franz, et al.: Management of flail chest without mechanical ventilation, *Ann. Thorac. Surg.,* **19**:355, 1975.

65 Visick, W. D., H. B. Fairley, and R. F. Hickey: The effects of tidal volume and end-expiratory pressure on pulmonary gas exchange during anesthesia, *Anesthesiology,* **39**:285, 1973.

66 West, J. B.: *Respiratory Physiology: The Essentials,* The Williams & Wilkins Company, Baltimore, 1974, p. 153.

67 Winter, P. M. and G. Smith: The toxicity of oxygen, *Anesthesiology,* **37**:210, 1972.

Chapter 23

Acute Renal Insufficiency Complicating Traumatic Surgery

Charles R. Baxter, M.D.

Acute, potentially recoverable loss of renal function is a formidable and frequent complication in trauma patients. The incidence of classical oliguric acute renal failure resulting from severe shock and blood transfusion reactions has decreased dramatically during the last 15 years as a result of rapid transportation of the severely injured, the improved treatment of shock, and the more knowledgeable intraoperative and postoperative fluid volume management. Over all, the incidence of renal damage with the acute care of major trauma has not decreased, but improved therapy has lessened the severity of the renal insult, resulting in a spectrum of renal insufficiency clinical states. Classic oliguric renal failure, the most severe experience of acute renal

insufficiency, is far less common than ever before. Nonoliguric acute renal failure has become the most common clinical form of renal damage diagnosed. Less severe, subclinical renal functional abnormalities which are important in the total management of surgical patients have been described.[6,27] The mortality rate for this spectrum of injury varies from 59 to 70 percent for oliguric renal failure to 15 to 18 percent for nonoliguric (high output) renal failure. Rarely does the "subclinical" variant result in loss of the patient, although management of the patient is more difficult. Renal insufficiency in the postoperative treatment period occurs as frequently as in the initial management phase. These cases result from the complications, particularly infection, and the therapy of infection and other complications.

Emphasis should be placed upon the prevention of renal damage, then upon early recognition of the varied clinical types of renal insufficiency, and finally, on the specifics of treatment of each type of clinical renal insufficiency necessary to minimize mortality and morbidity.

PATHOGENESIS OF ACUTE RENAL FAILURE (ARF)

The pathophysiology of acute renal insufficiency resulting from the severe trauma and shock is incompletely understood.

Experimentally, renal ischemia, per se, has been shown to produce nephron damage. The severity of injury depends upon the intensity and duration of the ischemic insult.[3] Renal blood flow is reduced disproportionately to the fall in cardiac output following hemorrhage.[25] Sudden hemorrhage with an acute reduction of blood pressure to one-half of control levels produces a virtual cessation of renal blood flow. Renal vasoconstriction persists for a considerable period after restoration of both blood volume and cardiac output following hemorrhage.[25] Decreased sodium delivery via the glomeruli to the proximal tubular fluid results in increased renin release, which produces intense afferent glomerular arteriolar constriction. This self-perpetuating mechanism of vasoconstriction (unproven in man) provides the rationale for blocking sodium reabsorption by the proximal tubule, thus increasing sodium delivery to the distal proximal tubular fluid, decreasing the stimulus for vasoconstriction. This postulated mechanism forms the basis for the use of potent tubular blocking agents (furosemide, ethacrynic acid) currently employed widely in the postoperative phase of the care of patients with trauma and shock.[28]

In addition to the severe arterial and arteriolar vasoconstriction occurring with shock, internal redistribution of blood flow may be of even greater significance. Cortical ischemia, with a relative increase in cortical medullary blood flow has been demonstrated experimentally in severe shock.[20] This mechanism accounts for the consistent observation that the most severe damage is to the nephrons of the cortex and that the medullary sodium depletion results from the disturbance of the countercurrent mechanism via the increase in medullary blood flow.[20]

In experimental animals reversible damage to the renal parenchyma similar to that found in posttraumatic renal insufficiency in humans can be consistently reproduced only when a volume deficit (blood volume or extracellular fluid volume deficit) and acidosis are both present prior to the administration of a nephrotoxic insult. An acute blood loss of more than 20 to 25 percent of the circulating blood volume produces a significant acidosis. With these preexisting conditions, a variety of circulating substances associated with shock, severe tissue trauma, or transfusion reaction (globin,[17] glycols,[10] methemoglobin,[7] or vasopressors[15]) will produce parenchymal renal damage. This mechanism emphasizes the role of tubular cast formation as a formidable factor and perhaps initiating event in the development of acute renal failure.[20]

Clinically, one or more of the causative factors may be present but not readily recognized. For example, volume replacement [both blood and extracellular fluid (ECF)] may be accomplished to the point of satisfying blood pressure (BP) and pulse (P) restoration with a modest urine volume (5 to 15 mL/h). In a fair number of such patients total renal blood flow and its distribution may be so deranged as to result in ARF.

The frequency of renal damage resulting from ARF occurs even more often during the postoperative course. Currently, more than one-half of all the cases of renal insufficiency result from these causes.

THE PREVENTION OF ACUTE RENAL INSUFFICIENCY

The majority of cases of acute renal insufficiency occur in association with injuries or operations producing severe or protracted blood loss or shock. The highest incidence is observed in cases of extensive intraabdominal or retroperitoneal injury, major blood vessel injury, and the multisystems traumatized patient. Less well recognized are the cases of incipient blood loss or incomplete replacement of volume deficits where compensatory mechanisms obscure the signs of hypovolemia and protracted renal ischemia. The use of vasopressors in the initial resuscitation of blood loss shock results in a very high instance of renal complications, so that their use has been virtually eliminated in the management of hemorrhagic shock.

Less frequently, renal insufficiency results from massive hemolysis of transfusion incompatibility or myoglobinuria from extensive muscle damage or ischemia.

Many cases of acute renal failure in these categories can be prevented or averted by several methods which are now routinely employed in the management of shock, trauma, and/or transfusion reactions.

The principles which seem to account for the reduction in the incidence of renal failure are the use of balanced salt solutions in addition to blood replacement in the initial resuscitation of hemorrhagic shock, the recognition and replacement of all fluid volume deficits incurred by injury to various organ systems, and an effective means of decreasing renal tubular metabolism with regional hypothermia when the rates of fluid losses exceed the capacity for immediate replacement.

Preoperative Prevention

Hemorrhagic shock has been shown to be associated with the functional loss of extracellular fluid in the cells. The initial resuscitation of most shock patients is begun with the administration of approximately 2000 mL of balanced salt solution, permitting time for the acquisition of type-specific blood in the majority of severe cases, and permitting time for accurate cross matching in most cases.

The use of balanced salt solution initially in the resuscitation of shock serves a dual function of correcting the isotonic sodium ion depletion resulting from movement of sodium into cells and often alleviating the shock by temporary plasma volume expansion for a sufficient period of time to permit the typing and cross matching of blood, thereby reducing the incidence of transfusion incompatibility.

Rapid and complete blood replacement is imperative in the management of trauma and shock. Equally important, however, is the replacement of the isotonic fluid sequestrations which occur as a result of soft tissue injury. Sequestration of large quantities of extracellular fluid results from the contusion of large muscle masses, soft tissue damage occurring with long bone fractures, or prolonged interruption of vascular supply to the extremities. Either direct trauma or operative injury to visceral organs, particularly the small bowel, produce rather large intraluminal and intramural collections of extracellular fluid as well as the chemical peritonitis produced by the intraabdominal spillage of digestive fluids.

It is often difficult to accurately estimate the volume of fluid losses which have occurred in these situations. The return of normal blood pressure and pulse in patients in the supine position may occur when replacement is deficient by as much as a liter of blood or several liters of extracellular fluid. The serial monitoring of urine volumes, central venous pressure, pulmonary wedge pressure, and the cardiac output in response to initial resuscitation, fluid replacement under anesthesia, and in the postoperative state is necessary to evaluate the adequacy of fluid replacement.

The most important treatment of hemolytic transfusion reactions is the established presence of adequate urinary volume at the time of the reaction. The maintenance of an already established diuresis when transfusion reactions occur markedly reduces the incidence of heme pigment precipitation and the formation of protein casts in the renal tubules. The existing adequate urine output is enhanced by the administration of one-sixth molar sodium lactate solution given rapidly until a urine volume of over 100 mL/h is maintained. Mannitol in doses of 12.5 g/h is reserved for those cases in which such a diuresis (100 mL/h) cannot be produced by the administration of adequate alkalinizing volume.[22,23] In 28 consecutive cases of mismatched transfusion reactions in patients with an established diuresis, no renal failure has occurred.

Myoglobinuria, occurring as the initial manifestation of severe muscle damage or later as a result of reestablishing flow after the prolonged interruption of major arterial supply to large muscle masses, has been associated with a high instance of renal failure. Employing sufficient isotonic fluid volume therapy to replace the losses of fluid that are occurring into the damaged area, alkalinizing the urine with 1 M sodium bicarbonate in sufficient quantities to produce an alkaline pH (usually between 40 to 80 meq/h) and prevent the precipitation of acid hematin, followed by the administration of mannitol at a rate of 12.5 g/h has virtually eliminated renal failure as a complication of this entity.[4]

Intraoperative Prevention

The highest incidence of renal insufficiency occurs when there is severe or continuing blood loss. Renal ischemia, particularly cortical hypoxia, may be severe and prolonged.

The well-documented evidence of the efficacy of protecting the kidney from ischemic damage by hypothermia[24] is utilized during operation when shock is severe or prolonged or when shock recurs during an operative procedure, and in special instances, such as temporary clamping of the aorta or renal arteries.

When laparotomy is required, adequate protection can be afforded the kidney by regional hypothermia carried out by sluicing the peritoneal cavity with a cold isotonic solution (4°C) at 1- to 1½-h intervals throughout the operative procedure.[3] Approximately 2 L is poured into the open abdominal cavity at logical intervals during the procedure, allowed to remain in contact with the upper retroperitoneal area for 5 min, and then withdrawn by suction.

Employing this method, a rapid decrease in the core temperature of the kidney occurs when renal blood flow has been significantly decreased (Fig. 23-1). Patients with hypotension and some decrease in renal blood flow are cooled less rapidly, and significant cooling does not occur when renal blood flow is normal. No detrimental effect on the kidney per se has occurred nor have postoperative complications been observed with an extensive use of this procedure.

Significant protection is afforded an ischemic kidney by reducing the intrarenal temperature by 8 to 10°C (Fig. 23-2). This effective, safe, and rapid method of cooling can be readily available in all operating rooms. Normal saline cooled to 4°C in a readily available refrigerator is used for cooling.

More recently, defective oxygen delivery at the tissue level has been emphasized in the routine management of patients. The quantity of oxygen delivered to the tissues is dependent upon the hemoglobin concentration, the cardiac output, and the ability of the blood to release oxygen at the tissue level. Deficits of 2,3-DPG in stored blood, hypothermia, and alkalosis result in the shift of the oxygen dissociation curve to the left and hence a

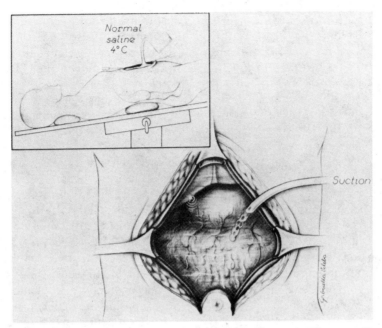

Figure 23-1 Technique of regional abdominal hypothermia. One or two liters of 4°C isotonic saline (refrigerator temperature) and slurred onto the upper retroperitoneal area; the operating table is lowered to keep the solution over the kidney fossa for 3 to 5 min.

decreased tissue oxygen delivery. In recent experiments by Canizaro et al.,[27] the progressive addition of anemia, 2,3-DPG deficiency, hypothermia, and respiratory alkalosis resulted in a progressive shift of the oxygen dissociation curve to the left. The P-50 in these experimental animals was observed to be below the critical tissue oxygen tension of most of the vital organ systems, including the kidney.

Figure 23-2 Regional hypothermia in patients. Renal core temperature measured in 10 patients with varying degrees of hypotension shock during laparatomy for trauma, compared to 10 elective surgical patients with normal blood pressure.

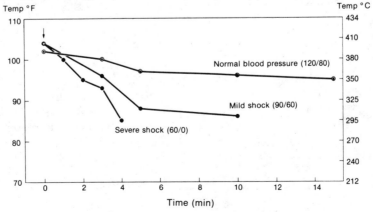

Similar changes may be prevented clinically by the use of whole blood preserved by dextrose-citrate-phosphorous (CPD) anticoagulants which maintain a satisfactory level of 2,3-DPG for 7 days. Fresh blood should be given as often as possible, preferably every third pint. Maintaining a normal core temperature with external heating devices and warming of blood and the intravenous fluids decreases hypothermic components of the O_2 dissociation curve shift. Nonhyperventilating techniques are currently being more widely employed in patients and intraoperative monitoring of pH and blood gases used as a guide to prevent significant pH changes.

With massive blood replacement, calcium (1 gr) is given to ensure citrate neutralization and augment cardiac function. Again, sufficient restoration and maintenance of cardiac output can be ascertained only by direct measurement. Potent tubular blocking agents (furosemide, ethacrynic acid) have been recommended for routine use in traumatized and surgical patients[28] during operation. Since the incidence of renal damage associated with even emergency surgery is less than 1 percent,[27] and even lower in elective surgery, the use of such drugs seems prohibitive. Moreover, the assessment of circulatory stability under anesthesia is difficult when the rate of urine formation, a good index of organ perfusion, is no longer reliable. With the use of these diuretics, urine may be produced when cardiac output is diminished or one of the above tissue oxygen delivery factors is deficient.

Anesthetic agents such as methoxyflurane (Penthrane) are now known to be definitely nephrotoxic when used in high concentrations, over long periods of time, in patients with diminished renal reserves (patients over 50 years of age)[4,8] or in patients with shock.

Postoperative Prevention

As previously stated, over one-half of the cases of renal insufficiency occur during the posttraumatic postoperative phase of the clinical course. These cases most often result from sepsis, the treatment of sepsis, or corrected fluid volume and specific electrolyte problems.

Systemic sepsis, usually with gram-negative organisms, often complicates the postoperative course. Endotoxemia and/or septicemia with these organisms first produces relative polyuria with an increase in free H_2O excretion. Usually hyponatremia accompanies this sign, representing an intracellular movement of Na^+ ion. Within 1 to 3 days, azotemia and/or a rising creatinine occurs. Oliguria is noted only after signs of vascular instability are manifest. Effective treatment is limited to treatment of the sepsis and early dialysis to prevent azotemia renal acidosis from further compromising the patient.

The treatment of overt systemic sepsis usually includes potentially nephrotoxic drugs. Prolonged use and/or high dosage regime of aminoglycosides are most frequently implicated as causative agents. In general, "up-limit" dose schedules for 48 h and the reduction to minimal therapeutic dose for 8 to 12 days virtually eliminate the renal toxicity. Therapeutic effectiveness is enhanced by the addition of carbenicillin to the treatment regime. Combinations of drugs such as Keflin plus an aminoglycoside are avoided when possible because of the associated renal insufficiency.

Careful management of fluid volumes, acid-base balance, and specific electrolyte concentrations avert renal insufficiency. Hypokalemic necropathy can be rather rapidly produced by uncorrected hypokalemia. ECF volume deficits, sodium loading, or alkalosis enhances renal potassium losses and should be avoided.

DIAGNOSIS

Early diagnosis of acute renal failure prevents life-endangering circulatory overloads, alerts one for the rapid development of hyperkalemia and acidosis common to all types of posttraumatic renal insufficiency, and permits time for the arrangement for the definitive specialized care necessary for the best survival.

The problems of diagnosis are commonly encountered in four categories: the acutely oliguric patients; patients with declining urine volumes during the first several days following injury; those with normal or high urine volumes who develop progressive azotemia; and finally patients with evidence of prolonged retention of sodium and H_2O in the postoperative state.

When the circulation has been stabilized and oliguria persists, the diagnosis of acute renal failure can often be made by the examination of urinary sediment[18] and determination of the blood-urine urea ratio.[21] In practice, abnormalities of the urinary sediment are more often related to injury involving the excretory system. The presence of red blood cells and a small quantity of albumin in urine with a specific gravity of 1.015 or less may indicate some renal damage if direct genitourinary tract injury can definitely be ruled out.

The most reliable test available in establishing the diagnosis of acute renal failure is the blood-urine urea nitrogen ratio. Normally the urine contains more than 30 times the blood concentration of urea. Following trauma, surgical intervention, or with prerenal deviations, this ratio drops as low as 1:15, and with aging or previously damaged kidneys, a ratio of 1:10 may occur. When the ratio is below 1:5, renal failure is most surely established *if* clinical shock is not present and vasopressors are not being used. All vasopressors are capable of reducing the ratio to this level.

When the diagnosis of acute renal failure is suspected early after a surgical procedure, the initial determination of the blood-urine urea nitrogen ratio will most often range between 1:15 and 1:8. The rapid administration of 1000 mL of crystalloid solution will change the ratio toward normal if hypovolemia (i.e., prerenal deviation) is the cause and will produce no change, or a decrease, in the ratio if renal failure is present. In several hundred such situations, this test has not failed to differentiate correctly renal failure from other causes of oliguria. Creatinine ratios (blood:urine) on clearance is unreliable in the immediate (1- to 48-h) postoperative period. Later, either determination accurately diagnoses degrees of renal insufficiency if the patient has circulatory stability.

Such findings as increased urinary sodium excretion, glycosuria in response to 50% dextrose administration, and urinary sediment abnormalities occur from a variety of causes and therefore are often misleading. Mannitol has been employed by some as a diagnostic test for the presence of acute renal failure.[2] Its administration may produce small increases in urine formation regardless of the cause of urinary suppression, but it will not prevent the development of renal failure and has not been shown in critical studies to increase renal blood flow or decrease renal vascular resistance.[30] Hypertonic mannitol (25 g) results in a significant (17 percent) increase in plasma volume, which probably explains its major physiologic effect. Tubular blocking agents (Lasix or erythcrinic acid) may occasionally be effective, particularly in converting an oliguric state to HOARF (High Output Acute Renal Failure). However, when given in the immediate postoperative phase, it is seldom effective and further lowers the GFR (Glomerular Filtration Rate).

The majority of patients with acute renal failure resulting from hypoxia damage are not acutely .anuric and seldom severely oliguric after surgery, but show a decreasing daily urine volume during the first several days after injury.[31,33] These patients have an adequate urine volume (500 mL to 1000 mL/day) on the day of the surgical procedure, 500 mL or less the following day, 250 mL the second day, etc., despite all modes of therapy. In these patients, the blood-urine urea ratio is initially below 1:10 and decreases daily toward a 1:1 ratio.

The third and most common form of renal dysfunction requiring diagnosis is progressive azotemia without oliguria (high output acute renal failure). The diagnosis is usually first suspected from the azotemia and confirmed by low (below 1:5) blood-urea ratio of normal or excessive urinary volumes.

Finally, the failure to excrete normally the sodium and water administered during the acute phase of treatment may be due to renal tubular damage. Edema or pulmonary congestion on the second to fourth postoperative day raises the suspicion of renal damage. When the low glomerular filtration rates characteristic of these patients is present, the BUN/UUN ratio is below 1:30.

RENAL RESPONSES FOLLOWING SURGERY AND TRAUMA

The spectrum of renal damage following surgery and/or trauma can be appreciated from studies which identify the normal and the abnormal responses to surgery. In a recent study, 40 severely injured trauma patients were selected for study from 1000 cases of operated trauma. Serial renal function studies were carried out under as controlled conditions as possible in such a clinical study.[6,27] This study showed that graded renal damage occurs in association with systemic injury and that identification of patients with subclinical, mild, and severe renal damage is important to their postsurgical care.

SUBCLINICAL RENAL DAMAGE FOLLOWING INJURY AND SHOCK

Comparison of the renal function studies in the 40 patients cited above identified a group (30 patients) who were considered to show normal renal response to trauma, 8 patients

with subclinical renal function, and 2 patients with nonoliguric progressive azotemia (Fig. 23-3 A and B).

There were no discernible differences between the two groups (normal and subclinical renal dysfunction group) in age, type of injury, length of hypotensive episodes, fluid and electrolyte requirements for resuscitation,

Figure 23-3 (A) Typical course of high output renal failure. The spectrum of clinical expression extends from BUNs of 60 to 350 g per 100 mL during the first week; urine volumes may reach 5 to 6 L/day. (B) Renal function after trauma: blood urea nitrogen values.

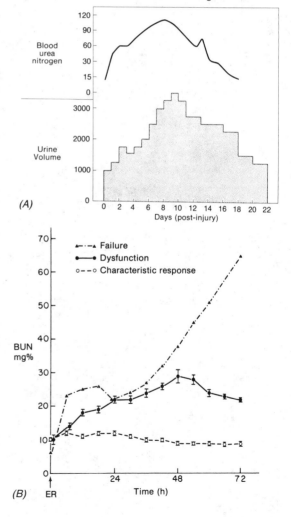

postoperative intravenous fluid administration, positive pressure ventilation, nephrotoxic antibiotics, blood volume, urine volume, or Pa_{O_2} or pH. The subclinical renal dysfunction group was characterized by GFRs that were approximately 30 percent of normal and remained at that level throughout the 72-h study (Fig. 23-4). The urea urine-to-plasma ratios remained below 30:1 but above 20:1 in this group (Fig. 23-5). Tubular reabsorption of water (TC H_2O) was significantly different in the two groups only at 18 and 24 h after admission. The trend in group 1 was toward excretion of free water, while the trend in the dysfunction group was toward continued retention of free water.

Sodium clearances were similar in the two groups until after 12 h following admission. Subsequently, C Na fell in group 2. Postoperative sodium balance (represented by the difference between daily sodium intake and urinary sodium excretion) was different in the two groups. Group 1 showed positive sodium balance during the first day, a zero balance during the second day, and negative balance during day three. In group 2, the dysfunction

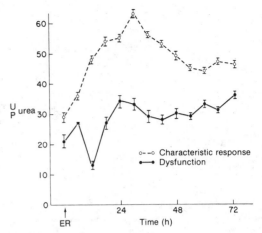

Figure 23-5 Renal function after trauma: urine-plasma urea ratio.

group, increasing sodium retention occurred during each of the three days of study.

The documentation of this renal abnormality, undetectable by usual clinical criteria for diagnosis, explains the tendency toward circulatory overloads encountered in the patients who have had severe stress when large quantities of fluid become available for excretion. It is apparent that even minimal persistent elevations of BUN are uniformly associated with significant renal dysfunction and are associated with sodium and water retention. Identification of such patients can readily be accomplished by serial evaluation of renal metabolism of urea or sodium. Careful management will minimize the circulatory overload which may occur on the third to fifth day from the large volume of administered fluids being mobilized which cannot be rapidly excreted.

HIGH OUTPUT (NONOLIGURIC) RENAL FAILURE

Progressive uremia occurring without a period of oliguria and accompanied by a daily urine volume of greater than 1000 to 1500 mL/day is now recognized as the most frequently diag-

Figure 23-4 Renal function after trauma: glomerular filtration rate determined by iothalamate ^{125}I constant infusion method.

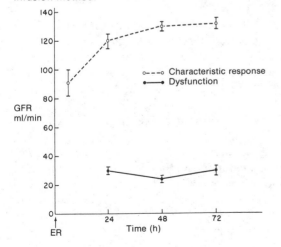

nosed clinical varient of renal failure occurring in association with surgery and trauma. Recognition of this entity has established the variable severity of renal damage and has indicated the frequency with which some renal damage occurs as a complication of trauma, shock,[5,13] infection, and nephrotoxic drug administration.[8]

The incidence of high output renal failure is between 5 and 10 times more frequent than oliguric renal failure.

The importance of this clinical entity lies in the fact that it is generally a milder form of renal insufficiency which, if diagnosed early and managed correctly, is not usually fatal.

The mean values for the typical clinical course of such patients is shown in Fig. 23-6. There is mounting azotemia for usually 10 days or more with progressive decrease toward normal for the next 10- to 12-day period. The azotemia is accompanied by urine volumes which generally increase daily, reaching their height at the peak of the azotemia and then gradually returning to a normal range.

In a series of 27 trauma patients, the spectrum varied from very mild elevations of blood urea nitrogen of 50 to 70 mg per 100 mL

Figure 23-6   Renal function after trauma: sodium clearance.

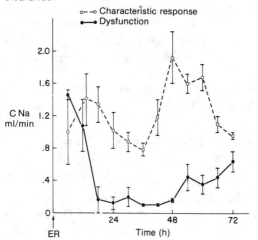

up to severe azotemia of 240 to 250 mg per 100 mL urea nitrogen. The wide spectrum of the severity of damage in this type of renal failure suggests that it is a less severe form of a similar process which produced oliguric renal failure. The principles of management are: (1) early recognition of the complication by observing azotemia without a low urinary volume, (2) withholding electrolytes, particularly K^+, (3) replacing the large volume of urea with electrolyte-free 5% dextrose in water when solute excretion is virtually absent, (4) control of acidosis with small increments of sodium lactate or bicarbonate, (5) use of dialysis only when the urea is above 180 g per 100 mL, severe acidosis or hyperkalemia become uncontrolled.

Serial measurements of blood urea nitrogen, potassium, O_2 combining power, and chlorides permit intelligent chemical and fluid management.

The mortality rate for high output ARF in this series is 18.5 percent[5] as opposed to the extremely high mortality for oliguric renal failure. The causes of death were thought to result from complications of the injury and are, in general, not related to the renal failure. However, deaths from infection constitute the most frequent cause of death in these patients as well as in patients with oliguric renal insufficiency.

This type of renal failure is not specific for traumatic injury. It frequently occurs in association with elective surgical procedures, in nonelective surgical illnesses usually involving infection or shock,[5] and with the administration of nephrotoxic agents such as methoxyflurane,[8] outdated tetracycline, and aminoglycosides.[15]

The increased recognition of this entity has resulted in the implication of many nephrotoxic factors which produce some degree of renal damage. Fortunately, most of these agents are weak (mild) nephrotoxic agents, and careful use minimizes this danger. For example, lowering the daily dose of gentamicin from 4 g/kg per day after 48 h of use to one-half that dose virtually eliminates nephrotoxicity.

OLIGURIC RENAL FAILURE

Oliguric renal failure is the most severe renal lesion in the spectrum of renal damage. Profound oliguria (urine volumes of 100 to 200 mL/day) do not usually occur abruptly except in instances of transfusion reaction or myoglobinuric nephrosis. Most often, urine volumes are between 400 to 700 mL/24 h on the first day, then progressively decrease over the next 2- to 4-day period, becoming fixed at 50 to 200 mL/day. Early diagnosis (using the UUN-to-BUN ratio) is important to prevent excessive fluid overloads, avoid potassium administration, and curtail protein intake in order to minimize the rapid rise in potassium and urea which usually occurs very rapidly in the early oliguric period.

Prophylactic dialysis offers great advantage in patient salvage over dialysis based on either clinical deterioration or chemical signs of severe uremia, acidosis, or hyperkalemia.

The choice of dialysis procedure should be individualized. Peritoneal dialysis is preferable when abdominal surgery has not been performed. It is also employed preferentially when the circulation is unstable, since hemodialysis under these circumstances often produces uncorrectable shock. Hemodialysis is selected for all patients with previous abdominal surgery or those with a suspicion of intra-abdominal complications. Arteriovenous shunts (Scribner) are placed 12 to 24 h prior to the initial dialysis procedure, and regional heparinization is employed in cases where bleeding may be produced by anticoagulation.

Prophylactic daily dialysis, using ultrafiltration, permits greater fluid intake since the excess fluid may be removed by daily dialysis. Fluid volumes of 1000 to 1200 mL/day are utilized for the administration of essential amino acid solutions and large glucose and insulin intakes. Total caloric intake of 2000 cal/day suppresses the rate of BUN rise in the plasma, presumably by decreasing gluconeogenesis from endogenous protein.

Awareness of the fact that acute renal failure patients seldom show the usual diagnostic signs of infection, inflammation, or pain will often permit early diagnosis of intervening complications. For example, perforated ulcers occur without pain, and peritonitis may manifest only by ileus.

Surgical procedures are hazardous in acute renal failure patients, but are required often for a variety of complications. Similarly, chronic renal failure patients present similar problems in surgical management for intercurrent illnesses. A high rate of infection and wound-healing failures follow such surgical procedures. Preoperative dialysis restoring all parameters of acid-base and electrolyte disequilibria and lowering of the BUN and creatinine improve the risk considerably. Extensive drainage is routinely employed, and all wounds are managed with through-and-through closure techniques.

Peritoneal dialysis may be safely employed after laparotomy in these patients for 48 to 72 h in most instances, even when spillage of visceral contents or bacterial peritonitis complicates its use. Appropriate antibiotics are added to the dialysis fluid, but in low doses since the transperitoneal absorption of all antibiotics are virtually complete and excretion via the kidneys is very low.

The survival rate of oliguric acute renal failure postsurgical patients is over 55 percent despite close adherence to the rigid requirements of total care and dialysis outlined.

BIBLIOGRAPHY

1 Baker, C. R. F., Jr., C. R. Baxter, and G. T. Shires: The evaluation of renal function follow-

ing severe trauma, Program of 1970 Annual Meeting of the *Am. Assn. for Surg. of Trauma,* p. 32 (abstract), 1970.

2 Balslov, J. T. and H. E. Jorgenson: A survey of 499 patients with acute anuric renal insufficiency: Causes, treatment, complications, and mortality, *Am. J. Med.,* **34**:753, 1963.

3 Barry, K. G. and J. P. Malloy: Oliguric renal failure: Evaluation and therapy by the intravenous infusion of mannitol, *J. Am. Med. Assoc.,* **179**:510, 1962.

4 Baxter, C. R. et al.: A practical method of renal hypothermia, *J. Trauma,* **3**:349, 1963.

5 ——— and D. R. Maynard: Prevention and recognition of surgical renal complications, *Clin. Anesth.*

6 ———, W. H. Zedlitz, and G. T. Shires: High output acute renal failure complicating traumatic injury, *J. Trauma,* **4**:567, 1964.

7 Carey, L. C. et al.: Serum protein changes in shock patients resuscitated with crystalloid solutions, *J. Trauma,* **9**:514, 1969.

8 Crandell, W. B., S. G. Pappas, and A. Macdonald: Nephrotoxicity associated with methoxyglurane anesthesia, *Anesthesiology,* **27**:591, 1966.

9 Crenshaw, C. A. et al.: Changes in extracellular fluid during acute hemorrhagic shock in man, *Surg. Forum,* **13**:6, 1962.

10 Finckh, E. S.: The failure of experimental renal tubulonecrosis to produce oliguria in the rat, *Aust. Ann. Med.,* **9**:283, 1960.

11 ———: The pathogenesis of uremia in acute renal failure: Abnormality of intrarenal vascular tone as possible mechanism, *Lancet,* **2**:330, 1962.

12 Forland, M. M. and R. E. Easterling: A five year experience with prophylactic dialysis for acute renal failure, U.S. Army Surg. Res. Unit. Brooke Army Med. Center Ann. Res. Progr. Rept. June 30, 1964.

13 Graber, I. G. and S. Sevitt: Renal function in burned patients and its relationship to morphological changes, *J. Clin. Pathol.,* **12**:25, 1959.

14 Griesman, S. E.: The physiologic basis for vasopressor therapy during shock, *Ann. Intern. Med.,* **60**:1092, 1959.

15 Kumin, C. M. and M. Finland: Restrictions imposed on antibiotic therapy by renal failure, *Arch. Intern. Med.,* **104**:1030, 1959.

16 Maher, J. F. and G. E. Schreiner: Cause of death in acute renal failure, *Arch. Intern. Med.,* **110**:493, 1962.

17 Mason, A. D., J. Alexander, and P. E. Teschan: Studies in acute renal failure, I. Development of a reproducible lesion in experimental animals, *J. Surg. Res.,* **3**:430, 1963.

18 Meroney, W. H. and M. E. Rubin: Kidney function during acute tubular necrosis: Clinical studies and theory, *Metabolism,* **8**:1, 1959.

19 Merrill, J. P.: "Acute Renal Failure," C. P. Artz and J. D. Hardy (eds.), *Complications in Surgery and Their Management,* W. B. Saunders Company, Philadelphia, 1969.

20 Mueller, B. B. et al.: Glomerular and tubular influences on sodium and water excretion, *Am. J. Physiol.,* **165**:411, 1951.

21 Perlmutter, M. et al.: Urine-serum urea nitrogen ratio (simple test of renal function in acute azotemic oliguria), *J. Am. Med. Assoc.,* **170**: 1533, 1959.

22 Powers, S. R.: Maintenance of renal function following massive trauma, *Trauma,* **10**:554, 1970.

23 ———: Renal response to systemic trauma, *Am. J. Surg.,* **119**:603, 1970.

24 Schloerb, P. R., R. D. Waldorf, and J. S. Welsh: The protective effect of kidney hypothermia on total renal ischemia. *Surg. Forum,* **8**:633, 1957.

25 Selkurt, E. E.: Renal blood flow and renal clearance during hemorrhagic shock, *Am. J. Physiol.,* **145**:699, 1946.

26 Sevitt, S.: Distal tubular necrosis with little or no oliguria, *J. Clin. Pathol.,* **9**:12, 1956.

27 Shires, G. T., J. Carrico, and P. C. Canizaro: "Major Problems in Clinical Surgery," in *Shock,* W. B. Saunders Company, Philadelphia, 1973, vol. XIII.

28 Stahl, W. M. and A. M. Stone: Effect of ethacrynic acid and furosemide on renal function in hypovolemia, *Ann. Surg.,* **174**:1, 1971.

29 Snyder, R. D., D. M. McCall, and M. A. Hayes: Functional defect in post-operative polyuric renal failure, *Surg. Forum,* **17**:19, 1966.

30 Teschan, P. E., G. P. Murphy, and J. A. Gagnon:

Renal hemodynamic effect of mannitol in normotension and hypotension, *Surg. Forum,* **15**: 99, 1963.

31 ——et al.: Prophylactic hemodialysis in the treatment of acute renal failure, *Ann. Intern. Med.,* **53**:992, 1960.

32 Torpey, D. J., Jr.: Resuscitation and anesthetic management of casualties, *J. Am. Med. Assoc.,* **202**:955, 1967.

33 Vertel, R. M. and J. P. Knochel: Non-oliguric acute renal failure, *J. Am. Med. Assoc.,* **200**:598, 1967.

Chapter 24

Cardiovascular Problems in the Trauma Patient

Andreas P. Niarchos, M.D.

John H. Laragh, M.D., F.A.C.C.

GENERAL CONSIDERATIONS

Any patient with injury (trauma, burns, post-surgical) may have preexisting cardiovascular disease or may develop new acute injury-related complications from the cardiovascular system. Since, as will be mentioned later, the injury-related cardiovascular complications cover a large clinical spectrum (precordial pain; arrhythmias; acute murmurs due to traumatic valve rupture; nonspecific electrocardiographic abnormalities; acute, injury-related hypertension; etc.), it is very important to obtain a detailed cardiovascular history regarding known previously "innocent" murmurs, angina pectoris, abnormal electrocardiogram, organic valvular disease, or hypertension. In particular, previous chronic treatment with cardiovascular drugs which affect cardiac rhythm and rate or myocardial function should be sought out. Thus, preexisting heart disease or drug effects will not be mistakenly taken as the result of cardiac or generalized injury. This will allow the therapeutic effort to be directed toward the main injuries and will preclude procedures or treatment with cardiovascular drugs which may not be beneficial to the injured patient, at least during the acute phase following the injury. On the other hand, in the noninjured patient with preexisting heart disease even elective surgical procedures increase perioperative morbidity and mortality by 7 percent and 12 percent, respectively.[39]

As with any patient who is in risk of developing serious cardiovascular complications, continuous monitoring of the crucial hemodynamic variables (heart rate, arterial pressure, central venous pressure, urinary output, electrolyte and fluid balance) by using reliable equipment and accurate techniques will be required for the severely injured patient. In addition to the above "conventional" monitoring, the introduction into clinical practice of the thermodilution method for the determination of cardiac output practically at the bedside by using the Swan-Ganz flow-directed catheter[22] has made possible the continuous evaluation of cardiac function during various therapeutic interventions. Through the Swan-Ganz catheter the pulmonary artery pressure and pulmonary capillary wedge pressure can be recorded concurrently with the injection of saline for the measurement of cardiac output. The diastolic pulmonary artery pressure or pulmonary capillary wedge pressure closely approximates the left atrial pressure, and either one can be taken as the left ventricular filling pressure. Stroke volume can be derived from cardiac output and heart rate. By plotting stroke volume versus left ventricular filling pressure, left ventricular function curves can be constructed and myocardial performance can promptly be assessed under control conditions and during drug administration. Thus with the above techniques the main determinants of cardiac output (preload, blood pressure, and systemic arteriolar resistance) can instantaneously be monitored. However, since generalized infection may adversely affect the outcome of the severely injured patient, care should be taken to introduce and maintain monitoring catheters under sterile conditions. For the same reason, pulmonary complications[11] related to the Swan-Ganz catheter should be avoided, and the latter should not be introduced to the pulmonary circulation when contraindications exist (pulmonary rupture, pneumothorax, etc.).

Since sudden cardiac arrest may occur in the absence of heart disease or may be the result of a potentially reversible predisposing condition, such as a benign cardiac dysrhythmia (bradycardia or heart block) which may occur following head injury and endotracheal intubation, familiarity with the appropriate cardiovascular drugs, equipment, and procedures for cardiopulmonary resuscitation is required by all who take care of the patient with trauma. It has been estimated[52] that although about 50 percent of the patients who develop cardiac arrest are saved, still every year a great number of patients die of sudden cardiac arrest which otherwise could have been either prevented or successfully treated.

SPECIAL PROBLEMS

Heart Failure

Acute Left Ventricular Failure Acute left ventricular failure (acute pulmonary edema) may complicate preexisting nontraumatic cardiac disease such as aortic or mitral valve disease (mainly stenosis), chronic coronary artery disease, severe hypertension, cardiomyopathies, etc. Acute myocardial infarction and rapid supraventricular arrhythmias often occur during surgical procedures and generalized injury, and both conditions may lead to pulmonary edema. Fluid overload, especially in the presence of impaired renal function caused either by previous disease or renal trauma, may increase pulmonary congestion in the patient who has already compromised cardiovascular reserve. Acute traumatic heart disease (rupture of intraventricular septum, rupture of chordae tendineae or acute valvular rupture) are invariably complicated by acute pulmonary edema. Pulmonary edema may occur when intracranial pressure is increased,[17] as following head injury or intracerebral bleeding.

It is beyond the scope of this chapter to describe in detail the altered pathophysiology[5,35] of the clinical manifestations of acute left ventricular failure.[46] The most obvious symptoms and signs include sinus tachycardia (unless the cause of failure is a supraventricular arrhythmia), muffled heart sounds, a fourth or third sound gallop, orthopnea with cyanosis, and frothy pink sputum. Marked bronchospasm is often present. Signs of sympathetic overstimulation with peripheral vasoconstriction and diaphoresis are almost invariably present. If the reduction in cardiac output has resulted in decreased cerebral perfusion, signs of brain hypoxemia will be presend. Blood pressure may be elevated, normal, or low.

Regardless of the specific cardiac abnormality which leads to acute pulmonary edema, the final pathogenetic factor responsible for most of the above symptoms and signs is fluid accumulation in the pulmonary alveoli. Fluid initially escapes the alveolar capillaries because of an increase in hydrostatic pressure and increase in permeability through the capillary wall. The cause of these abnormalities is the rise in pulmonary venous pressure associated with a decreased inotropic state of the left ventricle. When fluid enters the alveoli, gas exchange is compromised and generalized hypoxemia occurs. Gas exchange is further worsened by the noncompliant congested lungs or abnormalities in breathing in the patient with chest injury. In some conditions complicated by acute pulmonary edema the inotropic state of the myocardium may be normal, either naturally so or by previous digitalization. Therefore, a cornerstone in the therapy of acute pulmonary edema is intravenous administration of the rapidly acting and relatively nontoxic loop diuretic furosemide or ethacrynic acid.[30,33] Concurrent rapid digitalization, oxygen administration, and morphine even in the absence of pain will bring symptomatic relief and maintain most patients until the primary myocardial defect or other precipitating factors are corrected. Intractable

pulmonary edema may respond to intermittent positive pressure ventilation (IPPV). Acute pulmonary edema complicating acute renal failure due to renal trauma or other causes may require peritoneal dialysis or hemodialysis.

Treatment of acute pulmonary edema should start as promptly as possible with the patient in a 45° head-up position. Furosemide 40 to 80 mg IV should be given. Digoxin, or especially the rapidly acting ouabain preparation, 0.25 to 0.5 mg may be given IV followed by 0.25 mg every 6 h until up to 1.5 mg has been given within the first 24 h. Morphine 5 to 10 mg can be given intravenously. Oxygen 100%, preferably by a face mask, should be administered, possibly with mild positive pressure. The airways should be kept open by aspirating excessive bronchial secretions. For this purpose tracheostomy may be indicated if prolonged (more than 24 h) intermittent positive pressure ventilation (IPPV) is anticipated as in the presence of recurrent intractable pulmonary edema.

Care should be taken to avoid digitalis toxicity (which is more likely to occur in the presence of hypokalemia, or an acute myocardial infarction). For this problem, plasma digoxin or digitoxin levels may be helpful in guiding therapy. Morphine may cause respiratory depression and apnea, especially in the presence of CO_2 retention, which may occur when marked and prolonged bronchospasm accompanies pulmonary edema or preexists as a result of chronic pulmonary disease or chest trauma. Morphine is contraindicated in unconscious patients or in patients with head injuries because it increases intracranial pressure and may mask injury-related signs from the central nervous system. Cardiogenic shock may be worsened by morphine. Likewise, IPPV may adversely affect cardiogenic shock, especially when high inspiratory pressure (greater than 20 cm of water) or high respiratory rate (over 24/min) is used, since these may impede venous return, increase pulmonary resistance, and further decrease the already low cardiac output.

Maintenance therapy with oral diuretics, digitalis, glycosides and possibly with potassium supplements and/or other drugs (antiarrhythmics) will be required in most patients who have recovered from acute pulmonary edema. However, since orally administered potassium salts may cause ileal ulceration[30] and the hypokalemia during chronic diuretic therapy may be caused by secondary overproduction of aldosterone, diuretics which antagonize the action of aldosterone in the distal renal tubules (i.e., spironolactone or triamterene) may be safer than potassium supplements for preventing or correcting the hypokalemia which may occur during chronic diuretic therapy.[30]

Acute Right Ventricular Failure (Acute Cor Pulmonale) The most common cause of acute right ventricular failure is massive pulmonary embolism with subsequent severe precapillary pulmonary hypertension. The sudden obstruction of a main pulmonary artery will decrease pulmonary and systemic blood flow, and the markedly increased resistance to right ventricular emptying can eventually lead to ventricular dilation and right heart failure.[49] In addition to the effects of acute pulmonary artery obstruction and decreased coronary blood flow, venous admixture due to intrapulmonary shunts and sytemic hypotension can result in global myocardial ischemia and decreased myocardial function. The pulmonary hypertension in acute massive pulmonary embolism is the consequence of the decrease in the cross-sectional area of the pulmonary vascular bed.

Massive pulmonary embolism is caused by large thrombi arising from the heart, the deep pelvic veins, and upper thigh veins[21] and occurs mainly in patients who were subjected to operative procedures in the pelvic area.

Thrombosis also may complicate fractures of the pelvic bones or femur. Prolonged recumbency, especially in the presence of paralyzed lower extremities or chronic cardiac failure, predispose to deep vein thrombosis and subsequent pulmonary embolism. Other causes of acute right heart failure, especially in the patient with acute injury, may include conditions which impede systemic venous return such as pericardial tamponade and tension pneumothorax.

Treatment of acute right heart failure should be aimed toward the correction of the primary mechanical abnormality (embolectomy, pericardial aspiration, etc.). Heparin or fibrinolytic agents such as streptokinase may prevent extension or even dissolve the pulmonary thrombus.[38] Digitalis and diuretics may be useful in some forms of acute right heart failure, but care should be taken to avoid digitalis intoxication since a decreased tolerance to the drug exists in these patients. (Deep vein thrombosis and pulmonary embolism are extensively discussed in Chaps. 28 and 29.)

Cardiogenic Shock Cardiogenic shock should be considered as the third syndrome of acute heart failure, but in this type of heart failure the clinical picture is dominated not only by the manifestations of the decreased pumping ability of the heart, but also by manifestations due to numerous peripheral compensatory mechanisms, especially extensive vasoconstriction and decreased organ perfusion.[50] Cardiogenic shock is caused by factors which impair either cardiac filling and/or ventricular ejection. In relation to the trauma patient, acute cardiac tamponade, tension pneumothorax, rupture of a chordae, papillary muscle, or valve cusp may all result in cardiogenic shock. Massive pulmonary embolism is usually complicated by cardiogenic shock. Other nontraumatic myocardial diseases (myocardial infarction, myocarditis, post cardiac surgery) or stenosis of any valve and atrial ball thrombus may be complicated by cardiogenic shock.

In cardiogenic shock the heart is unable to maintain an adequate output regardless of the level of the venous pressure. The decrease in cardiac output results in systemic hypotension, tachycardia, myocardial ischemia, and peripheral vasoconstriction. The vasoconstriction affects mainly the skin and splanchnic vessels (kidney, liver, intestine), but is minimal in the cerebral and coronary arteries so that flow to these vital organs is maintained. The vasoconstriction is achieved by activation of the sympathetic nervous system (catecholamine release)[7] and the renin-angiotensin-aldosterone system.[44] Oliguria or complete anuria may accompany cardiogenic shock.

Treatment of cardiogenic shock should be directed to the correction of the primary abnormality (correction of extreme bradycardia or tachycardia, pulmonary embolectomy, valvulotomy, aspiration or pericardial tamponade, or tension pneumothorax). When cardiogenic shock is due to primary myocardial failure, agents which increase cardiac inotropy (digitalis glycosides) may be of some value. Sympathomimetic agents (epinephrine, norepinephrine) may increase myocardial contractility and cardiac output, but at the expense of increasing heart rate and enhancing vasoconstriction.[23] Both tachycardia and vasoconstriction will further increase myocardial oxygen consumption and may worsen myocardial ischemia. Of the sympathomimetic agents isoproterenol[18] may be the most beneficial in some patients with shock because by stimulating the peripheral beta-adrenergic receptors it produces vasodilatation. Large doses of steroids have been advocated and probably have a beneficial effect.[16] Although total blood volume is normal in the initial stages of cardiogenic shock, in the later phase when shock is established (irreversible shock) with increased resistance to venous outflow, transudation of fluid out of the vascular compartment and red cell sludging in the microcirculation may lead to some degree of hypovolemia. Hemodynamic measurements (central venous or left ventricular filling pressure and cardiac output) will help to determine the role of hypovolemia in the maintenance of hypotension in cardiogenic shock. If hypovolemia is present and myocardial function is still adequate, an increase in venous filling pressure will increase cardiac output and improve peripheral organ perfusion. Increase in venous filling pressure during fluid administration without further considerable improvement in cardiac output is indicative of myocardial failure, and in this situation fluid overload will deteriorate the heart failure. Renal failure and hyperkalemia (>7 meq/L) will require peritoneal dialysis or hemodialysis.

The most common cause of cardiogenic shock is extensive acute anterior myocardial infarction (5 percent of patients). In Table 24-1 are shown the results of two different therapeutic regimens in cardiogenic shock following acute myocardial infarction. Patients who were treated with small (100 to 200 mL) repeated volume infusion[43] under central venous pressure (CVP) monitoring, large doses of steroids,[16] isoproterenol infusion, and digitalis had a better prognosis in comparison with those who received digitalis, dextrose infusions, and steroids but not isoproterenol.

Recently, dopamine[48] and dobutamine,[1] substances which increase myocardial contractility but which have a lesser effect on heart rate and arterial pressure, have been shown to be of value in the treatment of cardiogenic shock and heart failure. These agents also produce renal vasodilatation and improve renal function.

Chronic Congestive Cardiac Failure The most commonly encountered clinical syndrome of chronic congestive heart failure hemodynamically is characterized by a low cardiac output and pulmonary and/or systemic

Table 24-1 Treatment of Cardiogenic Shock Following Acute Anterior Myocardial Infarction

	Age, yrs	Total number of patients	Survived	Died	Treatment
Group 1	54–60	16	6	10	Digitalis, isoproterenol, steroids, volume expansion
Group II	58–71	13	1	12	Digitalis, steroids, volume expansion

venous congestion. As in cardiogenic shock, the clinical manifestations of chronic heart failure are attributed to a primary myocardial pumping failure and to the secondary compensatory mechanisms which come into play in order to maintain arterial pressure and redistribute blood flow to vital organs. Thus peripheral vasoconstriction and increase in venomotor tone,[57] renal vascular constriction with sodium retention,[28] secondary hyperaldosteronism,[31] and increase in total blood volume and total exchangeable sodium[14] contribute to the various symptoms and signs of chronic congestive heart failure. Vasoconstriction is caused by increased sympathetic nerve activity and high levels of angiotensin II.

The etiology of chronic congestive heart failure is similar to that of acute right or acute left ventricular failure. Failure may initially be confined to the right or left ventricle, but after a variable period of time left ventricular failure becomes eventually biventricular. In relation to the patient with injury, hemorrhage, chronic pericardial tamponade, left-to-right shunts induced by trauma to the heart, or hypervolemia due to excessive transfusions, all may lead to congestive heart failure. In addition, chronic systemic or pulmonary hypertension, coronary artery disease, (tachyarrhythmias), valvular heart disease, and cardiomyopathies may all be complicated by

congestive heart failure. The symptoms and signs of congestive heart failure are either due to the insufficient cardiac output (weakness, fatigue, oliguria, nocturia, systemic hypotension, pallor, diaphoresis, cyanosis) or are due to congestion of the pulmonary circulation (elevated pulmonary capillary pressure, dyspnea, cough, orthopnea, acute pulmonary edema, hydrothorax) or to congestion in the systemic venous circulation (elevated central venous pressure, peripheral edema, symptoms due to congestion of the abdominal viscera, ascites).

The treatment of chronic congestive cardiac failure should be directed toward the correction of the primary abnormality. Digitalis glycosides and diuretic administration constitute the cornerstones of supportive or main therapy if no correctable lesion is found. Factors that precipitate or intensify heart failure, such as infections (respiratory, bacterial endocarditis, rheumatic fever), recurrent pulmonary embolism or tachyarrhythmia or excessive intake or administration of salt and fluids, should be looked for and treated accordingly. Thyrotoxicosis, physical trauma (injury, surgical), and emotional stress may also precipitate heart failure. Inadequate digitalis and diuretic dosage may be responsible for what appears to be drug-resistant heart failure. In the patient with trauma, acute blood loss, hypoxia, pain, fever, renal failure, and fluid overload may precipitate heart failure. Heart failure in the injured patient who requires major surgery should be corrected promptly since operative mortality is considerably increased in the presence of heart failure. In order to avoid hypervolemia, transfusion of packed red cells is preferable to whole blood. During fluid administration constant CVP monitoring is useful,[55] but venous pressure readings may be misleading since acute left ventricular failure (pulmonary edema) may occur before any obvious rise in CVP. Therefore, adequate digitalization and continuous clinical observation are mandatory during fluid replacement.

Vasodilator Therapy in Congestive Heart Failure   As mentioned earlier in this section, during congestive heart failure the decrease in cardiac output results in peripheral venous and arteriolar vasoconstriction (increased afterload). The vasoconstriction is mediated via the sympathetic nervous system and by humoral and structural changes in the arteriolar beds. Left ventricular dilatation, which accompanies most forms of heart failure, increases further the already elevated afterload and, consequently, myocardial oxygen requirements. It is now recognized that although all these peripheral compensatory changes are useful in maintaining cardiovascular homeostasis in the early stages of heart failure, in the latter stages they may adversely affect ventricular function, especially when it is already impaired. In this setting "afterload" becomes a most important determinant of cardiac output. Increased venomotor tone will increase preload (left ventricular diastolic volume) and consequently myocardial systolic wall tension (afterload). Therefore a venodilator that reduces preload may also lower afterload by decreasing left ventricular volume without affecting systemic vascular resistance. Hence, a more desirable approach now seems to involve the use of agents that have their primary action on the resistance vessels such as nitroprusside, hydralazine, or alpha-adrenergic blocking agents.

Numerous recent studies have shown that a decrease in afterload, either by aortic counterpulsation[12] or by vasodilators,[10] improves myocardial function. Vasodilators can be used in both acute and chronic cardiac failure of any etiology (e.g., myocardial infarction, valvular regurgitation, cardiomyopathies), either intravenously or by the oral route, and not only in patients with heart failure associated with an elevated arterial pressure, but also in the presence of normotension. As might be expected, patients with an elevated left ventricular filling pressure prior to vasodilator administration appear to have a greater increase in cardiac output than patients with normal or low filling pressures. Hence excessive volume depletion with diuretics should be avoided when afterload reducing agents are used.

The main vasodilators which have been used for the treatment of heart failure are shown in Table 24-2. Undue hypotension and decreased organ perfusion may complicate intravenous vasodilator therapy, so that continuous blood pressure monitoring is necessary during their administration. It has been reported that the combined use of vasodilator drugs together with agents with a positive inotropic effect[45] (dopamine, dobutamine, digitalis) are more effective in heart failure than either form of therapy alone. The introduction into clinical practice of the angiotensin II antagonists (saralasin, tepromide) will afford a potent, more specific, and presumably safer form of vasodilator therapy in patients with hypertension and heart failure characterized by angiotensin II excess. Our initial results[47] indicate that these agents, being potent arteriolar dilators and weak venodilators, have hemodynamic effects comparable to phentolamine and nitroprusside. Tepromide especially increases stroke volume and cardiac output

Table 24-2 Vasodilators Used in the Treatment of Heart Failure

	Predominant site of action		Main hemodynamic effects*	
Vasodilator	Arterial	Venous	Heart rate	Cardiac output
Phentolamine	+		↑ or →	↑ or →
Hydralazine	+		↑ or →	↑
Nitroprusside	+	+	↑ or →	↑ or → or ↓
Trimethaphan	+	+	→	→
Minoxidil	+		↑	↑
Prazosin	+	+	→	↑
Nitroglycerin		+	↑ or →	→ or ↓
Isosorbide dinitrate		+	↑ or →	→ or ↓
Angiotensin II blockers (CEI)**	+		→	↑ or → or ↓

*↑, increase; →, no change; ↓, decrease.
**CEI = converting enzyme inhibitor.

without increasing heart rate despite a marked reduction in afterload.

Coronary Artery Disease

Angina Pectoris The term "angina pectoris" is usually used to describe a group of symptoms consequent to myocardial ischemia, the most prominent of which is some form of paroxysmal precordial pain. The pain may be associated with a feeling of oppression in the chest, shortness of breath, tachycardia, pallor, sweating, a tendency to faint, etc. Narrowing or complete occlusion of the arterial lumen of the coronary arteries by atherosclerosis is the pathologic basis for angina pectoris in up to 90 percent of cases. Other causes for coronary pain are severe aortic stenosis or regurgitation, tight mitral stenosis, pulmonary valve stenosis, and chronic pulmonary hypertension. Embolic or inflammatory occlusion of the coronary arteries may also occur. Recently, spasm of presumably normal coronary arteries has also been claimed to induce angina.[19]

In the patient with trauma, acute myocardial ischemia (tachycardia, traumatic aortic regur-gitation, acute cor pulmonale) may cause chest pain. The appearance of angina pectoris during trauma or in the postoperative period usually indicates that angina due to preexistent coronary occlusive disease has been precipitated by fever, tachycardia, anemia, or hypotension. Arterial hypertension may also exaggerate preexisting angina. Noncardiac pain (traumatic or originating from abdominal viscera) may aggravate and distort the pain of angina.

The diagnosis of angina pectoris is based on the presence of typical or atypical chest pain of cardiac origin (radiation pattern, precipitating factors and its relief by nitroglycerin). Angina pectoris has been classified into various forms (such as spontaneous, effort, emotional, prandial, or nocturnal) according to the timing of its occurrence; the predisposing factors; the duration, severity, and response of pain and other symptomatology to treatment. Intractable angina (status anginosus, crescendo, intermediate coronary syndrome, unstable or preinfarction angina, preinfarction syndrome, or impeding myocardial infarction) refers to paroxysmal ischemic pain which has almost become continuous, is resistant to treatment, and is associated with electrocardiographic changes or myocardial ischemia and elevated myocardial enzymes. This type of angina is due to extensive occlusive coronary artery disease and carries a high incidence of myocardial infarction and cardiac death. Another form of severe angina with spontaneous prolonged chest pain often occurring at rest and thought to have a grave prognosis is the Prinzmetal's variant form of angina. The characteristic electrocardiographic pattern in Prinzmetal's angina is the ST-segment elevation in lead II or leads II and III (or occasionally in the precordial leads) instead of the usual ST depression during the attack. The elevated ST segments return to normal after the chest pain has subsided. Recent reports suggest that this form of angina may result from spasm of presumably normal coronary arteries.[19]

The physical findings during an attack of angina include pallor, sweating, tachycardia, a muffled first heart sound, and a paradoxically split second sound. Gallop rhythm (atrial or ventricular) may also be present. Acute papillary muscle dysfunction is manifested by a midsystolic or late systolic apical murmur; pulsus (mechanical) alternans may occur if left ventricula dysfunction is present. The tachycardia and increase in blood pressure usually occur before the onset of pain in the spontaneous form of angina.

Before treatment is commenced, a comprehensive diagnosis of the pattern of angina should be attempted. The differential diagnosis of anginal pain, especially in the injured patient without a previous history of coronary artery disease, may be a difficult task. Pain caused by trauma to the chest, pneumothorax, pulmonary infarction, and myocardial contusion may be similar to the pain of spontaneous angina. Electrocardiographic abnormalities suggestive of myocardial ischemia may occur in most of these conditions. Aggravating factors (pain, tachycardia, anemia, fever, hypotension, etc.) should be corrected before any

drug treatment is commenced. The treatment of angina pectoris depends on the severity of the individual case. Sublingual nitroglycerin is usually effective in patients with mild angina. After the acute attacks become less frequent, sublingual nitroglycerin may be replaced by a less rapid and longer acting agent such as nitroglycerin paste or sublingual isosorbide dinitrate. The mechanism by which nitrates relieve anginal pain is still not absolutely certain. They are undoubtedly coronary vasodilators and peripheral arteriolar and venodilators; whether they have a vasodilatory effect on atherosclerotic coronary vessels is rather uncertain. These agents decrease both afterload (blood pressure) and the venous return to the heart (preload) and consequently decrease oxygen requirements by the ischemic myocardium. When angina is more severe and/or associated with tachycardia, hypertension, or other evidence of sympathetic overactivity, a beta-adrenergic blocking drug such as propranolol should be considered, starting with a small dose and increasing it gradually. Propranolol should be given with care in the injured patient, especially if abnormal ventricular function is present. However, properly used, this agent can improve myocardial performance and reduce pain by reducing heart rate and oxygen consumption while often lowering arterial pressure. Combination of propranolol with diuretics or digitalis may be more effective in some of these patients. In a susceptible few, especially those with a history of asthma, propranolol may cause bronchospasm and impair respiratory function.

After the patient has recovered from trauma (injury or postoperative) further diagnostic work-up will be indicated, especially if anginal pain is drug resistant. If extensive occlusive disease is documented by coronary angiography and myocardial function is still relatively preserved, saphenous vein bypass grafting may be undertaken. This operation is now most frequently performed in patients with unstable angina which is resistant to medical treatment. Preliminary results, however, indicate that the mortality rate is the same in the medically or surgically treated groups, but long-term relief of pain is better in the surgically treated group. In addition, the evidence suggests that surgery may improve mortality rate in patients with left main coronary artery disease, and perhaps also in those with triple vessel involvement.

Acute Myocardial Infarction Another major cardiac problem which may complicate trauma or any operative procedure is an acute myocardial infarction. As many as 2 percent of patients without previous evidence of coronary artery disease develop myocardial infarction during or immediately after a major surgical procedure.[13] In patients with a previous myocardial infarction, if operated within 6 months from the time of the infarct, a 55 percent recurrence rate was observed following surgery; if operated within less than 2 years from the timing of their first infarct a 46 percent recurrence rate was observed.[54] Most of such patients had electrocardiographic abnormalities prior to operation.[3] The mortality in patients with acute myocardial infarction is greatly increased after surgical procedures and/or trauma. A 40 percent mortality has been reported if surgery is performed within 3 months from the onset of infarction, and if the infarction occurs in the postoperative period, the mortality rate is increased to 70 percent.[2] Therefore surgery should be postponed if possible from 3 months to as long as feasible following acute myocardial infarction. In the trauma patient myocardial infarction may be produced by injury to the coronary artery or directly to the myocardium. Emotional stress and hypotension following trauma may precipitate acute myocardial infarction in the patient with severe atherosclerosis of the coronary arteries.

The diagnosis of acute myocardial infarction is based on the history of acute onset chest pain and associated symptoms and signs, on sequential electrocardiographic changes, and on the serial elevation and decline of myocardial enzymes in the serum. However, there are occasions where the clinical and laboratory findings are not typical. For instance myocardial infarction can occur without apparent chest pain, as in unconscious patients and during anesthesia. Moreover, painless infarctions can occur, especially in the diabetic and elderly patient. The classical electrocardiographic findings include the ST-segment and T-wave changes, with the appearance of Q waves if the infarct is transmural. Inverted T waves alone are suggestive of subendocardial infarction. The electrocardiographic diagnosis of an acute myocardial infarction cannot be accepted with certainty in the presence of a previous bundle branch block, the Wolff-Parkinson-White syndrome, and right or left ventricular hypertrophy. Acute pulmonary embolism, head injury, intracerebral hemorrhage, myocardial contusion, shock states, and numerous other conditions may be associated more transiently with electrocardiographic signs suggestive of acute myocardial infarction. The sudden appearance of an arrhythmia or heart block may be the only electrocardiographic manifestation of a recent infarction. In difficult cases serial electrocardiograms and comparison to the pre-injury or preoperative electrocardiograms will help to confirm the diagnosis. The physical examination (gallop rhythm, arrhythmias, pump failure, cardiac murmur, pericardial friction rub, acute embolic phenomena) can further support or establish the diagnosis of acute myocardial infarction. Nevertheless, similar findings may occur following nonpenetrating injury to the heart and great vessels (acute valve rupture, cardiac tamponade, aortic rupture), so that a careful differential diagnosis, especially in the trauma patient, will be required.

The heart muscle is rich in various enzymes, but only three of them have found clinical application in the diagnosis of acute myocardial infarction. These include the glutamic-oxaloacetic transaminase (GOT), the lactic dehydrogenase cardiac isoenzyme (a-LDH) and the creatine phosphokinase cardiac isoenzyme (CPK-MB). The serum activity of these enzymes is greatly increased following an acute transmural myocardial infarction. Unfortunately, serial measurements are required, and several pathological processes affecting organs other than the heart (liver, kidney, muscles, red cell, brain) and various interventions (surgery, injections, drugs) will likewise increase the serum levels of these enzymes, especially generalized injury or burns. Measuring the more specific myocardial isoenzymes improves the diagnostic accuracy of myocardial infarction, although even these isoenzymes are increased in myocarditis or following myocardial contusion. The activity of the SGOT is increased within 6 to 12 h, CPK is increased within 6 to 8 h, and LDH is increased within 24 to 28 h after acute myocardial infarction. The peak and duration of the elevated CPK in the serum is said to correlate with the size of the infarct, and therefore CPK changes have prognostic significance[51] following acute myocardial infarction. Other confirmatory laboratory findings (erythrocyte sedimentation rate, leucocytosis) may be abnormal in the postoperative period and during recovery from trauma, and therefore are not diagnostic for acute myocardial infarction.

The management of acute myocardial infarction is directed toward relieving pain and hypoxia and correcting the various complications. Transfer of the patient to the coronary care unit, where constant monitoring and medical attention is available, is most desirable. In the injured patient or following surgery, hemorrhage, hypovolemia, respiratory or renal failure, electrolytic or acid-base balance disturbances should also be treated promptly. Pain after acute myocardial infarction is relieved with intravenous morphine,

unless contraindications exist (CO_2 retention, head injury, severe bradycardia, and hypotension). In the presence of severe hypotension an attempt should be made to increase the arterial pressure by using vasopressors, and then morphine can be administered. Oxygen 100% administered by a face mask or nasal catheter will relieve hypoxia, but if respiratory failure due to injury (chest, head) is present, artificial ventilation will be required. Heart failure and cardiogenic shock complicating acute myocardial infarction should be treated as outlined in the section on heart failure. Pericarditis may occur in up to 20 percent of patients with myocardial infarction and usually has a benign prognosis unless it is complicated by cardiac tamponade.[41,42] Deep vein thrombosis and pulmonary embolism should be prevented,[25] but anticoagulants are contraindicated in the presence of injury and bleeding. Small, subcutaneous doses of heparin,[26] however, may prevent deep vein thrombosis during surgery, without increasing the risk of hemorrhage. Anticoagulants may have some therapeutic value in the younger male patient with acute myocardial infarction.[36] The management of arrhythmias which complicate acute myocardial infarction or which occur spontaneously following injury and operative procedures is discussed in the following section.

Cardiac Arrhythmias

Cardiac arrhythmias may occur during the operative period, or may complicate generalized injury or trauma to the cardiothoracic area. Arrhythmias may be the only manifestation of organic heart disease, or they can appear spontaneously, being precipitated by extracardial factors (anxiety, pain, anesthesia, hypoxemia, electrolytic imbalance, intracerebral bleeding, etc.). Direct trauma to the sinus node or to the myocardium and the contracting system of the heart may result in arrhythmias.

Abnormal cardiac rate, rhythm, and conduction patterns can compromise cardiac performance, especially in the presence of heart failure and cardiogenic shock, and can precipitate angina pectoris or pulmonary edema. The main mechanisms responsible for the adverse hemodynamic effects of cardiac arrhythmias are the abnormal heart rate per se, the loss of atrial contraction, and the ventricular asynchrony and dyssynergy occurring as a result of the arrhythmia. Additional, but less important, mechanisms include the direct effects of arrhythmias on myocardial contractility (the force-frequency relationship), the increase in the amount of valvular regurgitation, and effects of atrial arrhythmias (via the atrial stretch receptors) on peripheral circulatory reflexes and renal function. In the presence of normal cardiac function, heart rate (HR) and stroke volume (SV) are interrelated, and the decrease in HR is accompanied by an increase in SV and vice versa, so that cardiac output (cardiac output = HR $\times$ SV) is maintained throughout a wide range of cardiac rates. However, with extremely slow or rapid heart rates, compensatory mechanisms are unable to preserve cardiac output. Furthermore, an increase in heart rate may cause myocardial oxygen demands to exceed myocardial oxygen supply with the subsequent development of myocardial ischemia and ventricular dyssynergy. Cardial arrhythmias, by eliminating or disrupting the normal sequence of atrial contraction to ventricular contraction, may induce cardiac dysfunction, since the atrial transport function supports ventricular performance, especially in patients with organic heart disease, where as much as 25 percent of the cardiac output is maintained by the atrial "booster pump." Asynchrony of ventricular contraction with impaired ventricular function can also result from ventricular arrhythmias or rate-dependent conduction disturbances.

The diagnosis of cardiac arrhythmias is based on the clinical examination, and the particular type of the suspected arrhythmia is confirmed by electrocardiography, before any definitive treatment is administered. From the clinical standpoint arrhythmias are classified according to the site of their origin within the heart (sinus, atrial, atrioventricular, ventricular), the normalcy of the heart rate (bradyarrhythmias, tachyarrhythmias), and the regularity of the cardiac rhythm (regular, irregular). Heart block may be caused by lesions of the sinoatrial node, the atrioventricular node, the main bundle of His, or from lesions affecting the left or right bundle branches. Arrhythmias should be promptly treated,[24,29,56] especially when they cause subjective discomfort, and precipitate or complicate myocardial ischemia, myocardial infarction, and heart failure. Predisposing factors should be eliminated, whenever possible, before any specific antiarrhythmic is commenced. The drug treatment of arrhythmias is now more effective because the pharmacokinetics[56] of the older antiarrhythmic drugs are better understood and newer agents are becoming increasingly available.[40,56]

Sinus bradycardia is present when the heart rate is below 60 beats per minute. Chronic sinus bradycardia does not require treatment unless it is associated with symptoms (e.g., unconsciousness, fainting, etc.). Sinus bradycardia occurs after acute inferior myocardial infarction and is associated with frequent ventricular premature contractions and/or hypotension. It should be treated firstly with intravenous atropine (0.4 to 0.6 mg, up to 2 mg total dose). If atropine is not effective, then an infusion of isoproterenol can be tried (2 to 5 mg in 500 mL dextrose in water). The infusion rate may be increased up to 40 drops per minute, or until a steady heart rate is achieved. In resistant cases artificial pacing with a ventricular demand pacemaker will be required. Extreme, and occasionally lethal, sinus bradycardia may occur following head injuries, subarachnoid hemorrhage, and intracerebral hemorrhage.

Sinoatrial block may be transient and responsive to atropine. Isoproterenol is usually more effective, either by intravenous infusion, sublingually (10 to 15 mg every 4 to 6 h), or even orally, 15 to 30 mg every eight hours. Chronic sinoatrial block associated with syncope (Stokes-Adams attacks) or bradycardia alternating with tachycardia (the bradycardia-tachycardia syndrome) and Stokes-Adams attacks will require permanent ventricular or demand artificial pacing. Since pacing will prevent only the bradycardia, oral antiarrhythmic agents, especially digitalis and/or propranolol, may be required to prevent the recurrent atrial tachyarrhythmias.

Sinus tachycardia (usual heart rate 100 to 140 beats per minute, normal P wave on the ECG) may be caused by fever, anemia, hypo- or hypervolemia, or may be compensatory in the presence of heart failure and cardiogenic shock. Thyrotoxicosis and the hyperbeta-adrenergic circulatory state are characterized by sinus tachycardia. The treatment of sinus tachycardia is that of the underlying cause. Digitalis is not indicated unless acute or chronic heart failure is present. Propranolol is quite effective in the sinus tachycardia of the hyperbeta-adrenergic state and in thyrotoxicosis.

Atrial premature systoles may occur in any condition that causes atrial enlargement (mitral valve disease, chronic cor pulmonale) and in coronary or hypertensive heart disease. During surgical procedures, especially in the abdominal area or following injury to the abdominal viscera, vagal stimulation or visceral reflexes may cause premature systoles, tachyarrhythmias or bradyarrhythmias. Atrial premature systoles, although benign, may trigger supraventricular tachyarrhythmias with subsequent deleterious hemodynamic effects, and therefore should be treated, particularly when they are numerous, multifocal, associated with ventricular extrasystoles, or in the presence of organic heart disease. From the antiarrhythmic drugs, procainamide, quinidine, and propranolol are effective, usually in

that order. Digitalis is often effective, and it should be used if heart failure is present, or imminent, when propranolol alone is contraindicated. If the atrial premature beats are suspected to be digitalis-induced, the drug should be discontinued and propranolol or potassium salts (if there is hypokalemia) administered.

Paroxysmal supraventricular tachycardia (usual heart rate 160 to 220 beats per minute) is a reciprocating tachycardia initiated by a premature beat with prolonged conduction time. Various cardiac and extracardiac conditions may be complicated by atrial or atrioventricular junctional (nodal) tachycardia, and before treatment is commenced, the possibility of digitalis intoxication should first be ruled out. From the several maneuvers which increase vagal stimulation and have been advocated for the termination of the paroxysmal atrial tachycardia, carotid massage has proved to be the most effective. If carotid massage fails, digitalis is the antiarrhythmic drug of choice. A rapid-acting preparation like ouabain may be given first. The starting IV dose is 0.25 to 0.5 mg, followed by 0.25 mg after 4 to 6 h if the arrhythmia is not controlled. The oral maintenance dose is 0.25 mg twice daily. Digitalis is particularly indicated if supraventricular tachycardia is associated with heart failure. An alternative drug is IV propranolol, 0.5 mg every two minutes, until 5 to 10 mg is given within 10 to 15 min. If bradycardia or hypotension develops, it should be treated with an IV infusion of isoproterenol or atropine. Cardioversion may be effective if drug treatment fails; cardioversion may be preferable when heart rate is extremely rapid or hypotension is present. In the presence of hypotension, sympathomimetic drugs (phenylephrine) which increase blood pressure may also terminate the tachycardia, presumably by reflexly increasing vagal tone. Cardioversion is contraindicated if the patient is taking digitalis. For the chronic prophylaxis of supraventricular tachycardias, digitalis or propranolol (40 to 160 mg daily in divided doses) appears to be the drug of choice. Propranolol alone is contraindicated in heart failure, and it should not be given in bronchial asthma or obstructive lung disease. In heart block propranolol may be used if a pacemaker is in place.

Digitalis-induced supraventricular tachycardia (atrial tachycardia with varying degree of atrioventricular block) is treated by stopping digitalis and administering propranolol or potassium if hypokalemia is present.

The paroxysmal supraventricular tachycardia associated with the preexcitation syndromes (the Wolff-Parkinson-White and the Lown-Ganong-Levine syndromes) are treated with digitalis and/or propranolol. Quinidine and/or procainamide are also effective, but if drug therapy fails, cardioversion may be applied.

Paroxysmal nodal (AV junctional) tachycardia is another form of supraventricular tachycardia which is treated in the same manner as the other atrial arrhythmias.

Atrial fibrillation and atrial flutter can either be paroxysmal or chronic. In atrial fibrillation the atrial rate may be as high as 350 beats per minute and chaotic in nature, while in atrial flutter the atrial rate varies from 220 to 400 beats per minute when some degree of atrioventricular block is present. The acute forms of these arrhythmias usually occur after acute myocardial infarction, acute cor pulmonale (pulmonary embolism), and during operative procedures. In the chronic form, both arrhythmias may complicate mitral valve disease, ischemic or hypertensive heart disease, and chronic cor pulmonale. Lone (idiopathic) atrial fibrillation may occur in some patients without evident heart disease. Digitalis intoxication may also be manifested with atrial fibrillation. If the arrhythmias are not digitalis-induced, this agent is the drug of first choice for the treatment of both arrhythmias because it suppresses atrioventricular conduction and controls ventricular rate. In atrial

flutter, if conversion to sinus rhythm is desired, quinidine or procainamide should be used only after adequate digitalization has been achieved, because these agents may increase the ventricular rate. Acute rapid atrial fibrillation and particular atrial flutter can be terminated by electric countershock. Cardioversion can be tried before drug treatment is attempted. In the chronic form of the arrhythmias, in preparation for electric conversion antiarrhythmic coverage with quinidine 400 mg every 6 h or procainamide 500 mg every 6 h is administered, while the maintenance dose of digitalis is reduced or discontinued. Anticoagulation for a period of 3 weeks prior to cardioversion is recommended, especially in patients with rheumatic heart disease and history of previous embolism.

Chronic first-degree heart block (prolonged PR interval) is asymptomatic and does not ordinarily require treatment. *Second-degree heart block* may also be asymptomatic and transient in nature, especially following acute myocardial infarction, head injury, and intracerebral bleeding or during anesthesia. Occasionally both first- and second-degree heart block (Mobitz I type) may herald complete heart block, and both types of block, if persistent, should be treated with intravenous atropine or isoproterenol infusion in order to prevent the development of complete heart block or to improve the hemodynamic status of the patient if bradycardia and hypotension are present. Following acute myocardial infarction,[40] second-degree, 2:1 heart block with wide QRS and the Mobitz II–type second-degree block arise from lesions of the conducting system located below the atrioventricular (AV) node. In these cases temporary artificial pacing is indicated. In the Mobitz I type of second degree heart block and in complete heart block with normal QRS duration and ventricular rates above 50 beats per minute, the conduction defect is usually within the AV node as a result of ischemia after inferior wall infarction, and both conduction disturbances are transient and do not constitute an indication for routine pacing. On the other hand, complete heart block with wide QRS and/or complete block with symptoms of the Stokes-Adams syndrome should be paced in order to prevent ventricular asystole.

Bilateral bundle branch block (BBB) usually complicates acute anterior myocardial infarction, and this type of block, although asymptomatic, may herald sudden complete block or asystole without previous disturbance in AV conduction. In bilateral BBB or acute bifascicular and/or trifascicular block the insertion of a prophylactic temporary pacemaker is indicated.

Ventricular premature systoles may occur in the absence of organic heart disease, as with pain, during anesthesia, hypoxia, or severe hypokalemia. Coronary heart disease and digitalis intoxication are common causes of ventricular ectopic beats. The most common arrhythmia following acute myocardial infarction is ventricular extrasystoles. The criteria for treating this arrhythmia are now better defined and consist of one of the following: more than five ectopics per min, multifocal or bidirectional ectopics, ectopics occurring during or near the vulnerable period (the R-on-T phenomenon), and ectopics occurring in bursts of two or more consecutive beats (ventricular tachycardia). Certain characteristics accompanying the ventricular extrasystoles may be indicative of an impending myocardial infarction, and these include: abnormal QRS, ST depression, T wave in the same direction as the QRS comples, inversion of T in the first postextrasystolic beat, ectopics increasing with exercise, combination of ventricular and atrial ectopics, etc.

Ventricular extrasystoles with the above characteristics and appearing during the operative period and after injury should be treated even in the absence of organic heart disease, especially in the older patients, because they

may lead to a life-threatening arrhythmia such as ventricular tachycardia or ventricular fibrillation. Intravenous lidocaine is clearly the first choice for treating ventricular premature systoles following acute myocardial infarction, cardiac surgery, or cardiothoracic injury. Lidocaine is given as a bolus first, 1 mg/kg body weight, but the total bolus dose should not exceed 50 to 100 mg. If the arrhythmia persists, the dosage may be repeated after 20 to 30 min. If the arrhythmia is recurrent, a continuous intravenous infusion is begun at 2 to 3 mg/min. The infusion is tapered off within the next 24 to 36 h, and oral prophylaxis is begun with procainamide or quinidine. Diphenylhydantoin or propranolol may also be used, if contraindications to these agents do not exist. If the arrhythmia is resistant to lidocaine, intravenous procainamide in small or moderate doses or intravenous propranolol may be effective. In the presence of heart block with slow ventricular rates and frequent ventricular ectopic beats, antiarrhythmic drugs should be given after a pacemaker has been inserted in place. Digitalis-induced ventricular extrasystoles are treated by stopping the drug, and if the arrhythmia still persists, by administering potassium or propranolol.

Ventricular tachycardia may appear in short paroxysms or the arrhythmia may be more prolonged and resistant to treatment with grave hemodynamic consequences (decrease in cardiac output, hypotension, loss of consciousness). Prolonged ventricular tachycardia complicating acute myocardial infarction is often followed by ventricular fibrillation and cardiac arrest. Paroxysmal ventricular tachycardia responds best to intravenous lidocaine or procainamide. Occasionally other antiarrhythmic drugs (propranolol, diphenylhydantoin, bretylium tosylate) are also effective. Oral procainamide and/or quinidine (200 to 600 mg every 6 h) is primarily used for prophylaxis after the arrhythmia has been stopped. Quinide should not be used intravenously because it may induce ventricular asystole. Occasionally thumping the precordium with the fist may terminate ventricular tachycardia. Prolonged ventricular tachycardia may also be terminated with dc countershock. Paroxysmal ventricular tachycardia or fibrillation complicating heart block can usually be prevented by ventricular pacing. If after an unsuccessful attempt to reverse ventricular tachycardia loss of consciousness or ventricular fibrillation occurs, external cardiac massage and the other means of cardiopulmonary resuscitation should be started immediately in order to maintain the circulation until defibrillation using dc countershock is attempted.

Hypertension and Hypertensive Crisis

Increased arterial pressure may be due[34] to an increased cardiac output or to an increased total peripheral resistance, or to both (mean arterial pressure = cardiac output × total peripheral resistance). However, for most, increased resistance is the critical factor. Tachycardia (to a point) and hypervolemia increase blood pressure by increasing cardiac output, and hypervolemia alone can cause hypertension if the arterial tree is noncompliant. But this effect per se is a transient one, since normally the kidneys react to increased filling with natriuresis and correction of volume hypertension. Accordingly, severe sustained hypertension is usually caused by excessive vasoconstriction due to increased amounts of circulating angiotensin II, and/or catecholamines, a process in which renal vasoconstriction participates. When these humoral agents are not found to be elevated, severe hypertension may be maintained by an increased resistance caused by structural, arterial, and mainly arteriolar damage to the renal and systemic vasculature.

In the patient with trauma, hypertension may have preexisted or it may be acute and trauma-induced (Table 24-3). In patients with

Table 24-3 Causes of Trauma-induced Hypertension

Head injury
Cervical cord transection
Dissection or rupture of thoracic aorta
Renal artery thrombosis or stenosis
  Unilateral
  Bilateral
Renal parenchymal injury
Perinephric hematoma
Renal failure
Fluid overload
Postcoronary artery bypass hypertension

previous hypertension, acute elevation of pressure may occur during surgery or following trauma because their antihypertensive medications were omitted or withheld.[27] Thus, severe rebound hypertension, related to plasma catecholamine excess, has been reported to occur after sudden clonidine withdrawal,[6] especially when this antihypertensive agent was prescribed in large dosage. However, rebound hypertension may occur, but less frequently, when other agents[27] which suppress the sympathetic nervous system (reserpine, methyldopa, propranolol) are suddenly withheld.

Moreover, during surgery or trauma several factors (pain, anesthetic agents, etc.) producing sympathetic stimulation may operate to exaggerate preexistent hypertension. Posttraumatic hypertension may be transient or permanent depending on the particular pathogenetic mechanism. It is clear from Table 24-3 that three main mechanisms are involved in posttraumatic hypertension: volume excess, overproduction of renin (angiotensin II), or the hypertension is neurogenic in origin.

Hypertension occurring during surgery has been recently described in patients undergoing coronary artery bypass surgery.[20,47] A large proportion of these patients were hypertensive prior to the operative procedure, but in most of them hypertension develops in the absence of previous documented hypertension. The pathogenetic mechanism[47] of the post coronary artery bypass hypertension is mainly an increase in total peripheral resistance (e.g., vasoconstriction), but in some patients excessive fluid administration (volume factor) is also involved. The vasoconstriction is due to elevated levels of renin (angiotensin II) and catecholamines (epinephrine, norepinephrine).

Hypertensive crisis may complicate any kind of hypertension. This term implies a markedly elevated arterial pressure complicated by encephalopathy, left ventricular failure, acute renal failure, or impending myocardial infarction. Such severe hypertension may cause bleeding and contribute to suture rupture in patients with trauma or cardiovascular surgery, and therefore in this setting even moderate hypertension may constitute a crisis. Severe hypertension due to a pheochromocytoma, because of the abrupt changes in blood pressure, possible attendant hypovolemia, and the arrhythmogenic effects of catecholamines, has a grave prognosis during operative procedures or following injury, and therefore when identified should be treated intensively with combined alpha and beta blockade, even in the absence of complications.

The management of hypertensive crisis requires a prompt decrease of the elevated blood pressure and treatment of the specific complication. From the various antihypertensive agents which are used in the treatment of hypertensive emergencies[4,53] the most effective for lowering blood pressure immediately is sodium nitroprusside. Nitroprusside is infused intravenously, and the rate of the infusion can be regulated (50 to 150 μg/kg per min) according to the level of blood pressure. Nitroprusside is not only a potent arteriolar dilator, but also a venodilator, and therefore is most useful in patients with severe hypertension complicated by left ventricular failure. If

nitroprusside is not available, other vasodilators (diazoxide, hydralizine) or the ganglionic blocker, trimethaphan, are almost as effective and can be used instead. Phentolamine also can be tried, but it is mainly indicated in the treatment of hypertension of pheochromocytoma or in the rebound hypertension caused by clonidine withdrawal. The impending availability of the angiotensin II antagonists[8] (tepromide, saralasin) will offer a more rational physiological approach in the treatment of severe hypertension caused by excessive circulating levels of angiotensin II at the same time ruling in or out a renin factor in causation, often an important diagnostic advantage.

In the treatment of severe hypertension with any one of the above mentioned vasodilating agents, care should be taken to avoid the sudden decrease of blood pressure to hypotensive levels, since an abrupt fall in blood pressure may lead to cerebral or myocardial ischemia or renal shutdown, particularly in an elderly patient with extensive vascular disease. If there is occult preexisting hypovolemia, agents such as nitroprusside, by enlarging the arterial and venous beds, can lead to hypotension and shock and to a decreased cardiac performance even though afterload has been reduced. Accordingly, such agents should not be given together with diuretics at first, and saline infusions may be needed to support blood volume.

The newly developed angiotensin blocking drugs (saralasin, converting enzyme inhibitor) offer a special advantage in dealing with hypertensive crises because of their great potency and lack of side effects when given intravenously. Moreover, a positive response identifies renin excess as the culprit, thereby establishing that the hypertension is renal in origin and pointing the way to further appropriate diagnostic work-up. On the other hand, a negative response to angiotensin blockade suggests that the hypertension is either of catecholamine origin and should respond to Regitine or, more likely, it is due instead to volume excess and should be treated primarily by diuresis or dialysis instead of by agents intended to reduce peripheral vasoconstriction.[32,34]

BIBLIOGRAPHY

1 Andy, J. J., C. L. Curry, N. Ali, and P. P. Mehrota: Cardiovascular effects of dobutamine in severe congestive heart failure, *Am. Heart J.,* **94**:175, 1977.

2 Arkins, R., A. A. Smessaert, and R. G. Hicks: Mortality and morbidity in surgical patients with coronary artery disease, *J. Am. Med. Assoc.,* **190**:485, 1964.

3 Baer, S., F. Nakhjavan, and M. Kajani: Postoperative myocardial infarction, *Surg. Gynecol. Obstet.,* **120**:315, 1965.

4 Bhatia, S. K. and E. D. Frohlich: Hemodynamic comparison of agents useful in hypertensive emergencies, *Am. Heart J.,* **85**:367, 1973.

5 Braunwald, E. (ed.): *The Myocardium, Failure and Infarction,* H.P. Publishing Co., Inc., New York, 1974.

6 Brodsky, J. B. and J. J. Bravo: Acute postoperative clonidine withdrawal syndrome, *Anesthesiology,* **44**:519, 1976.

7 Byrne, J. J.: Symposium on shock, *Am. J. Surg.,* **110**:293, 1965.

8 Case, D. B., J. M. Wallace, H. J. Keim, M. A. Weber, J. I. M. Drayer, R. P. White, J. E. Sealey, and J. H. Laragh: Estimating renin participation in hypertension: Superiority of converting enzyme inhibitor over saralasin, *Am. J. Med.,* **61**:790, 1976.

9 Chamberlain, D. and R. Leinbach: Electrical pacing in heart block complicating myocardial infarction, *Brit. Heart J.,* **32**:2, 1970.

10 Chatterjee, K. and W. W. Parmley: The role of vasodilator therapy in heart failure, *Prog. Cardiovasc. Dis.,* **19**:301, 1977.

11 Chun, G. M. and M. H. Ellestad: Perforation of the pulmonary artery by a Swan-Ganz catheter, *N. Engl. J. Med.,* **284**:1041, 1971.

12 Clauss, R. H., W. C. Birtwell, G. A. Albertal, et al.: Assisted circulation: I. The arterial counter-pulsator, *J. Thorac. Cardiovasc. Surg.,* **41**:447, 1961.

13 Dawber, T. R. and H. E. Thomas, Jr.: Prevention of myocardial infarction, *Prog. Cardiovasc. Dis.,* **13**:343, 1971.

14 Davis, J. O.: Mechanisms of salt and water retention in cardiac failure, in *The Myocardium, Failure and Infarction.*

15 De Maria, A. N., L. A. Vismara, Z. Vera, R. R. Miller, E. A. Amsterdam, and D. T. Mason: Hemodynamic effects of cardiac arrhythmias, *Angiology,* **28**:427, 1977.

16 Dietzman, R. H. and R. C. Lillehei: The treatment of cardiogenic shock: V. The use of steroids in the treatment of cardiogenic shock, *Am. Heart J.,* **75**:224, 1968.

17 Ducker, T. B.: Increased intracranial pressure and pulmonary edema. Part I. Clinical study of 11 patients, *J. Neurosurg.,* **28**:112, 1958.

18 Elliott, W. C. and R. Gorlin: Isoproterenol in treatment of heart diseases: Hemodynamic effects in circulatory failure, *J. Am. Med. Assoc.,* **197**:315, 1966.

19 Endo, M., K. Hirosawa, N. Kaneko, K. Hase, Y. Inoue, and S. Konno: Prinzmetal's variant angina: Coronary arteriogram and left ventriculogram during angina attack induced by methaeholine, *N. Engl. J. Med.,* **294**:252, 1976.

20 Estafanous, F. G., R. C. Tarazi, J. F. Viljoen, and M. Y. Tawil: Systemic hypertension following myocardial revascularization, *Am. Heart J.,* **85**:732, 1973.

21 Fowler, E. F. and J. A. Bollinger: Pulmonary embolism: A clinical study of ninety seven fatal cases, *Surgery,* **36**:652, 1954.

22 Ganz, W., R. Donoso, H. Marcus, J. S. Forrester, and H. J. C. Swan: A new technique for measurement of cardiac output by thermodilution in man, *Am. J. Cardiol.,* **27**:392, 1971.

23 Goldberg, L. I.: Use of sympathomimetic amines in heart failure, *Am. J. Cardiol.,* **22**:177, 1968.

24 Hampton, J. R.: The management of cardiac arrhythmias, *Brit. J. Hosp. Med.,* **17**:160, 1977.

25 Handley, A., P. A. Emerson, and P. R. Fleming: Heparin in the prevention of deep vein thrombosis after myocardial infarction, *Brit. Med. J.,* **2**:436, 1972.

26 International Multicentre Trial, *Lancet,* **2**:45, 1975.

27 Katz, J. D., L. H. Croneau, and P. G. Barash: Postoperative hypertension: A hazard of abrupt cessation of antihypertensive medication in the preoperative period, *Am. Heart J.,* **92**:79, 1976.

28 Kilcoyne, M. M., D. H. Schmidt, and P. J. Cannon: Intrarenal blood flow in congestive heart failure, *Circulation,* **47**:786, 1973.

29 Killip, T.: Management of arrhythmias in acute myocardial infarction, in *The Myocardium, Failure and Infarction.*

30 Laragh, J. H.: "Diuretics in the Treatment of Congestive Heart Failure," in *Congestive Heart Failure: Mechanisms, Evaluation and Treatment,* Yorke Medical Books, New York, 1976, p. 143.

31 ———: Hormones and the pathogenesis of congestive heart failure: Vasopressin, aldosterone, and angiotensin II. Further evidence for renal-adrenal interaction from studies in hypertension and in cirrhosis, *Circulation,* **25**:1015, 1962.

32 ———: Modern system for treating high blood pressure based on renin profiling and vasoconstriction-volume analysis: A primary role for beta blocking drugs such as propranolol, *Am. J. Med.,* **61**:797, 1976.

33 ———: The proper use of newer diuretics: Diagnosis and treatment, *Ann. Intern. Med.,* **67**:607, 1967.

34 ———: Vasoconstriction-volume analysis for understanding and treating hypertension: The use of renin and aldosterone profiles, *Am. J. Med.,* **55**:261, 1973.

35 Mason, D. T.: *Congestive Heart Failure: Mechanisms, Evaluation and Treatment,* Yorke Medical Books, New York, 1976.

36 Medical Research Council: Report of the working party on anticoagulant therapy in coronary thrombosis, *Brit. Med. J.,* **1**:335, 1969.

37 Merrill, A. P., J. L. Morrison, and E. S. Brannon: Concentration of renin in renal venous blood in patients with chronic heart failure, *Am. J. Med.,* **1**:468, 1946.

38 Miller, G. A. H.: The management of acute pulmonary embolism, *Brit. J. Hosp. Med.,* **18**:26, 1977.

39 Nachas, M. M., S. J. Abrams, and M. M. Goldberg: The influence of arteriosclerotic heart disease on surgical risk, *Am. J. Surg.,* **101**:447, 1961.

40 Niarchos, A. P.: Disopyramide: Serum level and arrhythmia conversion, *Am. Heart J.,* **92**:57, 1976.

41 ———: Electrical alternans in cardiac tamponade, *Thorax,* **30**:228, 1974.

42 ——— and C. S. Mackendrick: Prognosis of pericarditis after acute myocardial infarction, *Brit. Heart J.,* **35**:49, 1973.

43 Nixon, P. G., H. Ikram, and S. Morton: Infusion of dextrose solution in cardiogenic shock, *Lancet,* **1**:1077, 1967.

44 Page, I. H.: "Some Neurohumoral and Endocrine Aspects of Shock," in S. F. Seeley and J. R. Weisinger (eds.), *Recent Progress and Present Problems in the Field of Shock, Fed. Proc.,* **20**:75, 1961.

45 Parmley, W. W. and K. Chatterjee: Combined vasodilatory and inotropic therapy: A new approach in the treatment of heart failure, in *Congestive Heart Failure: Mechanisms, Evaluation and Treatment,* Yorke Medical Books, New York, 1976, p. 93.

46 Perloff, J. K.: "The Clinical Manifestations of Cardiac Failure in Adults," in *Congestive Heart Failure: Mechanisms, Evaluation and Treatment,* Yorke Medical Books, New York, 1976, p. 93.

47 Roberts, A. J., A. P. Niarchos, D. B. Case, R. M. Abel, V. A. Subramanian, J. H. Laragh, and W. A. Gay, Jr.: Coronary artery hypertension: Comparison of responses to nitroprusside, phentolamine, and converting enzyme inhibitor (abstract), *Circulation,* Suppl. xxxxx 1978.

48 Robie, N. W. and L. I. Goldberg: Comparative systemic and regional hemodynamic effects of dopamine and dobutamine, *Am. Heart J.,* **90**:340, 1975.

49 Sasahara, A. A., J. J. Sidd, G. Tremblay, and O. S. Leland, Jr.: Cardiopulmonary consequences of acute pulmonary embolic disease, *Prog. Cardiovasc. Dis.,* **9**:259, 1966.

50 Silber, E. N. and L. N. Katz: "Heart Failure," in *Heart Disease,* Macmillan Publishing Co., New York, 1975, p. 108.

51 Sobel, B. E.: Serum creatinine phosphokinase and myocardial infarction, *J. Am. Med. Assoc.,* **229**:201, 1974.

52 Stephenson, H. E., Jr., L. C. Reid, and J. W. Hinton: Some common denominations in 1200 cases of cardiac arrest, *Ann. Surg.,* **137**:731, 1953.

53 Tarazi, R. C., H. P. Dustan, E. L. Bravo, and A. P. Niarchos: Vasodilating drugs: Contrasting hemodynamic effects, *Clin. Sci. Molec. Med.,* **51**:575s, 1976.

54 Topkins, J. M. and J. F. Artusio, Jr.: Myocardial infarction and surgery: A five year study, *Anesth. Analg.,* **43**:716, 1964.

55 Wilson, J. N., T. B. Grow, C. V. Demong, A. E. Prevedel, and J. C. Owens: Central venous pressure in optimum blood volume maintenance, *Arch. Surg.,* **85**:563, 1962.

56 Winkle, R. A., S. A. Glantz, and D. C. Harrison: Pharmacologic therapy of ventricular arrhythmias, *Am. J. Cardiol.,* **36**:629, 1977.

57 Zelis, R., J. Longhurst, R. J. Capone, and G. Lee: Peripheral circulatory control mechanisms in congestive heart failure, *Am. J. Cardiol.,* **32**:481, 1973.

Chapter 25

Postoperative Pancreatitis

G. Tom Shires, M.D.

One of the most lethal complications that a patient can develop postoperatively is acute pancreatitis. Not infrequently, the patient may demonstrate a rise in serum amylase following an upper abdominal surgical procedure but remain asymptomatic. The high mortality occurs in those patients who clinically demonstrate signs and symptoms of acute pancreatitis, and it is estimated to be 50 to 70 percent.[1,25] It is difficult to diagnose pancreatitis in a patient immediately after operation, since often some degree of abdominal pain and ileus is present. Acute postoperative pancreatitis characteristically occurs in the first 48 h after surgical intervention and is most frequently seen following a surgical procedure on the gastroduodenal and biliary tract. The symp-

tom most suggestive of this disease is pain out of proportion to the operation performed. Hypotension is frequently out of proportion to the amount of fluid lost during and following the operation. Fever, tachycardia, shock, ileus, and distention are the usual findings. Postoperative pancreatitis may follow splenectomy when a portion of the tail of the pancreas is accidentally removed, operations directly on the pancreas, and nephrectomy. The spleen, pancreas, or kidney may be injured following trauma to the abdomen.

One of the following operative errors is usually responsible for the pancreatitis when a surgical procedure has been performed on the stomach or the duodenum: (1) injury to the main pancreatic duct or pancreatic tissue; (2)

division or ligation of the accessory pancreatic duct; or (3) excessive handling of the pancreas during mobilization of the duodenum. Warren[28] has emphasized that the duct of Santorini is the most common place for injury following gastric resection. Schmeiden and Schering[22] found that 11 of 91 cases of acute pancreatitis following gastric surgical procedures were caused by ligation of the duct of Santorini. This duct drains a large portion of the pancreas in approximately 10 percent of the cases. It is located $2\frac{1}{2}$ to 3 cm proximal to the ampulla of Vater (Fig. 25-1). Duodenal ulcer disease may shorten the duodenum, thus making the duct of Santorini nearer the pylorus.[10]

Wallenstein[27] analyzed 1769 cases of Billroth II subtotal gastrectomies and found 12 cases of fatal postoperative pancreatitis. He reviewed 605 Billroth I anastomoses and found no cases of postoperative pancreatitis. Postoperative pancreatitis may occur from an afferent loop syndrome with increased intraluminal pressure which may give reflux of duodenal contents into the pancreatic duct, thus producing pancreatitis.[24] This could account for the increased incidence of postoperative pancreatitis following Billroth II anastomoses. If a penetrating ulcer is found in the head of the pancreas, it is usually left in situ rather

Figure 25-1 *(From Harkins, Henry N., and Nyhus, Lloyd M.: "Surgery of the Stomach and Duodenum," p. 547, Little, Brown and Company, Boston, 1962.)*

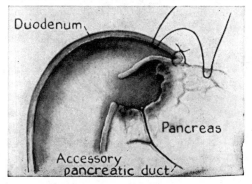

than attempting excision of the ulcer bed.[10] The duct of Santorini may empty into the base of the ulcer or nearby, and injury to this duct can result in fatal pancreatitis. Fatalities from pancreatitis occur in approximately 0.5 percent of all gastric surgical procedures, or in a ratio of 1:200 cases.

Since the common duct may be injured or explored during surgical intervention for trauma, it is interesting that pancreatitis following surgical procedures on the biliary tract is not an uncommon complication. In Bole's series,[3] acute pancreatitis was the leading cause of death in all patients undergoing cholecystectomy. All patients that died in this series had had either a common duct exploration or a sphincterotomy. Pancreatitis may result from manipulation of the pancreas or forceful dilatation of the sphincter of Oddi with trauma to the pancreatic duct.[2] It more commonly follows operations in which a common duct exploration was performed rather than a simple cholecystectomy. The mortality in the 75 patients having clinical pancreatitis following common duct exploration in the series of Thompson, Howard, and Vowles[25] was 77 percent. They also reviewed 17 cases of pancreatitis developing in patients in whom a long-arm T tube had been inserted through the common duct into the duodenum. Of these 17 patients, 16, or 95 percent died. Several cases of fatal postoperative pancreatitis have now been reported following the insertion of a long-arm T tube in the duodenum. In their series, only 9 percent of the patients developed an elevated serum amylase following cholecystectomy, whereas 29 percent developed an elevated serum amylase following common duct exploration. According to Bartlett and Carter,[2] the operative risk is increased in patients having common duct exploration, and so is postoperative acute pancreatitis. Direct duodenal approach to the common duct is a safer procedure than forceful manipulation from above. Ponka, Landrum, and Chaikof[20] reviewed 5747 cases of biliary tract and gastroduodenal surgical procedures. They found only 18 cases of pancreatitis, and only 8 of these were fatal. One in every 123 patients having gastroduodenal surgical procedures developed pancreatitis, but only one in every 371 cases ended fatally. They also noted that 55 percent of the patients developing postoperative pancreatitis had biliary tract disease if the surgical procedure was in an area remote from the pancreas. One patient of 1386 developed postoperative pancreatitis in which only cholecystectomy was done; however, one of every 301 patients who had common duct explorations developed postoperative pancreatitis. In Millbourn's series[17] of patients having subtotal gastrectomies, 35 percent had an elevated serum amylase postoperatively, but these patients did not necessarily have signs and symptoms of acute pancreatitis. In 9 percent of these patients the serum amylase was elevated to twice the normal level, but only one of these patients died.

In addition to these common causes, postoperative pancreatitis has been reported following surgical procedures on the colon, transuretheral resection, and umbilical herniorrhaphy.[1,20]

Many theories have been proposed as to the cause of postoperative pancreatis. Millbourn[17] and Dunphy[6] postulate that interference with blood supply to the pancreas may result from ligation of the gastroduodenal artery during subtotal gastric resection. This may be particularly true, as noted by Popper,[21] if there is pancreatic edema and may produce acute hemorrhagic pancreatitis in the aged. Other theories have been ligation of the duct of Santorini, direct trauma, and increased viscosity of pancreatic secretions during surgical procedures.[8]

The common channel theory has received wide acceptance as describing the cause of pancreatitis. This theory postulates that the pancreatic duct must empty into the common duct before entering the duodenum, thus forming a common channel. Pancreatic duct pressure is normally higher than common duct pressure. Pancreatic juice may therefore normally flow into the common duct. Obstruction near the ampulla secondary to stone, tumor, or stricture causes an increase in common duct pressure. After the pancreatic juice has incubated with bile in the common duct, the viscosity of the juice is less and the juice refluxes more easily into the pancreatic duct at low pressure. Elliott[7] has shown that the bile and pancreatic juice must incubate in the common duct before reflux into the pancreatic duct will produce pancreatitis (Fig. 25-2). The ratio of bile to pancreatic secretions in the incubated mixture determines the mortality from pancreatitis. Both must be present in about equal parts to produce a lethal lesion.

The diagnosis of postoperative pancreatitis at times is quite difficult to make because of the symptoms and findings which follow any abdominal operation. The early onset of pancreatitis aids in differentiating it from leakage of the duodenal stump or breakdown of an intestinal anastomosis, which characteristically occurs between the fifth and seventh day. Elevated serum amylase levels are known to occur with all these. The degree of elevation does not reflect the seriousness of the illness. The best means of diagnosis is determining the serum amylase level in all postoperative patients, which should be done at the end of 24 or possibly 48 h postoperatively. An elevation of the serum amylase may be the first finding in the development of postoperative pancreatitis.

PANCREATITIS FOLLOWING PANCREATIC INJURY

Patients rarely die as a direct result of a penetrating or blunt injury, such as gunshot wounds and knife injuries, to the pancreas. Death results from associated major vessel

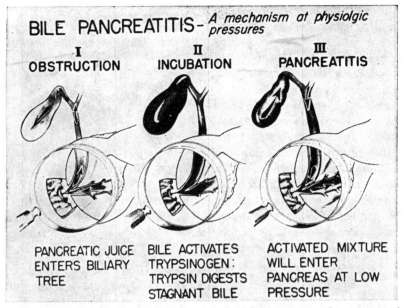

Figure 25-2 The mechanism suggested by which obstruction of a common channel can induce the regurgitation of bile into the pancreas and acute pancreatitis. *(Elliot, D. W., Williams, R. D., and Zollinger, R. M.: Alterations in the pancreatic resistance to bile in the pathogenesis of acute pancreatitis, Ann. Surg., 146:669, 1957.)*

injury.[11] Postoperative complications such as fistulas, pseudocysts, and pancreatic abscesses frequently develop. Following most pancreatic injuries there will be drainage of pancreatic secretions for several days. This rarely lasts for more than 1 month. Almost all fistulas will close and do not require definitive surgical treatment. Cultures from these areas usually reveal a mixed growth. The most common organism is *Staphylococcus,* with *Proteus, Pseudomonas,* and *Escherichia coli* being frequently noted.

In a series of patients with pancreatic injuries from blunt and penetrating trauma which were reviewed,[11] it was noted that almost every patient who had an elevated serum amylase level on more than one occasion had a fistula, an abscess, a pseudocyst, or a subphrenic collection. Of 12 patients with a pancreatic fistula, 11 had an elevated serum amylase level of several days to 1 month's duration. All patients with a pseudocyst had elevated serum amylase levels for 1 week or longer, and five of the six were elevated until the diagnosis was made. A serum amylase elevation in the presence of a pancreatic fistula should be of concern only if the patient is deteriorating. A consistently elevated serum amylase in the absence of a fistula usually indicates the formation of a pseudocyst. Of 17 patients with normal serum amylase levels, only two developed complications, and these were pancreatic abscesses. Therefore if the serum amylase level is consistently normal, the complication in question is usually not of pancreatic origin.

The treatment for postoperative acute pancreatitis is conservative and consists of the same treatment as that for acute pancreatitis. This consists of nasogastric suction to prevent gastric dilatation in the presence of ileus, which frequently occurs. It is also useful to decrease the amount of hydrochloric acid which spills into the duodenum, which in turn stimulates secretin and produces increased pancreatic secretions. The pain is managed with intramuscular meperidine (Demerol), although a sympathetic or epidural block is of benefit in patients with severe pain. Vagal blocking agents such as atropine and propantheline (Pro-Banthine) in high doses decrease the spasm of the sphincter of Oddi and decrease the production of hydrochloric acid, therefore decreasing the amount of pancreatic secretions. Antibiotics are routinely given, using penicillin for the gram-positive organisms and a broad-spectrum antibiotic for the gram-negative organisms. It has been shown that tetracycline is excreted in good concentration in the biliary tree but is excreted in low concentrations from the pancreas itself. Tetracycline or chloramphenicol may be used in conjunction with penicillin. The hypotension which occurs early in acute pancreatitis is probably due to the decreased blood volume and the loss of extracellular fluid into the retroperitoneal space. This is managed by utilizing a balanced salt solution such as Ringer's lactate and blood or plasma when indicated. Landrum[20] noted that all patients with postoperative pancreatitis who developed oliguria died. This frequently represents extracellular fluid deficit. No vasopressors should be used until volume is adequately replaced. Intravenous calcium may be necessary, although hypocalcemia is not often encountered.

BIBLIOGRAPHY

1 Artz, C. P. and J. D. Hardy: *Complications in Surgery and Their Management*, W. B. Saunders Company, Philadelphia, 1960.
2 Bartlett, M. K. and E. L. Carter: Special complications of gallbladder surgery, *Surg. Clin. North Am.*, 43:748, 1963.
3 Boles, E. T.: Postoperative pancreatitis, *Arch. Surg.*, 73:710, 1956.
4 Burton, C. C., W. G. Eckman, Jr., and J. Haxo: Acute postgastrectomy pancreatitis, *Am. J. Surg.*, 94:70, 1957.
5 DeJode, L. R. and J. M. Howard: The management of patients with acute pancreatitis, *Surg. Clin. North Am.*, 42:1494, 1962.
6 Dunphy, J. E., J. R. Brooks, and F. Achroyp: Acute postoperative pancreatitis, *N. Engl. J. Med.*, 248:445, 1953.
7 Elliott, Daniel W., Roger D. Williams, and Robert M. Zollinger: Alterations in the pancreatic resistance to bile in the pathogenesis of acute pancreatitis, *Ann. Surg.*, 146:681, 1957.
8 Ferris, D. O., T. E. Lynn, J. C. Cain, and A. H. Baggenstoss: Fatal postoperative pancreatitis, *Ann. Surg.*, 146:263, 1957.
9 Frieden, J. H.: Postoperative acute pancreatitis, *Surg. Gynecol. Obstet.*, 102:139, 1956.
10 Harkins, H. N. and L. M. Nyhus: *Surgery of the Stomach and Duodenum*, Little, Brown and Company, Boston, 1962, p. 697.
11 Jones, Ronald and G. Tom Shires: Management of pancreatic injuries, *Arch. Surg.*, 102:424–430, April 1971.
12 McCutcheon, A. D. and D. Race: Experimental pancreatitis: A possible etiology of postoperative pancreatitis, *Ann. Surg.*, 155:523, 1962.
13 ——— and ———: Experimental pancreatitis: Use of a new antiproteolytic substance, Trasylol, *Ann. Surg.*, 158:233, 1963.
14 McHardy, G., C. C. Craighead, L. Balart, H. Cradic, and C. LaGrange: Pancreatitis-intrapancreatic proteolytic trypsin activity, *J. Am. Med. Assoc.*, 183:527, 1963.
15 Mahaffey, J. H. and J. M. Howard: The Incidence of postoperative pancreatitis, *Arch. Surg.*, 70:348, 1955.
16 Marshall, S. F.: Special complications of gastric surgery, *Surg. Clin. North Am.*, 43:768, 1963.
17 Millbourn, E.: On acute pancreatic affections following gastric resection for ulcer or cancer and the possibilities of avoiding them, *Acta Chir. Scand.*, 98:1, 1949.
18 Nemir, P., Jr., J. Hoferichter, and D. Drakin: The protective effect of proteinase inhibitor in

acute necrotizing pancreatitis, *Ann. Surg.,* **158**: 655, 1963. (Discussion)

19 Perryman, R. G. and S. O. Hoern: Observations on postoperative pancreatitis and postoperative elevation of the serum amylase, *Am. J. Surg.,* **88**:417, 1954.

20 Ponka, J. L., S. E. Landrum, and L. Chaikof: Acute pancreatitis in the postoperative patient, *Arch. Surg.,* **83**:475, 1961.

21 Popper, H. L., H. Necheles, and K. C. Russel: Transition of pancreatic edema into pancreatic necrosis, *Surg. Gynecol. Obstet.,* **87**:79, 1948.

22 Schmeiden, V. and W. Schering: Surgery of the pancreas with especial consideration of acute pancreatitic necrosis, *Surg. Gynecol. Obstet.,* **46**:735, 1928.

23 State, D.: Immediate complications of gastric surgery, *Surg. Clin. North Am.,* **44**:374, 1964.

24 Stevens, L. W.: Subtotal gastrectomy for ulcer, *Surg. Clin. North Am.,* **42**:1423, 1962.

25 Thompson, J. A., J. M. Howard, and K. D. J. Vowles: Acute pancreatitis following choledochotomy, *Surg. Gynecol. Obstet.,* **105**:706, 1957.

26 Thorbjarnarson, B.: Complications of biliary tract surgery, *Surg. Clin. North Am.,* **44**:442, 1964.

27 Wallensten, S.: Acute pancreatitis and hyperdiastasuria after partial gastrectomy, *Acta Chir. Scand.,* **115**:182, 1958.

28 Warren, K. W., W. M. McDonald, and M. C. P. Veidenhumir: Trends in pancreatic surgery, *Surg. Clin. North Am.,* **44**:747, 1964.

Chapter 26

Nasogastric Suction

Malcolm O. Perry, M.D.

Nasogastric suction decompression has been widely accepted as an important part of the surgical treatment of intestinal obstruction. It has been of particular value in the postoperative patient in the prophylaxis and treatment of abdominal distention. The earliest use of nasogastric intubation apparently was by John Hunter in 1790.[6] He employed a tube made from fresh eel skin drawn over a whale probang. In 1874, Ewald and Oser developed a stomach tube of small-caliber, soft, pliable rubber, and demonstrated that no stylet was needed if the patient could cooperate.[19] In 1921, Levin introduced a small rubber tube with sufficient pliability that it could be passed with ease through the nose.[9] The technique of continuous gastric suction was demonstrated by Robertson Ward in 1925, and its beneficial effects in peritonitis, postoperative ileus, and intestinal obstruction were illustrated.[24] In 1931, Paine and Wangensteen advocated the use of nasogastric suction in patients with simple obstruction of the bowel or with postoperative adhesive obstruction.[15] Maddock, Bell, and Tremaine clinically and experimentally illustrated the harmful effects of aerophagia.[12] Their studies demonstrated that most of the air present in the bowel in abdominal distention was ingested, and they observed that apprehensive patients may swallow enormous amounts of air.

Suction decompression is of particular

value in patients with postoperative ileus, especially those in which the ileus follows compositional fluid derangements. Hypokalemia, hyponatremia, osmolar dilution, ketosis, or hypoxia may produce severe ileus. Abdominal decompression and correction of these aberrations result in restoration of bowel activity. The reflex ileus attending abdominal trauma, surgical or accidental, may require nasogastric suction for 3 to 5 days, and on rare instances as long as 10 days. It is difficult to separate this latter group of patients from those who have true mechanical intestinal obstruction due to fibrinous adhesions. These patients may respond to adequate decompression and not require surgical intervention, although certainly most patients with postoperative adhesive obstruction will eventually come to operation. The majority of these patients will show the classic features of intestinal obstruction, and when this persists beyond the twelfth postoperative day, surgical intervention should be considered. Any progression in severity of symptoms or indication of strangulation of bowel should be interpreted as a need for surgical decompression.

PATHOPHYSIOLOGY

Deleterious mechanical effects may follow the placement of a nasogastric tube, and these are generally related to pressure necrosis with subsequent ulceration and stricture. This is seen most often in the external nares, the hypopharynx, and in the upper portions of the esophagus. Overt perforation of the esophagus, stomach, or small intestine may occur after nasogastric intubation. Long or short tubes may become knotted.[10] This is particularly likely in the stomach rather than in other parts of the gastrointestinal tract, and usually occurs in patients in whom peristalsis has been reestablished. The inadvertent passage of a nasogastric tube into the tracheobronchial tree may produce mechanical injury or may directly inoculate the respiratory tract with pathogenic organisms.

Laryngeal damage may follow the placement of a nasogastric tube, and the area most vulnerable is at the cricoesophageal sphincter.[7] In this area, the circular muscle fibers of the esophagus together with the cricoid cartilage form a unique sphincter, one component muscular and the other cartilaginous. A nasogastric tube in the midline would thus be in a position for the pressure of the sphincter muscles to force the tube against the posterior border of the median ridge of the cricoid cartilage with subsequent ulceration of the very thin mucous membrane overlying the cartilage. With extension of infection to the deeper structures, perichondritis of the posterior aspect of the cricoid cartilage would occur, and subsequent acute subglottic stenosis or arytenoid fixation might supervene. Laryngeal abscess may be a concomitant complication which would enhance the severity of the damage.[5]

The nasogastric tube has been implicated as a factor in the production of damage to the distal esophagus with subsequent ulceration and stenosis.[1,2,3,14,19] Apart from the mechanical aspects of its presence, it is difficult to completely assess the exact role of the nasogastric tube in producing reflux of gastric juice into the distal esophagus. Nagler and Spiro studied esophageal pressures and esophageal pH in asymptomatic volunteer patients.[13] They were unable to define the mechanism by which gastric intubation produced gastric reflux into the distal esophagus. They could not demonstrate reflux of barium by cineradiography, nor could they detect changes in esophageal pressure to indicate disturbance of the intrinsic function of the inferior esophageal sphincter. They did illustrate a reduction in esophageal pH in the presence of gastric intubation. This was alleviated by removal or withdrawal of the tube into the esophagus. They concluded that with the patient supine, there was a lack of the gravitational force which normally returns regurgitated gastric contents to the stomach. This factor, combined with some degree of obstruction of the esophageal lumen produced by the tube was sufficient to maintain acid in the distal esophagus. Vinnik and Kern subsequently reported that in a study of patients with prolonged gastric intubation regurgitation into the distal esophagus did occur, and this was despite elevation of the head of the bed to 20°.[21] Removal of the gastric tube was followed by a return of the esophageal pH to normal. They could not demonstrate the symptoms of heartburn which had been described by Nagler and Spiro following their experimental procedures. They concluded that prolonged gastric intubation did induce reflux of gastric contents into the esophagus, probably as a result of functional alteration and incompetency of the cardioesophageal sphincter. Douglas indicated that a number of predisposing factors were often present which rendered the esophagus more vulnerable to trauma induced by an indwelling nasogastric tube.[2] He emphasized the association of vomiting and esophageal intubation and pointed out the difficulty of separating these particular factors. This was confirmed by the reports of Palmer.[16] The latter author also suggested that perhaps vomiting might remove protective esophageal mucus from the lower end of the esophagus and thus render it more vulnerable to mechanical trauma. Graham, Barnes, and Rubenstein suggested that esophageal mucus was altered and diminished by the avitaminosis and dehydration that often accompanied debility and senility.[3] They noted the frequent occurrence of these particular predisposing factors in patients who developed distal ulceration and stenosis of the esophagus. Bartels' survey of 6000 necropsies demonstrated 82 patients with ulcerative esophageal lesions, but only 30 had had gastric intubation.[1] Of these patients 67 percent were postoperative, and all the operations were considered to be difficult or the

patients were considered to be poor risks. No definite relation has been noted between the time that the tube is in place and the subsequent development of esophageal ulceration and stenosis. Palmer, however, suggested that the safe period is about 4 days in the presence of these conditions which might predispose to ulceration.

The nasogastric tube has been indicted as adversely affecting pulmonary ventilation and interfering with coughing, and this view was supported by Bevan.[11] The studies of MacKay, Aberd, and Matheson failed to show a significant reduction in vital capacity, peak expiratory flow rate, or forced expiratory volume.[11] They concluded that the deleterious effects were minimal, as measured by these parameters. The studies of Henley and Clausen demonstrated in a small group of patients that the nasogastric tube increased oral, pharyngeal, and bronchial secretions and, additionally, reflexly stimulated gastric secretion.[18] Although the experimental evidence is inconclusive, certainly the clinical impression that the presence of a nasogastric tube interferes with effective coughing and clearing of secretions is widely held.

Nasogastric suction may remove large amounts of fluid and electrolytes from the upper gastrointestinal tract, and the losses of chloride and hydrogen ions may be particularly high, and those of potassium will be less.[20] If the tube is inserted into the upper gastrointestinal tract beyond the pylorus, large amounts of alkaline secretions may be removed, and both volume deficit and compositional defects may ensue. If the patient is allowed to drink water, even in modest amounts, or ingest ice chips, the resultant ion loss may be magnified significantly.[17]

SPECIFIC COMPLICATIONS

The complications following nasogastric intubation are relatively uncommon but, nonetheless, quite serious when they occur. The following list illustrates some of the more significant problems which may arise:

1 Ulceration and/or abscess of the nasoseptum or the skin about the nares
2 Otitis media
3 Sinusitis
4 Hoarseness
5 Ulceration and stenosis of the esophagus
6 Ulceration and abscess of the larynx
7 Traumatic rupture of esophageal varices
8 Fluid and electrolyte depletion
9 Knotting of the tube and inability to withdraw the tube
10 Inadvertent intubation of the tracheobronchial tree with mechanical damage or inoculation of pathogenic organisms
11 Perforation of the esophagus, stomach, or gastrointestinal tract
12 Rupture of the esophagus by inflation of an indwelling catheter with an attached esophageal balloon
13 Nasal bleeding from trauma to the mucous membranes during passage of the tube

Wangensteen has noted that children particularly tolerate intubation very poorly, and not infrequently develop otitis media, and Harlow has reported nasoseptal abscess following nasogastric intubation.[23,4]

Iglauer and Molt reported 10 cases of severe injury to the larynx following use of the indwelling nasogastric tube, and 8 of their patients developed pharyngeal stenosis that required tracheostomy.[7] They discussed the mechanical factors present when the tube is lying in the midline separated from the cricoid cartilage by a very thin layer of mucous membrane. They noted that the average period of intubation in their cases was $8^{1}/_{2}$ days and that the signs of laryngeal involvement became manifest only after permanent removal of the duodenal tube. In their cases the early symptoms of laryngeal or esophageal injury were pain, dysphagia, blood-streaked sputum, hoarseness, croupy cough, and dyspnea. Hollinger and Loeb reported 24 cases of

stenosis of the larynx gleaned from the literature, added 4 cases of their own, and noted that in 3 patients tracheostomy was required following development of abscesses of the larynx.[5] They also recorded a stricture in the distal esophagus following intubation for 8 days.

The exact role of nasogastric intubation in the pathogenesis of esophageal ulceration and stenosis is difficult to assess, but Douglas, Olsen, Palmer, and Vinson in separate reports indicate that such a relationship may exist.[2,14,16,22] This relationship is further emphasized by Strohl, Hollinger, and Diffenbaugh.[19]

The withdrawal of large amounts of fluid and electrolytes from the upper gastrointestinal tract by nasogastric suction has been well documented by Taylor, and this has been confirmed by Smith and Farris.[18,20] Taylor demonstrated that suction may remove up to 180 meq of sodium chloride in a 24-h period. If water is given ad libitum, an even larger amount of chloride is lost. In these instances, a hypochloremic, hypokalemic alkalosis will supervene. This may be attended by significant volume depletion if a rigorous replacement schedule is not undertaken.

MANAGEMENT OF NASOGASTRIC INTUBATION

Successful, uncomplicated nasogastric intubation requires careful preparation of the tube and the patient, with meticulous attention to detail after placement of the indwelling tube. Initially, a sterile tube of proper size and sufficient resiliency should be selected. It should be well lubricated and inserted with care with adequate instruction to the patient to ensure the patient's cooperation. Recent studies indicate that siliconized tubes may be very useful. Inadvertent tracheobronchial intubation should be avoided, and traumatic passage of the tube through the nasal passages and the hypopharynx should be prevented. If a long duodenal tube is to be inserted, the stomach should be emptied prior to intubation, and separate measures should be undertaken to prevent gastric dilatation after passage of the tube into distal portions of the gastrointestinal tract. Once in place, the balloons should be deflated in order to prevent passage past the obstruction, avoiding the subsequent dangers of knotting, perforation, and pressure necrosis. If the balloon is in place during peristalsis, it should not be anchored to the nose, because ulceration and necrosis about the external nares may occur. Frequent examination of the patient should be made while the tube is in place; and complaints of nasal pain, hoarseness, sore throat, or pain in the ears are indications for removal and/or replacement of the tube. If at all possible, the opposite nares should be selected if the tube is to be reinserted. An attempt should be made to avoid placing the tube in the midline of the pharynx, thus inducing pressure on the posterior portion of the cricoid cartilage. Early removal of the tube is desirable; but if prolonged intubation is necessary, the tube should be frequently replaced.

The nasogastric tube is not a substitute for necessary surgical intervention and should not be used as definitive treatment for complete intestinal obstruction. If after placement of the nasogastric tube for intestinal obstruction undue delay occurs, strangulation and subsequent necrosis and gangrene of bowel may ensue. During the period of suction decompression, careful scheduling of fluid and ion replacement must be undertaken to prevent the deleterious effects of volume depletion and ion losses.

Frequent inspection and, if necessary, irrigation of the nasogastric tube must be performed to prevent blockage of the tube by mucus or blood clots or inadvertent placement of a clamp upon the suction apparatus. Blockage of an indwelling nasogastric tube may allow the patient to swallow large amounts of air about the tube and induce serious gastric dilation.

SUMMARY

Nasogastric intubation has gained wide acceptance in the surgical world and has proved to be a boon to the patient and the surgeon. There are certain potential hazards attending its use, but these may be minimized by careful attention to selection and placement of the tube, frequent examination of the patient, and meticulous replacement of the fluid and electrolytes withdrawn from the gastrointestinal tract.[8]

BIBLIOGRAPHY

1 Bartels, E. C.: Acute ulcerative esophagitis: A pathologic and clinical study of 82 cases observed at necropsy, *Arch. Pathol.,* **20**:369, 1935.
2 Douglas, W. K.: Esophageal strictures associated with gastroduodenal intubation, *Br. J. Surg.,* **43**:404, 1956.
3 Graham, J., N. Barnes, and A. S. Rubenstein: The nasogastric tube as a cause of esophagitis and stricture, *Am. J. Surg.,* **98**:116, 1959.
4 Harlowe, H. D.: Nasal septal abscess secondary to inlying duodenal tube, *Laryngoscope,* **58**:166, 1948.
5 Hollinger, P. H. and W. J. Loeb: Feeding tube stenosis of the larynx, *Surg. Gynecol. Obstet.,* **83**:253, 1946.
6 Hunter, John: *Proposals for the Recovery of Persons Apparently Drowned. Works of John Hunter,* Longmans, Green & Co., Ltd., London, 1837, vol. 4, p. 173.
7 Iglauer, S. and W. T. Molt: Severe injury to the larynx resulting from indwelling duodenal tube, *Ann. Otol. Rhinol. Laryngol.,* **48**:886, 1939.
8 Kleinsasser, L. J.: Complications of gastric and intestinal intubation, *Am. Practitioner Dig. Treat.,* **2**:221, 1951.
9 Levin, A. L.: A new gastroduodenal catheter, *J. Am. Med. Assoc.,* **76**:1007, 1921.
10 Lichtenstein, I. L.: Complications of intestinal intubation with report of two cases of unusual complications, *Calif. Med.,* **77**:192, 1952.
11 MacKay, W. D., M. D. Aberb, and N. A. Matheson: Nasogastric tube and pulmonary ventilation, *Arch. Surg.,* **87**:673, 1963.

12 Maddock, W. C., J. L. Bell, and M. D. Tremaine: Gastrointestinal gas: Observations on belching during anesthesia, operations, and pyleography, and rapid passage of gas, *Ann. Surg.*, **130**:512, 1949.

13 Nagler, R. and H. M. Spiro: Persistent gastroesophageal reflux induced during prolonged gastric intubation, *N. Engl. J. Med.*, **269**:495, 1963.

14 Olsen, A. M.: Esophagitis (editorial), *Surg. Gynecol. Obstet.*, **86**:372, 1948.

15 Paine, J. R. and O. H. Wangensteen: The history of the invention and development of the stomach and duodenal tubes, *Ann. Intern. Med.*, **8**:752, 1934.

16 Palmer, E. D.: *The Esophagus and Its Diseases,* Paul B. Hoeber, Inc., New York, 1952.

17 Shires, G. T.: Personal communication.

18 Smith, G. K. and J. M. Farris: Re-evaluation of temporary gastrostomy as a substitute for nasogastric suction, *Am. J. Surg.*, **102**:168, 1961.

19 Strohl, E. L., P. H. Hollinger, and W. C. Diffenbaugh: Nasogastric intubation: Indications, complications, safeguards and alternate procedures, *Am. Surg.*, **24**:721, 1958.

20 Taylor, F. W.: Electrolyte loss by postoperative nasal-gastric suction, *Arch. Surg.*, **66**:538, 1953.

21 Vinnik, I. E. and F. Kern: The effect of gastric intubation on esophageal pH, *Gastroenterology*, **47**:388, 1953.

22 Vinson, P. P.: *Diseases of the Esophagus,* Charles C Thomas, Publisher, Springfield, Ill., 1947.

23 Wangensteein, O. H.: The early diagnosis of acute intestinal obstruction with comments on pathology and treatment, *Tr. West. S. A.,* vol. 483, 1931.

24 Ward, R.: An apparatus for continuous gastric or duodenal lavage, *J. Am. Med. Assoc.*, **84**:1114, 1925.

Chapter 27

Catheter Care

Paul C. Peters, M.D.
Thomas C. Bright, III, M.D.

Since the thought-provoking editorial by Beeson regarding indiscriminate use of the urethral catheter published in 1958,[4] marked improvement in selection of patients for catheterization has occurred. Urologic attention has been directed toward elimination of the unnecessary indwelling catheter. At times the use of the indwelling catheter, even though temporary, simplifies the care of the patient, as following a cerebral vascular accident or head trauma; at times the indwelling catheter is therapeutic, as in the azotemic patient with obstructive uropathy; at times it is indispensable, as in the unconscious patient with multiple organ system injuries; and at times it is prophylactic against further injury, as in prevention of bladder distention in the acute

spinal cord injury patient. In the conscious traumatized patient with no neurologic injury, it is indeed rare to have to catheterize the patient simply to obtain a specimen for analysis. This practice should be condemned.

INSERTION OF THE INDWELLING CATHETER

The initial catheterization is of the utmost importance, and is unfortunately often the responsibility of the least medically trained individual in the unit. Data offered by Garibaldi suggest that the incidence of acquiring bacteriuria after catheterization is directly related to the professional status of the person inserting the catheter (Table 27-1).[5] The mea-

Table 27-1

Person performing catheterization	Number of patients	Patients with bacteriuria within 48 h
Licensed practical nurse	35	12
Registered nurse	62	13
Physician	99	10

tus is the narrowest point in the urinary tract, varying from 8 F (3 French = 1 mm) in the newborn male to 21 F in the adult male. In the female, the meatus will accommodate a 10 F catheter in the newborn and up to a 30 F in the adult. Prior to insertion of the catheter, the meatus should be thoroughly cleansed with an antiseptic solution such as Betadine or pHisoHex (hexachlorophene) and the tip of the catheter, not including the eye, coated with sterile lubricant. The prepuce should be retracted in the uncircumcised patient. An attempt should be made to insert the catheter centrally in the meatus ("dead center") and pass it cautiously into the bladder to sense any obstruction to passage. Three points of resistance are encountered in the normal urethra: (1) the meatus, (2) the urogenital diaphragm and verumontanum in the male, and (3) the bladder neck. Inability to pass [into the bladder a catheter that has already passed the meatus] usually indicates the presence of some kind of an urethral stricture, though inadequate lubrication and disruption of the urethra must also be considered. *Note:* In conscious patients when a history of blood at the meatus following injury has been obtained, the authors prefer urethrography with intravenous (sterile) contrast material prior to catheterization to avoid unnecessary manipulation of a rupture of the urethra at or below the urogenital diaphragm. Such patients often have swelling or discoloration in the perineum and scrotum.

When clear urine is obtained, a sample should be saved for culture and microscopic analysis and other indicated tests, i.e., myoglobin.

The catheter should then be advanced 2 or 3 cm if possible. Next, the balloon should be inflated to 5 mL capacity. Gentle traction should then be applied to the catheter to pull the balloon down to the vesical neck. If this can be easily accomplished, the attendant should then grasp the catheter as he would a fountain pen and see if he can advance it into the bladder again for a distance of 2 to 3 cm. If this can be accomplished, one can then be satisfied that the catheter is indeed in the bladder and that it is not inflated within the urethra or extrinsic to the urethra. When an indwelling catheter is necessary and the urine is clear, the authors prefer to use no larger than an 18F catheter in adults and the smallest appropriate to the size of the *meatus* in a child.

As soon as the catheter is properly positioned and draining, it should be immediately connected to a *closed dependent* drainage system. This connection, if not already fused to the catheter, should not be broken during the period of time that the catheter is needed except when it is anticipated that an unusually long period of catheter drainage will be needed, i.e., weeks, or when a defect is demonstrated in the closed drainage system necessitating its change.

CARE OF THE CATHETER

The occurrence of bacteriuria in patients initially abacteruric on *open* drainage *cannot be significantly prevented*, even with systemic antibiotics,[1,3] hence the authors' preference for a closed drainage system incorporating a valve in the dependent bedside collection bag. The valve, if effective in permitting rapid entry into the collection bag during periods of diuresis, will also prevent a siphoning effect on the bladder mucosa of a 3- or 4-feet-long dependent column of fluid (urine).

The use of an intraurethral lubricating catheter in an attempt to block ascending infection around the urethral catheter was not found to be advantageous in male patients having long-term catheter drainage in a controlled study by Kunin and Finkelberg. In female patients, the system did show some protection against infection during a 10-day period of catheter drainage, but placebo in the irrigant protected as well as polymyxin.[8]

A thin film of fluid separates the urethral catheter from the urethral mucosa within 24 h of the insertion of the catheter. This film, a combination of exudate and urine, serves to protect the mucosa from irritation by the indwelling catheter and products in its manufacture which may leach out over a period of days. This film may also serve as a medium by which bacteria may ascend from the skin, prepuce, and meatus to the urinary bladder.[7] To combat this possibility, the *meatus* and *catheter* at the point of entry into the meatus must be kept scrupulously clean with plain soap and water used at least twice a day. The authors do not favor the use of antibacterial ointments in this location, particularly in males. They are generally ineffective in reducing the incidence of bacteriuria after 10 days of catheter drainage (Table 27-2),[2] and they lull into complacency the attendants, including physicians, who forget to keep the meatus and adjacent urethral catheter scrupulously clean.

Although the use of a continuous wash of the bladder with an antibacterial agent (short term <10 days) might be preferable in certain cases, i.e., in an immunosuppressed patient,

Table 27-2 Acquisition of Bacteiruria after Indwelling Catheterization in Nonbacteruric Patients

Catheter groups (10 days or less)	Percent infection
Open drainage alone	100
Open drainage and saline	100
Open drainage and systemic antibiotics	75
Three-way catheter and acetic acid rinse	20
Three-way catheter and nitrofurazone	20
Three-way catheter and neosporin rinse	6

its long-term usage is not preferred because of the likelihood that a potentially dangerous and difficult to eliminate (drug-resistant) organism will ultimately be selected. The use of antibacterial rinses are ineffective in sterilizing the urine when bacteriuria existed prior to the insertion of the catheter (Table 27-3). The incidence of catheter-induced infections increases in patients with diseased urinary tracts.[9] Certain hazards may result from the use of antibacterial agents in a three-way irrigation system, particularly with long-term (>10 days) usage.

MANAGEMENT OF PATIENTS REQUIRING LONG-TERM INDWELLING CATHETERS

Prophylactic antibiotics are not used. If a closed system with an effective one-way valve is used so that reflux from the bag to the

Table 27-3

Antibacterial substance	Complication
Acetic acid rinse	Yeast infection
Neomycin-polymyxin	Candida, Proteus, or enterococcus infection
Nitrofurazone	Hematuria; resistant organisms; yeast infection
Distilled water	Hyponatremia; intravascular hemolysis

bladder does not occur and the bag is kept dependent by careful attendants, one still finds that the bag urine is infected 1 to 5 days before clinical infection of the patient's bladder is manifest. When the patient on closed-system valve bag-dependent drainage becomes infected, aspiration into a syringe by sterile technique of a sample of urine from the catheter is obtained for culture and sensitivity and appropriate antibiotic therapy given. Genital infections should be immediately sought, in the male particularly in the prostate, epididymis, or in the pendulous urethra. Abscesses discovered should be drained. Scrupulous cleansing of the catheter and adjacent meatus should be done 3 times daily with plain soap and water. In 30 percent of patients with an indwelling catheter who did not have prior bacteriuria, the urine can be rendered bacteria-free by colony count. At this point, the catheter and attached drainage system should be changed, a new catheter inserted under sterile technique, and specific antimicrobial therapy continued for a total of 10 days. The authors prefer to fill the urethra with a 1% neomycin solution at the time of insertion of a new catheter in the male. Female patients may have an ounce of 1% Neosporin placed in the bladder at the time of insertion of the new catheter.

At the time the catheter is finally removed, i.e., 10 days to infinity, a culture is taken and appropriate antimicrobial therapy is given to sterilize the urine in those patients who were not bacteriuric prior to insertion of the catheter and in those in whom no underlying urinary tract disease, such as urinary tract calculus, is present which would prevent effective sterilization of the urine.

In patients with urethral catheters or suprapubic tubes who require indefinite periods of (i.e., months or years) catheter drainage, periodic change of the catheter is necessary. This may be necessitated by plugging of the catheter by exudates or calcific material. One can rub the walls of the catheter between the thumb and forefinger to check for calcigerous material. If this is present, the catheter should be changed, even if it is draining well. One should be especially gentle in changing the catheter in such patients, as bacteremia may result from slight urethral mucosal trauma. Bacteremia may be reduced, though not eliminated, by the use of a single dose of 80 mg of Garamycin (gentamycin) given 1 h prior to the catheter change or by instilling 1 or 2 oz of neomycin into the bladder and/or urethra at the time of insertion of the new catheter. It has been the authors' experience that a urethral catheter may be left indwelling for 6 weeks without need for change, and a suprapubic tube often for 3 to 6 months without the need for change. In the authors' experience cranberry juice (30 oz daily) and vitamin C and Mandelamine in 1-g dosage qid. have been of little benefit in reducing the incidence of infection in patients requiring long-term catheter drainage. Sialastic coated catheters have shown the same propensity to calcification as latex catheters in those patients exhibiting the tendency, i.e., those patients with persistently alkaline urine and a urea splitting organism. The use of urease inhibitors, i.e., acetohydroxyamine, may play a role in reducing this tendency to calcification of the catheter.[6] At present, they are available on an experimental basis.

BIBLIOGRAPHY

1 Andriole, V. T.: "Care of the Indwelling Catheter," in D. Kaye (ed.), *Urinary Tract Infection and Its Management,* The C. V. Mosby Company, St. Louis, 1972.

2 ———: Hospital-acquired urinary infections and the indwelling catheter, *Urol. Clin. North Am.,* **2:**451–469, 1975.

3 ———, C. M. Kunin, T. A. Stamey, et al.: Preventing catheter-induced urinary tract infections, *Hosp. Pract.,* **3:**61, 1968.

4 Beeson, P. B.: The case against the catheter, *Am. J. Med.,* **24:**1, 1958.

5 Garibaldi, R. A., J. P. Burke, M. L. Dickman, et al.: Factors predisposing to bacteriuria during indwelling urethral catheterization, *N. Engl. J. Med.,* **29**:215–219, 1974.

6 Griffith, D.: "Medical Therapy of Urinary Stones," in G. D. Chisolm (ed.), *Tutorial Postgraduate Medicine: Urology,* 1977.

7 Kass, E. H. and L. J. Schneiderman: Entry of bacteria into the urinary tracts of patients with inlying catheters, *N. Engl. J. Med.,* **256**:556–557, 1957.

8 Kunin, C. M. and Z. Finkelberg: Evaluation of an intraurethral lubricating catheter in prevention of catheter-induced urinary tract infections, *J. Urol.,* **106**:928–931, 1971.

9 Stamey, T. A.: "Urinary Infections," in *The Diagnosis of Bacteriuria,* The Williams & Wilkins Company, 1972, pp. 1–30.

Chapter 28

Deep Vein Thrombosis

Malcolm O. Perry, M.D.

INTRODUCTION

In 1959 Sevitt and Gallagher found in an unselected series of fatally injured patients that 60 percent had deep venous thrombosis without pulmonary embolism, and that over 80 percent of elderly patients who died after having a fractured femur had this complication.[1,4,5] They subsequently demonstrated that deep venous thrombosis occurs in 30 to 60 percent of patients undergoing general surgical operations and in as many as 50 percent of patients undergoing orthopedic operations.[4] Pulmonary embolism is not only a frequent occurrence after surgery, but it is also one of the major causes of death after serious medical illnesses and is the greatest single cause of maternal deaths due to childbirth.[18]

Pathogenesis

Over 100 years ago Virchow suggested that thrombosis was the result of intimal damage, hypercoagulability, and stasis of blood. Subsequent studies suggested that two different types of thrombus occurred: one was composed primarily of erthyrocytes and fibrin characteristically formed in areas of venous stasis, and the other was a white thrombus which contained leucocytes, platelets, and fibrin and was found almost exclusively in areas adjacent to injured vessel walls or in association with rapid arterial flow.[4] Recent studies now strongly suggest that platelet activity may also trigger the formation of some venous thrombi, and that a small platelet nidus may precede activation of venous thrombosis. It now appears that thrombus formation begins when platelets adhere to an altered intimal surface or exposed collagen in a damaged vessel wall. Subsequent activation of the intrinsic clotting mechanism results in the formation of a thrombus in a progressive reaction.[13] There is persuasive evidence that this process may frequently begin in the valve cusps where there is relative stasis and less effect of dilutional factors. It is now apparent that changes in platelet adhesiveness occur during operation and after trauma, and some studies strongly suggest that the generation of deep venous thrombosis actually begins during the operative procedure.[7] Studies of deep venous thrombosis utilizing phlebography and ^{125}I-labeled fibrinogen have demonstrated the presence of thrombi early during the operation.[9]

Considerable controversy exists as to where deep venous thrombosis actually begins, but Kakkar and his associates have stated that it almost always starts in the tibial veins and soleal sinuses, and then extends proximally into popliteal and femoral veins.[9] A dissenting view is taken, however, by Mavor and co-workers who have suggested that about two-thirds of all pulmonary emboli arise from the iliofemoral segment, and they therefore consider these lesions to be primary.[10] In further studies of deep venous thrombosis based on ^{125}I fibrinogen scanning, Kakkar and his colleagues have demonstrated that about 35 percent of patients who have raised counts persisting for more than 72 h subsequently have extension of the clot into the popliteal and femoral veins. When this occurs, the chance in their study of the patient developing a pulmonary embolus was about 40 percent. In sharp contrast are those patients who have clots which reside only in the tibial or soleal veins and in whom pulmonary embolism is relatively rare. It would appear from these studies that deep venous thrombosis begins in the calf veins but does not pose great danger to the patient until it extends into the femoral and iliac veins. The difference in the viewpoints of these established investigators apparently revolves around the techniques of utilizing ^{125}I-labeled fibrinogen, which may not be incorporated into a thrombus which is either stationary or dissolving. It is therefore considered inappropriate by Kakkar to utilize this test to examine deep venous thrombosis under situations where the clots are already established.[9]

DIAGNOSIS

The unreliability of clinical examination in the detection of deep venous thrombosis is well known, but certain physical findings offer strongly suggestive evidence as to the presence of thrombosis. Swelling of the ankle and leg, tenderness of the calf and popliteal area, and a positive Homan's sign are characteristic of deep venous thrombosis. It is apparent that more than half of the patients with deep venous thrombosis diagnosed by other methods will be missed by clinical examination alone, and for this reason many studies have been proposed to aid in the early detection of venous thrombi.

Phlebography is the most sensitive and complete of the tests and can be utilized to visualize the entire venous system of the lower extremity. All other procedures used in the diagnosis of venous thrombosis are compared with phlebography as the standard, but because of the cost, risk, and time phlebography cannot be considered as a satisfactory screening technique. Many investigators believe that phlebography should be reserved for patients who have clinical signs and symptoms strongly suggestive of deep venous thrombosis and in whom other less specific tests are equivocal. Skillman has suggested that phlebography is particularly useful in separating cellulitis and hematomas, superficial phlebitis, and other conditions which do not require anticoagulation but cannot be easily excluded.[18] Mobin-Uddin and others believe that ascending phlebography should be used prior to operative procedures which include interrupting the vena cava.[11] These workers point out that phlebography may be used in these cases to establish the continuing presence of potentially lethal venous thrombi and may offer compelling indications for operative intervention. Complications of the method are few and are generally restricted to various allergic reactions to the contrast media, localized phlebitis and hematoma at the site of injection, and rarely deep vein phlebitis. Pulmonary embolism following ascending phlebography is apparently extremely rare.[18]

There are several noninvasive tests which have been used in the diagnosis of deep venous thrombosis, and these include impedance plethysmography, ultrasonic velocity flow detection, ^{125}I-labeled fibrinogen scanning, and radionuclide studies. Impedance plethysmography, described by Mullick and associates, is based on the principle that if the venous system in the lower extremity is patent, the venous blood volume and therefore the electrical impedance in the legs will change with respiration.[12] When the test is positive, compared with ascending phlebography, its reliability appears to be in excess of 90 percent, but unfortunately when it is negative, the accuracy has been reported to be only approximately 50 percent. Recent modifications in which external compression of the leg is utilized instead of respiratory excursions have been reported to increase the sensitivity and accuracy. Nevertheless, the number of false-negative and false-positive tests indicate that impedance plethysmography has significant limitations as a screening procedure.

The Doppler ultrasonic velocity flow detector has been advocated as useful in the detection of deep venous thombosis. Strandness and Sumner reported that this technique accurately predicted deep venous thrombosis in over 93 percent of 53 patients who subse-

quently had either venography or operation in order to confirm the diagnosis.[19] Sigel and his associates, however, report on utilizing Doppler ultrasonic examinations over 8500 times in over 5000 patients.[16] In 248 examinations concurrent phlebography was performed and the Doppler examination agreed with phlebography in approximately 75 percent of patients with limbs containing venous thrombosis. These authors concluded that the method could not detect clot when only tributary veins were involved and patent collateral veins were present. They also point out that error may arise because of improper positioning of the probe, emptying the veins by gravity or compression bandages, and therefore it is useful as a screening procedure only in conjunction with other examinations. They add that it is particularly useful in detecting thrombosis involving the femoral and iliac veins, especially when recent. From these reports it is apparent that the Doppler screening techniques have serious limitations and cannot be reliably employed as a solitary method of examination.[16]

The technique of scanning with fibrinogen tagged with ^{125}I has been advocated especially by Flanc, Kakker, and their associates.[6,9] The procedure requires that the radioactive fibrinogen be incorporated into newly forming thrombi, and then the activity is detected by scanning the leg and thigh with a portable scintillation counter. The test has proved to be extremely useful and very sensitive in the detection of patients with deep venous thrombosis, but is not completely reliable in patients with established clots because it depends on incorporation of labeled fibrinogen into the thrombus. It is also not useful for the detection of iliac and pelvic vein thrombosis and cannot be used immediately adjacent to areas of recent surgical wounds, such as those involving operations about the hip, because of pooling in hematomas near the operative incision. It is, however, the single most sensitive and useful noninvasive test in the diagnosis of deep venous thrombosis and has been widely employed in Europe. Because of limited access to hepatitis-free, labeled fibrinogen and because of the expense of the equipment it has not been employed as frequently in the United States.[18]

Pollak and his associates recently reported on studies of deep venous thrombosis in a series of patients in whom the labeled fibrinogen uptake test and a venous scan with technetium (^{99m}TC) sulfur was employed.[13] In this procedure microaggregates of albumin incorporating technetium (^{99m}TC) sulfur are prepared to form particles 10 to 50 μm in size and subsequently injected into dorsal veins of the foot. Isotope distribution in the legs and pelvis is detected by scintillation cameras and photographed. In the same patients autologous fibrinogen is secured and labeled with ^{125}I and injected into an antebrachial vein of each patient, and isotope uptake is monitored with scintillation counters. Technetium scan was performed in 77 patients and the fibrinogen uptake in 59 patients, and both were evaluated in a series of 89 patients. These authors indicated that an abnormal technetium scan is over 90 percent sensitive and approximately 80 percent reliable in separating patients with venous disease from those who do not have deep venous thrombosis. False positives may occur because any area of endothelial damage may trap the aggregates, and considerable skill is required to develop reproducible results. The fibrinogen uptake test is considered to be 100 percent sensitive in differentiating active recent thrombosis from longstanding venous obstruction in these patients. In these workers' opinion a combination of these two tests offers reliable evidence as to the presence of deep venous thrombosis and may obviate the necessity of ascending contrast phlebography.[13]

Cranley[3] and his associates developed a plethysmographic technique for the examination of thigh and calf volume changes in response to compression of the calf or foot. This method is called phleborheography, and after 4 years of testing in over 7000 extremities, a 98 percent correlation with 500 contrast phlebograms was found. These initial reports strongly suggest that this innovative technique will be of great value in the detection of deep vein thrombosis.

It is apparent from the foregoing discussion that numerous studies are available for the detection of deep venous thrombosis, and among these the fibrinogen uptake test is the most sensitive and the most reliable. When combined with radionuclide studies or Doppler ultrasonic examinations, the clinical evaluation is materially improved. At the present time all these tests are compared with ascending contrast phlebography as a standard, and it is apparent that despite its "invasive" nature phlebography may be required to resolve differences in interpretation of these various other tests.

PREVENTION OF DEEP VENOUS THROMBOSIS

The concept of the "peripheral heart" is central to the procedures developed to prevent deep venous thrombosis. Flanc and his associates have reported on an intensive program of prophylactic physical measures in a group of 67 patients who were instructed preoperatively in active leg exercises.[6] The diagnosis of deep venous thrombosis was based on the labeled fibrinogen uptake test. Of those elderly patients having major operations, the incidence of deep venous thrombosis was 61 percent in the control group and only 24 percent in the test group, a significant difference.

In a similar study Tsapogas, again utilizing labeled fibrinogen scans, reported that reduction of deep venous thrombosis by active exercises could be demonstrated.[20] In a randomized study reported by Rosengarten et al. compression stockings in a group of 50 patients undergoing elective operations could not be shown to be beneficial in the prevention of deep venous thrombosis.

Recent development of external pneumatic devices for intermittent rhythmic compression of the extremities as a substitute for the "soleal pump" strongly suggests that such procedures may be useful in preventing stasis and perhaps deep venous thrombosis. These reports, however, are related to experience and do not reflect controlled scientific data. It is reasonable to assume from the frequency of these studies that avoiding venous stasis during and immediately after an operation is an important concept and should be achieved if at all possible.[18]

PROPHYLACTIC DRUG THERAPY

According to Salzman several drugs are known to prevent thromboembolism in high-risk patients, and the evidence is most convincing in the case of warfarin and other oral anticoagulants.[8] Kakkar et al. have evidence that strongly suggests that low dose heparin may be useful in surgical patients of moderate risk.[9] Salzman and his associates have reported that clinically detectable thromboembolic complications can be significantly reduced in patients with fractures of the hip when prophylactic warfarin is administered. Harris, in a prospective randomized study of thromboembolic disease following total hip replacement in 227 patients, reported that warfarin sodium and dextran 40 were equally effective in preventing fatal pulmonary emboli.[7] There was no statistically significant difference between the two agents. In this high-risk group of patients clinically detectable thromboembolic disease occurred in approximately 10 percent.

Evarts, in reporting on a study of 514 patients, stated that low-molecular-weight dextran reduced an expected incidence of deep venous thrombosis of 50 percent to 4.3 percent.[5] Only 5 of the 514 patients developed nonfatal pulmonary emboli, an incidence of 1 percent. From these data Evarts suggested dextran is the agent of choice in these patients, but a dissenting view is taken by some investigators. Skillman and Salzman have indicated the complications and expense associated with use of dextran may detract somewhat from its usefulness.[18] Salzman states that "dextran produces allergic reactions frequently, anaphylactic reactions occasionally, and renal failure rarely."[8] From these data it is apparent that prophylactic administration of warfarin sodium and/or dextran are useful in the prevention and management of deep venous thrombosis related to high-risk patients, but certain undesirable side effects will be encountered with some frequency.

Kakkar, in an initial report concerning over 4000 patients admitted to a prospective controlled study, suggested that low dose heparin is the most effective prophylactic agent. In these patients 5000 U of heparin is administered subcutaneously 2 h before and immediately after surgery and two times a day thereafter.[8] The effect seems to be mediated through the activation of factor Xa, a naturally occurring anticlotting factor and does not depend on heparin's antithrombin activity. The regimen appears to be effective in patients undergoing general surgery, but has not been useful in high-risk patients with orthopedic procedures. The early results in approximately 4000 of the total of 20,000 patients in this study are encouraging in that only 1 case of fatal pulmonary embolism in the heparin-treated group has been reported, as compared with 12 in the control group.

ANTIPLATELET AGENTS

Salzman and his associates have reported on the prophylactic effect of dipyridamole, aspirin, and dextran in patients undergoing hip arthroplasty.[18] Dipyridamole was eliminated from the study early because of 34 patients being treated with this drug, 26 developed thromboembolic complications. The subsequent incidence of thromboembolism in the aspirin- and dextran-treated groups was approximately the same as in those treated with warfarin, and the conclusion was that in all of the patients significant protection was conferred by these drugs. In contrast was a report published by the National Research Council in Britain covering 303 patients undergoing elective operations. No protective effect of aspirin could be demonstrated utilizing labeled fibrinogen scans to detect deep venous thrombosis. Because of these discrepancies the pyrimdopyrimidine compounds and the nonsteroidal antiinflammatory agents such as aspirin cannot be recommended as effective prophylactic antithrombotic measures under currently employed protocols.

Conflicting reports as to the efficacy of these prophylactic measures are difficult to reconcile, but appear to be the result of varying methods of study, different dosage schedules, nonstandardized methods of detecting deep venous thrombosis, and inadequately controlled data. From these many reports certain conclusions seem warranted. It is apparent that older patients or those who have a history of deep venous thrombosis or pulmonary embolism or have varicose veins, obesity, or malignancy are likely to develop deep venous thrombosis. In these high-risk patients prophylactic low dose subcutaneous heparin or prophylactic warfarin may be indicated. When contraindications to prophylactic anticoagulation are present, the fibrinogen scanning technique is useful in the early detection of deep venous thrombosis in this group of high-risk patients.

SUPERFICIAL PHLEBITIS

Patients with phlebitis confined to the superficial venous system, the greater and lesser saphenous vein, rarely require anticoagulant therapy. Elevation, rest, and compression will usually be successful in the management of these patients. Once superficial phlebitis extends above the knee, it has been suggested by Cranley and others that ligation of the saphenous vein at its entrance into the common femoral vein is indicated.[2] This procedure will often produce early resolution of the process and prevent thrombotic extension into the deep venous system. The procedure may be performed under local anesthesia and often reduces pain and morbidity within the first 48 h after the procedure.

DEEP VEIN THROMBOSIS

Deep vein thrombosis is best treated by a regimen of continuous intravenous heparin. In the regimen described by Dale 5000 IU of aqueous heparin are administered by intravenous push, and following this, a patient of average weight would receive approximately 12,500 units of heparin in 500 mL of 5% dextrose solution every 8 h.[8] A continuous infusion pump is desirable, and levels of heparin activity are monitored measuring activated partial thromboplastin time or recalcification time at least once a day during therapy. Heparin sensitivity increases as the drug is continued, and it is often necessary to subsequently readjust the dose to a lower level. Most investigators maintain an activated partial thromboplastin time of approximately 2 times the normal level.

Salzman and Hume and others suggest that the patient with deep venous thrombosis initially receive warfarin sodium concomitantly with heparin administration and slowly be brought under control with this oral anticoagulant.[8] The usual practice is to give both for 10 days, and then subsequently the oral medication is continued for several months, if predisposing conditions leading to the deep venous thrombosis cannot be eliminated. Prothrombin time is initially checked every day during the first week, and after that 2 or 3 times a week is satisfactory. A separate view is taken by Dale, who does not use oral anticoagulants concomitantly with heparin, nor does he use warfarin in patients who cannot be followed very carefully. He indicates that the risk of dangerous bleeding is significant and adds that he has seen acute exacerbations of venous thrombosis and even fresh clots in patients who were adequately anticoagulated with warfarin.

It is apparent that anticoagulants following a major surgical procedure must be given judiciously. Most workers indicate that anticoagulants may be safely started within 6 to 12 h after the operation is successfully concluded. This may not be true in patients who have had orthopedic procedures, radical prostatectomies, or in whom significant danger of retinal or intracranial hemorrhage is present. Most surgeons combine anticoagulant therapy with elevation and in some instances elastic stockings or bandages if venous abnormalities are present in the lower extremities. Ambulation is begun as soon as symptoms permit. It is desirable to return the venous circulation to normal as soon as possible, while the patient is under the protection of intravenous heparin. Once the swelling has resolved and the pain permits, full ambulation is begun, but it is important to initially stage the convalescence in order to prevent a recurrence of swelling. Usually by the tenth day the patients are able to be fully ambulatory and leg swelling has decreased sufficiently to permit measurements for a custom fit elastic stocking.

THROMBOLYTIC AGENTS

Streptokinase and urokinase have been utilized in a cooperative control study in the evaluation of pulmonary embolism and have been shown to hasten the lysis of clots in patients with established pulmonary emboli.[17] Morbidity and mortality were not significantly changed, but these thrombolytic agents may shorten the course of venous occlusion and perhaps reduce postphlebitic phenomena. Silver has demonstrated that when heparin is given in sufficiently large amounts, clotting is inhibited and thrombolysis is augmented. Because of accelerated lysis such agents may therefore be important adjuncts in the management of patients with deep venous thrombosis and massive pulmonary embolism. Unfortunately, they cannot be administered in the immediate postoperative period in patients who have sustained serious trauma or after extensive surgical procedures.

OPERATIVE PROCEDURES

Iliofemoral venous thrombectomy was a popular procedure during the past decade, and as originally described by Mahorner, Haller, and others is very useful in patients with phlegmasia cerulea dolens. Patients with this massive iliofemorovenous outflow blockade face a 30 percent chance of amputation, and mortality of approximately 1 in 4 is reported. It has been repeatedly demonstrated that in patients with massive thrombosis in whom there is no threat to viability of the extremity, elevation, rest, and heparin administration are quite effective and surgery may be avoided. When there are contraindications to the administration of anticoagulants, or there is threatened tissue loss, iliofemoral venous thrombectomy may be very useful and often evokes a dramatic response. Some workers suggest that vena caval interruption should accompany this operation, but others believe that if complete thrombectomy is performed early in the disease thromboembolic phenomena are very uncommon.

Phlebographic studies reported at varying intervals following iliofemoral venous thrombectomy have revealed that in many instances the operation has failed and the operative segment has reclotted. In addition, the aim of preserving valvular function by early operation has not consistently been accomplished. In fact, late phlebographic studies reveal that the incidence of postphlebitic problems, destruction of valves, and recurrent thrombosis are quite similar in patients treated with heparin or with operation. For these reasons most surgeons limit this procedure to patients threatened with loss of life or limb.[1]

CAVAL INTERRUPTION

Utilizing continuous infusion of intravenous heparin, Silver in his report shows the documented recurrence of pulmonary emboli to be 3 percent, a rate of recurrence which compares favorably with those results obtained with caval interruption.[17] Most investigators believe that caval interruption should be undertaken only in those patients who exhibit a failure on heparin therapy, cannot tolerate anticoagulation because of concomitant illnesses such as bleeding ulcers, recent operations upon the brain or retina, or recent orthopedic procedures. Documented recurrent pulmonary embolization on adequate heparin therapy is generally considered by most surgeons to be an indication for caval interruption, and recurrence of small emboli under adequate therapy is also considered an indication for caval ligation. Septic emboli are usually treated by the combination of heparin and antibiotics, as ligation procedures have demonstrated a failure to completely trap these very small emboli which are able to traverse collaterals and eventually reach the pulmonary circulation.[8]

Numerous methods of caval interruption have been proposed, including ligature, encircling teflon clips, compartmentalization or plication and construction of a filtering grid across the lumen of the cava. More recently, intracaval techniques have been introduced in the form of fenestrated catheters, balloon catheters, metal cones for trapping clots, and an umbrella designed by Mobin-Uddin which has been extensively employed over the past few years.[11] In this latter procedure a fenestrated or solid sialastic umbrella may be inserted into the infrarenal cava through the ipsilateral internal jugular vein. This may be done under local anesthesia, and with phlebographic and fluoroscopic control it can be accurately positioned. The procedure is less difficult than some of the other methods and does not require a major operative procedure. Although slow progressive occlusion of the cava is supposed to ensue following insertion of the umbrella, on occasion abrupt occlusion does occur, and in other instances clots have been demonstrated on the cardiac side of the umbrella. Erosion out of the cava into the ureter or other viscera or into other vessels has also occurred on rare occasions. In most centers when the indications for caval interruption arise, insertion of the Mobin-Uddin umbrella is considered an extremely useful method which carries with it lower morbidity and mortality than direct operative intervention. Mobin-Uddin has suggested, however, that before the umbrella is placed, ascending contrast phlebography should be performed to be certain that the continuing risk of pulmonary emboli is present, because although this procedure is less risky than other operations, it is attended by a significant number of complications.[11]

BIBLIOGRAPHY

1 Coon, W.: Operative therapy of venous thromboembolism, *Mod.* Concepts *Cardiovas. Dis.,* **18:**71–75, February 1974.
2 Cranley, John J.: Venous stasis (Letters to the Editors), *Surgery,* **77:**730–734, May 1975.
3 Cranley, J. J., A. J. Canos, W. J. Sull, and A. M. Grass: Phleborheographic techniques for diagnosing deep venous thrombosis of the lower extremities, *Surg. Gynecol. Obstet.,* **141:**331–340, 1975.
4 Evarts, C. McCollister: Thromboembolic disease in orthopedic patients, *Contemp. Surg.,* **6:**65–68, March 1975.
5 ———: Thromboembolic disease in orthopedic patients: Prophylaxis and treatment, *Contemp. Surg.,* **6:**57–60, April 1975.
6 Flanc, C., V. V. Kakkar, and M. D. Clarke: The

detection of venous thrombosis of the legs using ^{125}I-labeled fibrinogen, *Br. J. Surg.*, **55**:742, 1968.

7 Harris, William H., Edwin W. Salzman, Roman W. DeSanctis, and Richard D. Coutts: Prevention of venous thromboembolism following total hip replacement: Warfarin vs dextran 40, *J. Am. Med. Assoc.*, **220**:1319–1322, June 1972.

8 Hume, M., W. A. Dale, E. W. Salzman, and A. Ochsner: A spectrum of viewpoints on managing thromboembolism, *Contemp. Surg.*, **6**:82–107, March 1975.

9 Kakkar V. V.: The diagnosis of deep vein thrombosis using the ^{125}I fibrinogen test, *Arch. Surg.*, **104**:152, 1972.

10 Mavor, G. E., R. G. Mahaffy, M. G. Walker, et al.: Peripheral venous scanning with ^{125}I-tagged fibrinogen, *Lancet*, **1**:551, 1972.

11 Mobin-Uddin, K., G. M. Callard, H. Bolooki, et al.: Transvenous caval interruption with umbrella filter, *N. Engl. J. Med.*, **286**:55, 1972.

12 Mullick, S. C., H. B. Wheeler, and G. P. Songster: Diagnosis of deep venous thrombosis by measurement of electrical impedance, *Am. J. Surg.*, **119**:417, 1970.

13 O'Brien, J. R.: The mechanisms of venous thrombosis, *Mod. Concepts Cardiovas. Dis.*, **42**:11–15, March 1973.

14 Pollak, Erich W., Milo M. Webber, Winona Victery, and Earl F. Wolfman, Jr.: Radioisotope detecting of venous thrombosis: Venous scan vs fibrinogen uptake test, *Arch. Surg.*, **110**:613–616, May 1975.

15 Sevitt, S., N. G. Gallagher: Prevention of venous thrombosis and pulmonary embolism in injured patients, *Lancet*, **2**:981, 1959.

16 Sigel, Bernard, W. Robert Felix, Jr., George L. Popky, and Johannes Ipsen: Diagnosis of lower limb venous thrombosis by Doppler ultrasound technique, *Arch. Surg.*, **104**:174–179, February 1972.

17 Silver, Donald, David C. Sabiston: The role of vena caval interruption in the management of pulmonary embolism, *Surgery*, **77**:1–10, January 1975.

18 Skillman, John, J.: Postoperative deep vein thrombosis and pulmonary embolism: A selective review and personal viewpoint, *Surgery*, **75**:114–122, January 1974.

19 Strandness, D. E., D. Sumner: Ultrasonic velocity detector in the diagnosis of thrombophlebitis, *Arch. Surg.*, **104**:180–183, February 1972.

20 Tsapogas, Makis J., Haider Goussous, Richard A. Peabody, Allastair M. Karmody, and Charles Eckert: Postoperative venous thrombosis and the effectiveness of prophylactic measures, *Arch. Surg.*, **103**:561–567, November 1971.

Chapter 29

Pulmonary Embolism

Watts R. Webb, M.D.

William A. Cook, M.D.

Pulmonary embolism constitutes a most important and dreaded complication. Pulmonary emboli have been found at autopsy in approximately 10 percent of general hospital patients and in even a higher percentage of institutional patients or those with known heart disease. Although in a large series of sudden deaths 40 percent may be due to myocardial infarcts and only 5 percent due to pulmonary emboli, under many circumstances the emboli form an aggravating or accelerating factor. The postoperative mortality from pulmonary embolism for most reported hospital series has usually been 5 to 6 percent. Autopsy studies have shown that pulmonary emboli cause or contribute to the deaths of 40 to 50 percent of elderly patients with long bone fractures.[27]

Perhaps most importantly from the surgical standpoint, a patient having one pulmonary embolus has a 30 percent chance of having a second embolus and an 18 percent chance of having a subsequent fatal embolus.[1]

ETIOLOGY AND SOURCES OF THE EMBOLI

In at least 20 percent of the patients no source will be discovered at autopsy, and in a similar number multiple sources will be found. If one includes medical cases, thrombi from the heart will constitute nearly 40 percent. McLachlin and Paterson[21] found that of 32 patients with evidence of venous thromboses, of whom 19 had pulmonary emboli, 73 percent had the thrombi in the thigh and pelvic veins.

Fowler and Bollinger[9] reported 97 patients with pulmonary embolism; 39 percent originated from the heart, 26 percent in the pelvis, and 20 percent in the thigh and leg, but no definite source was found in 13 percent. Very large emboli can develop when long, thin sticky clots are tumbled within the heart and "ballup" into clots of much greater diameter.

Most patients even in a surgical series do not have evidence of antecedent venous thrombosis, and in 70 to 80 percent the pulmonary embolism will be the first sign of the thromboembolic process.[9] Most pulmonary emboli occur from the fourth to the fourteenth postoperative day, the peak incidence being between the fifth and ninth day. Although the incidence of fatal pulmonary emboli rises with progressive age, emboli nonetheless do occur in children.

PREVENTION

The incidence of thromboembolism should be minimized by measures which reduce venous stasis, intimal damage, and hypercoagulability. The elderly, obese smoker with trauma, malignancy, or heart failure is particularly prone to venous thrombosis.

Elevation of the legs to at least 15°, as shown by McLachlin[20] and Tsapogas,[36] and intermittent pneumatic external compression of the legs have proved effective in preventing venous stasis and reducing the incidence of deep venous thrombosis. Both of these methods can be used in the posttrauma patient.

While not applicable to the trauma patient, since they must be started preoperatively, most studies of prophylactic anticoagulation have demonstrated a reduced incidence of thromboembolism in the treated group. Recent reports have indicated that intermittent subcutaneous heparin can also be effective. Kakkar[17] noted a 42 percent incidence of thrombosis in the control group, but only 8 percent in the heparinized group without an

increase in surgical bleeding. Gallus and his associates[10] reduced the incidence of venous thrombosis from 48 to 13 percent in patients with hip fractures by administering 5000 U of heparin subcutaneously within 12 h of admission. This modality has not been extended to other groups of trauma patients.

PATHOPHYSIOLOGY

In a massive embolism when the pulmonary arteries are suddenly blocked, acute cor pulmonale, or strain of the right side of the heart, occurs. Experimental studies in dogs have shown that in a previously healthy cardiorespiratory system the blockage must be at least 70 percent before producing death.[14] In patients with severely limited cardiorespiratory reserve, much smaller decreases in pulmonary arterial circulation may be fatal. Knisely and his coworkers[18] in summarizing the work on vasospastic reflexes indicate that no such reflex mechanisms exist. Ozdemir, Webb, and Wax[24] confirmed the lack of reflex hemodynamic changes in blood clot embolism since denervated reimplanted lungs had the same hemodynamic changes as normal lungs. Clot infusion into the proximally occluded right pulmonary artery produced severe hemodynamic changes in the left pulmonary vascular bed. This clearly demonstrated humoral effects due to vasoactive substances, probably most importantly serotonin, and this could be reduced by large doses of heparin. There were, however, some reflex changes in ventilation, but these appeared to be minor.

With obstruction of the pulmonary arterial bed, there is an acute rise in right ventricular, right atrial, and peripheral venous pressures. Cardiac output is drastically reduced, with a fall in pulse pressure and the cardinal signs of peripheral vascular collapse. While the work of the right ventricle is increasing enormously, along with right ventricular O_2 consumption, the coronary blood supply is decreased because the blood cannot get through the lungs. This leads to acute ischemia of the right ventricle that may be irreversible even if the clots break up and move peripherally. Thus digitalization as well as vasopressors should be considered in this disease to close the peripheral vascular beds and preserve normal organ perfusion. Cyanosis may be extreme, primarily because of venous desaturation from the low cardiac output since the arterial saturation usually is above 85 percent. Robin and his coworkers[25] demonstrated that the carbon dioxide concentration in the alveoli becomes much lower than that in the systemic arterial bed since portions of the lung are well ventilated but not perfused because of the pulmonary embolus. The nonperfused areas quickly wash out their carbon dioxide, and these areas dilute the CO_2 of the normal alveoli. Sabiston has utilized the increased dead space ventilation as a method of diagnosis.

DIAGNOSIS

Patients with minor emboli may have no clinical signs, whereas sudden death may follow a massive embolus. Infarction of the lung need not occur because of the dual circulation of the lungs (pulmonary and bronchial), and many feel that infarction takes place only with infection or when pulmonary circulation is already compromised. Similarly, embolic occlusion of the medium and small vessels of the lungs presents an extremely varied picture, ranging from severe peripheral collapse to the so-called "silent" embolism. Diagnosis may be simple when the textbook picture of dyspnea, cough, hemoptysis, and sudden chest pain appear; but this is not the usual picture, and the diagnosis is completely missed in at least half the fatal cases. The clinical picture often reflects the effects of reduced cardiac output with weakness, sweating, syncope, apprehension, restlessness, and peripheral collapse.

The differential diagnosis must include pneumonia, pleurisy, spontaneous pneumothorax, angina pectoris, myocardial infarction, and the various acute upper abdominal catastrophes.

Gorham[11] has emphasized the value of 12 physical signs which may give important clues to the diagnosis. The signs of pulmonary artery distention include: pulsation in the second left interspace, an accentuated P_2 which is greater than A_2, and a pseudopericardial or pleural pericardial friction rub. The signs caused by the embolus itself include a systolic murmur and thrill at the second left interspace, probably caused by partial stenosis of the pulmonary artery. If the embolus extends through the pulmonic valve, the diastolic murmur of pulmonary insufficiency may likewise be heard. An interscapular bruit and unilateral expansion lag of the chest may be present. The signs of pulmonary hypertension include: increased cardiac dullness on the right as the right ventricle enlarges, distended neck veins, enlarged liver, and gallop rhythm. The sign of movement of the embolus is a "red arterial wave" (die rote Blutwelle) passing over the patient's face as part of the obstructing embolus is dislodged temporarily to allow increased passage of blood through the lung. The triad of enzyme changes of elevated LDH and bilirubin and normal serum glutamic oxaloacetic transaminase (SGOT), though reported as being useful in establishing the diagnosis of pulmonary embolism,[37] occurs so infrequently or so late as to be very rarely helpful in establishing the diagnosis.[34] In the patient who has had an embolus, or even seems a strong candidate for one, a survey of the veins by ultrasonic probe techniques may be very helpful in identifying thrombi still present and potentially dangerous.

Laboratory Diagnosis

Pulmonary embolism is suggested electrocardiographically by evidence of acute cor pulmonale, which classically includes a deep S wave in lead I, a deep Q wave in lead III, depressed ST segments in leads I and II, and inverted T waves in leads II and III and in the precordial leads over the right ventricle. Israel and Goldstein[16] reported significant changes in the electrocardiogram in 70.7 percent of 75 patients who had at least two electrocardiograms made after a pulmonary embolism. Differential diagnoses include myocardial infarction, dissecting aneurysm, pneumonitis, hemorrhage, and acute electrolyte imbalance.

Radiologic Studies

Arendt and Rosenberg[3] found that less than 50 percent of all patients clinically suspected of pulmonary emboli develop an infarction that can be demonstrated by a plain chest x-ray. The most common abnormalities are pleural effusion and, less frequently, infiltrations consisting of linear, patchy, wedge-shaped, or homogenous densities or diaphragmatic elevation and cavitation. Stein et al.[32] were able to suggest the diagnosis of pulmonary embolism in only 54 percent of a series of 72 cases. Davis[8] places great emphasis on an increase in size in the diameter of the right and left descending pulmonary arteries as measured in the eighth posterior intercostal space. The upper limits of normal in men is 16 mm on the right and 17 mm on the left, and in women 15 mm on the right and 16 mm on the left. Small or microscopic emboli do not cause measurable increases in the descending pulmonary artery diameters. This Roentgen sign is of particular value because it can be obtained on critically ill patients without risk.

The pulmonary perfusion scan, since its introduction in 1964, is the most widely utilized diagnostic procedure for evaluating pulmonary embolism.[26] It may be performed rapidly, with minimal risk, and is not only useful in establishing the diagnosis, but subsequent scans are of great value in monitoring resolution of an embolus or in detecting new emboli. Since any other lesion in the lung such as

pneumonia, atelectasis, or cysts can also produce hypoperfusion, the scan is diagnostic only when there is decreased perfusion in areas of the lung which appear normal on the chest x-ray. False-positive and false-negative scans are relatively frequent, but correlation with angiograms, particularly in a pertinent clinical situation, is quite good.

Ventilation scanning increases the accuracy of perfusion scanning. A scan that shows decreased ventilation and perfusion in the same lung area indicates airway or parenchymal disease, and a normal ventilation scan with an abnormal perfusion scan suggests pulmonary embolism.[19] Pulmonary angiography remains the most valuable and reliable modality for establishing the diagnosis of pulmonary embolism. It is most reliable if performed immediately after the embolization, and becomes less reliable in a few days because of the rapid thrombolysis that occurs in the pulmonary circulation.[7]

THERAPY

The patient with a suspected pulmonary embolus should have blood drawn immediately for a baseline Lee-White clotting time and a prothrombin level. Heparin has become the agent of choice for the management of most patients with pulmonary thromboembolism. In 1964, Bauer treated 59 patients with pulmonary embolism with intravenous heparin without a single death from embolization.[4] In the series of Herman, Davis, and Holdham, 35.5 percent of the patients receiving no anticoagulation therapy had subsequent fatal emboli, whereas only 4.7 percent of those patients treated with heparin died.

In adequate amounts, heparin can completely inhibit coagulation and permit thrombolysis to occur; larger doses of heparin may augment fibrinolytic activity and help lyse the embolus. Heparin also interferes with the release or the action of serotonin and other bioactive amines in the thromboembolus and thus reduces their effects of bronchoconstriction and vasoconstriction in the lung.[24,38] Our preference is to administer heparin intravenously instantly when the diagnosis is strongly suspected so that propagation of the embolus can be inhibited during the time required for diagnostic studies. Large doses of heparin are required to inhibit coagulation and platelet aggregation; probably 60,000 to 100,000 U during the first 24 to 48 h.[4,29] Silver recommends 600 U of heparin/kg as an initial rapid intravenous injection, and a similar amount is given as a continuous intravenous infusion during the first 24 h. After 24 h, the heparin infusion is regulated to maintain the Lee-White clotting time at 30 min. Heparin is continued for 10 to 14 days and discontinued only when the prothrombin time is prolonged to therapeutic levels. This regimen has reduced the death from massive pulmonary embolism to about 5 percent.[29,34] Warfarin (Coumadin) is continued for a minimum of 3 and usually 6 months when it is gradually tapered and then discontinued. We then ask the patient to take 600 mg aspirin daily for at least a year to interfere with platelet aggregation. The patient is also asked to wear elastic stockings and avoid positions of stasis indefinitely.

Although much embolic material may be cleared and blocked arteries recanalized, often the end result is pulmonary hypertension. Obviously, the preferred treatment is removal of the pulmonary embolus. This was suggested by Trendelenburg[35] in 1908; it was first successfully performed by Kirschner in 1924, but not in the United States until 1958.[31] The problems of exact diagnosis and the limitations of time in a moribund patient have made the Trendelenburg procedure hazardous and of limited application. Allison[2] in 1960 removed an embolus 13 days after its occurrence, utilizing total hypothermia to usher in the modern era of pulmonary embolectomy. Since February 1961, when Sharp[28] first removed an embolus utilizing the pump oxygenator, this procedure has been performed successfully in many different centers throughout the world.

The decision to operate on a particular patient requires first of all a firm diagnosis and secondly the facilities for immediate institution of circulatory support, since the patients most urgently requiring operation are those dying within a few hours after embolization. Those patients dying of acute massive emboli can be saved only by immediate surgical intervention, but because of the frequency of confusion with myocardial infarctions or other major catastrophes, a pulmonary embolectomy should never be attempted without a definitive diagnosis by an arteriogram. The patient can be supported by femorofemoral bypass during the period of radiologic confirmation and for anesthetization in the early stages of the operation. With the use of a plastic disposable oxygenator, using glucose or electrolyte prime, cardiopulmonary bypass can be instituted within a very few minutes. A femoral artery and vein are cannulated prior to opening the chest to institute partial circulatory support since deterioration and death frequently occur with the induction of general anesthesia. Partial bypass improves the circulatory status and allows adequate time for vena caval cannulation and institution of complete bypass. The pulmonary artery is opened and the emboli removed. Cooley has demonstrated that opening both pleural cavities and manual compression of the lungs may be helpful for removing smaller clots from the periphery.[6] This maneuver is continued until only liquid blood can be aspirated through the pulmonary arteriotomy. Passage of a Fogarty balloon-tipped catheter may also be helpful in removing peripheral clots.

Pulmonary embolectomy is probably indicated only if the patient demonstrates shock, unconsciousness, convulsions, right ventricular failure, or severe abnormalities in the ECG with the initial embolus and if these abnormalities are not immediately corrected with a massive dosage of heparin. Certainly, in a clinical situation with persistent or progressive changes in the ECG or x-ray, immediate surgical intervention should be considered. Nonetheless, with early aggressive heparin therapy, the need for pulmonary embolectomy has become extremely infrequent.

Another innovation in a nonoperative approach to pulmonary emboli is that of Greenfield, who inserts a directionally steerable catheter through the femoral vein and guides it into the pulmonary artery under fluoroscopic control. Suction is applied to the distal vacuum cup to remove emboli. Multiple emboli can be removed from either branch of the pulmonary artery as directed by the pulmonary angiogram and small injections of radiopaque mediums during the procedure.[12] This technique proved to be successful in eight out of nine patients.[13] Two of these patients later died of recurrent emboli, which has motivated him to recommend insertion of a filter device into the inferior vena cava at the time of catheter embolectomy.

Investigations of platelet inhibiting agents, prothrombinopenic agents, and the fibrinolytic activators—streptokinase and urokinase—have not shown any superiority over heparin in most situations.[33] In the patient with massive pulmonary embolism and cardiopulmonary decompensation the fibrinolytic agents may lyse the clot more rapidly and thus be beneficial.

VENA CAVAL INTERRUPTION

In many instances, inferior vena cava ligation may be required with or without pulmonary embolectomy. These include (1) recurrent pulmonary embolism despite "adequate anticoagulant" therapy, (2) presence of active bleeding, (3) contraindication to the use of heparin such as following a transurethral resection or

in the presence of an active duodenal ulcer, and (4) septic pelvic thrombophlebitis, in which the ovarian veins should also be ligated since these patients die of sepsis rather than of massive embolism.[5]

Inferior vena cava ligation probably should be done for emboli recurrent after discontinuing anticoagulation, after thrombectomy of the femoral veins for phlegmasia cerulea dolens, and certainly in the presence of progressive peripheral vein thrombosis on full heparinization. In most instances if a pulmonary embolectomy has been performed, vena cava interruption is performed to prevent a subsequent fatal pulmonary embolus. In addition, interruption is indicated by ligature rather than by clip or filter if recurrent small emboli have produced pulmonary hypertension either at rest or during exercise and if the pulmonary angiocardiograms or physiologic studies indicate that more than 50 percent of the pulmonary arterial bed has been occluded.

Following vena cava ligation, care of the legs is very important. This includes bandaging and the use of diuretics, low-salt diet, and elastic stockings or pants to create a pneumatic squeezing of the legs. In general, the long-term sequelae of vena cava ligation will be dependent on the status of the leg veins before ligation, but the use of a fenestration technique which allows continuing blood flow through the cava—whether with suture, plastic clip, or intraluminal sieve or umbrella—appears to be less incapacitating and equally effective.[13,22,30] Vena cava interruption procedures have not reduced the mortality or the occurrence rate of pulmonary embolism below that of a good anticoagulant or fibrinolytic-anticoagulant program.

REHABILITATION

Houk and his coworkers reviewed 250 reported cases of chronic thromboembolic obstruction of major pulmonary arteries.[15] The diagnosis had been established in only six prior to death, and direct surgical therapy had been attempted in only three. In one case, utilizing cardiopulmonary bypass, Houk was able to remove the thrombotic casts which almost completely occluded the right pulmonary artery and a small branch of the left pulmonary artery. Subsequent studies demonstrated that the patient's gas exchange had returned to normal, with the alveolar arterial carbon dioxide tension gradient having been reduced to 7 mmHg compared with 27 mmHg prior to operation. Subsequent experience has suggested that late embolectomy should be attempted only if there is occlusion of one main pulmonary artery.[23] Removal of multiple distal clots has not proved feasible and has carried a high mortality rate, primarily from pulmonary hemorrhage, in attempted cases.

BIBLIOGRAPHY

1 Allen, E. V., N. W. Barker, and E. A. Hines, Jr.: *Peripheral Vascular Diseases,* 2d ed., W. B. Saunders Company, Philadelphia, 1955, p. 524.

2 Allison, P. R., M. S. Dunnill, and R. Marshall: Pulmonary embolism, *Thorax,* 15:273, 1960.

3 Arendt, J. and M. Rosenberg: Thromboembolism of the lungs, *Am. J. Roentgenol. Radium Ther. Nucl. Med.,* 81:245, 1959.

4 Bauer, G.: Clinical experiences of a surgeon in the use of heparin, *Am. J. Cardiol.,* 14:29–35, 1964.

5 Collins, C. G., R. O. Norton, E. W. Nelson, E. W. Weinstein, B. B. Weinstein, J. H. Collins, and H. D. Webster, Jr: Suppurative pelvic thrombophlebitis, *Surgery,* 31:528, 1952.

6 Cooley, D. A. and A. C. Beall, Jr.: Surgical treatment of acute massive pulmonary embolism using temporary cardiopulmonary bypass, *Dis. Chest,* 41:102, 1962.

7 Dalen, J. E., J. S. Banas, Jr., H. L. Brooks, G. Evans, J. A. Paraskos, and L. Dexter: Resolution rate of acute pulmonary embolism in man, *N. Engl. J. Med.,* 280:1194–1199, 1969.

8 Davis, C. W.: Immediate diagnosis of pulmonary embolus, *Am. Surg.,* 30:291, 1964.

9 Fowler, E. F. and J. A. Bollinger: Pulmonary embolism: A clinical study of ninety-seven fatal cases, *Surgery,* 36:650, 1954.

10 Gallus, A. S., J. Hirsh, R. J. Tuttle, R. Trebilcock, S. E. O'Brien, J. J. Carroll, J. H. Minden, and S. M. Hudecki: Small subcutaneous doses of heparin in prevention of venous thrombosis, *N. Engl. J. Med.,* 288:545, 1973.

11 Gorham, L. W.: A study of pulmonary embolism, *Arch. Intern. Med.,* 108:76, 1961.

12 Greenfield, L. J.: Pulmonary embolism: Diagnosis and management, *Curr. Probl. Surg.,* 13:1, April 1976.

13 ———, R. C. Elkins, and P. P. Brown: Treatment of acute massive pulmonary embolism by transvenous catheter embolectomy and a new filter device, *Bull. Soc. Int. Chir.,* XXXIV:57–60, 1975.

14 Holden, W. D., B. W. Shaw, D. B. Cameron, P. J. Shea, Jr., and J. H. Davis, Jr.: Experimental pulmonary embolism, *Surg. Gynecol. Obstet.,* 88:23, 1949.

15 Houk, V. N., C. A. Hufnagel, J. E. McClenathan, and K. M. Moser: Chronic thrombotic obstruction of major pulmonary arteries, *Am. J. Med.,* 35:269, 1963.

16 Israel, H. L. and F. Goldstein: The varied clinical manifestations of pulmonary embolism, *Ann. Intern. Med.,* 47:202, 1957.

17 Kakkar, V. V., J. Spindler, P. T. Flute, T. Corrigan, D. P. Fossard, and R. Q. Crellin: Efficacy of low doses of heparin in prevention of deep-vein thrombosis after major surgery, *Lancet,* 2:101, 1972.

18 Knisely, W. H., J. M. Wallace, M. S. Mahaley, and W. M. Satterwhite, Jr.: The cause of death in pulmonary embolization, *Am. Heart J.,* 54:483, 1957.

19 Loken, M. K.: Camera studies of lung ventilation and perfusion, *Semin. Nucl. Med.,* 1:229–245, 1971.

20 McLachlin, A. D., J. A. McLachlin, T. A. Jory, and E. G. Rawling: Venous stasis in the lower extremities, *Ann. Surg.,* 152:678, 1960.

21 McLaughlin, J. and J. C. Patterson: Some basic observations on venous thrombosis and pulmonary embolism, *Surg. Gynecol. Obstet.,* 93:1, 1951.

22 Mobin-Uddin, K., G. M. Callard, H. Bolooki,

R. Robinson, D. Michie, and J. R. Jude: Transvenous caval interruption with umbrella filter, *N. Engl. J. Med.*, **286**:55–58, 1972.

23 Moor, G. F. and D. C. Sabiston, Jr.: Embolectomy for chronic pulmonary embolism and hypertension, *Circulation*, **41**:701, 1970.

24 Ozdemir, I. A., W. R. Webb, and S. D. Wax: Effect of neural and humoral factors on pulmonary hemodynamics and microcirculation in pulmonary embolism, *J. Thorac. Cardiovasc. Surg.*, **68**:896–904, 1974.

25 Robin, E. D., D. G. Julian, D. M. Travis, and C. H. Crump: A physiologic approach to the diagnosis of acute pulmonary embolism, *N. Engl. J. Med.*, **260**:586, 1959.

26 Sabiston, D. C., Jr. and H. N. Wagner, Jr.: The diagnosis of pulmonary embolism by radioisotope scanning, *Ann. Surg.*, **160**:575, 1964.

27 Sevitt, S. and N. G. Gallagher: Prevention of venous thrombosis and pulmonary embolism in injured patients, *Lancet*, **2**:981–989, 1959.

28 Sharp, E. H.: Pulmonary embolectomy: Successful removal of a massive pulmonary embolus with the support of cardiopulmonary bypass, *Ann. Surg.*, **156**:1, 1962.

29 Silver, D.: Pulmonary embolism: Prevention, detection and nonoperative management, *Surg. Clin. North Am.*, **54**:1089–1106, 1974.

30 Spencer, F. C., J. K. Quattlebaum, J. K. Quattlebaum, Jr., E. H. Sharp, and J. R. Jude: Plication of the inferior vena cava for pulmonary embolism: A report of twenty cases, *Ann. Surg.*, **155**:827, 1962.

31 Steenburg, R. W., R. Warren, R. E. Wilson, and L. D. Rudolph: A new look at pulmonary embolectomy, *Surg. Gynecol. Obstet.*, **107**:214, 1958.

32 Stein, G. H., J. T. Chen, F. Goldstein, H. L. Israel, and A. Finkelstein: The importance of chest roentgenography in the diagnosis of pulmonary embolism, *Am. J. Roentgenol. Radium Ther. Nucl. Med.*, **81**:255, 1959.

33 The urokinase pulmonary embolism trial: A National Cooperative Study: *Circulation (Suppl. 2),* **47**, 1973.

34 Thomas, D. P.: "The Anticoagulant Therapy of Venous Thromboembolism," in J. M. Moser and M. Stein (eds.), *Pulmonary Thromboembolims,* Year Book Medical Publishers, Inc., Chicago, 1973, pp. 271–279.

35 Trendelenburg, F.: Ueber die Operative Behandlung der Embolie der Lungenarterie, *Arch. Klin. Chir.*, **86**:686, 1908.

36 Tsapogas, M. J., H. Goussous, R. A. Peabody, A. M. Karmode, and C. Eckert: Postoperative venous thrombosis and the effectiveness of prophylactic measures, *Arch. Surg.*, **103**:561, 1971.

37 Wacker, W. E. C. and P. H. Snodgrass: Serum LDH activity in pulmonary embolism diagnosis, *J. Am. Med. Assoc.*, **174**:2142, 1960.

38 Webster, J. R., Jr., G. B. Saadeh, P. R. Eggum, and J. R. Suker: Wheezing due to pulmonary embolism, *N. Engl. J. Med.*, **274**:931–933, 1966.

Chapter 30

Stress Gastroenteropathy ("Stress" Ulcers)

Joel Horovitz, M.D.

INTRODUCTION

Acute mucosal bleeding from the upper gastrointestinal (GI) tract (stomach and duodenum) is a distressing complication seen in patients being treated for other serious surgical problems who develop complications (particularly septic) in the postoperative period. Advances in the general care of the injured patient have led to increasing survival of more seriously ill patients and the unmasking of several serious complications in the recovery period. This accounts for the prominence achieved recently by pulmonary insufficiency in the severely injured patient. Similarly, the emergence of gastric mucosal bleeding is a manifestation of improved resuscitation and postoperative care.

A plethora of names has been used to describe the entity of stress enteropathy, e.g., hemorrhagic gastritis, acute gastroduodenal erosions, superficial gastric erosions, and stress gastritis. The term "stress gastroenteropathy" (SG) was chosen because it avoids the use of the words ulceration (not uniformly present) and gastritis (inflammation is not a prominent part of the syndrome). Most authors would agree that although the term "stress" may not be entirely accurate, there is little doubt that all of these patients have some form of physiologic stress applied to them which is associated with the development of acute gastroduodenal mucosal changes.

It is helpful to consider a simple classification of SG which is relevant to patient identification and management. Such a scheme is outlined in Table 30-1. This classification differs from previous classifications in several respects. First, the acute gastroduodenal changes associated with thermal burn injury (Curling's ulcer) are now known to have the same etiology as the remaining entities subsumed under the rubric of ischemic SG. Second, the question of the role of steroid administration in the production of gastroduodenal ulceration has recently undergone reevaluation. Conn's thorough evaluation of the literature indicates that there is no convincing evidence for the role of steroids in the production of peptic ulcer disease or SG.[10]

Accurate estimates of the incidence of SG are difficult to make. There is a wide variability among authors' experience with the most common manifestation of the syndrome, i.e., gross gastrointestinal hemorrhage. McNamara and Stremple reported an overall incidence of 3 percent GI bleeding due to SG occurring in 2297 instances of combat trauma in Viet Nam.[46] This is the same incidence reported by Girvan and Passi in a civilian population of 980 patients with upper gastrointestinal bleeding.[15] Other authors have noted higher incidences of GI bleeding and SG. Stremple and Elliott described a 20 percent incidence of erosive gastritis among 796 GI bleeders treated at their institution.[45] Czaja et al. from the

Brooke Army Medical Center reported a 22 percent incidence of GI bleeding after thermal injury in 1974.[13] The same authors reported an 11.1 percent incidence of gastric hemorrhage in 54 burn patients reported the following year.[12] It is probable that from 3 to 20 percent (average 5 to 10 percent) of all severely injured patients will develop obvious upper gastrointestinal hemorrhage in the recovery course of their illness. The widespread use of the fiberoptic panendoscope has shown, however, that a much higher percentage of severely injured patients will develop acute mucosal changes in the stomach and duodenum. Major body surface area burns (i.e., 50 percent and greater) were shown to be associated with an 84 percent incidence of erosive changes in the stomach and a 63 percent incidence of similar changes in the duodenum.[12] Lucas et al. showed endoscopic changes in the mucosa of the fundus and body of the stomach in all 42 patients they studied by serial endoscopy.[27] It is apparent, therefore, that the majority of severely ill patients will develop subclinical SG and a significant number of these will go on to frank GI bleeding. The mortality rate of this complication varies from 10 percent to 95 percent in the reported literature, with a median mortality of 35 to 50 percent.[29] Perforation is relatively uncommon in SG. These figures point out the importance of the early identification and treatment of the patient with SG.

Table 30-1   Classification of Stress Gastroenteropathies

Iatrogenic
Alcohol
Aspirin
Butazolidin
Cushing's ulcer
(CNS)
Ischemic
Burns (Curling's ulcer)
Hypovolemia
Sepsis
Cardiogenic shock

ETIOLOGY AND PATHOGENESIS

Considerable controversy exists as to the single most important etiologic factor in the development of SG. Table 30-2 lists the factors implicated in the development of acute mucosal gastroduodenal changes in both animal and human studies. Undoubtedly no single factor can fully explain the diverse experimental findings reported. It appears that the basic abnormality involves a change in gastric mucosal barrier function, first described by

Table 30-2 Etiology of Stress Gastroenteropathy

Mucosal ischemia
Sepsis
Gastric acid hypersecretion
Back diffusion of gastric acid
Regurgitation of duodenal contents
Coagulopathy

Teorell in 1947.[49] As noted in the classification of SG given in Table 30-1, mucosal damage may arise from (1) iatrogenic factors (the administration of various drugs), (2) persistent hypersecretion of gastric acid, and (3) direct ischemic damage.

Much of the controversy has arisen over the variable findings of gastric acid secretion.[29] Early in the poststress period the hydrogen ion concentration (H^+) in gastric juice is low or normal, and two to three days later may rise to the high normal or elevated range in the injured patient. Silen and Skillman have shown that SG is associated with an increase in back diffusion of H^+ through the gastric mucosa.[42] Therefore, the absolute level of H^+ in gastric juice is not important. However, there is a correlation between the severity of injury and the level of gastric acid.[44] One injury has been associated with persistent hypersecretion of acid: central nervous system trauma.[33,52] Furthermore, it has been shown that anticholinergics are able to reverse the high level of gastric acid in these patients. Recently, however, Stremple reported normal acid levels in 15 patients with cranial trauma in the absence of other severe injury.[44] It appears that gastric hypersecretion is not a primary factor in the development of SG.[27] Similarly, there is little evidence that defects in the amount or quality of mucus are important. The role of bile acids in the pathogenesis of SG has been extensively debated. It is probable that acid is necessary for the destructive effect of duodenal contents.[41]

Although its exact role is unclear, sepsis is an important etiologic factor in the development of SG. Altemeier et al. reported 54 patients with proven septicemia and GI hemorrhage.[2] Fifty-five percent had diffuse gastric erosions. Sepsis was associated with abnormal prothrombin times and thrombocytopenia in the majority of these patients. Experimental studies have shown that (1) endotoxin causes maximal ischemia in the body of the stomach,[40] (2) direct application of endotoxin to the mucosa produces pallor and mottling,[9] and (3) sepsis caused erosive gastritis in the body and fundus, sparing the antrum.[24] LeGall et al. reported a prospective study of 30 patients admitted to an intensive care unit and followed by serial gastroscopy.[21] Of the 14 patients with sepsis, 71 percent developed mucosal changes which correlated with the severity of sepsis. By day 6 all in the septic group had hemorrhagic erosions. In contrast, none of the 16 patients without sepsis developed acute ulceration. There is ample evidence that sepsis plays an important role in SG, probably mediated via mucosal ischemia.

Another factor of importance in the development of SG may be a coagulopathy. This may be a complication of shock, multiple transfusions, or sepsis. Nilsson et al. described four patients with a primary coagulopathy as a cause of erosive gastritis.[32] All patients had increased fibrinolytic activity in their gastric juice coupled with decreased factor XIII blood levels. Successful treatment was achieved with factor XIII and ε-aminocaproic acid (Amicar).

The major abnormality leading to the development of SG appears to be a decrease in mucosal blood flow (ischemia), which causes disruption of the barrier. Experimentally, ulcers are not produced without the presence of gastric acid. This includes the iatrogenic induction of ulcers by acetylsalicylic acid, ethanol, Butazolidin and bile salts. Therefore, the adage "no acid, no ulcer" remains valid for

SG. Damaged mucosal cells then allow the back diffusion of H^+, which leads to further mucosal cell destruction and mast cell degranulation. This is associated with the release of seratonin and other vasoactive amines. The role of seratonin and other amines in human SG has not been well delineated.

Lucas et al. provided the first description of the development of stress gastroenteropathy by the prospective study of 42 trauma patients by serial endoscopy and biopsy.[27] All patients developed changes in the gastric mucosa within 24 h of having sustained severe injury. The first signs were focal areas of pallor surrounded by hyperemia, usually confined to the fundus and body of the stomach. By 24 h superficial mucosal erosions were noted, and these progressed in depth down to but not through the level of the muscularis mucosa. There were no reported instances of isolated antral involvement, although the disease progressed to that level in severe cases. Microscopically the first changes noted in the mucosa were patchy edema which became widespread and was associated with diapedesis of red cells, mucosal hemorrhage, and necrosis leading to gross ulceration. There was little or no evidence of acute inflammation in any of the microscopic sections. An identical pattern of evolution has been reported in the burn population.[12]

TREATMENT

Prevention

It is likely that advances in postoperative management have led to a decrease in the incidence of severe SG. However, it still remains a significant problem which is far better prevented than treated. Table 30-3 outlines several preventive steps which have been shown to be beneficial. Clearly, the early identification of high-risk patients is of the utmost importance so that early prophylactic measures can be instituted. Patients at great-

Table 30-3 Prevention of Stress Gastroenteropathy

Early identification of high-risk patients
Prophylactic gastric alkalinization
Anticholinergics in CNS trauma
Provide adequate nutrition

est risk for stress bleeding are those recovering from major abdominal surgery or who have sustained the following injuries: major intracranial injuries, extensive thermal burns, and severe thoracoabdominal injuries. Both renal and respiratory insufficiency are also associated with an increased incidence of SG. Perhaps the single most prevalent factor is the presence of systemic sepsis as discussed above. All of the high-risk individuals should have a nasogastric tube inserted both for gastric decompression and for the installation of antacids. Scant information is available in the literature concerning the benefit of prophylactic antacid therapy. A small number of patients given prophylactic antacids were reported by McAlhany et al. in 42 burn victims who underwent gastric mucosal permeability tests utilizing the lithium ion.[28] Twenty-one of the 42 patients demonstrated increased permeability to lithium ion and seven of those were given prophylactic antacids. None of the antacid group developed any GI complications. In an untreated control group of 14 patients, 42 percent developed gastrointestinal complications.

The method of gastric alkalinization is important and usually involves more than the standard 30 to 60 mL of antacid hourly through the nasogastric tube. The initial gastric aspirate is tested with nitrazine pH paper and usually measures less than pH 5. The initial antacid dose should be 60 mL instilled into the nasogastric tube, which is then clamped for 15 min. At this time another sample of gastric juice is aspirated and tested for pH. If the pH remains below 7, an additional aliquot of 30 mL of antacid is again dripped through the nasogastric tube and the testing procedure repeated in 15 min. This procedure allows the rapid identification of the amount of antacid to be given on an hourly basis which will maintain the pH at or above 7. It has been found that most patients require 60 to 180 mL of antacid/h to maintain gastric neutrality.[43]

Black et al. were the first to describe the H_2-receptor antagonist drugs, i.e., those able to block gastric acid secretion without having systemic antihistaminic properties.[5] The first such pharmacologic agent available was metiamide. It was found to be an effective inhibitor of gastric acid secretion in patients with duodenal ulcer disease.[30] Metiamide was found to cause agranulocytosis in some cases and was, therefore, replaced by cimetidine. Clinical studies with this drug showed that basal acid secretion could be abolished for up to 5 hours after a single dose in duodenal ulcer patients.[16,23] Cimetidine is apparently free of serious side effects and has recently been cleared for clinical use by the Federal Drug Administration (FDA). There are no reported clinical studies on the effectiveness of the H_2-receptor blockers in SG. However, there is experimental evidence that high doses of metiamide protect against the development of ulcers in the rat restraint model.[6] Given the currently available number and type of antacids, it would appear that cimetidine will become the drug of choice in the prophylaxis of SG.

It is known that the gastric mucosa renews itself every few days. This process of mucosal regeneration requires energy and amino acid substrate. Experimental evidence indicates that the incidence of SG can be greatly diminished by proper attention to adequate nutrition. Mullane et al. showed an increase in the incidence of gastric ulceration in the rat restraint model when the animals were starved compared with the controlled group.[31] In another study using the murine model, it was found that the use of intravenous essential amino acid solutions prevented the appearance of gastric erosions compared with a group of animals treated with intravenous dextrose and water.[35] It is probable that the more widespread use of total parenteral nutrition and greater emphasis on caloric intake coupled with the common use of prophylactic antacid therapy has led to a decrease in the complications of SG, particularly massive gastrointestinal hemorrhage requiring surgery.

The use of vitamin A, a substance required for mucosal regeneration in the stomach, is more controversial. Chernov et al. reported a high incidence of vitamin A deficiency in their burn and trauma population.[8] They studied 52 patients divided into two groups: control and those given vitamin A in a dosage of 100,000 U twice a day. A marked diminution in the number of patients demonstrating ulceration (18 percent in the vitamin A group versus 63 percent in the control group) was shown. None of the ulcerations was verified by endoscopy. Eighteen of the control patients developed upper gastrointestinal tract bleeding. This represented 60 percent of the patients at risk and is the highest reported in literature. Subsequent studies from the Brooke Army Medical Center have failed to corroborate the importance of vitamin A administration.

Management of the GI Bleeder

Resuscitation The majority of patients with SG who develop gastrointestinal bleeding will be recovering from a recent operation. In the absence of an antecedent history of peptic ulcer disease or esophageal varices, the differential diagnosis of the cause of hemorrhage will be relatively limited. Quite commonly, the patient will have had a complicated septic course with the development of renal and/or pulmonary insufficiency. If a nasogastric tube is present, it will first be noted that there is a change in the character of the aspirate: flecks of "coffee ground" material appear which progress to frank red blood. If nasogastric suction is not being utilized, the first indication of gastrointestinal hemorrhage will be tachycardia, hypotension, and oliguria. The basic steps in the treatment of gastrointestinal hemorrhage are outlined in Table 30-4. The initial priority is the prompt and effective resuscitation of hypovolemic shock. While awaiting properly typed and cross-matched whole blood, the patient is given an infusion of balanced salt solution as a temporary extracellular fluid expander. Close monitoring of the vital signs during the early phases of resuscitation is important. The adequacy of tissue perfusion is best gauged by the half-hourly urine output in the early phases of the resuscitation effort. A complete discussion of hemodynamic monitoring techniques is contained in Chap. 31.

If a nasogastric tube is not present, a large-caliber tube should be passed as soon as possible. Vigorous iced saline lavage through the nasogastric tube will result in cessation of bleeding in a significant number of patients. It has been shown experimentally that saline at 6° to 8° Centigrade instilled into the stomach achieves a 60 percent reduction in gastric blood flow.[51] Iced saline irrigations will also dilute and remove any hydrochloric acid and pepsin present in gastric juice and facilitate removal of gross blood clots from the stomach. Once the bleeding has been slowed or totally controlled, then expeditious definite diagnosis of the bleeding site can be carried out.

The prompt resuscitation of hypovolemic shock and the early institution of iced saline lavage should result in the cessation of bleeding in 50 to 80 percent of patients with SG. Because of the high mortality associated with

Table 30-4 Treatment of GI Hemorrhage

Resuscitation of hypovolemic shock
Iced saline lavage
Diagnosis of bleeding site
Topical therapy

surgery in these critically ill patients, other nonoperative means of control of hemorrhage should be utilized first. Most of the adjunctive methods for nonoperative control of bleeding are only effective in hemorrhage complicating SG. Therefore, it is mandatory that an accurate diagnosis of the site of bleeding be made early in the course of the disease.

Diagnosis of Site of Bleeding The easiest and most reliable way to determine the site of bleeding is the early use of the fiberoptic endoscope. Sugawa and his coworkers performed endoscopic examination in 188 bleeding patients with a 97 percent success rate.[47] Sixty percent of the patients were found to have a bleeding site originating in the stomach, two-thirds of these being acute erosive gastritis. All patients had follow-up barium contrast studies of the upper GI tract, which showed a lesion in only 34 percent of the cases. Allen et al. endoscoped 101 patients with GI bleeding and found a 90 percent diagnostic accuracy if done early in the course of the disease.[1] They found that barium x-rays only revealed a possible cause of bleeding in 54 percent of patients and actually identified the bleeding site in 32 percent. In a subgroup of 18 patients with hemorrhagic erosions of the stomach, 11 were found to have a totally normal barium GI study. In this series only 6 of the 101 patients were unable to undergo endoscopy, 4 because of technical factors and 2 because of massive exsanguinating hemorrhage. Villar et al. recently reported a series of 192 patients that underwent emergency diagnosis of upper GI bleeding by fiberoptic endoscopy with an accuracy rate of 96 percent.[50] Hemorrhagic gastritis was found in 18.2 percent of the patient population. This paper provides a good description of the technique of endoscopy and contains photographs of various bleeding lesions.

It is well established that prompt fiberoptic endoscopy is the procedure of choice in the diagnosis of upper gastrointestinal hemorrhage. If carried out by a qualified and experienced individual, the incidence of complications is extremely low. The most serious complication is perforation of the esophagus. This is a rare occurrence with the modern, flexible endoscopes. An additional potentially serious complication is that of aspiration of blood and gastric juice into the tracheobronchial tree. Therefore, there are certain contraindications to the use of endoscopy, and these include (1) massive exsanguinating hemorrhage, (2) unconsciousness, (3) unresponsive shock, and (4) acute alcoholic intoxication. This latter contraindication is unlikely to be present in the vast majority of patients that develop SG in the absence of iatrogenic causes.

As soon as it is determined that SG is the cause of upper GI bleeding, iced saline lavage should be continued. With severe gastric involvement in SG this is unlikely to be effective however. The physician then has the choice of several other nonoperative measures to control bleeding.

Nonoperative Control of Hemorrhage It has already been stated that antacid therapy is thought to be important in the prevention of GI bleeding in SG. Simonian and Curtis have recently advocated the use of antacids for the treatment of GI bleeding and hemorrhagic gastritis.[43] They studied 49 patients with documented erosive bleeding, sepsis being responsible in 68 percent of the cases and alcoholic gastritis in 32 percent. Using a rigorous method of gastric alkalinization, they reported an 89 percent success rate in the control of hemorrhage. Only five patients required emergency surgery to control bleeding, and only three patients had rebleeding within 7 days after gastric acid neutralization was discontinued. In spite of the successful management of the GI bleeding nonoperatively, these patients had a 25 percent mortality rate. The importance of this study is that it points out the importance of complete and early gastric acid neutralization. Antacid therapy is unlikely to be beneficial in severe bleeding complicating SG.

In 1972 LeVeen et al. proposed the use of levarterenol (Levophed) administered via the intragastric or the peritoneal route as an effective means of controlling gastric bleeding from erosions.[22] Their preliminary report of 18 patients treated in this manner indicated that 12 of the 18 had control of hemorrhage. Five patients had rebleeding with cessation of therapy. Kiselow and Wagner found that Levophed gastric lavage was very effective in the treatment of hemorrhagic gastritis.[20] Five out of the six patients treated with Levophed had permanent control of their bleeding. The author has had a very favorable personal experience with the use of intragastric Levophed in the control of SG bleeding. The recommended dose is 8 mg of Levophed in 100 mL of normal saline. This is injected through the nasogastric tube, which is then clamped for one half-hour. The same procedure may be repeated at hourly intervals and is usually successful after two or three attempts. Failure to significantly slow or stop the bleeding after several attempts is an indication to abandon the use of Levophed. There is some theoretical concern in utilizing a mode of therapy which produces gastric mucosal ischemia (believed to be an important precipitating cause of SG). In the limited number of cases in the literature, there are no reports of serious sequelae. Because of the ease and rapidity of this technique it seems to be an ideal choice following iced saline lavage.

In recent years the use of selective visceral angiography with the infusion of vasopressin has become more popular in the treatment of gastrointestinal hemorrhage.[3,4,11,18,38] A compilation of the results of recent studies utilizing Pitressin for bleeding gastritis is shown in Table 30-5. Of the total number of cases reported, control of bleeding was achieved in

Table 30-5   Pitressin Control of Stress Bleeding

Series*	Number of patients	Number controlled
38	6	4
4	9	6
11	37	31
18	5	?
19	18	9
Total	75	50

*Reference number.

approximately 66 percent. Unfortunately, most of the data was obtained in an uncontrolled fashion. There has been only one controlled clinical trial comparing the effectiveness of conventional therapy with intraarterial vasopressin.[11] Conn studied 13 patients with proven gastric erosions, of which 5 were assigned to the vasopressin group. No data was given referable to the efficacy of this technique in diffuse gastric bleeding. This study did show that the Pitressin group required less blood transfusion.

Other pharmacologic adjuncts to control GI hemorrhage from diffuse mucosal disease have been advocated. It has been shown experimentally that pretreatment of the rat stress-ulcer model with pharmacological doses of dexamethasone prevented the development of stress ulcers.[19] Similarly, Norton et al. reported that both cholestyramine and methylprednisolone given early protected animals against the development of gastric ulceration.[34] The first report of clinical success using steroid therapy for SG was published by Proudfoot et al.[37] They treated 14 patients with massive bleeding secondary to SG. Eleven of the 14 patients stopped bleeding within 3h of receiving the first dose of dexamethasone (8 to 12 mg intravenously). Patients were then given progressively smaller doses of dexamethasone over the ensuing 7 days. A more recent report concerning the incidence of SG

associated with steroid therapy in various shock states did not demonstrate any beneficial effect with pharmacological doses of steroids given over a short period of time.[17] Although these authors reported a marked and significant diminution in the incidence of SG, there were no differences in mortality rates between the group given pharmacological doses of steroids versus that given therapeutic doses of steroids versus that given no steroids at all. There have been no clinically controlled trials of pharmacologic doses of steroids versus conventional means of therapy for SG bleeding.

Several mechanical means of control of hemorrhage from the gastric mucosa have recently been described. Papp treated 38 patients by means of an electrocautery introduced through the suction port of a fiberoptic endoscope.[36] He only reported one patient successfully treated that had diffuse mucosal disease. This relatively simple mode of therapy has a great deal of appeal in the patient with focal gastric involvement. However, it is unlikely to be successful in the massively bleeding patient with diffuse disease. Yellin et al. reported on the use of an argon laser beam introduced via an endoscope for the control of bleeding gastric lesions.[54] Several other authors have documented the effectiveness of this approach in the experimental laboratory. There are, however, significant technological problems which must be overcome before adequate clinical trials can be undertaken.

The author's approach to the patient with bleeding SG is outlined in Fig. 30-1. Following early endoscopic diagnosis and correction of any coagulation defects, all patients are treated with iced saline lavage. If this is successful in either markedly slowing or totally stopping the bleeding, the patients are treated further with vigorous gastric alkalinization, as outlined above. If significant bleeding persists in spite of the saline lavage, a trial of intragastric Levophed is undertaken. Plans for emergency

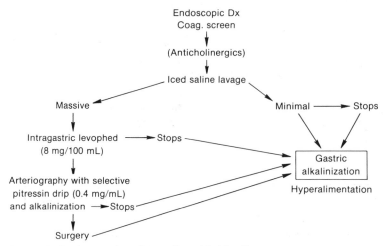

Figure 30-1 Approach to "stress" gastric bleeding.

arteriography are made concurrently, and if bleeding persists, selective catheterization of the left gastric artery with infusion of Pitressin appears to be an effective course. It is stressed that gastric alkalinization must be continued throughout all of these nonoperative manipulations. The net result of this therapeutic regimen is successful control of bleeding in 80 to 90 percent of patients.

If significant bleeding persists or exsanguinating hemorrhage is present, then prompt emergency surgery must be undertaken. In spite of the fact that most of these patients have severe multisystem problems, the indications for surgical intervention in this group are the same as any other patient with gastrointestinal hemorrhage. If more than 4 or 5 U of blood are required to achieve resuscitation and bleeding continues in spite of the nonoperative measures taken, then emergency operation is indicated.

Operative Management Because of the clinical setting in which it occurs, uncontrollable bleeding from SG disease presents a formidable operative risk. Review of the literature does not demonstrate a clear superiority

for any single operative procedure. Table 30-6 was compiled by reviewing all English language reports from 1949 to the present.[2,6,7,36,49] Of the nearly 500 cases reported, the overall mortality rate was 33 percent with a postoperative rebleeding rate of 36 percent. These statistics, as presented, are somewhat misleading. The major cause of death in all series was a complication of the primary problem leading to SG: renal failure, respiratory failure, or sepsis. Relatively few patients died as a direct result of GI bleeding, even though one in three did rebleed postoperatively. The majority of cases of postoperative bleeding can be controlled by blood transfusion alone.

Sullivan et al. first described the beneficial effects of vagectomy in bleeding SG.[48] It is thought that vagectomy produces its effect by opening submucosal arteriovenous shunts. Experimentally, this effect has been shown to be a transient one, most marked under general anesthesia. Coupled with systematic suture ligation of visible erosions, vagectomy and a drainage procedure appears to be the operation of choice. Wilson et al. reported a decrease in rebleeding from 47 percent to 9.5 percent by adding ligation to vagotomy and

Table 30-6   Operative Results in "Stress" Bleeding*

Procedure	Number of patients	Patients rebleeding	Mortality rate
Exploration only	26	15 (58%)	12 (46%)
Subtotal gastrectomy	122	58 (47%)	54 (44%)
Vagectomy and gastrectomy	90	18 (20%)	28 (31%)
Vagectomy and drainage	243	87 (36%)	67 (28%)
Total gastrectomy	12	0	1 (8%
Total	493	178 (36%)	162 (33%)

*Compilation of cases reported in references 45, 27, 53, 26, 7, and 48.

drainage.[53] This was achieved with a mortality rate of 24 percent.

The author's plan for operative management of these cases is illustrated in Fig. 30-2. If the patient must be taken to surgery without having had diagnostic endoscopy, this can be done in the operating room under anesthesia. Lucas and Sugawa reported an 88 percent success rate in diagnosis at laparotomy.[25] This procedure obviates multiple gastrotomies in search of the source of bleeding. Most cases of SG are confined to the body and fundus of

Figure 30-2   Operative management of "stress" bleeding.

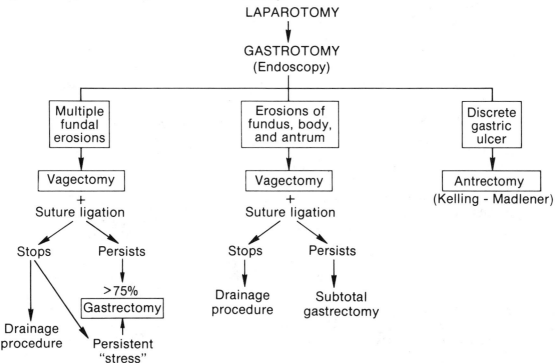

the stomach. Vagectomy usually results in an immediate blanching of the mucosa with cessation of bleeding. Suture ligature with nonabsorbable material is used to oversew all visible erosions or ulcers. If bleeding perists after these maneuvers, then a gastric resection must be done. Immediate and vigorous antacid therapy is mandatory postoperatively.

Vagectomy, pyloroplasty, and suture ligation is a reasonable procedure of first choice, especially when the "stress" can be limited, e.g., drainage of an abscess or discontinuance of a drug. Recently, the results of a salvage procedure for SG bleeding were reported by Richardson and Aust.[39] They performed total gastric devascularization in 21 patients (9 alcoholic, 8 septic, 4 steroids) with massive hemorrhagic gastropathy with total success. The rebleeding rate was only 9 percent, but the operative mortality was 38 percent. These authors did not comment on any long-term consequences of vascular interruption of the stomach. This would seem to be a definite hazard since gastric gangrene has been reported to follow intraarterial embolization procedures for control of hemorrhage.

SUMMARY

Stress gastroenteropathy is a diffuse mucosal disease caused by mucosal ischemia with disruption of barrier function. Subclinical involvement is present in over 80 percent of severely injured patients. Patients who develop complications (GI bleeding and perforation) usually have had an episode of shock or sepsis. The key to successful management is prevention by (1) effective resuscitation of shock, (2) prophylactic gastric alkalinization, and (3) maintenance of adequate nutrition. GI hemorrhage can usually be managed nonoperatively by iced saline lavage, topical vasoconstrictors, or intraarterial vasopressin. Failure of conservative therapy necessitates emergency surgery to control bleeding. This is associ-

ated with an average mortality rate of 33 percent. Vagectomy, suture ligation, and a drainage procedure is the preferred operative approach.

BIBLIOGRAPHY

1 Allen, H. M., M. A. Block, and B. M. Schuman: Gastroduodenal endoscopy: Management of acute upper gastrointestinal hemorrhage, *Arch. Surg.,* **106**:450, 1973.
2 Altemeier, W. A., W. D. Fullen, and J. McDonough: Sepsis and gastrointestinal bleeding, *Ann. Surg.,* **175**:759, 1972.
3 Athanasoulis, C. A., B. Brown, and J. H. Shapiro: Angiography in the diagnosis and management of bleeding stress ulcers and gastritis, *Am. J. Surg.,* **125**:468, 1973.
4 ———, S. Baum, A. C. Waltman, et al.: Control of acute gastric mucosal hemorrhage: Intra-arterial infusion of posterior pituitary extract, *N. Engl. J. Med.,* **290**:597, 1974.
5 Black, J. W., A. M. Duncan, and C. D. Durant, et al.: Definition and antagonism of histamine H_2-receptors, *Nature (London),* **236**:385, 1972.
6 Bodily, K. and R. P. Fischer: The prevention of stress ulcers by Metiamide, an H_2-receptor antagonist, *J. Surg. Res.,* **20**:203, 1976.
7 Byrne, J. J. and V. A. Guardione: Surgical treatment of stress ulcers, *Am. J. Surg.,* **125**:464, 1973.
8 Chernov, M. S., F. B. Cook, M. Wood, and H. W. Hale: Stress ulcer: A preventable disease, *J. Trauma,* **12**:831, 1972.
9 Cheung, L. Y., L. W. Stephenson, F. G. Moody, et al.: Direct effects of endotoxin on canine gastric mucosal permeability and morphology, *J. Surg. Res.,* **18**:417, 1975.
10 Conn, H. O. and B. L. Blitzer: Nonassociation of adrenocorticosteroid therapy and septic ulcer, *N. Engl. J. Med.,* **294**:473, 1976.
11 ———, G. R. Ramsby, E. H. Storer, et al.: Intra-arterial vasopressin in the treatment of upper gastrointestinal hemorrhage: A prospective controlled clinical trial, *Gastroenterology,* **68**:211, 1975.
12 Czaja, A. J., J. C. McAlhany, W. A. Andes, and

B. A. Pruitt: Acute gastric disease after cutaneous thermal injury, *Arch. Surg.,* **110**:600, 1975.

13 ——, —— and B. A. Pruitt: Acute gastroduodenal disease after thermal injury: An endoscopic evaluation of incidence and natural history, *N. Engl. J. Med.,* **291**:925, 1974.

14 Drapanas, T., W. C. Woolverton, J. W. Reeder, et al.: Experiences with surgical management of acute gastric mucosal hemorrhage: A unified concept in the pathophysiology, *Ann. Surg.,* **173**:628, 1971.

15 Girvan, D. P. and R. B. Passi: Acute stress ulceration with bleeding or perforation, *Arch. Surg.,* **103**:116, 1971.

16 Henn, R. M., J. I. Isenberg, V. Maxwell, and R. A. L. Sturdevant: Inhibition of gastric acid secretion by cimetidine in patients with duodenal ulcer, *N. Engl. J. Med.,* **293**:371, 1975.

17 Jama, R. H., M. H. Perlman, T. Matsumoto: Incidence of stress ulcer formation associated with steroid therapy in various shock states, *Am. J. Surg.,* **130**:328, 1975.

18 Johnson, W. C. and W. Widrich: Efficacy of selective splanchnic arteriography and vasopressin perfusion in diagnosis and treatment of gastrointestinal hemorrhage, *Am. J. Surg.,* **131**: 481, 1976.

19 Kawarada, Y., R. Weiss, and T. Matsumoto: Pathophysiology of stress ulcer and its prevention, *Am. J. Surg.,* **129**:249, 1975.

20 Kiselow, M. C. and M. Wagner: Intragastric instillation of levarterenol, *Arch. Surg.,* **107**:387, 1973.

21 LeGall, J. R., F. C. Mignon, and M. Rapin, et al.: Acute gastroduodenal lesions related to severe sepsis, *Surg. Gynecol. Obst.,* **142**:377, 1976.

22 LeVeen, H. H., C. Diaz, G. Falk, et al.: A proposed method to interrupt gastrointestinal bleeding: Preliminary report, *Ann. Surg.,* **175**: 459, 1972.

23 Longstreth, G. F., V. L. W. Go, and J-R Malagelada: Cimetidine suppression of nocturnal gastric secretion in active duodenal ulcer, *N. Engl. J. Med.,* **294**:801, 1976.

24 Lucas, C. E., T. Ravikant, and A. J. Walt: Gastritis and gastric blood flow in hyperdynamic septic pigs, *Am. J. Surg.,* **131**:73, 1976.

25 —— and C. Sugawa: Diagnostic endoscopy during laparotomy for acute hemorrhage from the upper part of the gastrointestinal tract, *Surg. Gynecol. Obst.,* **135**:285, 1972.

26 ——, ——, W. Friend, and A. J. Walt: Therapeutic implications of disturbed gastric physiology in patients with stress ulcerations, *Am. J. Surg.,* **123**:25, 1972.

27 ——, ——, and J. Riddle et al.: Natural history and surgical dilemma of "stress" gastric bleeding, *Arch. Surg.,* **102**:266, 1971.

28 McAlhany, J. C., A. J. Czaja, and B. A. Pruitt: Antacid control of complications from acute gastroduodenal disease after burns, presented at the AAST, Scottsdale, Arizona, September 11, 1975.

29 McClelland, R. N.: "Acute Gastroduodenal Stress Ulceration," in M. H. Sleisenger and J. S. Fordtran (eds.), *Gastrointestinal Disease,* W. B. Saunders Company, Philadelphia, 1973, Chap. 53.

30 Mainardi, M., V. Maxwell, A. L. Sturdevant, and J. I. Isenberg: Metiamide, an H_2-receptor blocker, as inhibitor of basal and meal-stimulated gastric acid secretion in patients with duodenal, *N. Engl. J. Med.,* **291**:373, 1974.

31 Mullane, J. F., R. L. Pyant, R. G. Wilfong, and W. Dailey: Starvation, glucose and stress ulcers in the rat, *Arch. Surg.,* **109**:416, 1974.

32 Nilsson, I. M., S. E. Bergentz, O. Wiklander, and U. Hedner: Erosive hemorrhagic gastroduenitis with fibrinolysis and low factor XIII, *Ann. Surg.,* **182**:677, 1975.

33 Norton, L., J. Greer, and B. Eisenman: Gastric secretory response to head injury, *Arch. Surg.,* **101**:200, 1970.

34 ——, D. Mathews, L. Avrum, and B. Eisenman: Pharmacological protection against swine stress ulcer, *Gastroenterology,* **66**:503, 1974.

35 Oram-Smith, J. C. and E. F. Rosato: The effects of semistarvation and parenteral nutrition on the gastric mucosa of rats, *Surgery,* **79**:306, 1976.

36 Papp,, J. P.: Endoscopic electrocoagulation of upper gastrointestinal hemorrhage, *J. Am. Med. Assoc.,* **236**:2076, 1976.

37 Proudfoot, W. H., R. Bolick, R. D. Schoffstall, et al.: Dexamethasone therapy for "stress ulcer," *Am. Surg.,* **638**, 1972.

38 Rav, R. R., R. J. Thompson, C. R. Simmons, et al.: Selective visceral angiography in the

diagnosis and treatment of gastrointestinal hemorrhage, *Am. J. Surg.,* **128**:160, 1974.

39 Richardson, J. D. and J. B. Aust: Gastric devasculatization: A useful salvage procedure for massive hemorrhagic gastritis, *Ann. Surg.,* **185**:649, 1977.

40 Richardson, R. S., L. W. Norton, J. E. L. Sales, and B. Eisenman: Gastric blood flow in endotoxin-induced stress ulcer, *Arch. Surg.,* **106**:191, 1973.

41 Ritchie, W. P.: Bile acids, the "barrier" and reflux-related clinical disorders of the gastric mucosa, *Surgery,* **82**:192, 1977.

42 Silen, W. and J. J. Skillman: Stress ulcer, acute erosive gastritis and the gastric mucosal barrier, *Adv. Int. Med.,* **19**:195, 1974.

43 Simonian, S. J. and L. E. Curtis: Treatment of hemorrhagic gastritis by antacid, *Ann. Surg.,* **184**:429, 1976.

44 Stremple, J. F.: Prospective studies of gastric secretion in trauma patients, *Am. J. Surg.,* **131**:78, 1976.

45 ——— and D. W. Elliott: Hemorrhage due to diffuse erosive gastritis, *Arch. Surg.,* **110**:606, 1975.

46 ———, H. Mori, R. Lev, and G. B. Jerzy Glass: The stress ulcer syndrome, *Curr. Probl. Surg.,* **4**, 1973.

47 Sugawa, C., M. H. Werner, D. F. Hayes, et al.: Early endoscopy: A guide to therapy for acute hemorrhage in the upper gastrointestinal tract, *Arch. Surg.,* **107**:133, 1973.

48 Sullivan, R. C., B. B. Rutherford, and W. R. Waddell: Surgical management of hemorrhagic gastritis by vagotomy and pyloroplasty, *Ann. Surg.,* **159**:554, 1964.

49 Teorell, T.: Electrolyte diffusion in relation to the acidity regulation of the gastric juice, *Gastroenterology,* **9**:425, 1947.

50 Villar, H. V., H. R. Fender, L. C. Watson, and J. C. Thompson: Emergency diagnosis of upper gastrointestinal bleeding by fiberoptic endoscopy, *Ann. Surg.,* **185**:367, 1977.

51 Waterman, N. G. and J. L. Walker: Effect of a topical adrenergic agent on gastric blood flow, *Am. J. Surg.,* **127**:241, 1974.

52 Watts, C. and K. Clark: Effects of an anticholinergic drug on gastric acid secretion in the comatose patient, *Surg. Gynecol. Obst.,* **130**:1, 1970.

53 Wilson, W. S., T. Godacy, C. Olcott, and F. W. Blaisdell: Superficial gastric erosions: Response to surgical treatment, *Am. J. Surg.,* **126**:133, 1973.

54 Yellin, A. E., R. M. Dwyer, J. R. Craig, et al.: Endoscopic argon-ion laser phototherapy of bleeding gastric lesions, *Arch. Surg.,* **111**:750, 1976.

Chapter 31

Monitoring the Injured Patient

Joel H. Horovitz, M.D.
Charles J. Carrico, M.D.

Patients sustaining severe injury and undergoing major fluid and operative resuscitation are at risk for developing several serious postoperative complications. Inadequate tissue perfusion, resulting from hemorrhage and hypovolemia, is the primary predisposing factor. Major organ dysfunction with attendant high morbidity and mortality may be delayed in appearance in the convalescent period and may begin with surprisingly subtle signs. Therefore, close monitoring of the injured patient is mandatory. Early diagnosis and the institution of early aggressive therapy may ameliorate many of these complications.

In this chapter, the use of the common methods for assessing cardiovascular stability will be discussed, particularly as they relate to hemodynamic, renal, and gastric complications in the postinjury period. Pulmonary monitoring is considered in Chap. 32. Although recent technical advances will be mentioned, emphasis will be placed on the use of widely available clinical techniques.

The verb "monitor" means to observe without influencing the system under observation. Ideally, the instrumentation should be noninvasive and unobstrusive. Unfortunately, the present state of the art does not allow reliable and accurate measurement of many functions without direct access to the system under consideration. Any invasive technique has the potential for giving rise to complications, some avoidable and some not. Therefore, the risk-to-benefit ratio must be evaluated by the physician prior to insertion of intravascular catheters, sensors, etc. If the patient's condition warrants the risk of possible complications from instrumentation, the benefits to be derived must outweigh the risks.

An important principle of monitoring is that it should not decrease the frequency of contact between patients and the medical and paramedical personnel involved in their care. The most sophisticated electronic devices cannot take the place of clinical judgment and examination. Effective monitoring, therefore, is only an adjunct to accurate clinical assessment.

In general, the postoperative trauma patient requires more careful monitoring than the average surgical patient. Certain postinjury patients are at high risk for developing severe complications postoperatively. These patients should be admitted to an intensive care unit (ICU) and carefully monitored. The following factors should alert the physician to the need for monitoring in an ICU:

1 Severe multisystem injury
2 Prolonged hypotension
3 Multiple transfusions
4 Septic complications
5 Direct pulmonary injury
6 Aspiration
7 Moderate to severe preexisting cardiovascular, respiratory, or renal disease in conjunction with the above entities

BASIC HEMODYNAMIC MONITORING

It is customary after all operative procedures to assess hemodynamic stability. This is traditionally done by the frequent recording of the heart rate, systemic blood pressure, electrocardiogram, and urine output. These basic measurements are very valuable but have limitations. Their chief advantage is that they can be obtained without invasion of the vascular system. However, these measurements

may be inadequate when needed most, e.g., in the complicated shock or fluid problem. Under these circumstances, more sophisticated and invasive monitoring devices are required. These are listed in Table 31-1.[15]

Arterial Catheter

Arterial cannulation has become a relatively commonplace technique in the modern ICU. It is useful for obtaining continuous blood pressure readings as well as arterial blood for blood gas determination and the measurement of cardiac output. Rarely is the insertion of an arterial line justified on the basis of arterial pressure study alone. However, it may be very useful in the unstable patient because it is frequently impossible to obtain accurate arterial pressure measurements or reliable arterial blood in the patient who may suddenly become hypotensive. Frequent arterial punctures may cause greater patient discomfort than arterial cannulation. An arterial cannula allows repeated arterial sampling without disturbing the steady state, and so avoids the acute changes in blood gas tensions which may confuse the interpretation of results obtained by intermittent puncture. The importance of obtaining pure arterial blood has been demonstrated by Doty and Mosely.[15] Because of the shape of the oxyhemoglobin dissociation curve, admixture of a small volume of venous with arterial blood may produce a disproportionately large drop in the partial pressure of oxygen (Pa_{O_2}). For example, 0.5 mL of venous blood with a Pa_{O_2} of 31 mmHg, mixed with 4.5 mL of arterial blood with a

Table 31-1 Hemodynamic Monitoring

Arterial catheter
Central venous pressure catheter
Pulmonary artery catheter
Cardiac output
Blood volume

Pa_{O_2} of 86 mmHg, will result in a final mixture with a Pa_{O_2} of 56 mmHg.

There are several options available in choosing the site of cannulation and the method of insertion of the catheter. Commonly used arteries for long-term cannulation include the radial, brachial, and femoral vessels. It is the opinion of the authors that the radial artery is the vessel of choice for continuous arterial cannulation. The risk of accidental obstruction of the blood supply to the hand is minimal if certain simple precautions are taken. Fixation of the catheter is secure, and it is easy to apply effective pressure to the puncture site to minimize hematoma formation. Table 31-2 details the most common complications associated with the use of a radial artery catheter. Major complications occur infrequently, with an overall incidence of less than 1 percent. Mortensen reported no major complications in 500 cases.[37] Minor complications, predominately hematoma formation and a decrease in peripheral pulsation, occur quite commonly.[2,6,7,36,49] Atherosclerosis, hypertension, the use of anticoagulants, and failure to adhere to simple guidelines predispose to both major and minor complications.[36]

At present the material of choice for the arterial catheter is Teflon.[5] Bedford has recently published a study comparing polypropylene and Teflon catheters. He found that only 10 percent of Teflon catheters resulted in prolonged arterial occlusion, versus 70 percent of polypropylene catheters over the same period.[2] Chemically, Teflon is the most inert and least likely to cause tissue reaction.[26,31] An Allen test should be performed to assess the ulnar palmar circulation prior to catheter insertion.[25] The test is performed by compressing the radial artery at the wrist while the patient forcibly opens and closes the hand a few times. Normally, a slight transitory ischemia will be seen which disappears quickly when the hand is kept still and compression maintained. When the ulnar artery does not adequately support the palmar circulation, persistent signs of ischemia will be seen. During the final part of the examination, the fingers should not be hyperextended, since this may result in a false-positive reaction.[14,40] If a Doppler instrument is available, it may be used to test the completeness of the palmar circulation.[38]

Whether percutaneous or cut-down techniques are used for insertion of the catheter, aseptic technique is mandatory. If the palmar arch is intact, the diameter of the catheter is probably not critical. However, a small catheter size relative to the artery is probably associated with a lower risk of thrombus formation.[16,22] Intermittent high-volume irrigation of radial artery catheters may result in distal and proximal (even cerebral) embolization and should be avoided. With continuous low flow irrigation, distal emboli to the terminal digital vessels are less likely[16] and proximal embolization to the central circulation is not possible.[5,9,33,35] Removal of the cannula should be followed by compression of the puncture site for 5 to 10 min. During unexplained septic periods, the cannula should be removed and the tip cultured.[12,22,34] With meticulous care, the arterial catheter may be safely kept in for at least 48 to 72 h. Since thrombotic complications increase with time

Table 31-2 Complications of Radial Artery Catheterization

Major	Minor
Local obstruction with distal ischemia	Pain
External hemorrhage	Ecchymosis (common)
False aneurysm	Temporary loss of pulse
Massive ecchymosis	(Arteriospasm)
Dissection	Infection (rare)

after 30 h, the catheter should be removed as soon as it is no longer necessary.

Central Venous Catheter

Central venous pressure (CVP) monitoring has been the most widely accepted guide for the regulation of fluid and blood replacement in the seriously ill patient. It may be a valuable technique if measuring error or misinterpretation are avoided. Table 31-3 lists the normal values for pressure measurements on both sides of the circulation. A properly positioned CVP catheter should be within the superior vena cava (SVC). This may be inserted either through an antecubital fossa vein or into the subclavian or internal jugular veins and advanced to the SVC. Proper placement must be verified by a chest roentgenogram prior to fluid administration. It is important to establish a zero reference level (midaxillary line–right atrium) and to use this level for all subsequent measurements.

The CVP reading is a reflection of right ventricular end-diastolic pressure and is related to the efficacy of the right ventricle in handling the venous return presented to it. Since the CVP is a measure of the dynamic interrelationship between myocardial contractility, vascular resistance, and blood volume, it is obvious that one cannot determine a patient's volume status from a CVP measurement. In the case of nondisparate ventricular function, serial CVP readings are valuable in assessing the patient's response to a fluid challenge. A rising CVP is an indication that the right ventricle is absolutely or relatively overloaded. Table 31-4 outlines several common causes of incorrect CVP values. In general, all measurements of filling pressure should be obtained off the ventilator if the patient's condition permits. Most inaccuracies can be obviated by attention to the technical details of measurement. Table 31-5 outlines several guidelines to the safe use of the CVP catheter.

Pulmonary Artery Catheter

Swan and his associates have introduced a method for measuring the pulmonary artery pressure (PAP) and pulmonary capillary wedge pressure (PCWP) for routine clinical use.[46] This catheter is shown schematically in Fig. 31-1. Insertion into the pulmonary artery (PA) is accomplished by inflating a soft latex balloon at the catheter tip, which allows the flow of blood to carry it through the central veins and heart (see Table 31-3 for normal pressures). The catheter can be easily positioned with the aid of a pressure monitor, oscilloscope, and ECG. With the balloon inflated and the catheter advanced to a "wedge" position, a static column of blood is created which allows estimation of the pressure level and pressure changes in the left atrium. In the absence of mitral valvular disease the PCWP will be a good estimate of left ventricular

Table 31-3 Normal Systemic and Pulmonary Pressures

	Systolic	End diastolic	Mean
Right atrium	—	—	4
Right ventricle	25	0–4	15
Pulmonary artery	25	8–10	15
Pulmonary artery (wedge)	—	—	8
Left atrium	—	—	8
Left ventricle	90–140	0–5	—
Aorta	90–140	60–90	—

Table 31-4 Causes of Inaccurate CVP Readings

Incorrect zero reference
Change in position of patient
Coughing, straining during a reading
Positive pressure ventilation
Incorrect placement of catheter

end-diastolic filling pressure.[13,18,19,23] The criteria for wedging of the catheter include (1) recording a mean pressure less than mean PAP, (2) the characteristic change in wave form which varies with respiration, and (3) the presence of arterialized blood in a withdrawn sample.

In diseases characterized by differences in function of the two ventricles, disparities between CVP and PCWP should be anticipated. Forrester and coworkers[20] studied patients after myocardial infarction and found that the CVP did not correlate well with left ventricular filling pressure, PCWP, or x-ray evidence of congestive heart failure. Rapaport and Scheinman[41] found CVP values less than 10 cmH$_2$O in 30 percent of postinfarction patients with acute left ventricular failure and

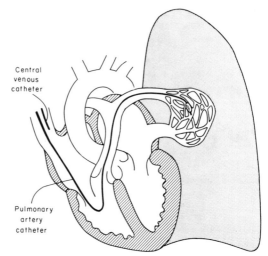

Figure 31-1 Pulmonary artery catheter.

pulmonary edema. Referring to Fig. 31-1, it may also be seen that if pulmonary vascular resistance is abnormally elevated, PCWP has the advantage of measuring left atrial pressure more accurately than the CVP. In patients with normal cardiac reserve and normal pulmonary vascular resistance, however, the CVP will reflect the ability of the myocardium to pump the volume presented to it. Properly

Table 31-5 Guidelines to the Safe Use of the CVP Catheter

Carry out surgical skin preparation for all cannulations.

Assure proper adapter-catheter fit prior to insertion.

Place the patient's head down when inserting subclavian or jugular catheters to avoid air embolism.

When subclavian puncture is unsuccessful, obtain x-ray of chest before attempting puncture on the contralateral side.

Use only radiopaque catheters. Do not bevel catheter tips. Remeasure after removal.

Whenever the catheter does not advance through the needle with ease, remove needle and catheter together. Never attempt to withdraw the catheter through the needle.

Obtain chest x-ray routinely after catheter insertion to assure location of catheter tip and the absence of a pneumothorax.

Remove catheter for unexplained fever, local inflammation, or at the earliest date that catheter does not contribute to patient's care.

Submit the distal catheter tip for culture.

Expend every effort to locate and retrieve lost catheters.

Table 31-6 Indications for Pulmonary Artery Catheters

Increased pulmonary resistance (chronic obstructive lung disease)

Coronary artery disease requiring complicated intravenous fluid regimen

Cardiac surgery and trauma

Decreased left ventricular function secondary to anoxia, acidosis, or electrolyte imbalance

Decompensated cirrhosis, severe pancreatitis, generalized peritonitis and severe multisystem trauma

Massive transfusions

High CVP in the presence of underperfusion of peripheral tissues

Suspected disparate ventricular function

applied, the CVP remains a useful clinical tool.

The advantages of using a pulmonary artery catheter must be weighed against the added risk to the patient. Table 31-6 lists those patients in whom the authors feel the risk-to-benefit ratio justifies its use. Other uses of the Swan-Ganz catheter are listed in Table 31-7. Individually, these uses rarely serve as an adequate indication for the insertion of a PA catheter. The importance of obtaining true mixed venous blood for the assessment of the shunt fraction has been demonstrated.[27] If central venous blood is used in critically ill patients, it will lead to an overestimation of the shunt fraction.

Table 31-8 lists the complications associated with both central venous and pulmonary artery catheters. The same guidelines of safety for CVP catheters are applicable to the PA catheter. In addition, during and after insertion, repeated evaluation of the character of the pressure tracing is important. Loss of the characteristic pulse may indicate unintentional catheter wedging,[11,42] with the possibility of pulmonary infarction.[10] Frequent chest films in the first 24 h should be obtained to detect tightening of the catheter loop, which indicates peripheral movement.[17] In the original description of the flow-directed balloon-tipped catheter, Swan and coworkers suggested advancing the catheter 1 to 3 cm further after the initial wedge position had been obtained.[47] It is now felt that this could lead to rupture of a pulmonary artery in some patients.[17,24,30] If, on repeated balloon inflations, a wedge pressure is obtained with less than the recommended volumes (0.8 cm³, No. 7 French), it is probable that the catheter has advanced too far and should be partially withdrawn.[17] Before wedge determinations, withdrawal of the catheter a short distance and inflation of the balloon in small increments will minimize the chances of perforation of the PA. If the pulmonary artery end-diastolic pressure is less than 20 mmHg and pulmonary edema is not present, a wedge

Table 31-7 Additional Uses of Pulmonary Artery Catheters

Bedside pulmonary angiogram in cases of pulmonary emboli

Mixed venous blood sampling

Injection of indicators for cardiac output study and determination of pulmonary venous resistance

Administration of medication

Table 31-8 Complications of CV and PA Catheters

Both CV and PA	PA only
Infection	PA perforation
Loss of catheter	Ischemic lung lesion
Thromboembolism	Catheter kinking
Perforation right ventricle	Heart murmurs

pressure is not necessary, since mean left atrial pressure is almost certain to be lower than pulmonary artery end-diastolic pressure.[43] Intracardiac knotting of the catheter can be prevented by allowing the catheter to advance itself while the tip remains in the right atrium or ventricle.[11] Continuous dilute heparin infusions should be used to maintain patency in all intravenous monitoring cannulas. By adhering to these guidelines, the incidence of complications can be minimized.

The use of positive end-expiratory pressure (PEEP) affects the PCWP measurement.[51] Up to levels of 10 cmH$_2$O of PEEP, the PCWP accurately reflects the left atrial pressure (LAP). Higher PEEP levels will compress the pulmonary capillary bed, collapsing the vessels distal to the balloon. Above 15 cmH$_2$O of PEEP, the PCWP will overestimate the true LAP. If possible, wedge pressure measurements should be done at zero end-expiratory pressure.

Cardiac Output

The determination of cardiac output (CO) flow is valuable but not essential in the postoperative management of the injured patient. Methodology is more cumbersome and expensive than the previously outlined hemodynamic tests. The dye dilution technique has been the most common method for measuring CO, although more recent techniques are gaining in popularity. Indocyanine green dye estimations of cardiac output are subject to a minimum 10 to 15 percent error under most conditions, this being increased by extremely low or high

CO.[51,8] Ganz et al.[21] have simplified the thermal dilution method of CO measurement by incorporating thermistors in a pulmonary artery catheter. This allows measurement of a change in temperature of a bolus of cold saline injected into the SVC and sampled in the PA. The CO is then inversely proportional to the fall in temperature. The advantages of this method are: (1) a "physiologic" indicator is used, (2) blood withdrawal is not required, and (3) no recirculation of the indicator occurs (a pure right heart CO is obtained). Extensive use of this method in patients has recently been reported.[21]

Another modification of the Swan-Ganz catheter has allowed a virtually continuous estimate of the cardiac output without the use of an indicator or sampling. A small fiberoptic oximeter attached to the tip of a PA catheter is able to measure oxygen saturation in the mixed venous blood. Mixed venous oxygen saturation is directly proportional to the CO if oxygen consumption is unchanged and the position of the hemoglobin-oxygen dissociation curve is constant. This method is still experimental, but does have a great deal of appeal because of its simplicity. The range of error in human work done to date is about the same as that for the dye-dilution method.[50]

Blood Volume

A direct measure of the circulating blood volume may be very helpful in the management of fluid balance problems. To date, these measurements have remained almost exclusively a research tool. The indicator dilution principle is utilized, the marker most commonly used being a radioactive-tagged element of the blood. Swan and Nelson have written an excellent review of the theory and practice of blood volume determinations.[28] Using chromium-tagged erythrocytes, the red blood cell mass can be measured. Total blood volume can be determined either by adding the estimated plasma volume (^{131}I-labeled albumin) or by using the corrected hematocrit. The red cell volume is the most accurate because the label resides exclusively in the intravascular fluid space. A commercially available device (Volemetron) is available for clinical measurement of blood volume. Its major disadvantages are that its error increases during acute changes in volume status and "normal" values are subject to wide individual variation.

The use of cardiac output and blood volume estimates depends upon the financial and technical resources of the hospital. Effective hemodynamic monitoring can be done without these measurements. However, cardiotonic and vasoactive drugs are administered only after an accurate hemodynamic assessment has been made. This approach avoids the administration of drugs deleterious to a particular patient's circulation and organ perfusion in the treatment of complicated circulatory problems.

RENAL FAILURE

Damage to the kidney may result from ischemia, the extent of damage varying with the severity and duration of the insult.[48] The incidence of primary acute oliguric renal failure has decreased secondary to improved fluid resusciation and immediate corrective surgery.[3,44] Less severe forms of renal failure, with normal or increased urine output are now recognized as being a more frequent occurrence in the injured patient. Awareness of these forms of renal dysfunction is important in the management of the postoperative trauma patient (see Chap. 23).

Table 31-9 lists the time-honored classification of renal failure. Adequate monitoring must supply information as to the effective plasma volume perfusing the kidneys. Similarly, any suggestion of postrenal obstruction must be investigated by means of retrograde

Table 31-9 Causes of Renal Failure

Type	Cause
Prerenal	Decreased effective plasma volume
Renal	Intrinsic disease or ischemia
Postrenal	Obstruction

pyelography. A useful bedside test for the quick differentiation of prerenal and renal failure is the measurement of urine electrolyte concentration and specific gravity. In renal failure, the urine sodium concentration is usually greater than 20 meq/L, and the specific gravity is less than 1.018 and fixed.[4] These easily obtained measurements may be very useful in the rapid differentiation between prerenal and renal dysfunction when more elaborate tests are unavailable.

The blood urea nitrogen (BUN) and serum creatinine are considered the preferred methods for assessing glomerular function.[32] Tissue trauma and multiple transfusions do not lead to azotemia or hypercreatinemia in patients with normal renal function. Persistent minimal elevations of BUN or serum creatinine are uniformly associated with a significant loss of renal function (at least 70 percent).[32,45] Normal tubular function alters the amount of water and the concentration of dissolved materials in the urine, making it different from plasma. Urine-to-plasma concentration ratios approaching unity, therefore, are diagnostic of tubular damage (acute tubular necrosis).

Table 31-10 lists those measurements which have been proposed as good determinants of renal damage in the postoperative trauma patient. Studies in the injured patient have demonstrated two- and three-fold increases in endogenous creatinine clearances (C_{cr}). Because of changes in muscle metabolism following severe trauma, increased loads of

Table 31-10 Test of Renal Function

Urine sodium concentration

Urine specific gravity

C_{cr} (clearance creatinine)

C_{urea} (clearance urea)

C_{osm} (osmolar clearance)

U/P* urea ratio

U/P creatinine

U/P osmolality

Free water clearance

*Urine to plasma.

creatinine are presented to the kidney. Apparently normal values of C_{cr} may lead to a false sense of security, when, in fact, the glomerular filtration rate may be reduced by a factor of 2 to 3. Free water clearance, calculated as the difference between urine output and osmolar clearance, has been proposed as a useful test of early renal impairment.[45] The complete loss of concentrating ability of the kidney is characterized by free water clearance values near zero. The return of free water clearance toward normal marks the functional recovery of the tubular cells. However, in a recent study, patients with the most severely damaged kidneys demonstrated positive free water clearances, as did septic patients.[48] Therefore, care must be taken in interpreting the results of positive free water clearance in the postinjury patient.

Simultaneous measurement of urine and plasma concentration of solutes is important. Clearance studies in the trauma patient tend to be difficult because of the need for prolonged urine collections.[32] Because of the variability of individual dissolved materials, one of the most useful measurements appears to be the urine-to-plasma osmolar ratio.[48] This method indicates the ratio of the concentrations of all dissolved materials in the urine. If an osmometer is not readily available, the urine-to-plasma urea ratio may be determined. The finding of identical concentrations of dissolved material in both plasma and urine is proof of a loss of the concentrating ability of the kidney and substantiates the diagnosis of acute renal failure.

Oliguric renal failure is a well recognized complication of trauma. It is less well recognized that renal failure may occur without an observed period of oliguria.[48] Renal insufficiency without oliguria is important from the standpoint of recognition. Table 31-11 lists the main features of the two syndromes. The chief danger in the nonoliguric type of renal failure lies in failure of recognition. This may allow the rapid progression of hyperkalemia from the administration of potassium salts with the threat of cardiac arrest. In addition, mild azotemia may be converted to severe renal failure by the inadvertent administration of nephrotoxic drugs. Similarly, drugs that normally do not demonstrate toxicity may do so in the face of reduced renal function.

In summary, the monitoring of renal function requires an assessment of the adequacy of plasma volume, specific renal function tests, and the exclusion of obstruction. Table 31-12 lists the tests that should be routinely

Table 31-11 Types of Renal Failure

Oliguric	Nonoliguric
Persistent oliguria after circulatory stabilization	Normal or increased urine output
Chemical evidence or uremia	Chemical evidence of uremia
Progressive rise in urine volume after several days to several weeks	
Gradual restoration of excretory plus concentrating functions of the kidney	

Table 31-12 Tests for Monitoring Renal Function

General	Specific renal function
Arterial pressure	Urinalysis
Central venous pressure	Specific gravity
ECG	Urine electrolytes
Strict intake and output	Urine-plasma osmolar ratio
Serum electrolytes	Serum BUN and creatinine

performed in the postinjury patient to assure adequate renal function and to alert the physician that alterations in therapy may be required.

SUMMARY

This review has focused on several aspects of monitoring postinjury patients. A few of the more commonly used monitoring devices have been discussed to emphasize that their use carries some risk. Because of this, proper indications, based on the benefit to be achieved, must be available before they are used (Table 31-13). Guidelines for the safe use of these devices have been outlined.

The postoperative injured patient is at risk for developing certain complications dependent upon the magnitude of the injury. This

Table 31-13 Patients at Greatest Risk for Stress Bleeding

Trauma

Major general surgery

Major intracranial injury or surgery

Hypovolemic shock

Burns

Sepsis

Renal insufficiency

Respiratory insufficiency

Table 31-14 Prevention of Stress Ulceration in Postinjury Patients

Nasogastric tube

Antacids

Anticholinergics

Coagulation studies

Careful monitoring for precipitating causes:
  Infection
  Renal or respiratory insufficiency

Support for healing or protective processes:
  Hyperalimentation
  Vitamin A

review has dealt with assessment of cardiovascular and renal function. Guidelines have been presented to aid in the prevention, early diagnosis, and management of these problems (Table 31-14). Pulmonary failure is discussed in Chap. 32.

BIBLIOGRAPHY

1 Baek, S. M., R. S. Brown, and W. C. Shoemaker: Early predicition of acute renal failure and recovery, *Ann. Surg.,* **177**:253, 1973.

2 Barr, P. O.: Percutaneous puncture of the radial artery with a multipurpose Teflon catheter for indwelling use, *Acta Physiol. Scand.,* **51**:343, 1972.

3 Baxter, C. R. and D. R. Maynard: Prevention and recognition of surgical renal complications, *Clin. Anesthesiol.,* **3**:322, 1968.

4 ———, W. H. Zedletz, and G. T. Shires: High output acute renal failure complicating traumatic injury, *J. Trauma,* **4**:567, 1964.

5 Bedford, R. E.: Percutaneous radial-artery cannulation: Increased safety using Teflon catheters, *Anesthesiology,* **42**:220, 1975.

6 Berneus, B., A. Carlsten, A. Holmgren, et al.: Percutaneous catheterization of peripheral arteries as a method for blood sampling, *Scand. J. Clin. Lab. Invest.,* **6**:217, 1954.

7 Brown, A. E., D. B. Sweeney, and J. Lumley: Percutaneous radial artery cannulation, *Anesthesia,* **24**:532, 1969.

8 Carey, J. S. et al.: Accuracy of cardiac output computers, *Ann. Surg.*, 174:762, 1971.

9 Chernov, C. S., F. B. Cook, M. Wood, et al.: Stress ulcer: A preventable disease, *J. Trauma*, 12:831, 1972.

10 Chun, G. M. H. and M. H. Ellestad: Perforation of the pulmonary artery by a Swan-Ganz catheter, *N. Engl. J. Med.*, 284:1041, 1971.

11 Civetta, J. M. and J. C. Gabel: Flow-directed pulmonary artery catheterization in surgical patients, *Ann. Surg.*, 176:753, 1972.

12 Control of infections from intravenous infusions: *Med. Lett. Drugs Ther.*, 15:105, 1973.

13 DeLaurentis, D. A., M. Hayes, T. Matsumoto, et al.: Does central venous pressure accurately reflect hemodynamic and fluid volume patterns in the critical surgical patient?, *Am. J. Surg.*, 126:415, 1973.

14 DeGowin, E. L. and R. L. DeGowin: *Bedside Diagnostic Examination*, 3d ed., The Macmillan Company, New York, 1976.

15 Doty, D. B. and R. V. Mosely: Reliable sampling of arterial blood, *Surg. Gynecol. Obstet.*, 219:701, 1970.

16 Downs, J. B., A. D. Rackstein, and E. F. Klein: Hazards of radial artery catherization, *Anesthesiology*, 38:283, 1973.

17 Foote, G. A., S. I. Schabel, and M. Hodges: Pulmonary complications of the flow-directed balloon-tipped catheter, *N. Engl. J. Med.*, 290:927, 1974.

18 Forrester, J. S.: Pulmonary arterial catheterization, *Geriatrics,* 76:65, 1971.

19 ———, G. Diamond, V. Ganz, et al.: Right-and-left-heart pressures in the acutely ill patient, *Clin. Res.*, 18:306, 1970.

20 ———, T. J. McHugh, et al.: Filling pressure in the right and left sides of the heart in acute myocardial infarction, *N. Engl. J. Med.,* 285:190, 1971.

21 Ganz, W. et al.: A new technique for measurement of cardiac output by thermodilution in man, *Am. J. Cardiol.*, 27:392, 1971.

22 Gardner, R. M., R. Schwartz, H. C. Wong, et al.: Percutaneous indwelling radial artery catheters for monitoring cardiovascular function, *N. Engl. J. Med.*, 290:1227, 1974.

23 Gold, H. K.: Wedge pressure monitoring in myocardial infarction, *N. Engl. J. Med.*, 285:230, 1971.

24 Golden, M. S., T. Pinder, Jr., W. T. Anderson, et al.: Fatal pulmonary hemorrhage complicating use of a flow-directed balloon-tipped catheter in a patient receiving anticoagulant therapy, *Am. J. Cardiol.*, 32:865, 1973.

25 Greenlow, D. E.: Incorrect performance of Allen's test: Ulnar artery flow erroneously presumed inadequate, *Anesthesiology,* 37:356, 1972.

26 Harrison, J. H., D. S. Swanson, and F. A. Lincoln: A comparison of the tissue reaction to plastic materials, *Arch. Surg.*, 74:139, 1957.

27 Horovitz, J. H., C. J. Carrico, and G. T. Shires: Venous sampling sites for pulmonary shunt determinations in the injured patient, *J. Trauma*, 11:911, 1971.

28 Johnson, C. C.: Fiberoptic probe for oxygen saturation and dye concentration monitoring, *Biomed. Sci. Instrum.*, 10:45, 1974.

29 Kassirer, J. P.: Clinical evaluation of kidney function glomerular function, *N. Engl. J. Med.*, 285:385, 1971.

30 Lapin, E. S. and J. A. Murray: Hemoptysis with flow-directed cardiac catheterization, *J. Am. Med. Assoc.*, 220:1246, 1972.

31 LeVeen, H. H. and J. R. Barberio: Tissue reaction of plastic used in surgery with special reference to Teflon, *Ann. Surg.*, 129:74, 1949.

32 Levinsky, N. G.: Acute renal failure, *N. Engl. J. Med.*, 274:1016, 1966.

33 Lowenstein, E., J. W. Little, III, and H. H. Lo: Prevention of cerebral embolization from flushing radial artery cannulas, *N. Engl. J. Med.*, 285:1414, 1971.

34 Maki, D. G., D. A. Goldmann, and F. S. Rhame: Infection control in intravenous therapy, *Ann. Intern. Med.*, 79:867, 1973.

35 Meguid, M. and R. Bevilacqua: Management of arterial cannulas, *N. Engl. J. Med.*, 286:376, 1972.

36 Moran, F., A. R. Lorimer, and G. Boyd: Percutaneous arterial catheterization for multiple sampling, *Thorax*, 22:253, 1967.

37 Mortensen, J. D.: Clinical sequelae from arterial needle puncture cannulation and incision, *Circulation*, 25:1118, 1967.

38 Mozersky, M. C., C. J. Budkley, C. O. Hagood,

et al.: Ultrasonic evaluation of the palmar circulation: A useful adjunct to radial artery cannulation, *Am. J. Surg.*, **126**:810, 1973.

39 Oriol, A., et al.: Limitations of indicator-dilution methods in experimental shock, *J. Appl. Physiol.*, **23**(4).605, 1967.

40 Paaby, H. and F. Stadil: Thrombosis of the ulnar artery, *Acta Orthop. Scand.*, **39**:336, 1968.

41 Rapaport, E. and M. Scheinman: Rationale and limitation of hemodynamic measurements in patients with acute myocardial infarction, *Mond. Conc. Cardiovasc. Dis.*, **38**:55, 1969.

42 Scott, M. L., D. R. Weber, J. F. Arers, et al.: Clinical applications of a flow-directed balloon-tipped cardiac catheter, *Am. Surg.*, **38**:690, 1972.

43 Sharefkin, J. B. and J. D. MacArthur: Pulmonary artery pressure as a guide to the hemodynamic status of surgical patients, *Arch. Surg.*, **105**:699, 1972.

44 Shires, G. T., C. J. Carrico, and P. C. Canizaro: "Shock," in *Major Problems in Clinical Surgery*, W. B. Saunders Company, Philadelphia, vol. XIII, 1973.

45 Stahl, W. M. and A. M. Stone: Prophylactic diuresis with ethacrynic acid for prevention of postoperative renal failure, *Ann. Surg.*, **172**:361, 1970.

46 Swan, H. J. C., W. Ganz, J. Forrester, et al.: Catheterization of the heart in man using a flow-directed balloon-tipped catheter, *Nineteenth Annual Scientific Session of the American College of Cardiology*, New Orleans, 1970.

47 ———, ———, J. Forrester, et al.: Catheterization of the heart in man with the use of a flow-directed balloon-tipped catheter, *N. Engl. J. Med.*, **283**:447, 1970.

48 ——— and A. W. Nelson: Blood volume, *Ann. Surg.*, **173**:481, 1971.

49 Ward, R. J. and H. D. Green: Arterial puncture as a safe diagnostic aid, *Surgery*, **57**:672, 1965.

50 Weisel, R. D. et al.: Measurement of cardiac output by thermodilution, *N. Engl. J. Med.*, **292**:682, 1975.

51 Woods, M. et al.: Practical considerations for the use of a pulmonary artery thermistor catheter, *Surgery*, **79**:469, 1976.

Chapter 32

Postinjury Acute Pulmonary Failure

Charles J. Carrico, M.D.

Joel H. Horovitz, M.D.

INTRODUCTION

Acute pulmonary failure following injury has been described intermittently since the early 1880s. Laennec's writings on massive pulmonary collapse contained descriptions compatible with this entity.[59] Reports of fulminant pneumonia in World War I casualties appeared in the medical literature in the early 1900s.[17,30] During World War II Burford described patients who developed pulmonary failure following chest trauma and named this syndrome "traumatic wet lung."[14] Since that time this clinical entity has been variously referred to as shock lung, adult hyaline membrane disease, adult respiratory insufficiency syndrome, Da Nang lung, hemorrhagic atelec-

tasis, posttraumatic pulmonary insufficiency, progressive respiratory distress, stiff lung, wet lung, traumatic wet lung, and white lung syndrome. The most commonly used term at present is the "adult respiratory distress syndrome" (ARDS).

Several recent developments have allowed posttraumatic respiratory failure to gain widespread clinical recognition. Among these are improved techniques and methods of resuscitation from shock of all forms and the development and clinical application of devices for accurately measuring arterial blood gas concentration.

The Viet Nam war, with its rapid evacuation of the injured soldier and the application of sophisticated resuscitative methods, allowed the emergence and study of a large "at risk" population. The compilation of data from Viet Nam gave some estimate of the overall incidence of the problem. In 1968, in response to a rising clinical interest, a symposium on pulmonary insufficiency following nonthoracic trauma was convened under the auspices of the National Science Foundation.[29] The largest series presented at this conference indicated that the overall incidence of isolated ARDS was about 1 percent of the severely wounded.[71] Approximately the same incidence of ARDS has been found in a large civilian population sustaining blunt and penetrating trauma admitted to Parkland Memorial Hospital.[54] However, retrospective studies of patients who died in intensive care units have shown that as many as 50 percent of such patients have had pulmonary failure, and may have died from it. Therefore, although the overall frequency of occurrence of ARDS is low in the total trauma population, it affects a significant number of those who ultimately die of their injury.

Extensive study of the pulmonary response to major injury is taking place throughout the country. Available evidence now suggests that rather than being a distinct clinical entity, ARDS is the end result of many noxious stimuli applied to the pulmonary apparatus.[2,9,22,35,91]

CLINICAL PRESENTATION

The syndrome of ARDS may occur under a variety of circumstances and result in a spectrum of clinical severity from mild dysfunction to progressive eventually fatal, pulmonary failure. Fortunately, with proper management, the latter type is far less frequent than a milder type of abnormality.[54]

For descriptive purposes the clinical picture may be divided into arbitrary stages.[72] The first stage (injury, resuscitation, and alkalosis) immediately follows initial injury and is characterized by spontaneous hyperventilation with *hypocarbia,* diminished pulmonary compliance, mixed metabolic and respiratory alkalosis, and a normal chest x-ray. After apparent stabilization of vital signs and adequate tissue perfusion, the patient enters stage 2 (circulatory stability and beginning respiratory difficulty). This may persist for several hours to days. Persistent *hyperventilation,* progressive hypocarbia, increased cardiac output, progressive decrease in compliance, falling oxygenation and increasing pulmonary shunt fraction, all indicate that progressive pulmonary insufficiency will predominate in the subsequent clinical course. Stage 3 (progressive pulmonary insufficiency) and stage 4 (terminal hypoxia with asystole) complete the syndrome.

The hallmarks of the clinical syndrome are:

1 Hypoxemia which is relatively unresponsive to elevations of inspired oxygen concentration (indicating ventilation-perfusion imbalance and shunting).
2 Decreased pulmonary compliance (progressively increased airway pressure required to achieve adequate tidal volume).
3 Chest x-ray changes are characteristically minimal in the early stages. With progression of the syndrome interstitial edema and diffuse infiltrates appear, which may progress to widespread areas of consolidation.

Minor criteria for diagnosis include hyperventilation, increased cardiac output, and a history of nonthoracic trauma. The diagnostic criteria are summarized in Table 32-1.

PATHOPHYSIOLOGY

A review of a basic terminology is shown in Table 32-2.

The prominent derangements in pulmonary function associated with ARDS are: (1) hypoxia which is unresponsive to increased in-

Table 32-1 Diagnostic Criteria in Postinjury Pulmonary Insufficiency

Major
  Hypoxemia (unresponsive)
  Stiff lung (low compliance)
  ↓ Resting volume (functional residual capacity)
  X-ray (diffuse interstitial pattern)
  ↑ Dead space ventilation

Minor
  ↑ Cardiac output
  Hyperventilation
  Nonthoracic trauma

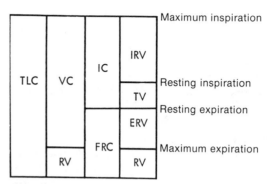

Figure 32-1 Lung volumes and capacities: TLC, total lung capacity; VC, vital capacity; IC, inspiratory capacity; FRC, functional residual capacity; RV, residual volume, ERV, expiratory reserve volume; TV, tidal volume; IRV, inspiratory reserve volume.

spired oxygen concentrations, (2) decreased pulmonary compliance (compliance is defined as the amount of volume increase in the lungs obtained by a given change in pressure), which clinically appears as "stiff lungs," and (3) a fall in resting lung volume, specifically a fall in the functional residual capacity. The functional residual capacity as shown in Fig. 32-1 is the amount of air remaining in the lungs after a normal expiration.

The possible causes of hypoxemia (assuming an adequate inspired O_2 concentration) are shown in Table 32-3. Although all clinicians are familiar with hypoventilation as a cause of hypoxia, such as is seen in the recovery room, it is unlikely that hypoventilation is responsible for the hypoxia in this syndrome. Hypo-

ventilation significant enough to result in hypoxia is associated with a rise in the P_{CO_2}. These patients, however, have abnormally low P_{CO_2}'s.

Although diffusion defects can theoretically result from interstitial edema and thickening, diffusion defects should respond to the administration of 100 percent oxygen. Such is not the case in the patients in question, so that diffusion defects would appear to be unlikely causes of the clinical syndrome.

Ventilation-perfusion inequalities could explain the hypoxia seen in these patients, and shunting represents the ultimate ventilation-perfusion abnormality. This statement deserves further explanation. Normally, there is autoregulation of ventilation and perfusion within the lung so that a balance exists between ventilation and perfusion of alveolar

Table 32-2 Basic Terminology and Symbols

VO_2	Oxygen consumption
CO	Cardiac output
VD/VT	Physiologic dead space ventilation as a fraction of tidal volume
Qs/Qt	Venous admixture as a fraction of total cardiac output
D(A-a)	Alveolar arterial gradient
FI_{O_2}	Fraction of inspired O_2
V/Q	Ratio of ventilation to perfusion

Table 32-3 Causes of Hypoxemia

Hypoventilation

Diffusion defects

V/Q abnormalities

Shunting

groups. Compensatory mechanisms exist so that when a group of alveoli become nonventilated or have a decreased alveolar P_{O_2} (PA_{O_2}), there is a decrease in blood flow around these alveoli. This, in its extreme, results in no ventilation and no perfusion to that alveolar unit; thus no abnormality in terms of dead space ventilation or shunting occurs. The effects of loss of this normal balance or loss of compensatory mechanisms are shown in Fig. 32-2. On the left, alterations in blood flow are demonstrated. It can be seen that a progressive decrease in blood flow with continued ventilation has little effect on arterial oxygenation. This can be defined as high ventilation-to-perfusion ratio and is usually reflected by increases in dead space ventilation. Such changes do not result in hypoxemia. On the right side of Fig. 32-2 is shown the

effect of reduction in ventilation while perfusion is maintained. It can be seen that progressive lowering of ventilation can result in hypoxemia until the ultimate reduction, i.e., nonventilation, occurs. In theory, as long as any ventilation of the alveolus occurs, the hypoxia should be responsive to oxygen. This then is generally referred to as a ventilation-perfusion abnormality characterized by a low V/Q ratio. When complete alveolar collapse or nonventilation occurs for any reason, the hypoxia secondary to this is no longer responsive to oxygen, and this is defined as a *shunt*.

Causes of pulmonary shunting are shown in Fig. 32-3. Shunting normally takes place to the extent of about 3 percent of the cardiac output. This is through both intrapulmonary and extrapulmonary routes. Although pathologic shunts occur from extrapulmonary causes,

Figure 32-2 Diagrammatic representation of ventilation-perfusion ratio (V/Q) abnormalities.

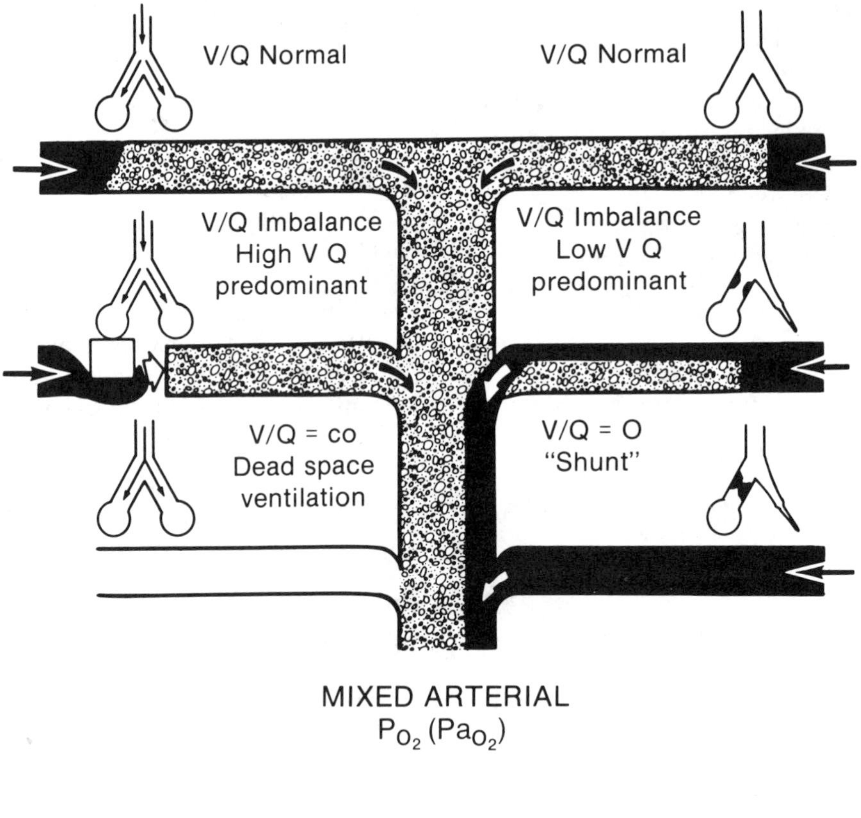

V/Q Normal

V/Q Normal

V/Q Imbalance
High V Q
predominant

V/Q Imbalance
Low V Q
predominant

V/Q = co
Dead space
ventilation

V/Q = O
"Shunt"

MIXED ARTERIAL
P_{O_2} (Pa_{O_2})

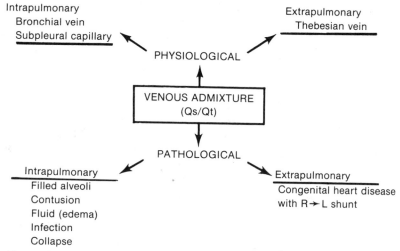

Figure 32-3 Mechanisms of arteriovenous admixture.

intrapulmonary shunting appears to be the problem in posttraumatic pulmonary insufficiency. Basically, there is perfusion of alveoli which are collapsed or for other reasons cannot be ventilated. The alveoli, for example, may be filled with secretions, exudate, blood, edema, or protein.

Whatever the cause, the clinical picture appears to result from a distortion of the normal ventilation-perfusion balance. This concept is shown in Fig. 32-4. In some areas of the lung there appears to be perfusion with poor ventilation, and in other areas there is ventilation of nonperfused alveoli. This combination of abnormalities will produce decreased resting lung volume, or functional residual capacity (FRC), shunting, and increased dead space ventilation.

The common denominator producing the abnormalities in ventilation and perfusion and other abnormalities seen in ARDS is thought to be injury to the alveolar-capillary membrane. This injury results in loss of integrity of the membrane with increased permeability to albumin. The consequent leak of protein-rich fluid leads to *interstitial pulmonary edema* and decreased pulmonary compliance. With con-

tinued leakage, the alveolar units become fluid-filled, and hypoxemia (shunting) ensues. Thus the entire clinical picture of ventilation of poorly perfused segments (capillary injury), decreased compliance (interstitial edema), perfusion of poorly ventilated segments, and loss of lung volume (partial and complete fluid-filled alveoli) appears to result from capillary injury with a "capillary leak."

The majority of the causative factors listed

Figure 32-4 Diagrammatic representation of mismatched ventilation and perfusion.

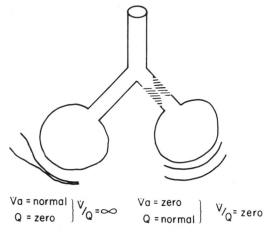

in the next section cause such an alveolar-capillary injury.

ETIOLOGY

The etiology of posttraumatic respiratory failure remains unsettled. It appears that a variety of noxious stimuli may result in a common clinical picture. Table 32-4 lists the factors that are now considered to be of primary and secondary importance as causes of this syndrome. As a group, these factors appear to have in common the ability to damage the pulmonary capillary endothelium. The importance of recognizing possible etiologic factors rests in the early identification of high-risk patients who may benefit from early intensive treatment. Many of these etiologic factors are apparent immediately upon presentation of the case or very shortly thereafter.

Hemorrhagic Shock (Ischemic Pulmonary Injury)

Pulmonary failure is commonly seen in severely injured patients, many of whom have been in shock. It is natural to assume that at least part of the respiratory failure noted is the result of an ischemic injury to the lung. Support for this hypothesis came from early studies in animals and in humans. Retrospective reports implied a correlation between shock and pulmonary failure.[10,69,84,85] Hemorrhage and congestion were noted in canine and human lungs after hemorrhagic shock and resuscitation.[28,69,100,108] Shock is a primary factor in the etiology of this syndrome. Studies in dogs, primates, and other experimental animals continue to show anatomic lesions of varying degree associated with hemorrhagic shock, but do not demonstrate any measurable functional defect in the lung. No significant or progressive hypoxia occurs.[13,79,81,103] In fact, several studies have shown a decrease rather than an increase in pulmonary shunt fraction. Adequate arterial oxygenation has been maintained during and up to several days following hypovolemic shock.[37,52,116,121]

Only extreme severe hemorrhagic shock preparations, lasting more than several hours, have been able to demonstrate preterminal decreases in arterial oxygen concentration concomitant with generalized circulatory collapse.[58] This is in contradistinction to sepsis and septic shock, in which hypoxia has been demonstrated to occur regularly.[42] Recent clinical studies have confirmed this finding. The highest incidence of pulmonary dysfunction is noted in those patients with sepsis, irrespective of the presence or absence of shock.[35,54] The results of one prospective study are shown in Table 32-5. Thus, while hemorrhagic shock may compound other pulmonary injuries, it does not appear to be a primary cause of respiratory failure following trauma.

Table 32-4 Etiology of Posttraumatic Respiratory Failure

Primary	Secondary
Sepsis, systemic infection	Ischemic pulmonary injury, i.e., hemorrhagic shock
Fat embolism	Pulmonary infection
Microembolization	Fluid overload (crystalloid or colloid)
Soft tissue trauma	Microatelectasis
Multiple transfusions	Recumbency
Intravascular coagulation	Operation
Aspiration	Anesthesia
Oxygen toxicity	Narcotics
Direct pulmonary injury	
Massive CNS injury, hypoxia	

Table 32-5 Incidence of Pulmonary Failure After Injury

Group	Total number	Significant pulmonary number	Dysfunction, %
All patients operated upon for trauma	978	21	2.1
Patients selected for study	49	21	43
Shock (all types)	28	11	39
Patients with no shock	21	10	48
Septic patients	10	8	80
Nonseptic patients	39	13	33

The lungs have a limited number of ways of responding to any injury. The existence of hemorrhagic shock may make the lungs more vulnerable to other injurious agents. For example, it has been shown that the combination of shock and fat embolism is much more damaging to the lung than is either alone.[26]

Pulmonary Infection

Pulmonary infection is eventually present in virtually all patients succumbing to respiratory insufficiency. It is usually clinically apparent during the later stages of the syndrome.[7,101] Prophylactic broad-spectrum antibiotics fail to prevent this complication.[3] Although this can certainly compound the syndrome and produce further hypoxia and decreased compliance, it is probably a secondary event and not the initiating cause of the entire clinical picture.[22]

Ventilators and other respiratory equipment may be a source of bacterial contamination in these patients. Appropriate measures should be taken so that the equipment being used for treatment does not contribute to the incidence of bacterial pneumonia.[89]

Aspiration

The syndrome produced by severe aspiration with subsequent pneumonia can resemble the clinical picture described. In a small but significant number of patients, aspiration, recognized or unrecognized, does occur and may occasionally be the causative factor producing posttraumatic pulmonary insufficiency.[15,45]

Fat Embolism

The syndrome associated with multiple long bone fractures, which appears to be related to embolization of fat, can produce a clinical picture similar to that described above. Although mild x-ray differences may occur, these patients are diffult to separate from the remainder of patients with pulmonary insufficiency after injury.[72] Fulminant fat embolism has been described in combat casualties.[66] There is evidence that a more subtle form may occur in less severely injured patients, especially after significant soft tissue trauma and long bone fractures.[23,46] Again, the mechanism remains to be defined.

Oxygen Toxicity

Prolonged use of high oxygen concentrations can result in a clinical picture and pathologic findings identical to those seen in ARDS.[40,57] Ventilation with high concentrations of oxygen is thought to poison cell enzyme systems and disrupt membrane integrity.[110] It has been shown to significantly reduce mucociliary clearance in the tracheobronchial tree.[98,120] The critical level appears to be between 25 and 40% oxygen.[61,99] There is also a time factor involved, so that the higher the oxygen tension, the less time is required to produce symptoms and evidence of damage.[110] A conscientious attempt to limit inspired oxygen tension should be made. If oxygen concentration and bacterial contamination are controlled, "respirator lung" should no longer occur.[82,89] It seems unlikely that oxygen toxicity is a major factor in the etiology of ARDS, although it may compound the problem if given in high concentrations.

Microatelectasis

Microatelectasis can result from recumbancy, sedation, operation, and anesthesia. Although not the primary factor responsible for the clinical picture, it may contribute to the hypoxia seen in these patients.

Direct Pulmonary Injury

There is little doubt that direct pulmonary injury can produce the progressive syndrome previously outlined.[94] Although most patients considered to have this syndrome are thought to have nonthoracic injury, unrecognized injury may well have occurred.[56] A force applied to an animal's abdomen comparable to that of a steering wheel blow received during a head-on collision, results in raising the diaphragm to the level of the second intercostal space.[83] Thus, abdominal trauma may produce tremendous compressive pulmonary injury, which may not be immediately apparent.

Cerebral Injury

Massive head injury has been associated with acute pulmonary edema, and laboratory evidence of a cause-and-effect relationship exists.[27,104] The progression of acute pulmonary edema to the clinical syndrome under discussion has not been established. Moss has proposed a centrineurogenic basis for progressive pulmonary insufficiency.[74] He has presented evidence that cerebral hypoxia in animals without direct head injury can produce the syndrome. The clinical significance of these observations has not been established.

Sepsis

Significant extrapulmonary infection with systemic sepsis appears to be a constant finding in a number of clinical studies of ARDS.[5,10,22,35,54,84,88] Acute respiratory failure is the first manifestation of sepsis in approximately 40 percent of surgical patients.[35,112] Excluding patients with burns, intracranial lesions, and pulmonary contusion, the syndrome is rarely seen without severe sepsis.[49] The concept that sepsis is an important causative agent is supported by a significant amount of laboratory evidence. A variety of septic insults, including injection of *Escherichia coli* endotoxin, live *E. coli* organisms, and peritonitis-induced septicemia, produce both physiologic and anatomic derangements.[19,31,41,42,48]

The specific mechanism of septic lung damage is still speculative, but a number of factors appear to be operative:

1 Direct endothelial damage to the pulmonary capillaries with resultant loss of integrity and alveolar injury[1,20,21,41,118]

2 Gross disturbances in the clotting mechanism as well as the release of a variety of vasoactive and bronchoconstrictive substances[20,41,118]

3 Decrease in activity and/or amount of surfactant[97]

Whatever the mechanism, available information supports the hypothesis that sepsis produces pronounced changes in vascular resistance, airway resistance, direct alveolar and vascular injury, interstitial and intraalveolar edema, hemorrhage, changes in surfactant, and progressive hypoxia. The association of sepsis and acute respiratory failure appears clear. The underlying mechanism of pulmonary damage, however, remains obscure.

Microembolization

Microemboli of various sorts, with their attendant release of vasoactive substances, injury to pulmonary capillaries and adjacent alveoli, and hemodynamic effects, may produce defects in pulmonary function. A number of theories exist as to the origin and clinical significance of these microemboli.

One source of microemboli appears to be stored blood.[73] Changes in screen filtration pressure as a result of particulate material in stored, banked blood have been reported. Several series have demonstrated a rough correlation between the number of transfusions and the incidence of pulmonary insufficiency.[3,16,65,82,93] There is a growing body of evidence supporting the use of Dacron-wool filters in patients receiving massive transfusions as a possible means of decreasing the incidence of pulmonary failure.[24,50,95] The precise role of such filters remains to be established.

A second source of microemboli appears to be the formation of intravascular microaggregates. These have been demonstrated in the venous return following release of a cross-clamped aorta[62] and following massive soft tissue injury.[106] Recently they have been demonstrated in the venous effluent of limited nonhypotensive soft tissue injuries[6] and in hypovolemic, nonhypotensive states.[24] It now appears that arterial hypotension, hypovolemia, low flow states, and trauma may all lead to the formation of microemboli. A third source of microembolism is disseminated intravascular coagulation.[44] Progressive changes in the clotting mechanism correlates with the development of significant pulmonary dysfunction. Thrombocytopenia appears to precede full development of the pulmonary disturbance.[70]

In summary, many of these mechanisms appear to be operative in the trauma patient who develops pulmonary failure. However, the value of specific therapy in preventing or treating each entity has not been determined.

Fluid Overload

The role of fluid administration in the production of ARDS has created great controversy. It has been proposed that, in the severely injured patient, a point is reached at which maintenance of renal function and restoration of adequate tissue perfusion are gained at the cost of significant fluid overload to the detriment of pulmonary function.[4,43]

Animals massively transfused with balanced electrolyte solutions develop fulminant pulmonary edema. However, they respond briskly to assisted ventilation, and ventilatory therapy prevents hypoxia. Those that survive the insult clear the edema rapidly and do not develop progressive pulmonary failure characteristic of the clinical syndrome.[39,109] Similarly, clinical studies show no correlation between the amounts of fluids received and the development of pulmonary insufficiency.[16,93,101]

Although there is little question as to the deleterious effects of massive fluid overload, its role in the production of this syndrome remains questionable. Excessive "drying out" of the lungs may be dangerous. If excessive fluid restriction results in a fall of cardiac output, then the degree of hypoxia resulting from any pulmonary damage will be compounded.[92] At present the most reasonable course appears to be to maintain fluid balance as close to normal as possible.

Type of Resuscitative Fluid

An even more controversial subject is that of the administration of colloid versus crystalloid solutions in the production of the syndrome. If the pulmonary vasculature is normal, a fall in the serum oncotic pressure renders the lungs more susceptible to pulmonary edema. Some authors reason that if crystalloid solutions are used in resuscitation, a fall in oncotic pressure might occur and cause or compound a pulmonary abnormality. If this were the case, the administration of colloid might be potentially beneficial to these patients. Clinical reports on the use of colloid solutions in the therapy of this condition are scanty and the results difficult to evaluate.[32,38,105] They do not conclusively demonstrate the clinical effectiveness of colloid and/or diuretic therapy in decreasing extravascular lung water and restoring normal serum oncotic pressure.

The available evidence implies that the pulmonary capillary membrane is abnormal. Therefore, colloids administered intravenously may gain access to the pulmonary interstitium and could potentially increase the interstitial oncotic pressure. This conceivably could compound the pulmonary problem in the healing phase.[96]

Unfortunately, few experimental data are available at present to resolve these conflicting hypotheses. A reliable experimental model of the syndrome is lacking. A large number of studies have evaluated pulmonary capillary permeability in hemorrhagic shock.[47,52,78,90,102,114] Little change in permeability or in interstitial ultrastructure as a result of shock alone has been shown. Although large amounts of colloid have been shown to produce some changes in interstitial ultrastructure, the clinical importance of such changes remains debatable. Trunkey et al. have demonstrated a greater increase in lung water after resuscitating animals with colloids than were seen after resuscitation with electrolyte solutions.[51] The concept that colloid solution administration is unlikely to be beneficial (and may be harmful) in the face of a "capillary leak" is supported by the extensive studies of Staub and others.[11,107,113] However, a number of other animal and clinical studies have demonstrated no significant difference in pulmonary function after resuscitation from hemorrhagic shock with either crystalloid or colloid solution.[2,50,53,63,75,76,77]

It is unlikely that the type of resuscitative fluid plays a primary role in the etiology of the syndrome. Hypervolemia produced by either type of fluid may produce pulmonary edema, but this responds quickly to standard treatment and should not be confused with the syndrome being described. Attempts at "drying out" the lung may be dangerous because a decrease in cardiac output secondary to hypovolemia may compound any pulmonary functional defect present.

ANATOMIC CHANGES

The pathologic changes in the lungs in most cases of ARDS are similar, regardless of the etiology. They depend predominately on the severity and duration of the disease.[60] In the early stages, the lungs may appear normal or show petechial hemorrhages and edema on cut section. With progression, the lungs become congested and hemorrhagic. Fibrinous exudates may develop on the pleural surface. As bronchopneumonia commonly supervenes, purulent bronchial secretions or frank abscesses may be present.

Microscopically the early signs are subtle. Fibrin and platelet microemboli filling pulmonary arterioles have been described.[7] This is followed by vascular congestion, interstitial edema, atelectasis, hypertrophy of alveolar lining cells, and later hemorrhage and intra-alveolar edema. Eventually, hyaline membranes appear and become the predominant lesion, while the changes of hemorrhage and congestion decrease in prominence. After a few days, bronchopneumonia is usually superimposed on the changes described.

TREATMENT

The concepts presented above will continue to be modified, as the pathophysiology of ARDS has yet to be completely delineated. For example, intrapulmonary shunting measured using a single inert gas consistently yields a lower value than that obtained by the oxygen inhalation method.[53] This implies that there are areas of the lung with very low ventilation-to-perfusion ratios which are not atelectatic but are behaving as a shunt. Studies using alveolar-arterial nitrogen gradients suggest the same possibility.[68] Recently West and Wagner using six inert gases have demonstrated such very low V/Q segments in patients with ARDS.[115] The common pattern, however, appears to be alveolar-capillary membrane injury with a pulmonary capillary protein leak. This results in interstitial pulmonary edema and subsequent derangements of the distribution of ventilation and perfusion.

Thus, therapeutic maneuvers could theoretically be directed at (1) manipulating pulmonary blood flow to increase the perfusion of well ventilated units and decrease the perfusion of poorly ventilated units; (2) directly reducing the capillary leak by reversing the membrane injury; (3) indirectly reducing the interstitial edema; or (4) improving ventilation of poorly ventilated segments and preventing further alveolar filling or collapse. The one which is most practical and which is most often used clinically is the latter. This involves using respiratory techniques designed to support and increase alveolar volume (PEEP or CPAP). These are described in Chap. 22.

There is a general impression that the earlier in the course such therapy is applied, the more successful it is likely to be. Thus it is important to identify and closely monitor patients at high risk for developing ARDS after injury. Table 32-6 indicates patients in the high-risk category. Of these five groups, patients who have either systemic and/or pulmonary sepsis are most likely to develop acute respiratory failure. They should be admitted to the intensive care unit for repeated evaluation of pulmonary function. Appropriate respiratory support and other therapy (as indicated below) is begun as early as significant abnormalities in

Table 32-6 Patients at Greatest Risk for Postinjury Respiratory Failure

Sepsis (systemic and pulmonary)

Massive soft tissue injury with or without long bone fractures

Direct pulmonary injury

Massive transfusion of whole blood

Aspiration of gastric contents

pulmonary function are detected by careful monitoring.

Monitoring Pulmonary Functioning

Assessment of the adequacy of pulmonary function should begin immediately postoperatively in those patients at risk for developing ARDS. Endotracheal tubes inserted for airway control during surgery should not be removed prematurely. In many patients an additional 4 to 6 h of intubation postoperatively will be sufficient to allow the physician to determine that ARDS is not a threat. Extubation is not considered until adequate lung function has been demonstrated (described below). If several days of intubation are contemplated, a nasotracheal tube may be substituted for the endotracheal tube in the operating room. This will allow for greater patient comfort and acceptance.

A prerequisite for optimal lung function is a normal cardiovascular status. Hemodynamic monitoring, therefore, should be instituted routinely. This would include recording of heart rate, arterial pressure, electrocardiogram, central venous pressure, and pulmonary artery pressure if indicated. Serial body weight, intake and output balance, bacteriologic studies, coagulation profile, and chest x-rays are important data to be obtained. A more thorough discussion of hemodynamic monitoring is contained in Chap. 31.

Monitoring of pulmonary function can be conveniently divided into three general areas: evaluation of oxygenation, ventilation, and lung-thorax mechanics. Table 32-7 details the most easily obtained tests with normal values included. As a general principle, isolated determinations are not as valuable as serial measurements obtained at regular intervals. Hypoxemia is often detected in apparently normal patients who appear to be doing well clinically.

The partial pressure of oxygen in the arterial blood (Pa_{O_2}) is the hallmark of determining the adequacy of oxygenation. This must be

Table 32-7 Assessment of Pulmonary Function

Function	Acceptable	Consider institution of therapy*
Oxygenation		
Partial pressure oxygen arterial blood	$Pa_{O_2} > 90$ mm on 40% $F_{I_{O_2}}$	<90 mm Hg on 40% $F_{I_{O_2}}$ or decreasing
Partial pressure oxygen arterial blood to fraction inspired oxygen ratio ($Pa_{O_2}/F_{I_{O_2}}$)	$Pa_{O_2}/F_{I_{O_2}} > 350$	<300
Alveolar-arterial oxygen gradient (breathing 100% O_2 for 10 to 15 min)	50-200 mmHg	>200 mmHg or increasing
Ventilation		
Partial pressure carbon dioxide arterial blood	35-40 mmHg	30 or decreasing
Minute volume	<12 L/min	Increasing
Mechanics		
Rate	12-25/min	25 or increasing
Effective compliance	50 cm³/cmH₂O	50 or decreasing

*Trends over a period of time are useful in marginal situations.

considered in the light of the inspired oxygen concentration ($F_{I_{O_2}}$). A simple means of establishing a measurable relationship between Pa_{O_2} and $F_{I_{O_2}}$ is their ratio ($Pa_{O_2}/F_{I_{O_2}}$). Ratios between 350 and 500 are considered adequate, while a value of less than 300 is frequently associated with continued deterioration of pulmonary function. This ratio provides the clinician with a gross estimation of the efficacy of oxygenation at the bedside during rapid changes in therapy. It appears to be most reliable when the $F_{I_{O_2}}$ is between 0.2 and 0.6.

The alveolar-arterial oxygen difference $D(A-a)_{O_2}$ with the patient breathing pure oxygen for 10 to 15 min, may allow rapid differentiation of the cause of hypoxemia. Of the four causes of hypoxemia (hypoventilation, diffusion defects, ventilation-perfusion abnormalities, and pulmonary shunt) only the intrapulmonary shunt is theoretically refractory to O_2

administration. In general, this relationship holds true. However, the $D(A-a)_{O_2}$ is affected by cardiac output, O_2 consumption, the position of Hgb-O_2 dissociation curve and the magnitude of the pulmonary shunt. If the three other variables are constant, then the $D(A-a)_{O_2}$ is a good reflection of the amount of pulmonary shunting. Characteristically, the patient with ARDS will have hypoxemia resistant to oxygen administration and therefore an elevated shunt fraction.

The adequacy of ventilation is determined by the arterial partial pressure of carbon dioxide (Pa_{CO_2}). By definition, hypoventilation occurs when the Pa_{CO_2} is elevated. Postinjury pulmonary failure is usually associated with hypocarbia (hyperventilation). The patient in such a situation, with both a decreased Pa_{CO_2} and Pa_{O_2}, probably has ARDS. Tidal volume (V_T) (the amount of air breathed during one respiratory cycle) is another indication of the adequacy of ventilation. This is readily measured with a modestly priced respirometer. VT multiplied by the respiratory rate is called the minute ventilation. This value is easily derived, but by itself is only a rough guide to adequate ventilation. In many postinjury patients high minute ventilations are recorded. It is not established whether this is a compensatory response or an indicator of pathology.

The effective compliance (C_{eff}) may be quite valuable as an assessment of the ease of distensibility of lung and thoracic cage. This derived value is obtained by dividing the VT by the airway pressure required to hold the lungs inflated. C_{eff} indicates the "stiffness" of the lungs, i.e., how difficult they are to ventilate (low C_{eff} means increased stiffness). A decreased C_{eff} may indicate increased extravascular lung water, airway constriction, or increased chest wall resistance (impaired bellows activity). Low values are usually found in patients with ARDS.

An adequate assessment of pulmonary function can be achieved by serial measurement of arterial blood gases, tidal volume minute ventilation, and the effective compliance. Several other monitoring devices have been advocated. Of these, the work of breathing is almost always increased in ARDS. This value is a measure of the mechanical cost of achieving adequate ventilation. Peters et al. have reported on the efficacy of the work of breathing measurement in predicting the need for ventilatory support.[86] The major disadvantage of this test is that it requires an intraesophageal balloon to measure transthoracic pressure and the availability of an analogue computer for usable results.[84] Although highly desirable, the work of breathing is difficult to obtain in the critically ill patient.

Although sophisticated and expensive equipment is available to continuously monitor arterial and venous blood gases and other pulmonary function tests, they have not been shown to significantly improve patient survival.[25,87,111]

Ventilatory Support

There are no universal guidelines for the institution of ventilatory support. The guidelines outlined in Table 32-7 have been found to be reliable in treating a large number of patients. The most common indication for beginning ventilatory therapy is hypoxemia. Initial management should be to increase the $F_{I_{O_2}}$ both as a diagnostic test and to temporarily relieve hypoxemia if the Pa_{O_2} is less than 65 mmHg. For effective therapy, control of the airway must be achieved. The most rapid and reliable way to do this is the insertion of an endotracheal or nasotracheal tube. Mechanical ventilation may then be applied. Since a defect in the matching of ventilation to perfusion is present, this therapy is directed at trying to maintain ventilation to marginally ventilated alveoli and the recruitment of collapsed or partially occluded alveoli. This will directly increase the FRC of the lungs. In general, respiratory support (PEEP, CPAP, ↑VT) is initiated when the parameters listed in Table 32-7 fall outside the acceptable ranges. As described in Chap. 22, progressively more vigorous ventilatory support is employed until "acceptable" levels of oxygenation and ventilation are obtained.

Oxygen Carrying Capacity of Blood

Although the Pa_{O_2} can be increased by higher levels of $F_{I_{O_2}}$, it is the red blood cell that carries almost all the O_2 to the tissues. One unit of packed red cells carries more O_2 than plasma exposed to pure O_2 at hyperbaric pressure. Therefore, the hemoglobin (Hgb) concentration should be maintained between 12 and 14 g per 100 mL. Attention should also be given to the acid-base status of the patient. Both acidosis and alkalosis produce shifts of the Hgb-O_2 dissociation curve which can affect the ability of Hgb to off-load O_2 at the tissue level (see Chap. 22).

Diuretics

Administration of diuretics has been proposed as a method for indirectly decreasing the amount of interstitial edema. However, reports in the literature that claim a therapeutic role for diuretics in treating ARDS are not conclusive.[33,36] There is no study which has randomly and prospectively shown that diuretics are as effective or more effective than ventilatory therapy alone. Our practice is to give small doses of furosemide *when hemodynamic studies indicate that fluid overload has occurred*, e.g., an elevated pulmonary artery wedge pressure. No attempt is made to "dry out" the patient by the long-term administration of diuretics. There is no solid evidence to suggest that lowering fluid volumes below normal will decrease the leak from injured capillaries. Such decreases in volume may have a serious deleterious effect if they result in a decreased cardiac output.[64]

Fluid Management

As noted in the discussion of the etiology of ARDS, there is much debate concerning proper fluid management. It is our opinion that maintenance of normal fluid balance is important. This will obviate any deleterious effects of hypovolemia on the Pa_{O_2} and minimize any decrease in cardiac output which may occur with PEEP administration. We rarely administer colloids for reasons previously discussed.

Steroids

Despite extensive interest in their use, there is no conclusive proof that pharmacologic doses of steroids should be part of the specific therapy of the ARDS syndrome.[12,34,55,80,119] Data do exist to indicate that steroids may be effective in treating pulmonary fat embolism, septic shock, and aspiration of gastric acid.

Thus, we reserve high-dose steroid therapy of short duration for those clinical entities.

Heparin

If intravascular coagulation can be shown to be a problem in the postinjury patient with ARDS, then appropriate heparin therapy may be of benefit.[8,85] Heparin is associated with significant side effects and should not be used indiscriminately in the patient who has recently sustained a traumatic injury.

Antibiotics

Prophylactic use of broad-spectrum antibiotics has no place in the primary therapy of ARDS. Indiscriminate use of these agents may allow the emergence of resistant strains of bacteria which are very difficult to treat. Many patients will already have been given antibiotics because of certain types of injury. Specific antibiotics are used to treat pulmonary sepsis. Their choice is determined by serial cultures of the sputum.

Ancillary Pulmonary Care

Patients treated in the ICU tend to be bound to the bed by numerous tubes, wires, and catheters. Change in position then becomes a difficult problem. It has been shown, however, that significant improvement in oxygenation can result from frequent position changes.[18] Maintenance of one position is likely to compound pulmonary abnormalities.[117]

Routine pulmonary toilet, suctioning with sterile technique, and attempts to prevent pulmonary infection are very important. These must all be done on a routine basis.

SUMMARY

The syndrome of acute pulmonary failure, as it occurs in the injured patient, has many possible causes. The definable causes are amenable to specific modes of therapy. The chief functional defect, hypoxemia unresponsive to increased $F_{I_{O_2}}$, is treated with ventilatory therapy $\pm$ PEEP on an empiric basis.

With early aggressive ventilatory support, morbidity and mortality may be minimized. Adjunctive therapy may play a significant role when specific indications exist.

BIBLIOGRAPHY

1 Ashbaugh, D. G. et al.: Continuous positive-pressure breathing (CPPB) in adult respiratory distress syndrome, *J. Thorac. Cardiovasc. Surg.,* 57:31, 1969.

2 ――――, D. B. Bigelow, T. L. Petty, and B. E. Levine: Acute respiratory distress in adults, *Lancet,* 2:319, 1967.

3 ―――― and T. L. Petty: Sepsis complicating acute respiratory distress syndrome, *Surg. Gynecol. Obstet.,* 135:865, 1972.

4 Bave, A. E.: The pushmi-pullyu syndrome, *Surgery,* 72:655, 1972.

5 Berke, J. F., H. Pontopiddan, and C. E. Welch: High output respiratory failure: An important cause of death ascribed to peritonitis and ileus, *Ann. Surg.,* 158:581, 1963.

6 Berman, I. R. et al.: Pulmonary microembolism after soft tissue injury in primates, *Surgery,* 70:246, 1971.

7 Blaisdell, W. F.: Pathophysiology of the respiratory distress syndrome, *Arch. Surg.,* 108:44, 1974.

8 ―――― and F. R. Lewis: "Etiologic Factors in the Respiratory Distress Syndrome," in *Respiratory Distress Syndrome of Shock and Trauma,* W. B. Saunders Company, Philadelphia, 1977.

9 ―――― and R. M. Schlobohm: The respiratory distress syndrome: A review, *Surgery,* 74:251, 1973.

10 Bredenberg, C. E. et al.: Respiratory failure in shock, *Ann. Surg.,* 169:392, 1969.

11 Brigham, K. L., W. C. Woolverton, L. H. Blake, et al.: Increased sheep lung vascular permeability caused by *Pseudomonas* bacteria, *J. Clin. Invest.,* 54:792, 1974.

12 Brothers, J. R., G. Olsen, and H. C. Polk, Jr.: Enhancement of infection by corticosteroids, *Surg. Forum,* 14:30, 1973.

13 Buckberg, G. D. et al.: Pulmonary changes following hemorrhagic shock and resuscitation in baboons, *J. Thorac. Cardiovasc. Surg.,* 59: 450, 1970.

14 Burford, T. H. and B. Burbank: Traumatic wet lung: Observations on certain physiologic fundamentals of thoracic trauma, *J. Thorac. Surg.,* 14:415, 1945.

15 Camerson, J. L. et al.: Aspiration pneumonia: A clinical and experimental review, *J. Lung Res.,* 7:44, 1967.

16 Carey, L. C. et al.: Hemorrhagic shock, *Curr. Probl. Surg.* January 1971.

17 Churchill, E. D.: Pulmonary atelectasis with special reference to massive collapse of lung, *Arch. Surg.,* 11:489, 1925.

18 Clauss, R. H. et al.: Effects of changing body position upon improved ventilation-perfusion relationships, *Circulation, Suppl. II,* 37, 38:214, 1968.

19 Clowes, G., Jr. et al.: Circulatory factors in the etiology of pulmonary insufficiency and R heart failure accompanying severe sepsis (peritonitis), *Ann. Surg.,* 171:663, 1970.

20 ――――: The nonspecific pulmonary inflammatory reaction leading to respiratory failure after shock, gangrene and sepsis, *J. Trauma,* 8:899, 1968.

21 Coalson, J. J. et al.: The pulmonary ultrastructure in septic shock, *Exp. Mol. Pathol.,* 12:84, 1970.

22 Collins, J. A.: The causes of progressive pulmonary insufficiency in surgical patients, *J. Surg. Res.,* 9:685, 1969.

23 ―――― et al.: Inapparent hypoxemia in casualties with wounded limbs: Pulmonary fat embolism?, *Ann. Surg.,* 167:511, 1968.

24 Connell, R. S., R. L. Swank, and M. C. Webb: The development of pulmonary ultrastructural lesions during hemorrhagic shock, *J. Trauma,* 15:116, 1975.

25 Dardik, H. et al.: On-line in vivo measurements of partial pressures of oxygen and carbon dioxide of blood, tissue and respired air by mass spectrometry, *Surg. Gynecol. Obstet.,* 131:1157, 1970.

26 Derks, C. M. and R. M. Peters: Role of shock and fat embolus in leakage from pulmonary

capillaries, *Surg. Gynecol. Obstet.*, **187**:945, 1973.

27 Ducher, T. B.: Increased intracranial pressure and pulmonary edema, *J. Neurosurg.*, **28**:112, 1968.

28 Eaton, R. M.: Pulmonary edema: Experimental observation on dogs following acute peripheral blood loss, *J. Thorac. Surg.*, **16**:668, 1947.

29 Eisenman, B. and D. G. Ashbaugh: Pulmonary effects of nonthoracic trauma: Proceedings of a conference conducted by the Committee on Trauma, a division of Medical Sciences, National Research Council, *J. Trauma*, **8**, 1968.

30 Elliot, T. R. and L. A. Dingley: Massive collapse of the lungs following abdominal operation, *Lancet*, **1**:1305, 1914.

31 Farrington, G. H. et al.: Blood borne factors in the pulmonary response to sepsis (acute experimental peritonitis), *Surgery*, **68**:136, 1970.

32 Finley, R. J. et al.: Pulmonary edema in patients with sepsis, *Surg. Gynecol. Obstet.*, **140**:851, 1975.

33 Fleming, W. H. and J. C. Bowen: The use of diuretics in the treatment of early wet lung syndrome, *Ann. Surg.*, **175**:505, 1972.

34 Franz, J. L., J. D. Richardson, F. L. Grover, and J. K. Trinkle: Effect of methylprednisolone sodium succinate on experimental pulmonary contusion, *J. Thorac. Cardiovasc. Surg.*, **68**:842, 1974.

35 Fulton, R. L. and C. E. Jones: The cause of post-traumatic pulmonary insufficiency in man, *Surg. Gynecol. Obstet.*, **140**:179, 1975.

36 Geiger, J. P. and I. Gielchinsky: Acute pulmonary insufficiency, *Arch. Surg.*, **102**:400, 1971.

37 Gerst, P. H. et al.: The effects of hemorrhage on pulmonary circulation and respiratory gas exchange, *J. Clin. Invest.*, **38**:524, 1959.

38 Giordano, J. M. et al.: The management of interstitial pulmonary edema: Significance of hypoproteinemia, *J. Thorac. Cardiovasc. Surg.*, **64**:739, 1972.

39 Greenfield, L. J.: Pulmonary dysfunction in shock: The Fundamental mechanisms of shock, *Adv. Exp. Med. Biol.*, **23**:47, 1972.

40 —— et al.: Pulmonary oxygen toxicity in experimental hemorrhagic shock, *Surgery*, **68**:662, 1970.

41 Groves, A. C. et al.: Fibrin thrombi and the pulmonary microcirculation of dogs with gram negative bacteremia, *Surg. Gynecol. Obstet.*, **134**:433, 1972.

42 Guenter, C. A. et al.: Cardiorespiratory and metabolic responses to live *E. coli* and endotoxin in the monkey, *J. Appl. Physiol.*, **26**:780, 1969.

43 Gump, F. E. et al.: Pre and postmortem studies of lung volume and electrolytes, *J. Trauma*, **11**:474, 1971.

44 Hardaway, R. M.: Disseminated intravascular coagulation as a possible cause of acute respiratory failure, *Surg. Gynecol. Obstet.*, **137**:419, 1973.

45 Hedden, M. and G. J. Miller: Mendelson's syndrome and its sequelae, *Can. Anaesth. Soc. J.*, **19**:351, 1972.

46 Herndon, J. H. et al.: Fat embolism: A review of current concepts, *J. Trauma*, **11**:673, 1971.

47 Hillen, G. P., W. D. Gaisford, and G. G. Jenson: Pulmonary changes in treated and untreated hemorrhagic shock: Early functional and ultrastructural alterations after moderate shock, *Am. J. Surg.*, **122**:639, 1971.

48 Hinshaw, L. B. et al.: Cardiovascular responses of the primate in endotoxin shock, *Am. J. Physiol.*, **210**:335, 1966.

49 Hirsch, E. F., R. Fletcher, and S. Lucas: Hemodynamic and respiratory changes associated with sepsis following combat trauma, *Ann. Surg.*, **174**:211, 1971.

50 Holcroft, J. W. and D. D. Trunkey: Pulmonary extravasation of albumin during and after hemorrhagic shock in baboons, *Ann. Surg.*, **180**:408, 1974.

51 ——, ——, and R. C. Lim: Further analysis of lung water in baboons resuscitated from hemorrhagic shock, *J. Surg. Res.*, **20**:291, 1976.

52 Horovitz, J. H. and C. J. Carrico: Lung colloid permeability in hemorrhagic shock, *Surg. Forum*, **23**:6, 1972.

53 ——, ——, J. Maher, and G. T. Shires: Pulmonary shunt determination: A comparison between oxygen inhalation and Xe(133) method, *J. Lab. Clin. Med.*, **78**:785, 1971.

54 ——, ——, and G. T. Shires: Pulmonary response to major injury, *Arch. Surg.*, **105**:699, 1974.

55 Hughes, A. and R. S. Tonks: Lung and heart lesions from intravascular platelet clumping and its sequelae, *J. Pathol. Bacteriol.*, **95**:523, 1968.

56 Huller, T. and Y. Bazini: Blast injuries of the chest and abdomen, *Arch. Surg.*, **100**:24, 1970.

57 Kafer, E. R.: Pulmonary oxygen toxicity: A review of the evidence for acute and chronic oxygen toxicity in man, *Br. J. Anaesth.*, **43**:687, 1971.

58 Kim, S. I. et al.: Sequential respiratory changes in an experimental hemorrhage shock preparation designed to simulate clinical shock, *Ann. Surg.*, **170**:166, 1969.

59 Laennec, R. T. H.: De L'auscultation médiate ou traité du diagnostic des maladies des poumons et du coeur, fondé principalement sur ce nouveau moyen d'exploration, Paris, 1819.

60 Lamy, M., R. J. Fallat, E. Koeniger, et al.: Pathologic features and mechanisms of hypoxemia in adult respiratory distress syndrome, *Am. Rev. Respir. Dis.*, **114**:267, 1976.

61 Laurenzi, G. A., S. Yin, and J. J. Guarneri: Adverse effect of oxygen on tracheal mucus flow, *N. Engl. J. Med.*, **279**:333, 1968.

62 Lim, R. C. et al.: Pulmonary microvascular changes following regional shock: A clinical and experimental study, *Bull. Soc. Int. Chir.*, **1**:22, 1968.

63 Lowe, R., G. Moss, J. Jilele, et al.: Crystalloid versus colloid in the etiology of pulmonary failure after trauma, presented at the 38th Annual Meeting of the Society of University Surgeons, published in *Surgery*, 1977.

64 Lucas, C. E., J. G. Zito, K. M. Carter, A. Cortez, and F. C. Stebner: Questionable value of furosemide in preventing renal failure, *Surgery*, **82**:314, 1977.

65 McLaughlin, J. S.: Physiologic consideration of hypoxemia in shock and trauma, *Ann. Surg.*, **173**:667, 1971.

66 McNamara, J. J. et al.: Clinical fat embolism in combat casualties. *Ann. Surg.*, **176**:54, 1972.

67 ——: Screen filtration pressure in combat casualties, *Ann. Surg.*, **172**:334, 1970.

68 Marhello, R. et al.: Assessment of ventilation perfusion inequalities by arterial alveolar nitrogen differences in intensive care patients, *Anesthiology*, **37**:4, 1972.

69 Martin, A. M., Jr. et al.: Pathologic anatomy of the lungs following shock and trauma, *J. Trauma*, **8**:687, 1968.

70 Milligan, G. F. et al.: Pulmonary and hematologic disturbances during septic shock, *Surg. Gynecol. Obstet.*, **138**:43, 1974.

71 Mills, M.: The clinical syndrome, *J. Trauma*, **8**:651, 1968.

72 Moore, F. D. et al.: *Post-traumatic Pulmonary Insufficiency*, W. B. Saunders Company, Philadelphia, 1969.

73 Mosely, R. V. and D. B. Doty: Changes in the filtration characteristics of stored blood, *Ann. Surg.*, **171**:329, 1970.

74 Moss, G.: The role of the central nervous system in shock: The centrineurogenic etiology of the respiratory distress syndrome, Critical Care Medicine **2**:181, 1974.

75 —— et al.: Effect of hemorrhagic shock on pulmonary interstitial sodium distribution in the primate lung, *Ann. Surg.*, **177**:211, 1973.

76 ——: Effect of saline solution resuscitation on pulmonary sodium and water distribution, *Surg. Gynecol. Obstet.*, **136**:934, 1973.

77 ——: Effects of saline and colloid solutions on pulmonary function in hemorrhagic shock, *Surg. Gynecol. Obstet.*, **133**:53, 1971.

78 ——: Morphologic changes in the primate lung after hemorrhagic shock, *Surg. Gynecol. Obstet.*, **134**:3, 1972.

79 ——: Ventilatory response to hemorrhagic shock and resuscitation, *Surgery*, **72**:451, 1972.

80 Murray, J. F.: Conference report: Mechanisms of acute respiratory failure, *Am. Rev. Respir. Dis.*, **115**:1071, 1977.

81 Naimark, A. et al.: Regional pulmonary blood flow and gas exchange in hemorrhagic shock, *J. Appl. Physiol.*, **25**:301, 1968.

82 Nash, G. et al.: "Respirator lung": A misnomer, *Arch. Pathol.*, **21**:234, 1971.

83 Nichols, R. T. et al.: Effects of experimental pulmonary contusion on respiratory exchange and lung mechanics, *Arch. Surg.*, **96**:723, 1968.

84 Neely, W. A. et al.: Postoperative respiratory

insufficiency: Physiologic studies with therapeutic implications, *Ann. Surg.*, **171**:679, 1970.

85 Olcott, C., R. E. Barber, and F. W. Blaisdell: Diagnosis and treatment of respirator failure after civilian trauma, *Am. J. Surg.*, **122**:260, 1971.

86 Peters, R. M. et al.: Objective indications for respiratory therapy in post-trauma and postoperative patients, *Am. J. Surg.*, **124**:262, 1972.

87 —— and R. W. Stacy: Automatized clinical measurement of respiratory parameters, *Surgery*, **56**:44, 1964.

88 Petty, T. L.: *Intensive and Rehabilitative Respiratory Care*, 2d ed., Lea & Febiger, Philadelphia, 1974.

89 Pierce, A. K. et al: Long-term evaluation of decontamination of inhalation therapy equipment and the occurrence of necrotizing pneumonia, *N. Engl. J. Med.*, **282**:528, 1970.

90 Pinardi, G., E. Leal, A. Sallas Coll: Vascular permeability to red blood cells and protein in hemorrhagic shock, *Acta. Physiol. Lat. Amer.*, **17**:175, 1967.

91 Pontoppidan, H. et al.: Acute respiratory failure in adults, *N. Engl. J. Med.*, **287**:690, 1972.

92 ——, M. B. Laver, and B. Geffen: Acute respiratory failure in the surgical patient, *Adv. Surg.*, **4**:163, 1970.

93 Proctor, H. G. et al.: An analysis of pulmonary function following nonthoracic trauma with recommendations for therapy, *Ann. Surg.*, **172**:180, 1970.

94 ——: Analysis of pulmonary function following penetrating pulmonary injury with recommendations for therapy, *Surgery*, **68**:92, 1970.

95 Reid, S. et al.: Effect on pulmonary ultrastructure of Dacron-wool filtration during cardiopulmonary bypass, *Ann. Thorac. Surg.*, **15**:217, 1973.

96 Robin, E. D. et al.: Capillary leak syndrome with pulmonary edema, *Arch. Intern. Med.*, **130**:66, 1972.

97 Rubin, J. W.: Impaired pulmonary surfactant synthesis in starvation and severe nonthoracic sepsis, *Am. J. Surg.*, **123**:461, 1972.

98 Sachner, M. A. et al.: Pulmonary effects of oxygen breathing, *Ann. Intern. Med.*, **82**:40, 1975.

99 Sackner, M. A., J. A. Hirsch, S. Epstein, and A. M. Rywlin: Effect of oxygen in graded concentrations upon tracheal mucous velocity: A study in anesthetized dogs, *Chest*, **69**:164, 1976.

100 Sealy, W. C. et al.: Functional and structural changes in the lungs in hemorrhagic shock, *Surg. Gynecol. Obstet.*, **122**:754, 1966.

101 Shires, G. T., C. J. Carrico, and P. C. Canizaro: Shock: Major problems in clinical surgery, W. B. Saunders Company, Philadelphia, vol. XIII, 1973.

102 Siegel, D. C. et al.: The ventilatory response to hemorrhagic shock and resuscitation, *Surgery*, **72**:451, 1972.

103 Silvershmid, M., K. P. Szczepanski, and C. Lund: Normal lung function during experimental shock, *Eur. Surg. Res.*, **5**:1, 1973.

104 Simmons, R. L. et al.: Respiratory insufficiency in combat casualties: Pulmonary edema following head injury, *Ann. Surg.*, **170**:39, 1969.

105 Skilman, J. J. et al.: Pulmonary arterovenous admixture: Improvement with albumin and diuresis, *Am. J. Surg.*, **119**:450, 1970.

106 Stallone, R. J. et al.: Pulmonary changes following ischemia of lower extremities and their treatment, *Am. Rev. Respir. Dis.*, **100**:813, 1969.

107 Staub, N. C.: Pathogenesis of pulmonary edema, *Am. Rev. Respir. Dis.*, **109**:358, 1974.

108 Sugg, W. F. et al.: Congestive atelectasis: An experimental study, *Ann. Surg.*, **168**:234, 1968.

109 Terzi, R. G. and R. M. Peters: The effect of large fluid loads on lung mechanics and work, *Ann. Thorac. Surg.*, **6**:16, 1968.

110 Thomas, A. N. and A. D. Hall: Mechanism of pulmonary injury after oxygen therapy, *Am. J. Surg.*, **120**:255, 1970.

111 Turney, S. Z. et al.: Respiratory monitoring: Recent developments in automatic monitoring of gas concentration, flow, pressure and temperature, *Ann. Thorac. Surg.*, **16**:184, 1973.

112 Vito, L., R. C. Dennis, R. D. Weisel, and H. B. Hechtman: Sepsis presenting as acute respiratory insufficiency, *Surg. Gynecol. Obstet.*, **138**:896, 1974.

113 Vreim, C. E. and N. C. Staub: Protein compo-

sition of lung fluids in acute alloxan edema in dogs, *Am. J. Physiol.*, **230**:376, 1976.

114 Wagensteen, O. D., L. E. Sittmers, and J. A. Johnson: Permeability of the mammalian blood gas barrier and its components, *Am. J. Physiol.*, **216**:719, 1969.

115 Wagner, P. D., H. A. Saltzman, and J. B. West: Measurement of continuous distributions of ventilation-perfusion ratios: Theory, *J. Appl. Physiol.*, **36**:588, 1974.

116 Wahrenbrock, E. A. et al.: Increased atelectatic pulmonary shunt during hemorrhagic shock in dogs, *J. Appl. Physiol.*, **29**:615, 1970.

117 ———: The effect of posture on pulmonary function and survival of anesthetized dogs, *J. Surg. Res.*, **10**:13, 1970.

118 Walker, L. and B. Eisenman: The changing pattern of post-traumatic respiratory distress syndrome, *Ann. Surg.*, **181**:693, 1975.

119 Wilson, J. W.: Treatment or prevention of pulmonary cellular damage with pharmacologic doses of corticosteroid, *Surg. Gynecol. Obstet.*, **134**:675, 1972.

120 Wolfe, W. G., P. A. Ebert, and D. C. Sabiston, Jr.: Effect of high oxygen tension on mucociliary function, *Surgery*, **72**:246, 1972.

121 Wyche, M. Q. et al.: Lung function, pulmonary extravascular water volume and hemodynamics in early hemorrhagic shock in anesthetized dogs, *Ann. Surg.*, **174**:296, 1971.

Chapter 33

Nutritional Support of the Traumatized Patient

P. William Curreri, M.D.

During the past two decades hospital mortality, as a consequence of serious injury, has been markedly reduced. Increased survival during the early posttraumatic period has been noted, even though more seriously injured patients now reach the hospital emergency room as a result of consistent improvement in ground and air transportation systems and the development of sophisticated prehospital therapy by paramedical personnel. Undoubtedly the increased survival of massively traumatized patients is related to improved diagnostic and therapeutic modalities for the treatment of shock, pulmonary dysfunction, occult injury, and postoperative complications. In addition, the development of in-

house trauma teams consisting of specialized physicians, nurses, technicians, and other paramedical personnel has allowed the delivery of a high level of around-the-clock intensive care to patients with rapidly changing pathophysiological demands.

Nevertheless, late deaths are not uncommon among patients with severe trauma as a result of septic complications or failure of wound healing. Often the fatal complications are a manifestation of acute nutritional deficiency and may be successfully avoided if the nutritional requirements of the patient are met in the early postoperative period. For this reason it is important to emphasize the nutritional requirements of the seriously injured patient and to outline practical means of providing sufficient calories and nitrogen to ensure positive energy balance.

PHYSIOLOGICAL RESPONSE TO MAJOR INJURY

Although the metabolic response to injury has been comprehensively reviewed in Chap. 3, several principles require reemphasis in order to quantitate the nutritional requirement for the seriously injured patient. Major injury is characterized by a hypermetabolic response. Roe and Kinney[15,21] have demonstrated that the resting metabolic expenditure is increased in patients with major injury and that the magnitude and duration of the hypermetabolism is related to the severity of the sustained trauma. Patients with major thermal injury exhibit an exceedingly high resting metabolic expenditure, often reaching $1\frac{1}{2}$ to 2 times normal, a level which exceeds the metabolic rate of patients with severe thyrotoxicosis. Obviously, hypermetabolism of this magnitude is associated with markedly increased energy requirements.

The daily expenditure of energy in the seriously injured patient can be estimated by either direct or indirect calorimetry. Reiss,[20] utilizing oxygen consumption measurements, estimated the resting metabolic rate of the young adult patient with major burns to be approximately 1600 kcal/m² body surface per 24 h. Total daily energy consumption during the nonresting state in the severely injured patient may exceed 5000 kcal/day. Confirmation of such excessive energy consumption has been obtained by the direct measurement of heat loss (direct calorimetry) from severely burned patients.[2]

Wilmore[28] has recently reported detailed metabolic studies of 29 adults with major thermal burns, all of whom were evaluated in an environmental chamber at two or more temperatures ranging between 19 and 30°C at a constant vapor pressure. He noted a very close correlation between energy production and the rate of catecholamine secretion. The hypermetabolic response was blocked by the administration of alpha- and beta-adrenergic blocking agents. Likewise, the infusion of epinephrine was associated with an increased metabolic rate in unburned controls under the same experimental conditions. The hypermetabolic response was exaggerated by reducing the ambient temperature in the environmental chamber below 25°C or by the occurrence of a septic complication. However, the baseline metabolic response of injured patients under ideal environmental conditions remained elevated when compared to controls. Skin temperature of burned patients was elevated, indicating they were externally warm. These results suggest that the hypermetabolic response is secondary to alterations in central nervous system temperature control mediated via hypothalamic centers.

In addition to elevated energy requirements, a marked catabolic response accompanies severe trauma. This catabolic response to injury is associated with weight loss, retarded wound healing, and negative nitrogen, potassium, sulfur, and phosphorous balance. Again, many investigators have noted that both the magnitude and the duration of the catabolic response roughly parallels the severity of trauma. Up to 30 g of nitrogen/day may often be recovered from the urine of severely injured patients. If extraordinary means to provide excessive dietary nitrogen are not pursued, negative nitrogen balance may be observed for up to 40 to 60 days following the traumatic insult. However, protein catabolism does not proceed uniformly in all tissues. It is apparent that the structural and functional integrity of vital organs such as the heart and liver are maintained at the expense of muscle protein.[16]

It is known that posttraumatic negative nitrogen balance can be ameliorated if sufficient caloric and nitrogen intake is provided.[4,24,25]

However, practical and safe methods for achieving the required intake have not always been available to the practicing physician during the early postinjury period. Soroff[24] and his associates have calculated the nitrogen requirements following major thermal injury by regression analysis of urinary nitrogen excretion following various levels of nitrogen intake. More than 20 g of nitrogen/m^2 body surface per day are required during the first postburn month in order to maintain positive nitrogen balance. During the second postburn month, nitrogen intakes of 13 to 16 g of nitrogen/m^2 per day will maintain nitrogen equilibrium.

Though nitrogen excretion is markedly increased following trauma, muscle protein is not the only tissue catabolized as an energy source. Human studies of oxygen consumption, carbon dioxide production, and nitrogen excretion following various types of extensive trauma by Duke[12] and his coworkers would suggest that the caloric contribution of body fat stores to the elevated resting metabolic expenditure is approximately 80 percent as opposed to 20 percent of the calories supplied by endogenous protein.

Wilmore and his associates[27] have recently shown that plasma glucagon and catecholamine levels are strikingly elevated during the posttraumatic hypermetabolic response. On the other hand, plasma insulin levels are initially quite depressed and return toward normal only as glucagon and catecholamine levels fall. Human limb perfusion experiments by Cahill[6] have uncovered the importance of insulin in regulating the release of amino acids from muscle as a source of energy. Insulin deprivation is associated with mobilization of fatty acids from fat depots as a secondary source of energy. During brief fasting periods, the liver is rapidly depleted of its carbohydrate stores, i.e., glycogen. As blood glucose and insulin concentrations in the plasma decrease, amino acids are mobilized from muscle. These are converted in the liver to glucose via gluconeogenesis, and serve as a source of energy for the brain and hematopoietic tissues. After 3 to 4 days of fasting in normal, *uninjured* humans, keto acids, which result from the metabolism of fat, gradually replace glucose as a source of energy for the brain. However, in massively traumatized patients, metabolic products of fat oxidation are not utilized efficiently by the central nervous system as an energy source; therefore, there remains an obligatory requirement for the catabolism of lean muscle mass unless sufficient nitrogen is supplied exogenously. Cahill[7] has also demonstrated that the infusion of glucagon in human subjects results in increased glucose production, decreased concentration of glucogenic amino acids, and normal or slightly elevated levels of branched-chain amino acids. These observations support the contention that glucagon stimulates hepatic gluconeogenesis, whereas insulin stimulates amino acid uptake by muscle as well as increased protein synthesis. Blackburn[14] and his associates have extended these observations and have shown that the magnitude of the catabolic response may be decreased in starving humans for short periods of time by avoiding the intravenous infusion of isotonic solutions of glucose and, instead, substituting isotonic solutions of amino acids.

CLINICAL CONSEQUENCES OF INADEQUATE NUTRITIONAL REPLACEMENT

The body composition of a normal 70-kg male includes 48.7 kg of water and minerals, 0.3 kg of carbohydrates, 6 kg of protein, and 15 kg of fat. Total oxidation of such an individual would yield approximately 166,000 kcal. It is estimated that healthy individuals will tolerate acute losses of up to one-third lean body weight before death ensues. Thus, an extensively injured adult, with energy requirements of 5000 cal/day, becomes a severe nutritional risk in approximately 11 days, assuming no caloric intake.

Death, as a result of acute nutritional deficiency, can be insidious and masquerade in many clinical forms. However, since most of the kinetic energy requirements of the supine, bedridden patient are associated with the maintenance of normal respiratory function, the most common cause of death in these patients is pulmonary sepsis. An ineffective respiratory effort results in progressive atelectasis with subsequent lung infection by opportunistic pathogens.

It is clear that unless extraordinary means are taken to provide sufficient exogenous calories in order to prevent negative energy balance, weight loss will inevitably follow serious injury. In a retrospective study,[8] the Brooke Army Burn Unit showed an average weight loss of more than 25 percent of the preburn weight within the first 8 postburn weeks in patients with greater than 40 percent total body surface burns. These extraordinary examples of malnutrition occurred despite energetic attempts to provide the patients with high-caloric, nitrogen meals, as well as between-meal nutritional supplements. Voluntary intake of calories rarely exceeded preburn habitual caloric intakes, even in the most cooperative patients.

Not only was this profound weight loss associated with delayed reepithelialization of second-degree burn wounds and the development of unhealthy granulation tissue in areas of third-degree burn wounds, but in addition, the superior mesenteric artery syndrome was often observed in patients suffering the most pronounced weight loss.[19] This syndrome presents itself as a functional obstruction of the third portion of the duodenum and presumably results from the loss of fat in the retroperitoneum, with subsequent narrowing of the angle between the aorta and the superior mesenteric artery, through which the duode-

num must pass. With loss of the enteral route as a source of nutritional supplementation, negative nitrogen balance and weight loss became more pronounced.

In addition to the unfavorable physiological consequences of malnutrition outlined above, it has recently been demonstrated that the cellular metabolism of erythrocytes, isolated from severely burned patients maintained in negative energy balance for more than a week, is severely impaired.[9] Significant elevation of red blood cell intracellular sodium concentration is observed in these patients, whereas normal concentrations of intracellular sodium are maintained in those patients receiving enough exogenous calories to meet their nutritional needs. Further analysis of erythrocyte transmembrane sodium efflux and influx revealed that the increased intracellular sodium concentration in malnourished patients resulted from severe inhibition of the active transport (sodium pump) mechanism. Thus the metabolic performance of erythrocytes from malnourished, thermally injured patients mimics the "sick cell syndrome" observed in dying organs. Interestingly, the sodium pump defect could be reversed within 72 h when adequate exogenous caloric intake was reinstituted.

NUTRITIONAL MANAGEMENT OF THE SEVERELY INJURED PATIENT

Current nutritional management of the patient with severe injury should be directed in four principal areas: control of the external environment, early operative repair of injured organs with prompt wound closure, prevention of septic complications, and provision of adequate exogenous nutrition to prevent negative energy balance.

Since catecholamine secretion is markedly influenced by external stimuli, every effort should be made to modify the environment so as to minimize the hypermetabolic response resulting from excessive circulating catecholamines. This can be accomplished by alleviating patient discomfort associated with a cold environment. In addition, apprehension and pain should be treated appropriately with narcotics and tranquilizers, since both these stresses are known to potentiate the regulation of catecholamine secretion via the hypothalamus. Every effort should be made to effect early operative repair of major injury after fluid resuscitation has been established, for it has been well documented that amelioration of the catabolic and hypermetabolic responses occurs coincident with successful repair of major tissue injury. Only a few days of negative energy and nitrogen balance is observed in the patient with minor intraabdominal injury that has been completely repaired at exploratory laparotomy, while the patient with major intraabdominal injury and significant postoperative complications may display hypermetabolism and catabolism for several weeks. Normal metabolic rate and anabolism are not observed in patients with major burns until the eschar has been entirely removed and the wound covered with skin grafts (about 8 weeks).

The provision of adequate exogenous calories and nitrogen to prevent prolonged catabolism following major injury is obviously the cornerstone of nutritional management. Whenever possible, the gastrointestinal tract should be utilized for the administration of various dietary regimens designed to supply the nutritional needs of the patient during the postoperative period. Caloric requirements in the injured patient will obviously depend on body size as well as the severity of the injury. Approximately 25 kcal/kg of body weight is required to satisfy the normal nutritional requirements of the *uninjured* adult patient. An additional 5 to 60 kcal/kg of body weight is required for the injured patient, if negative energy balance is to be avoided. Although it is difficult to quantitate the severity of injury in most patients, and thus estimate the magni-

tude of the hypermetabolic response, patients with thermal injury can be precisely categorized, since the injury may be entirely visualized. The adult patient with major thermal injuries will require 25 kcal/kg of body weight, plus 40 kcal/percent total body surface burn.[10] Appropriate adjustments must be made for injured children, since their maintenance caloric requirements are much higher.

Maintenance of adequate nutrition is best monitored by accurate daily measurements of body weight. Postoperative weight loss of less than 10 percent is usually well tolerated providing the patient was not nutritionally depleted prior to the injury. On the other hand, weight loss of greater than 10 percent is often associated with an increased incidence of delayed wound healing, sepsis, and multiple organ failure.

Although nutritional supplementation via the gastrointestinal tract is preferred, it often becomes necessary to provide nutritional requirements entirely or in part by parenteral means in the massively injured patient. Such patients may exhibit postoperative paralytic ileus, intraabdominal abscesses, and postoperative fistula, all of which prevent sufficient utilization of the gastrointestinal tract for absorption of nutrients. One of the most frequent errors in surgical judgment results from the natural inclination of the physician to procrastinate during the postoperative period before instituting a parenteral nutritional program. Unfortunately such delays (often in an effort to avoid the known complications of parenteral hyperalimentation) frequently contribute to further septic or wound complications such as dehiscence, a leaking anastomosis, or pneumonia, which further interfere with the delivery of an adequate nutritional program. Therefore, it is imperative that the physician establish some guidelines to ensure that the patient has reached appropriate nutritional goals in a reasonable period of time. In most cases, patients who have demonstrated a

10 percent loss of preinjury weight, or in whom it has been impossible to establish a normal dietary intake by the seventh postinjury day, should be supplemented either parenterally or enterally, in order to prevent the complications associated with further nutritional deficiency. Once the caloric needs of the posttraumatized patient are established, the optimal amount of nitrogen administration can be estimated by providing a calorie-nitrogen ratio of approximately 150:1.

When the voluntary food intake of the injured patient is of insufficient quantity to provide for positive energy balance, the physician must intervene with forced feedings either by the parenteral or enteral route. Enteral feedings should be accomplished by the insertion of a small nasogastric feeding tube or the utilization of a feeding jejunostomy. Regardless of the means of delivery, feedings are most efficiently delivered and utilized when administered at a constant rate over each 24-h period. In order to ensure a uniform delivery rate of nutrients into the gastrointestinal tract, it is usually necessary to employ a constant delivery pump. The utilization of such pumps increases the volume of fluid which can be safely delivered into the stomach over a 24-h period without substantially increasing the risk of gastric distention, vomiting, and pulmonary aspiration.

Tube feedings are now available commercially in many different forms, and thus the physician may choose a diet which is compatible with the absorptive capabilities of the patient's gastrointestinal tract. When a patient with normal gastrointestinal function is unable to voluntarily ingest an adequate quantity of food, the physician ordinarily should utilize one of the complete, homogenized diets. However, in the presence of colocutaneous fistulas, malabsorption, or prolonged starvation, the patient may better tolerate a partially digested diet containing polypeptides, oligosaccharides, and medium-chain triglycerides.

Completely elemented diets, containing only simple sugars and amino acids, are also available for utilization as tube feedings in those patients with severe malabsorption syndromes, short bowel syndrome, or distal small intestinal fistulas.

It is important that tube feedings be diluted initially and administered in small volumes at a constant rate. The osmolality of the solution and the rate of infusion may be gradually increased as tolerance of the gastrointestinal tract is demonstrated. Attempts to immediately provide all of the caloric supplementation by tube feeding may result in gastric distention, profuse diarrhea, and dehydration.

Whenever positive energy balance is unobtainable by the utilization of gastrointestinal route alone, intravenous nutritional supplementation should be employed in order to avoid prolonged periods of malnutrition. The development of a safe method for the delivery of hypertonic solutions (containing glucose and a nitrogen source) directly into a central vein by Dudrick[11] has allowed the support of traumatized patients for long periods of time without any enteral administration of nutrients. These hypertonic solutions will support normal growth and development in infants and have been associated with the spontaneous closure of gastrointestinal fistulas, spontaneous regression of acute inflammatory disease of the small or large bowel, improved response to chemotherapy for malignancy, decreased catabolism in patients with acute renal failure, as well as long-term maintenance of body weight in patients with major burns and trauma.

All the intravenous hyperalimentation solutions produced in this country contain a carbohydrate source, usually glucose, which is mixed with a nitrogen source consisting of either crystalline amino acids or a protein hydrolysate. The final mixed solution of 25% glucose and between 2.5 to 5% amino acids contains about 1 kcal/mL. To this solution must be added appropriate minerals and vitamins in order to meet daily requirements.

All hypertonic glucose solutions readily support microbiological growth, and, therefore, they should be prepared in the hospital pharmacy by individuals familiar with the safety precautions required to maintain strict aseptic techniques. A clean air environment created by laminar air flow in the pharmacy preparation area is strongly encouraged. The solutions should be stored under refrigeration at 5°C following preparation until ready for utilization at the patient's bedside.

The clinician must be aware that the catabolic patient often has large total body deficits of the intracellular cations and anions as a result of prolonged breakdown of lean tissue mass. The principal intracellular cations and anions (potassium, magnesium, and phosphorus) are liberated into the extracellular fluid as lean tissue is consumed to supply endogenous energy. These cations and anions are excreted by the kidney, resulting in total body deficit, although plasma concentrations may remain relatively normal. When the patient has been converted to an anabolic state by the provision of exogenous calories, new cells are again synthesized and, unless the intracellular anions and cations are provided in excess, serious extracellular and plasma hypokalemia, hypophosphatemia, and hypomagnesemia result.

The hypertonic solutions must be administered through a central vein, e.g., the subclavian, in order that the hyperosmotic fluid may be quickly diluted and, thus, chemical phlebitis avoided. The physician should assure that the delivery rate is constant over a 24-h period and that the initial administration be modest enough to avoid serious hyperglycemia. In general most patients will tolerate between 1200 and 1800 mL during the first 24 h without evidence of glucosuria. Thereafter, the volume administered may be slowly increased each day until the desired caloric intake is reached. Should significant glucosuria be noted as the daily volume of fluid is increased, the administered volume should be held at a constant level for several days to allow the patient to respond with increased endogenous insulin output. The development of hyperglycemia or glucosuria in a patient who has been tolerant of a specific daily volume of hyperosmotic fluid for a long period of time suggests a septic complication causing carbohydrate intolerance.

In order to prevent serious metabolic or septic complications of parenteral hyperalimentation, it is necessary that each hospital develop a system to allow regular review of the preparation and delivery of such solutions within the hospital environment. Several protocols to standardize delivery practices have been published;[5,14,22,23] these can be modified for utilization in most general hospitals. It is obvious that the successful utilization of intravenous hyperalimentation requires the cooperative efforts of many professionals. In order to ensure safe and efficient administration of such solutions, many hospitals have developed an intravenous hyperalimentation team consisting of at least one interested physician, a nurse, and a pharmacist. The team is responsible for periodically reviewing the protocols utilized; for gathering in-hospital data which allows early identification of breaks in the protocol; for in-house education of physicians, nurses, and paramedic personnel; and for providing consultative services to those less familiar with the technique.

Safe delivery to the patient begins with percutaneous aseptic insertion of the catheter into the central vein. Such catheters should be inserted after surgical preparation of the skin. Personnel must utilize caps, masks, and gloves to prevent inadvertent contamination of the catheter. In most cases, fluid should be delivered by pumps capable of maintaining a constant rate of infusion. In-line micropore filters are generally required when intravenous hyperalimentation solutions are delivered to children and may be used in adult patients if adequate flow rates can be maintained. Solutions should not be allowed to hang more than 12 h, and the tubing between the solution and the catheter must be changed every 24 h to prevent colonization of the tubing with microorganisms.

The patient must be carefully monitored for initial response to the administration of the hypertonic solutions. Fractional urines should be obtained at least every 6 h, and blood sugar, plasma electrolytes, and arterial blood gases should be obtained daily until the patient has reached the desired caloric intake. Body weight and fluid input and output must be carefully recorded. In addition, a complete blood count, prothrombin time, creatinine, serum glutamic oxaloacetic transaminase, serum alkaline phosphatase, serum magnesium, and serum phosphorous should be periodically monitored several times a week. Adjustments in the mineral and vitamin contents of the solutions are regularly made after review of patient response as monitored above. It is important to note that iron, vitamin B_{12}, and folic acid are incompatible or unstable within these hyperosmotic solutions and must be provided separately in appropriate doses to provide maintenance requirements.

Complications of intravenous hyperalimentation are easily divided into three specific areas, namely, anatomical, septic, and physiological. Anatomical complications resulting from faulty insertion of the catheter have included pneumothorax, hemothorax, hydrothorax, catheter perforation of the right atrium, arterial and venous thrombosis, and catheter embolism. All can be prevented by the experienced clinician, provided careful attention is paid to anatomical landmarks and established, published techniques for insertion of central venous catheters[3,13,18] are not violated.

Septic complications of parenteral hyperali-

mentation may be held to a minimum by carefully following the protocol established for asepsis during preparation and delivery of solutions. Septic complications occur in only 4 to 5 percent of patients in hospitals with established hyperalimentation teams. If clinical signs of sepsis appear shortly after hanging a new bottle of solution, that bottle should be immediately removed and replaced with a freshly prepared bottle. The suspect bottle should be returned to the pharmacy for appropriate bacteriological and fungal culture, as well as for pyrogen analysis. Should the clinical signs of sepsis not disappear following this simple maneuver, the catheter should be immediately removed and a new catheter inserted in another central vein. In order to prevent infection of the catheter from the skin, the catheter must always be kept in an occlusive dressing. Dressings should be changed at least every 48 h, at which time the skin around the catheter should be surgically scrubbed with an appropriate antibiotic soap solution.

Numerous physiological complications have been reported as a result of inappropriate administration of hyperalimentation solutions. Probably the most common is hyperglycemia, glucosuria, osmotic diuresis, and dehydration, which usually results from too rapid an infusion of glucose, particularly in stressed or septic patients. A reduction in the rate of administration, as well as small supplemental doses of insulin, will usually correct this complication. Hyper- or hyponatremia may result when inappropriate amounts of sodium are infused in relation to the water intake. This complication is most prone to occur when the patient has large abnormal fluid losses, such as may occur from a gastrointestinal fistula. The complication can be readily corrected by adjusting the concentration of sodium added to the hyperalimentation solution. Hypokalemia, hypophosphatemia, and hypomagnesemia will result when inadequate concentrations of these minerals are added to solutions administered to patients who are converting from a catabolic to anabolic state. Hypercalcemia is infrequently observed when insufficient inorganic phosphate has been administered. Occasionally, congestive failure or pulmonary edema has resulted from excessively rapid infusion of hypertonic solutions, particularly in elderly individuals with previous cardiac insufficiency. This complication is usually avoided by more judicious attention to the rate of infusion. Both hyperammonemia and azotemia have been noted when excessive administration of amino acids has been delivered to newborn infants or patients with previous hepatic or renal disease. Anemia has occurred in patients in whom insufficient folic acid, vitamin B_{12}, or iron has been administered. Likewise, prolongation of the prothrombin time may occur in patients who do not receive maintenance doses of vitamin K. Hypervitaminosis A and D may result when excessive administration of these vitamins is provided in the solution as a result of errors in preparation of the solutions.

Patients receiving only parenteral nutrition with carbohydrate and amino acids for a period of several months often develop essential fatty acid deficiency. This syndrome is most readily recognized by the development of scaly lesions of the skin and loss of hair. The diagnosis can be confirmed by measurement of the triene:tetraene ratio of total serum fatty acids.[17] Simultaneously, the patients generally show an increase in plasma eicosatrienoic acid. Essential fatty acid deficiency may be avoided if small amounts of fat can be administered via the gastrointestinal tract. If the gastrointestinal tract cannot be utilized, essential fatty acid deficiency must be treated with the intravenous administration of a fat emulsion. The intravenous administration of fat emulsions by peripheral vein may also be used to supplement enteral caloric intake if necessary. However, total nutritional support via a peripheral vein is rarely possible, since the caloric requirements are so markedly elevated in posttraumatic patients. A solution providing a source of nitrogen should be simultaneously infused with the emulsion. Fat emulsion may not be premixed with amino acid solutions, since the emulsion is broken by the addition of water. Therefore, the solutions are delivered via separate tubing joined together by a Y connector at the intravenous catheter. Patients exhibiting abnormal fat metabolism or transport, liver disease, coagulopathy, serious pulmonary disease, or diabetes mellitus should not be administered fat emulsions, since inadequate clearance of fat from the bloodstream may cause additional hepatic or pulmonary dysfunction or may induce clinical bleeding.

Utilization of intravenous hyperalimentation in patients with major trauma or burns is often necessary if prolonged catabolism is to be avoided. Enteral administration of nutritives alone generally provides an inadequate caloric intake, since paralytic ileus secondary to the initial trauma and subsequent postoperative infectious complications very commonly occur, resulting in decreased bowel motility. The utilization of both oral and intravenous feeding programs in patients with major trauma has been shown to avoid the profound weight loss usually associated with massive injury when less vigorous nutritional programs are pursued[26] and has often resulted in spontaneous wound healing of damaged organs which might previously have required reoperation to effect repair. In addition, the maintenance of normal lean muscle mass allows more rapid rehabilitation and, thus, substantially reduces morbidity associated with major injuries of the extremities.

SUMMARY

Major trauma is characterized by a hypermetabolic response. Failure to provide injured patients with sufficient caloric and nitrogen intake results in pronounced weight loss, impaired wound healing, and cellular dysfunction. The clinician must direct therapy at preventing infection, accomplishing early operative correction of traumatic defects, and providing sufficient exogenous calories and nitrogen to prevent unnecessary catabolic sequelae.

During the past 10 years, great strides have been made in providing better nutritional maintenance of severely injured patients. These efforts have resulted in increased long-term survival and have markedly reduced the morbid complications of prolonged catabolism.

BIBLIOGRAPHY

1 Blackburn, G. L., J. P. Flatt, G. H. A. Clowes, Jr., et al.: Protein sparing therapy during periods of starvation with sepsis or trauma, *Ann. Surg.,* **177**:588, 1973.

2 Bradham, G. B.: Direct measurement of total metabolism of a burned patient, *Arch. Surg.,* **105**:410–3, Sept. 1972.

3 Brinkman, A. J. and D. O. Costley: Internal jugular venipuncture, *J. Am. Med. Assoc.,* **223**: 182, 1973.

4 Bull, J. P.: Nitrogen balance after injuries, *Proc. Nutr. Soc.,* **17**:114, 1958.

5 Burke, W. A.: "Preparation and Guidelines to Utilization of Solutions," in *Total Parenteral Nutrition,* Publishing Sciences Group, Inc. Acton, Mass. 1974, pp. 329–347.

6 Cahill, G. F.: Starvation in man, *N. Engl. J. Med.,* **282**:668, 1970.

7 Cahill, G. F., Jr. and T. T. Aoki: How metabolism affects clinical problems, *Res. Staff Phys.,* April 1973.

8 Curreri, P. W.: "Long-term Supranormal Caloric Dietary Programs in Extensively Burned Patients," in W. L. Scheetz and G. S. M. Cowan, Jr. (eds.), *Intravenous Hyperalimentation.* Lea & Febiger, Philadelphia, 1972, pp. 136–144.

9 ——, J. E. Hicks, R. J. Aronoff, et al.: Inhibition of active sodium transport in erythrocytes

from burned patients, *Surg. Gynecol. Obstet.,* **139**:538, 1974.

10 ——, D. Richmond, J. A. Marvin, and C. R. Baxter: Dietary requirements of patients with major burns, *J. Am. Diet. Assoc.,* **65**:415, 1974.

11 Dudrick, S. J., D. W. Wilmore, and H. M. Vars: Long-term total parenteral nutrition with growth, development, and positive nitrogen balance, *Surgery,* **64**:134, 1968.

12 Duke, J. H., S. B. Jorgensen, J. R. Broell, et al.: Contribution of protein to caloric expenditure following injury, *Surgery,* **68**:168, 1970.

13 Feiler, E. M. and W. E. de Alva: Infraclavicular percutaneous subclavian vein puncture, *Am. J. Surg.,* **118**:906, 1969.

14 Goldmann, D. A. and D. G. Maki: Infection control in total parenteral nutrition, *J. Am. Med. Assoc.,* **223**:1360, 1973.

15 Kinney, J. M.: "Calories: Nitrogen: Disease and injury relationships," in *Total Parenteral Nutrition,* Publishing Sciences Group, Inc. Acton, Mass., 1974, pp. 81–91.

16 Levenson, S. M. and D. L. Watkin: Protein requirements in injury and certain acute and chronic diseases, *Fed. Proc.,* **18**:1155, 1959.

17 Meng, H. C.: "Fat Emulsions," in *Total Parenteral Nutrition,* Publishing Sciences Group, Inc. Acton, Mass., 1974, pp. 178–179.

18 Moosman, D. A.: The anatomy of infraclavicular subclavian vein catheterization and its complications, *Surg. Gynecol. Obstet.,* **136**:71, 1973.

19 Reckler, J. M., H. M. Bruck, A. M. Munster, P. W. Curreri, and B. A. Pruitt, Jr.: Superior mesenteric artery syndrome as a consequence of burn injury, *J. Trauma,* **12**:979, 1972.

20 Reiss, E., E. Pearson, and C. P. Artz: The metabolic response to burns, *J. Clin. Invest.,* **35**:62, 1956.

21 Roe, C. F. and J. M. Kinney: The caloric equivalent of fever: Influence of major trauma, *Ann. Surg.,* **161**:140, 1965.

22 Ruberg, R. L.: "Hospital Practice of Total Parenteral Nutrition," in *Total Parenteral Nutrition,* Publishing Sciences Group, Inc. Acton, Mass., 1974, pp. 349–355.

23 Schaffner, W. F.: "Problems in Preparation and Handling of Solutions," in *Total Parenteral Nutrition,* Publishing Sciences Group, Inc. Acton, Mass., 1974, pp. 313–317.

24 Soroff, H. S., E. Pearson, and C. P. Artz: An estimation of the nitrogen requirements for equilibrium in burned patients, *Surg. Gynecol. Obstet.*, **112**:263, 1961.

25 Troell, L. and A. Wretlind: Protein and caloric requirements in burns, *Acta. Chir. Scand.*, **122**:15, 1961.

26 Wilmore, D. W., P. W. Curreri, K. W. Spitzer, et al.: Supranormal dietary intake in thermally injured hypermetabolic patients, *Surg. Gynecol. Obstet.*, **132**:881–886, 1971.

27 ———, C. A. Lindsey, J. A. Moylan, Jr., G. R. Fallona, B. A. Pruitt, Jr., and R. H. Unger: Hyperglucoganemia in burns, *Lancet,* **1**:73, 1974.

28 ———, J. M. Long, A. D. Mason, Jr., R. W. Skreen, and B. A. Pruitt, Jr.: Catecholamines: Mediator of the hypermetabolic response to thermal injury, *Ann. Surg.*, **180**:653, 1974.

Index